Scott-Brown's Otolaryngology

Sixth edition

Rhinology

Scott-Brown's Otolaryngology

Sixth edition

General Editor

Alan G. Kerr FRCS

Consultant Otolaryngologist, Royal Victoria Hospital, Belfast and Belfast City Hospital;
Formerly Professor of Otorhinolaryngology, The Queen's University, Belfast

Other volumes

1 **Basic Sciences** *edited by* Michael Gleeson

2 **Adult Audiology** *edited by* Dafydd Stephens

3 **Otology** *edited by* John B. Booth

5 **Laryngology and Head and Neck Surgery** *edited by* John Hibbert

6 **Paediatric Otolaryngology** *edited by* David A. Adams and Michael J. Cinnamond

Rhinology

Editors

Ian S. Mackay FRCS

Consultant Otorhinolaryngologist, The Royal Brompton Hospital, London and
Charing Cross Hospital, London

T. R. Bull FRCS

Consultant Surgeon, Royal National Throat, Nose and Ear Hospital, London and
Charing Cross Hospital, London

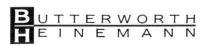

Butterworth-Heinemann
Linacre House, Jordan Hill, Oxford OX2 8DP
A division of Reed Educational and Professional Publishing Ltd

℞ A member of the Reed Elsevier plc group

OXFORD   BOSTON   JOHANNESBURG
MELBOURNE   NEW DELHI   SINGAPORE

First published 1952
Second edition 1965
Third edition 1971
Fourth edition 1979
Fifth edition 1987
Sixth edition 1997

British Library Cataloguing in Publication Data
A catalogue record for this book is
available from the British Library

Library of Congress Cataloguing in Publication Data
A catalogue record for this book is
available from the Library of Congress

ISBN 0 7506 0595 2 (Volume 1)
         0 7506 0596 0 (Volume 2)
         0 7506 0597 9 (Volume 3)
         0 7506 0598 7 (Volume 4)
         0 7506 0599 5 (Volume 5)
         0 7506 0600 2 (Volume 6)
         0 7506 1935 X (set of six volumes)
         0 7506 2368 3 (Butterworth-Heinemann International Edition, set of six volumes)

Printed and bound in Great Britain by Bath Press, Bath

Contents

Colour plates in this volume

Contributors to this volume

Carsten Bindslev-Jensen MD, PhD
Head, Food Allergy Department, National University Hospital, Copenhagen, Denmark

David Brain FRCS
Formerly Consultant ENT Surgeon, The University Hospital, Birmingham

T. R. Bull FRCS
Consultant Surgeon, Royal National Throat, Nose and Ear Hospital, London and Charing Cross Hospital, London

Charles B. Croft MB, FRCS, FRCS(Ed)
Consultant Otolaryngologist, Royal National Throat, Nose and Ear Hospital, London

J. Paul Dilworth MA, DM, MRCP
Consultant Physician, Royal Free Hospital, London

A. B. Drake-Lee MB, ChB, FRCS
Consultant ENT Surgeon, The University Hospital, Birmingham

S. R. Durham MA, MD, FRCP
Reader in Allergy and Clinical Immunology; Honorary Consultant Physician, National Heart and Lung Institute, London

Charles East FRCS
Consultant Surgeon, Royal National Throat, Nose and Ear Hospital, London

Ronald Eccles BSc, PhD, DSc
Reader in Physiology and Director, Common Cold and Nasal Research Centre, University of Wales College of Cardiff

Michael Gleeson MD, FRCS
Professor of Otolaryngology, UMDS, Guy's Hospital; Consultant Otolaryngologist and Skull Base Surgeon to Guy's, St Thomas' and Kings College Hospitals, London

D. G. Golding-Wood FRCS
Senior Registrar, The Royal Free Hospital, London

Colin Hopper FDS, FRCS
Senior Lecturer/Honorary Consultant, Eastman Dental Hospital, London

David Howard BSc, MB BS, LRCP, FRCS, FRCS(Ed)
Honorary Consultant ENT Surgeon, Royal National Throat, Nose and Ear Hospital, London; Senior Lecturer in Laryngology, The Institute of Laryngology and Otology, University of London

A. S. Jones MD, FRCS
Professor of Otolaryngology and Head and Neck Surgery, University of Liverpool

N. S. Jones BDS, FRCS
Consultant Otorhinolaryngologist, Department of ENT, Queen's Medical Centre, Nottingham

Anne Kobza Black MD, FRCP
Consultant Dermatologist and Senior Lecturer, St John's Institute of Dermatology, St Thomas' Hospital, London

V. J. Lund MSc, FRCS
Professor of Rhinology, Royal National Throat, Nose and Ear Hospital, London

I. S. Mackay MB, BS, FRCS
Consultant Otorhinolaryngologist, The Royal
Brompton Hospital, London and Charing Cross
Hospital, London

Philip McLoughlin FRCS
Consultant Oral and Maxillofacial Surgeon,
Chesterfield

C. A. Milford BSc, FRCS
Consultant Surgeon in Otolaryngology, Radcliffe
Infirmary, Oxford; Clinical Lecturer, University of
Oxford

David M. Mitchell MA, MD, FRCP
Consultant Physician, St Mary's Hospital, London

Victoria L. Moore-Gillon FRCS
Consultant Otolaryngologist, St George's Hospital,
London

Brigid F. O'Donnell MRCPI
Senior Registrar, St John's Institute of Dermatology,
St Thomas' Hospital, London

P. D. Phelps MD, FRCS, FFR, FRCR, DMRD
Consultant Radiologist, The Royal National Throat,
Nose and Ear Hospital, London

Michael B. Pringle FRCS
Senior Registrar, Royal Devon and Exeter Hospital,
Exeter

J. C. Watkinson MSc, MS, FRCS, DLO
Consultant Otolaryngologist and Head and Neck
Surgeon, The University Hospital, Birmingham

N. Weir MB, BS, FRCS
Consultant Ear, Nose and Throat Surgeon, Royal
Surrey County Hospital, Guildford; Honorary
Consultant Neuro-otologist, St George's Hospital,
London

R. A. Williams MA, MB BChir, FRCS, FRCSE
Emeritus Consultant ENT Surgeon, Middlesex
Hospital and King Edward VII Hospital for Officers,
London

Introduction

When I started work on this Sixth Edition I did so in the belief that my experience with the Fifth Edition would make it straightforward. I was wrong. The production of the Fifth Edition was hectic and the available time short. The contributors and volume editors were very productive and in under two and a half years we produced what we, and happily most reviewers, considered to be a worthwhile academic work. On this occasion, with a similar team, we allowed ourselves more time and yet have struggled to produce in four years. One is tempted to blame the health service reforms but that would be unfair. They may have contributed but the problems were certainly much wider than these.

The volume editors, already fully committed clinically, have again been outstanding both in their work and in their understanding of the difficulties we have encountered. Once again there was an excellent social spirit among the editors. They have been very tolerant of the innumerable telephone calls and it has always been a pleasure to work with them. The contributors have also been consistently pleasant to deal with, even those who kept us waiting.

There have been technical problems in the production of this work and I want to pay tribute to the patience of all those who suffered under these, not least the publishing staff at Butterworth-Heinemann. One of the solutions to the problems has been the use of a system of pagination that I consider to be ugly and inefficient for the user and I wish to apologize in advance for this. Unfortunately anything else would have resulted in undue delay in the publication date.

Medicine is a conservative profession and many of us dislike change. Some will feel that we have moved forward in that most Latin plurals have been replaced by English, for example we now have polyps rather than polypi. We have also buried acoustic neuromata, with an appropriate headstone, and now talk about vestibular schwannomas. It has taken about two decades for this to become established in otological circles and may take even longer again, to gain everyday usage in the world of general medicine.

I am pleased with what has been produced. Some chapters have altered very little because there have been few advances in those subjects and we have resisted the temptation of change for change's sake. There have been big strides forward in other areas and these have been reflected in the appropriate chapters.

Despite, and because of, the problems in the production of these volumes, the staff at Butterworth-Heinemann have worked hard and have always been pleasant to deal with. I wish to acknowledge the co-operation from Geoff Smaldon, Deena Burgess, Anne Powell, Mary Seager and Chris Jarvis.

It would be impossible to name all those others who have helped, especially my colleagues in Belfast, but I want to pay tribute to the forbearance of my wife Paddy who graciously accepted the long hours that were needed for this work.

As I stated in my introduction to the Fifth Edition, I was very impressed by the goodwill and generosity of spirit among my Otolaryngological colleagues and am pleased that there has been no evidence of any diminution of this during the nine years between the editions. I remain pleased and proud to be a British Otolaryngologist and to have been entrusted with the production of this latest edition of our standard textbook.

Alan G. Kerr

Preface

We were pleased to be invited to edit the Rhinology Volume for this, the Sixth Edition of *Scott-Brown's Otolaryngology*. The past decade has seen radical changes in our specialty and nowhere has this been more noticeable than in rhinology.

Major changes were made to this volume in the last edition, with still more being made in this to cover such topics as endoscopic sinus surgery, nasal mucociliary clearance, local and systemic immune deficiency, food allergy and intolerance, the relationship of the upper and lower respiratory tract and two additional chapters covering odontogenic lesions and CSF rhinorrhoea.

Special thanks go to all the contributors to this volume who have worked so hard to ensure that their chapters are both comprehensive and up-to-date. It has been a pleasure to work with such an excellent team.

We are indebted to Alan Kerr, the General Editor, for his constructive comments and constant encouragement, to the Butterworth-Heinemann team for all their sterling work, to Amanda Laman for her secretarial help and to Julian Rowe-Jones for his editorial assistance.

Ian S. Mackay
T. R. Bull

1

Examination of the nose

Charles East

Nasal symptoms are the commonest reason for adult referral to an otolaryngological clinic in the UK, and for complete assessment, the rhinologist needs to be able to evaluate both the functional and aesthetic aspects. This requires knowledge of the anatomy of nose and paranasal sinuses, orbit, an understanding of pathophysiology of the respiratory tract, and appreciation of ethnic and racial perceptions of the nose. There are few structures in the body that can match the diverse social, cultural and emotional as well as functional attention attracted by the nose. It has been said that the nose is man's most paradoxical organ – it has its root above, its back in front, its wings below, and one likes best of all to poke it into places where it does not belong (Diffenbach, 1845).

Functional assessment

To some extent functional and aesthetic assessments are intertwined particularly in the damaged nose.

A complete nasal examination includes an external evaluation, and an intranasal assessment using specialized instruments. External examination should start with an overall assessment of the nasal form noting obvious irregularities or asymmetries of the pyramid. Swellings should be palpated, and the presence of tender areas, cysts and scars should be noted: the latter may be difficult to see without good lighting, and therefore particular attention should be paid to the areas around the inner canthus, the eyebrows, and the alar bases.

Palpation of the bony and cartilaginous vaults will reveal useful information disguised by the skin and subcutaneous tissues. It is helpful to perform this initial examination from both the front and the side. By asking the patient to raise the chin, the columella and nasal base can be assessed. The condition of the skin, shape of the nostrils, and position of the caudal septum with respect to the columella can easily be evaluated. At this point if the patient is asked to take a steady breath in through the nose, some evidence of patency is obtained, and any inspiratory collapse of the ala is revealed. Elevation of the nasal tip with the thumb allows further assessment of the membranous septum, nasal floor and valve region before inserting a nasal speculum. The examination so far requires no special instruments, and can be carried out with a simple light. Intranasal examination needs adequate instruments and lighting (Table 1.1).

It is important that a comfortable position is adopted by the patient and examiner, who should both be at roughly the same height. A headmirror or headlight is necessary to leave both hands free for instruments.

A nasal speculum allows a clear view of nasal septal deformities to the mid-cavity and is good for assessing the gently curving septum, a feature which may be missed by endoscopy. Various speculae are available. The Thudicum is widely used in the UK with the longer bladed Killian or Cottle as alternatives. Speculae should be introduced gently into the nasal vestibule, and the blades opened sufficiently to obtain a view of the nasal fossae. Pressure medially

Table 1.1 Instruments required for intranasal examination

Nasal speculum
Decongestant
Headmirror/light
Blunt probe
Endoscope – rigid/flexible
Microscope
Suction

on the nasal septum is quite uncomfortable. The condition of the nasal valve region, i.e. the area bounded by the limen nasi laterally, the nasal septum medially and the inferior border of the pyriform aperture below, is probably best examined with an endoscope, as any manipulation of the nasal tip will distort this area. A speculum introduced to the valve area which relieves the sensation of nasal block is however diagnostic of valvular insufficiency. The heads of the inferior and middle turbinates are usually visible, and the anterior parts of the corresponding meatus examined. This is best done after decongestion of the mucosa, particularly when there is a prominent tuberculum of the septum. The state of the overlying mucosa, which is normally pink and moist is noted; abnormal secretions or crusting should be removed or collected for analysis. Gross anterior nasal disease, e.g. polyposis or a distorted septum can easily be diagnosed (see Plate 4/1/I). Examination of the choanal opening of the nose may be performed with a mirror (posterior rhinoscopy). Although occasionally useful, this examination has been largely replaced by endoscopy, which gives a far superior all round view of the area.

The operating microscope is useful for manipulations in the anterior nasal cavities with the patient recumbent where two hands are required, e.g. removal of fine sutures from the columella.

Endoscopic examination

Nasal endoscopy is now the standard by which other visual examinations are judged. Endoscopes may be of glass rod design with various deflection angles (rigid endoscope) or fibreoptic (flexible) (see Plate 4/1/II). Although modern endoscopy has been available for nearly 30 years, its application to the assessment of nasal and sinus disease remained with a few clinical groups until the mid-1980s. Messerklinger (1978), Draf (1983), Stammberger (1985) developing the work of Messerklinger, Wigand (1981, 1990) and Kennedy (1985) are responsible for the recent enthusiastic interest in the use of endoscopy for diagnosis and surgery.

Rigid instruments are preferred (4 mm or 2.7 mm, 0° or 30°) because of the superior image quality, and angular viewing ability. To look at an angle with a flexible scope involves bending the tip, which effectively almost doubles the working diameter and is a significant disadvantage when attempting to inspect under the middle turbinate.

Technique

The nasal mucosa is prepared with a local anaesthetic/vasoconstrictor spray. If there is an obvious spur narrowing the airway, an additional pledget of cotton wool with local anaesthetic is placed in the area where the endoscope may press. It is preferable that the patient is recumbent or semirecumbent with the examiner seated on the right. This position provides a stable base for the head, allows the patient to be relaxed and permits use of suction or gentle manipulations, avoiding mucosal injury. It is possible to endoscope the nose with the patient sitting.

A 30° 4 mm (or 2.7 mm if the nose is narrow) telescope is introduced. The wide field of vision is such that a straight ahead view is still possible in the direction of insertion. The nasal vestibule is inspected first, followed by the floor of the nose, the inferior meatus, the nasopharynx and the eustachian tube orifice as the patient swallows. On this pass it is important to note a previous nasoantral window (see Plate 4/1/III) and any abnormal secretions passing around or over the eustachian tube. Not infrequently, several large submucosal vessels are seen at the posterior edge of the hard palate on the nasal floor, which may be significant in recurrent posterior epistaxis. The telescope is then withdrawn and advanced medial to the middle turbinate. Rotation allows examination of the sphenoethmoidal / superior nasal recess. Often the sphenoid sinus ostium is visible medially, close to the insertion of the nasal septum. An abnormal mucus trail traced back to this area indicates disease in the posterior ethmoid/sphenoid sinus group, thus endoscopic assessment provides a degree of topographic diagnosis which is not achieved by anterior or posterior rhinoscopy.

The middle turbinate head is easily examined from the front. The uncinate process may be visible, and occasionally part of the ethmoid bulla (see Plate 4/1/IV). Variations of the middle turbinate (pneumatization of the head, reversed curvature, may obscure any view, but sometimes gentle medial displacement of the head allows entry of the endoscope anteriorly. If the lateral nasal wall around the lacrimal eminence is prominent it is extremely difficult to introduce the telescope or any instruments. However, the easiest way to assess the middle meatus is to start posteriorly at the widest point by rotating the telescope under the free margin of the middle turbinate, allowing inspection of the posterior basal lamella, ethmoid bulla, hiatus semilunaris and uncinate process as the 'scope is withdrawn. If the telescope is not pushed out of the middle meatus by the middle turbinate head, upward movement allows a view of the frontal recess. The middle meatus is the area where most pathology will be identified in inflammatory sinonasal disease. Abnormal purulent secretions, inflammatory oedema, polypoidal changes and fungal accumulations should be recorded. Frequently ostia are visible in the lateral wall, and may be sufficiently large to inspect the maxillary antrum. These are openings in the anterior or posterior nasal fontanelle, and are invariably accessory ostia and not the natural ostium of the maxillary sinus which is found in the lateral

Colour plates

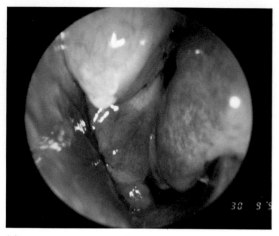

(a)

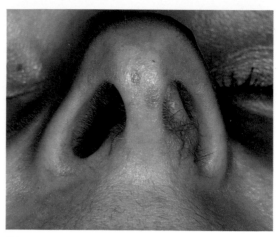

(b)

Plate 4/1/I (*a*) Extensive nasal polyps

(*b*) Caudal dislocation of the nasal septum

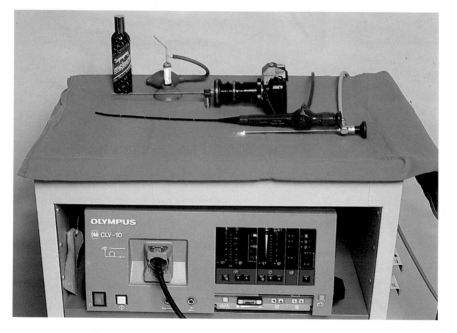

Plate 4/1/II Rigid and flexible endoscopes with light source
for daylight colour film

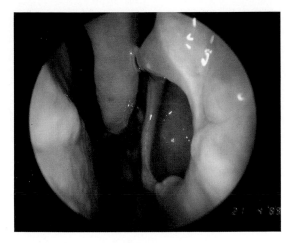

Plate 4/1/III Patent left inferior meatal antrostomy

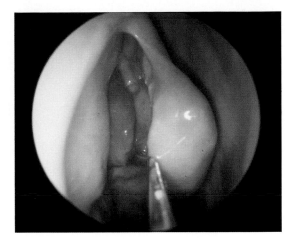

Plate 4/1/IV Middle turbinate retracted displaying uncinate process and ethmoidal bulla

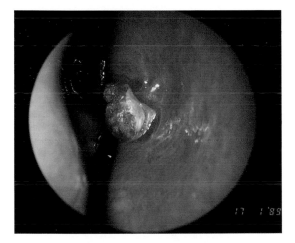

Plate 4/1/V Capillary haemangioma of the nasal septum

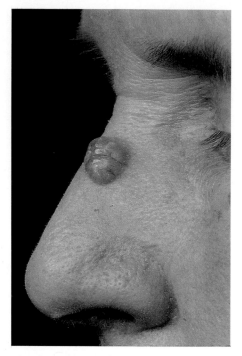

Plate 4/2/I Typical basal cell carcinoma on the nose – the pearly papule. (Courtesy of St John's Institute of Dermatology)

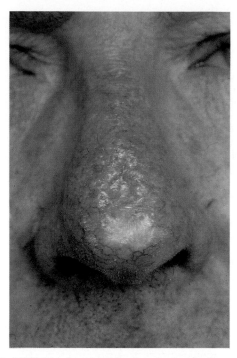

Plate 4/2/II Morphoeaform or sclerosing basal cell carcinoma. Such lesions are deceptively extensive. (Courtesy of St John's Institute of Dermatology)

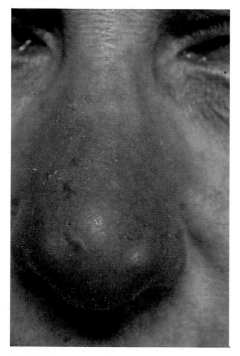

Plate 4/2/III Lupus pernio. (Courtesy of St John's Institute of Dermatology)

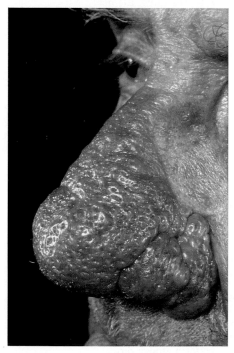

Plate 4/2/IV Rhinophyma. (Courtesy of St John's Institute of Dermatology)

wall of the infundibulum, guarded by the uncinate process. Mucus loops passing between the natural and accessory ostia are believed to be important in the transfer of pathogenic organisms from the nose to the maxillary sinus during acute upper respiratory infections, but may be asymptomatic (Stammberger, 1991).

Both sides of the middle turbinate should be examined – polyps arising from the medial aspect of the turbinate or the olfactory region will produce an obstructive anosmia. These need careful attention to avoid damage to the olfactory epithelium and cribriform plate which is very thin and fragile. Rarely, the nasal septum is so displaced that even a 2.7 mm telescope cannot be passed. Evaluation in this case is based on radiology or at the time of septal correction.

Not every patient requires nasal endoscopy, but where the history suggests possible sinusitis endoscopic assessment is recommended even if there is an obvious anatomical abnormality, e.g. a deviated septum. With experience of endoscopy, it is surprising how often further inflammatory changes are found. This is particularly relevant as the diagnosis will change and hence the treatment.

Endoscopic assessment of the *paranasal sinuses* became common in the late 1970s, and usually preceded a traditional radical operation. As the knowledge of secretion transport within the nose and paranasal sinuses was understood, and with the advent of high resolution CT scanning, the need for direct endoscopy of the sinuses is limited to only a few special instances, e.g. an opaque antrum on CT. The most satisfactory route of access is via the canine fossa. Using a 4 mm trocar and cannula the antrum is punctured at the thinnest point on the front wall. This is usually between the fourth and fifth teeth, high up and lateral to avoid the infraorbital nerve. As the trocar is rotated the finger and thumb of the opposite hand should be resting on the edge of the pyriform aperture and the infraorbital rim. The advantage of this route is that only 0° and 30° endoscopes are required to examine the whole of the antrum including the ostium, as the cannula can be rotated through a large arc. Under vision, manipulations within the antrum are possible with curved instruments introduced via the middle or inferior nasal meatus, or guided biopsies can be performed through the cannula with suitable long cupped forceps. Conditions where endoscopy contributes to diagnosis and management are listed in Table 1.2 and an example is shown (see Plate 4/1/V).

Endoscopy forms an important part of post-surgical assessment and monitoring – both in the management of inflammatory and neoplastic conditions. It is often combined with other diagnostic or therapeutic procedures, e.g. removal of a polyp or biopsy, which are easy to perform under direct vision. Regular endoscopic follow up is likely to improve the management of sinonasal disease. Monitoring key areas such as the frontal recess, and maxillary sinus ostium is vital

Table 1.2 Conditions where endoscopy contributes to diagnosis and management

Congenital atresia
Cleft palate
Septal perforations
Adhesions
Sinusitis
Polyps
Neoplasms
Foreign bodies
CSF leaks
Recurrent epistaxis
Eustachian dysfunction
Documentation
Fungal sinus disease

in preventing late sinus obstruction. This is particularly so in the management of allergic fungal sinus disease which requires continued and meticulous endoscopic cleaning.

Endoscopic documentation

Good endoscopic photographs are difficult to obtain and require dedicated telescopes preferably not the wide angle types, because the light coverage is not adequate. A constant light source of suitable colour temperature for daylight film, with the endoscope mounted on a telezoom adapter and a centre weighted or spot metering camera is probably the easiest method. Commercial flash generators with dedicated systems are available, but expensive. Video-capture of an image onto computer software with 35mm slide generation is likely to replace standard photography in future.

For further detail on endoscopic assessment of the nose the reader is referred to other texts by Messerklinger (1978), Stammberger (1991) and Wigand (1990).

Examination of infants and children

Neonates are obligate nasal breathers, and have to learn to breathe through their mouths. Complete nasal obstruction (bilateral choanal atresia) is a surgical emergency but lesser degrees of block can interfere with feeding. Bubbles in nasal mucus or movement of a whisp of cotton wool held in front of each nostril will confirm an airway, which may only require topical nasal decongestants. Where there is still doubt, a soft rubber catheter should be passed into the pharynx to exclude an atretic palate. The nose is aspirated as the catheter is withdrawn to clear inspissated mucus. Failure to pass a catheter requires endoscopic and radiological evaluation.

In young children, it may not be possible to examine the nose with instruments but, with a careful approach, anterior rhinoscopy may be performed by elevating the nasal tip with the thumb. Alternatively a battery auriscope with speculum can be used. It may be necessary for a nurse to hold a child firmly, particularly when attempting to remove a foreign body, and if this fails it is simpler to resort to examination under anaesthetic, than persevere with an increasingly fractious patient.

Trauma

The nose is the most commonly damaged facial structure due to its prominent position, and it is almost inevitable that injury will be sustained at some time – usually in childhood and commonly as an adult. Domestic injuries and sport are the commonest childhood causes. Violence and contact sports are the usual adult aetiology, there being a dramatic reduction in damage from road traffic accidents since compulsory use of seat belts and crash helmets.

A damaged nose can be assessed immediately after the injury, before haematoma formation disguises any deviation. This is rarely possible and it is better to allow oedema and haematoma formation to subside enough for assessment of the external pyramid. Normally 4–5 days are adequate but it is vital to exclude a haematoma of the nasal septum as soon as possible because this requires drainage to prevent avascular necrosis of cartilage or abscess formation. CSF rhinorrhoea may follow nasal injury and is usually obvious, although a post-traumatic rhinitis can cause confusion. Where doubt exists, glucose estimation of the fluid or analysis for $\beta2$ transferrin will confirm CSF (see Chapter 14).

Clinical examination is sufficient in simple nasal trauma, and plain X-rays are not useful in routine management (Clayton and Lesser, 1986), although they are still sometimes performed for medicolegal reasons. There is evidence that in adults a septal fracture may exist with a nasal fracture when there is a deviation of more than half the bridge width of the nose. Therefore it is important that the septum be examined as the results of manipulation of fractured nasal bones in these cases may be better if the septal deformity is simultaneously corrected.

Childhood nasal trauma is easily overlooked, particularly neonatal injuries and the degree of injury is difficult to evaluate even to the experienced observer. Children's noses are predominantly cartilaginous and soft tissue swelling may conceal a significant deformity. Where doubt exists examination under anaesthetic is recommended. Thirty to 50% of children with non-accidental injury suffer a facial injury which should be remembered if the clinical findings do not match the history.

Radiology

Imaging of the nose and paranasal sinuses can be by plain X-ray, CT scan, or MRI. With the advent of computerized multiplanar imaging the detailed anatomy of the nose and sinuses, particularly the ethmoid, the skull base and orbit has become of paramount importance. Plain X-rays are of negligible value in examination of the nose or nasal fractures. Their role in assessment of the paranasal sinuses is also of limited value for diagnosis, unless combined with endoscopic examination of the nose. Various authors have shown the poor correlation between X-ray and the antroscopic findings. Draf (1983) reported complete agreement in only 42%, and no agreement in 22% of cases. Pfleiderer, Croft and Lloyd (1986) reported correlation in 44% with a false-positive rate of 35% and a false-negative rate of 9%. Two recent studies comparing high kV lateral plain films (145 kV) with CT have shown a high correlation with respect to ethmoid opacification. This is a simple examination, but does not give information about laterality of disease. In the study by Roberts *et al.* (1995) evaluating the investigations for the primary diagnosis of inflammatory sinus disease there was a clinical correlation of up to 92% using plain X-rays and endoscopy when compared with CT scanning. Diagnosis depended on the level of experience of the clinician performing the endoscopy.

CT scanning and MRI provide the most superior and versatile imaging, and for many conditions are complementary. CT has the advantage of delineating fine bony architecture and soft tissue and is the preferred imaging technique for detailed anatomy, particularly in relation to the skull base, orbits, and carotid vessels. The major disadvantages are ionizing radiation, especially to the lens and the limitation to two scanning planes. Recently, 3-D reconstructed images have been produced, although their clinical use appears limited. MRI scanning gives some information about tissue characterization. It is possible to distinguish between retained secretions and soft tissue. MRI is an important investigation where disease extends outside the nasal cavity and sinuses, e.g. into the anterior cranial fossa. In cases of angiofibroma it has largely replaced angiography for diagnosis. Subtraction MRI scanning to evaluate sinus neoplasia is a new technique undergoing evaluation, and is likely to add to the already high standards of nasal and sinus imaging now available.

These developments therefore raise the question whether plain X-rays should be abandoned. There is no doubt that CT and MRI are vastly superior and are the imaging techniques of choice, but this is probably the council of perfection, as availability of scanning and cost containment still limit access in many units. The commonest reason for imaging of the nose and sinuses is inflammatory sinus disease and, in those units where access to scanning is limited, the use of nasal endoscopy and properly executed plain films, including the high kV lateral will provide a high diagnostic yield in the *primary* investigation of sinusitis. CT is requested if the patient is to undergo surgery, to delineate the local anatomy, or if the diagnosis is still in doubt with a patient who has a convincing story, but negative endoscopic findings.

Allergy testing

Allergic rhinitis affects between 10 and 15% of the population. The prevalence of allergic rhinitis has increased in recent years and is a significant cause of nasal morbidity. The recognition of an allergic basis for nasal symptoms is important for long-term management, particularly if surgery is being considered. In routine clinical work, a good clinical history supported by skin prick testing will identify the majority of allergic patients, assuming they have not recently taken antihistamines (especially astemizole, which has a long half-life). Where skin tests are negative, but clinical suspicion remains high, cytology of the nasal secretions can be examined for eosinophils, and the radio-allergosorbent (RAST) test performed. Direct measurement of specific IgE is unaffected by anti-allergy drugs. The common allergens which can practically be controlled are house dust, pets, feathers, and pollens. The effect of the ubiquitous house dust mite can be reduced by the use of acaricides, wet dusting, vacuuming using a filter to prevent dust recirculation and special bedding covers (Intervent, Alprotec).

Olfaction

This neglected sense cannot be easily examined and as yet there is no ideal clinical test. The standard methods of examination are mainly qualitative, inaccurate and have very little value, e.g. smell bottles. Commercial kits are available to quantify smell using dilutions of pyridine or *n*-butyl alcohol. The UPSIT scratch and sniff cards also quantify loss and can detect malingerers. Evoked response olfactometry is still an experimental and research investigation. Olfaction is detailed in Chapter 5.

Mucociliary and ciliary function tests

Examination of nasal clearance, i.e. testing the mucociliary mechanism can simply be performed in the clinic using a particle of saccharine placed on the lateral nasal wall 1 cm behind the anterior end of the inferior turbinate. The time taken until the patient tastes the sweetner gives a rough estimate of nasal transport time. Ideally the test should be carried out in a controlled environment as temperature and humidity variation will alter the result. The transport time in normal individuals is usually less than 20 minutes. Abnormal results require testing the other nostril and, if necessary, testing the patient's ability to taste saccharine.

Other mainly research methods for *in vivo* assessment include an india ink drop in the anterior nares, or radiolabelled discs, using a gamma camera to measure the rate of clearance. Direct measurements are invasive and alter the nasal environment, and so are unreliable. *In vitro* measurement of ciliary activity from brushings along the inferior turbinate using phase contrast microscopy will detect ciliary dyskinesias. The normal frequency is 12–15 Hz. This also provides a useful research model to study pharmacological agents and toxins.

Nasal airway assessment

Subjective assessment of the nasal airway is a poor guide to the state of patency of the nasal airways, but is the most commonly relied on symptom in recommending surgical treatment. In attempting to quantify measurements the following have been used, but all have their limitations:

1 Peak nasal inspiratory flow. Using a modified peak flow meter, inspiratory flow levels can be measured in the clinic. This measurement is limited as nasal valvular collapse can occur, particularly after turbinectomy, when the point of maximal nasal resistance moves forward.
2 Rhinomanometry. The measurement of nasal resistance is an important objective assessment of the nasal airway. Unfortunately in such a dynamic structure this has proved difficult to achieve reliably. Also, there appears to be no correlation between the patient's symptoms and the rhinomanometric findings (Jones *et. al.*, 1987; Jones, Willat and Durham, 1989). Anterior and posterior rhinomanometry is not easy to perform, and its use is mainly in research establishments.
3 Acoustic rhinometry, however, gives an accurate measurement of the cross-sectional area of the airway from the nasal vestibule to the nasopharynx. The technique is non-invasive and easy to perform without distorting the nasal architecture. It still has to be validated as a technique but it should provide a much more objective measurement, particularly in the evaluation of surgery for nasal obstruction.

Nasal aesthetic assessment

Assessment of the cosmetic aspects of the nose should not be limited to physical examination, but should include psychological, social and sexual factors. However, it is important to have a guide to 'ideal' proportions so that recording of deformities and their planned correction is facilitated, rather than relying on the 'cosmetic eye' – something that may take several years to acquire. Nasal deformities may be obvious to the patient and surgeon particularly after trauma and the only record needed is a clinical photograph, and discussion of the operative procedure. Definition of the nasal deformities one intends to correct, in agreement with the patient, is the key to a satisfied patient and a successful outcome.

Nasal deformities require assessment against the face as a whole, and there are four major areas to consider: the forehead, eyes, lips and chin. In general, female noses are smaller and narrower both across the bridge and lobule. Males may have a convexity to the nasal dorsum, a feature often disliked by females. The angle between the columella and the upper lip (nasolabial angle, an evaluation of tip rotation) has a normal range of 90–120°. Powell and Humphries (1984) have suggested various triangles based on established cephalometric points to evaluate the face and nose. These are based on standardized photographs of the face particularly the lateral view which should be taken with the head in the Frankfurt horizontal plane (a horizontal line joining the top of the tragus with the infraorbital rim). In practice it can be difficult to identify the infraorbital rim on a photograph and a good compromise is for the eyes to be parallel to the floor (Figure 1.1). Good quality photographs are a

minimum requirement for corrective nasal surgery, and copies should be kept in the patient's notes. It is recommended that written consent be obtained. Four views are recommended: frontal, lateral (or profile), three-quarter where the nasal tip is aligned with the cheek, and the basal or columella view (Figure 1.2). There are many published articles on photographic techniques, and for further details the reader is referred to the text-reference (Schwartz and Tardy, 1991).

The 35mm SLR camera is the standard body, and a 105 mm lens gives an undistorted view of the face. An electronic flash is important for even illumination and correct colour temperature of light so that daylight film can be used. If a single flash source is used,

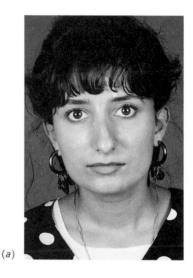

(*a*)

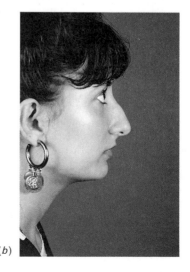

(*b*)

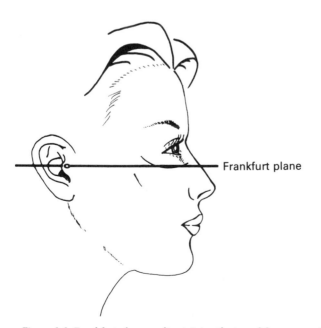

Figure 1.1 Frankfurt plane – a line joining the top of the tragus and the infraorbital rim

Figure 1.2 Standard rhinoplasty views. (*a*) Frontal; (*b*) lateral (or profile)

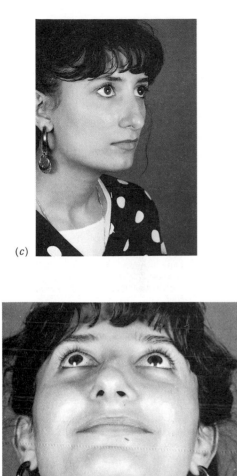

(c)

(d)

Figure 1.2 *continued:* Standard rhinoplasty views. (*c*) three-quarter; (*d*) basal or columella

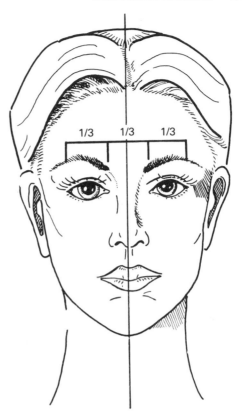

Figure 1.3 The outer canthal distance is divided roughly into thirds. The nasal width is measured at the alar margins

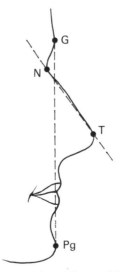

Figure 1.4 Facial points relating the nasal dorsum to the glabella and chin. G = glabella; N = nasion; T = tip; Pg = pogonion

particularly if it is mounted on the camera hot shoe, in the lateral view the flash should be arranged so as not to produce a background shadow. For colour photographs a light blue background is suitable. By reference to these hard copies using an overlay of tracing paper, a systematic examination of the external nose can be followed using fixed landmarks. These include the nasion (N), tip (T), columella break-point (C), subnasale (SN), upper lip (LS), alar crease (AC), and pogonion (Pg). From the front, the face is divided roughly into thirds between the hairline, glabella area, subnasale and menton. Most of the published data relate to the Caucasian nose and allowance needs to be made for racial variation. The width of the nose at the ala should be in line with the medial canthus and be equivalent to the width of the eyes (Figure 1.3). On the profile view, by drawing lines between the various points, the proportions of the face can be related (Figure 1.4). This exercise brings to attention the most important areas namely the nasolabial angle, the angle of the dorsum to the face and the position of the chin, setting the basis for discussion with the patient. It is also important for teaching and training purposes. The following is a brief account of the important nasal measurements in relation to the face, and for further detail the reader is referred to the description by Powell and Humphries (1984).

Nasolabial angle (Figure 1.5). This has a normal range of 90–120° with males at the more acute end. This angle may change when the patient smiles if the tip is pulled down.

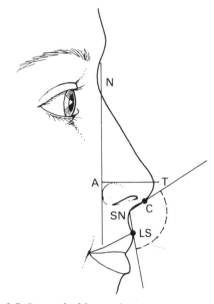

Figure 1.5 One method for nasal tip projection measurement. The ratio of the length A–T to N–T is roughly 0.55–0.6. The nasolabial angle is measured between the most convex part of the columella (C), the subnasal point (SN) and the upper lip (LS). N = nasion; A = alar groove; T = tip

Tip projection. From a line joining the nasion and the alar groove a perpendicular measurement to the tip point is measured.

Nasal length. The distance between the nasion and the tip. This measurement divided by the previous distance is expressed as a ratio with a normal range of 0.55–0.6.

Nasofacial angle. This is taken from a line joining the glabella point and pogonion and the intersection of a line along the nasal dorsum. The range is between 30–40°. This aspect is discussed further in Chapter 17.

Glossary of facial anthropomorphic points

Glabella (G): most prominent point in the middle of the forehead

Nasion (N): deepest depression at the root of the nose

Pogonion (Pg): most anterior part of the chin

Subnasale (Sn): point at which the columella merges with the upper lip

Tip (T): most anterior projected point of the nasal tip

Upper lip (Ls): vermilion border of the upper lip

Alar groove (A): attachment of the ala to the face

Mentum (M): lowest point of the chin.

References

CLAYTON, M. and LESSER, T. (1986) The role of radiography in the management of nasal fractures. *Journal of Laryngology and Otology*, **100**, 797–801

DIEFFENBACH, J. F. (1845) *Die operative chirurgie*. Liepzig: F. A. Brockhaus

DRAF, W. (1983) *Endoscopy of the Paranasal Sinuses*. Berlin: Springer-Verlag

JONES, A. S., WILLAT, D. J. and DURHAM, L. M. (1989) Nasal airflow: resistance and sensation. *Journal of Laryngology and Otology*, **103**, 909–911

JONES, A., LANCER, J., STEVENS, J. and BECKINGHAM, E. (1987) Nasal resistance to airflow. *Journal of Laryngology and Otology*, **101**, 800–808

KENNEDY, D. W. (1985) Functional endoscopic sinus surgery. *Archives of Otolaryngology*, **111**, 643–649

MESSERKLINGER, W. (1978) *Endoscopy of the Nose*. Munich: Urban and Schwarzenberg.

PFLEIDERER, A., CROFT, C. and LLOYD, G. (1986) Antroscopy: its place in clinical practice: a comparison of antroscopic findings with radiological appearances of the maxillary sinus. *Clinical Otolaryngology*, **11**, 455–461

POWELL, N. and HUMPHRIES, B. (1984) *Proportions of the Aesthetic Face*. New York: Theime-Stratton Inc.

ROBERTS, D., HAMPLE, S., EAST, C. and LLOYD, G. (1995) The diagnosis of sinonasal disease. *Journal of Laryngology and Otology*, **109**, 27–30

SCHWARTZ, M. and TARDY, M. E. (1991) Standardised photo-documentation in facial plastic surgery. *Facial Plastic Surgery*, **7**, 1–12

STAMMBERGER, H. (1985) Endoscopic endonasal surgery – concepts in treatment of recurring rhinosinusitis. Part I and part II. *Otolaryngology – Head and Neck Surgery*, **94**, 143–156

STAMMBERGER, H. (1991) *Functional Endoscopic Sinus Surgery. The Messerklinger Technique*. Philadelphia: B. C. Decker

WIGAND, M. E. (1981) Transnasal ethmoidectomy under endoscopical control. *Rhinology*, **19**, 7–15

WIGAND, M. (1990) *Endoscopic Surgery of the Paranasal Sinuses and Anterior Skull Base*, Stuttgart; Thieme

2

Conditions of the external nose

Brigid F. O'Donnell and Anne Kobza Black

The nose and nasal vestibules are covered with skin and may be involved in most dermatoses affecting the facial skin. However, a number of cutaneous and systemic conditions show a predilection for the nose, e.g. sarcoidosis and lupus vulgaris. As a consequence of various disease processes the nose may develop a characteristic deformity, e.g. the saddle nose of congenital syphilis or Wegener's granulomatosis and the beaked nose of scleroderma. A peculiar shape of nose may indicate a genetic syndrome like the pointed nose of Bloom's syndrome, while nasolabial angiofibromas are pointers to tuberous sclerosis.

As the nose occupies a prominent anatomical position on the face, early diagnosis and treatment of any scarring or ulcerative lesion is imperative. Centrofacial ulcerations present a particular challenge, since similar clinical and microscopic findings can result from many diverse causes. In this chapter we deal with conditions affecting the nose and adjacent skin under the headings of acute infections, chronic infections, neoplasms, sarcoidosis, connective tissue diseases, and other disorders affecting the external nose.

Acute infections

The flora of the nose consist of prominent corynebacteria, staphylococci (*Staphylococcus aureus* and *Staphylococcus epidermidis*) and streptococci. The nose should be examined as a possible source of infection in institutional outbreaks and in recurrent staphylococcal infections in the individual or in the family.

Furunculosis

A furuncle or boil is an acute infection of a hair follicle with *Staphylococcus aureus*. The hair-bearing area of the nasal vestibule is a vulnerable site due to the strong hairs and mechanical trauma to this area. The furuncle commences as a hard tender red nodule which enlarges and becomes more painful and fluctuant. The majority of vestibular furuncles discharge into the vestibule and resolve. A serious and fortunately now very rare complication of nasal furunculosis is the spread of infection via the valveless facial veins and superior ophthalmic veins to the cavernous sinus. Cavernous sinus thrombosis produces a severe illness with fever, vomiting, prostration and convulsions. Local changes include oedema with cyanosis of the eyelids and base of the nose and chemosis, due to obstruction of the ophthalmic veins. Ophthalmoplegia and pupillary changes (dilated or small and immobile) are common. Retinal haemorrhages and papilloedema are late events.

Squeezing of nasal furuncles is to be avoided to reduce the risk of blood-stream spread. Local application of moist heat will enhance the localization of infection and promote drainage. Systemic antibiotics are mandatory for all but very rapidly resolving nasal furuncles. Patients with larger boils or with surrounding cellulitis should be treated with parenteral antibiotics and observed closely.

Vestibulitis

Nasal vestibulitis describes inflammation of the vestibule with recurrent crusting and pain, usually due to infection with *Staphylococcus aureus*. It may also be caused by an irritant dermatitis-type reaction such as occurs in acute coryza, due to watery rhinorrhoea and rubbing. Alternatively, it may be part of an atopic diathesis. It may be treated with a mild topical corticosteroid ointment or with an antibiotic ointment in cases of infection.

Unilateral vestibulitis in a child or mentally impaired person should raise suspicion of a foreign body. The tell-tale malodour and offensive discharge are further strong evidence.

Erysipelas

Erysipelas is a bacterial infection of the dermis and upper subcutaneous tissues usually caused by group A streptococci. It most commonly affects infants, young children and older adults. The process may begin as a small break in the skin and the patient becomes febrile. There may be a frank rigor. The affected skin has a characteristic swollen, indurated or *peau d'orange* appearance and spreads peripherally. It is bright red, hot and shiny with a sharp border. Small vesicles and bullae may develop as may petechiae or ecchymoses. Occasionally erysipelas involves the bridge of the nose and one or both cheeks in a 'butterfly' distribution. The diagnosis of erysipelas is a clinical one as bacteriological isolation of the offending organism from the skin is unusual. However, blood cultures should be taken and, in the case of facial infections, pathogens should be sought from the nose, throat, conjunctiva and sinuses. The diagnosis may later be supported by evaluating paired sera for antistreptolysin (ASO) from days 1 and 14. Treatment is with benzyl penicillin for presumed streptococcal infection, administered intravenously in the more severe cases. Mild cases may be adequately treated with oral antibiotics.

Cellulitis

Cellulitis is an acute spreading inflammation of the skin involving the deeper subcutaneous tissues, most commonly caused by group A streptococci and *Staphylococcus aureus*. It resembles erysipelas, but as the inflammation is deep the margins tend to be ill-defined, in contrast to the sharp margins of erysipelas. Facial cellulitis extending to involve the periorbital and orbital areas may be complicated by cavernous sinus thrombosis.

Impetigo

Impetigo is a contagious superficial infection of the skin, which may affect any part of the body, but particularly the face. The bullous variety is caused by *Staphylococcus aureus* and non-bullous impetigo may be caused by *Staphylococcus aureus*, streptococcus or both together. Bullous impetigo is characterized by tense bullae 1–2 cm in diameter or larger, which contain clear fluid initially. After rupture, flat brownish crusts are formed. In non-bullous impetigo small pustules enlarge and rupture to form the typical honey-coloured crusts. Except for the very localized cases impetigo should be treated with systemic antibiotics (flucloxacillin or erythromycin).

Herpes simplex

Herpes simplex type 1, the 'cold sore' or 'fever blister' most commonly affects the face (lips, perioral area, cheeks and nose) and neck. After a prodrome of stinging or burning tiny grouped vesicles develop on normal or slightly red skin. The vesicles, initially clear become cloudy and purulent, dry and crust and heal within 7–10 days. As herpes virus persists in sensory nerve ganglia the patient may suffer recurrent episodes arising in the same area. Recurrences may be triggered by trauma, dental manipulation, strong sunlight, febrile illnesses, upper respiratory tract infections, menses and stress. Mild uncomplicated herpes simplex requires no treatment. Topical acyclovir improves recurrent cutaneous infections.

Patients with atopic dermatitis may develop widespread cutaneous infection with herpes simplex particularly after primary exposure (eczema herpeticum). Patients with eczema herpeticum should receive intravenous acyclovir as early as possible.

Herpes zoster

The nasal skin is involved in herpes zoster of the maxillary division of the trigeminal nerve when vesicles develop on the cheek, nose, nasal vestibule, nasal mucosa and palate. Lesions on the tip of the nose herald involvement of the nasociliary branch of the ophthalmic division of the trigeminal nerve, implying a strong possibility of concomitant keratoconjunctivitis. Severe pain may precede the eruption and in the maxillary division may be mistaken for sinus or dental disease. Erythematous macules, papules and plaques are seen first. Grouped vesicles and blisters appear within 24 hours, become purulent, crust and fall off in 1–2 weeks. Patients with severe disease show haemorrhagic, bullous and infarctive lesions which heal slowly with scarring. Patients with herpes zoster require adequate analgesia and skin care. Those with involvement of the nasal tip should be urgently referred to an ophthalmologist. Patients who are seen early in the course of their illness may benefit from oral acyclovir, which will lessen zoster pain during treatment.

Warts

Warts or verrucae are benign epithelial proliferations of the skin and mucosae caused by infection with papillomaviruses. The common wart is caused by types 2 and 4 and are rough papules. Some exhibit a distinctive filiform surface. Patients with warts on the nose are likely to request treatment for cosmetic reasons and liquid nitrogen cryotherapy is usually effective.

Molluscum contagiosum

Molluscum contagiosum is a common benign viral (poxvirus) disease of the skin and mucous membranes that predominantly affects children. Individual lesions usually 3–6 mm in size, are characteristic pink or flesh-coloured dome-shaped papules with central umbilication. Patients with atopic dermatitis and those who are immunosuppressed may develop persistent and extensive lesions. In the majority of immunocompetent patients the condition is self-limiting but resolution may be aided by liquid nitrogen cryotherapy or by curettage.

Chronic infections

Lupus vulgaris

Lupus vulgaris describes post-primary cutaneous infection with *Mycobacterium tuberculosis*. Although relatively rare it represents the most common form of cutaneous tuberculosis in Europe (Marcoval *et al.*, 1992). It originates from tuberculosis elsewhere in the body by haematogenous, lymphatic or contiguous spread. It is possible that organisms disseminated at the height of a previous infection can remain latent in the skin for many years, to be activated later by various stimuli (Ustvedt and Ostensen, 1951). Rarely lupus vulgaris may follow primary inoculation tuberculosis or BCG vaccination.

The lesions are usually solitary but two or more sites may be involved simultaneously. Lupus vulgaris shows a predilection for the head and neck with 90% of lesions being found at these sites. The initial lesion starts on the nose or cheek and slowly extends into the adjacent areas. The early lesion is a reddish-brown papule with a gelatinous consistency. This gradually extends and becomes more infiltrated. The typical appearance later is of an irregular reddish-brown nodular plaque with a scaly surface. When pressed with a glass slide (diascopy) the brown nodules, referred to as 'apple jelly nodules', are more easily seen. The natural course of these lesions is slow peripheral extension. In *ulcerative* lupus vulgaris the underlying tissue may be affected by progressive necrosis, and, if the nasal or auricular cartilage is involved, extensive destruction takes place. *Scarring* is a prominent feature of lupus vulgaris. Atrophic scars occur subsequent to or independent of ulceration, and new 'apple jelly' nodules develop within the scarred areas.

Diagnosis

Histopathology of the skin shows typical tubercles with sparse caseation necrosis. However, secondary changes may be superimposed and necrosis and ulceration are usually accompanied by non-specific inflammatory reactions that may conceal the tuberculous structures. Differentiation from sarcoidosis may be very difficult, but the reticulin staining seen in sarcoidosis is not a feature of lupus vulgaris. Special stains for acid-fast bacilli may not demonstrate the organisms which are present in small numbers. A positive culture for *Mycobacterium tuberculosis/bovis* will confirm the diagnosis in less than 10% of cases. The Mantoux test is strongly positive. The patient should be investigated for an underlying focus of tuberculosis in other organs.

Course and prognosis

The natural course of lupus vulgaris is slow progression which may be continuous or intermittent. Spontaneous resolution may eventually occur leaving scarring contractures and tissue destruction. There is a risk that aggressive squamous cell carcinomas or, less commonly, basal cell carcinomas and rarely sarcomas will develop in the scar tissue (Sehgal and Wagh, 1990).

Treatment

Antituberculous chemotherapy is indicated, usually for 9 months. The clinical response to treatment is usually satisfactory. However, there may be residual atrophic scarring and hyperpigmentation.

Syphilis

The characteristic lesion of primary syphilis, the chancre, is a painless firm button-like nodule occurring at the site of treponemal penetration. Extragenital chancres usually occur on or close to the lips and may very rarely involve the nose or nasal vestibule. Untreated chancres persist for 3–6 weeks while, with treatment, they resolve in 1–2 weeks. The lesions of secondary syphilis are papular and involve the trunk, limbs, palms and soles. They may become quite scaly and resemble psoriasis, pityriasis rosea or even lupus erythematosus. Annular lesions are common in Black patients and late lesions show a predilection for the corners of the mouth and angles of the nose.

The lesion of tertiary syphilis, the gumma, is a mass of syphilitic granulation tissue. It is a painless nodule which breaks down to leave a 'punched out' ulcer with a ragged necrotic floor. It heals with scarring and tissue destruction. 'Snuffles' or syphilitic rhinitis is an early and important sign of congenital syphilis. Fissures or 'split' papules may develop at the angles of the mouth or lateral to the external nares. Late congenital syphilis produces the classical stigma of saddle-nose deformity.

Yaws, leprosy, leishmaniasis and rhinosporidiosis are discussed in Chapter 8.

Neoplasms

Basal cell carcinoma

Synonym: basal cell epithelioma, rodent ulcer.

Basal cell carcinoma (BCC) is a malignant tumour of the skin that arises from the basal cell layer. Lesions most commonly affect the face and in one study of 1620 basal cell carcinomas 25% involved the nose (Roenigk *et al.*, 1986). A typical basal cell carcinoma is a shiny papule with a pearly translucent surface traversed by telangiectasia (Plate 4/2/I). The typical pearly feature may be accentuated by either compressing or stretching the surrounding skin and viewing the lesion with the aid of a side lamp. Differentiation of basal cell carcinoma from a dermal naevus is aided by history of a long-standing lesion and static size in the case of the latter. When the basal cell carcinoma becomes ulcerated (rodent ulcer) the raised rim of the tumour retains the typical pearly telangiectatic features. A pigmented basal cell carcinoma may be difficult to distinguish from melanoma, but it tends to retain a shiny translucent appearance. Basal cell carcinomas are typically slow growing. If neglected they may be destructive and locally invasive, but very rarely metastasize.

Small basal cell carcinomas involving the nose may be effectively treated by curettage and cautery, excision or radiotherapy. It is important that surgically removed specimens include an adequate margin of normal skin to reduce the risk of local recurrence. The relative risk for recurrence of tumour on the nose is particularly high compared to other locations (Roenigk *et al.*, 1986). Ulcerative and morphoeaform (sclerosing) (Plate 4/2/II) lesions may be deceptively extensive, and those extending inside the nose should ideally be managed by Mohs' microscopically controlled surgery.

Actinic/solar keratoses

Actinic or solar keratoses are areas of dysplastic epithelium arising in sun-damaged skin. They are ill-defined red or pink scaly patches which are rough to touch. They have a predilection for the forehead, temples, tip of the nose, vermilion of the lower lip and dorsa of the hands. They are premalignant, progressing to low grade invasive squamous cell carcinomas in approximately 10% of cases. Actinic keratoses respond well to treatment with liquid nitrogen cryotherapy.

Bowen's disease

Bowen's disease refers to squamous cell carcinoma in situ and is characterized clinically by a well-defined red scaly plaque. It responds to treatment with liquid nitrogen cryotherapy or topical 5-fluorouracil.

Squamous cell carcinoma

Squamous cell carcinoma (SCC) is a malignant proliferation of the keratinocyte. It arises in a precursor lesion, for example actinic keratosis, Bowen's disease or scar or de novo. Clinically it presents as a hypertrophic actinic keratosis, a warty growth, a keratoacanthoma (see below), an indurated nodule or an ulcerating nodule. Squamous cell carcinomas have metastatic potential. In a population-based study of invasive squamous cell carcinoma (Chuang *et al.*, 1990) metastases occurred in 3.6% of patients. Treatment of the primary cutaneous lesion is by excision or radiotherapy.

A subgroup of mid-facial basal cell carcinomas and squamous cell carcinomas behave aggressively and invade extensively into the surrounding soft tissues and even bone and cartilage. In a retrospective study of 147 patients (Teichgraeber and Goepfert, 1990) requiring full-thickness nasal resections, 68 (46.3%) required a hemi- or complete rhinectomy. Lesions requiring extensive surgery usually involved the ala or were recurrent multicentric squamous cell carcinomas greater than 4 cm.

Keratoacanthoma

Keratoacanthoma is a rapidly evolving benign tumour which most commonly affects the central part of the face – nose, cheeks, eyelids and lips. It commences as a papule or 'pimple' and enlarges rapidly to a typical dome-shaped nodule with a central keratotic plug, which may mimic a large molluscum contagiosum.

After rapid growth over a number of weeks the lesion resolves spontaneously. Keratoacanthomas may be difficult to distinguish from squamous cell carcinomas on clinical and histological grounds. A history of rapid growth is suggestive of keratoacanthoma and spontaneous healing confirms the diagnosis. Treatment with curettage and cautery or excision produces a better cosmetic result than waiting for spontaneous resolution which is associated with scarring.

Fibrous papule of the nose

This benign papule develops slowly in middle-aged persons as a dome-shaped flesh-coloured, pink or pigmented lesion which is usually sessile. It occurs as a single lesion on the nose, but occasionally there are multiple papules which involve other parts of the face. Most are asymptomatic and may be removed by excision or 'shave' removal for cosmetic reasons or because of bleeding. Diagnosis may be confirmed by the histological findings which are characteristic.

Angiofibromas

Firm discrete telangiectatic papules with a predilection for the nasolabial furrows and chin and usually developing in childhood or adolescence should raise the possibility of tuberous sclerosis (epiloia). The presence of other stigmata of this autosomal dominant condition like periungual fibromas or ash-leaf macules makes the diagnosis easier, but there is a range of severity and the condition may remain latent until adult life. Mental deficiency is present in 70% of cases and epilepsy is also common. Angiofibromas may be few in number or numerous and conspicuous. They may be confused clinically with other benign growths with a similiar distribution, e.g. tricho-epitheliomas. In cases of diagnostic doubt a skin biopsy should be carried out. The cosmetic appearance of angiofibromas may be improved by the use of diathermy or laser. Lesions tend to recur after dermabrasion.

Naevi

Compound, junctional and dermal naevi may involve the nose.

Lentigo maligna

Lentigo maligna most commonly affects the cheek in elderly persons. Clinically it is a flat pigmented patch with various shades of brown and an irregular edge. Its importance lies in its potential to develop into invasive melanoma, usually after many years.

Melanoma

Melanoma, a malignant proliferation of melanocytes, affects the head and neck in 10–20% of cases. The commonest type is the superficial spreading melanoma which manifests as a pigmented lesion with colour variegation and an irregular edge. However, unusual and some non-pigmented melanomas (desmoplastic and amelanotic) may particularly affect the head and neck. Urgent referral or biopsy is warranted for such lesions. Primary cutaneous melanoma is treated by excision. The margin size is dictated by tumour thickness (Breslow thickness) and anatomical constraints. Special techniques are often required to

perform successful reconstruction of the nose. Primary closure is not usually possible and the best reconstructions are performed with the use of local flaps.

Kaposi's sarcoma

Kaposi's sarcoma is a multifocal neoplasm originating from the vascular endothelium. It may involve the nose in patients with acquired immune deficiency syndrome (AIDS). The early lesions are macules with a reddish-salmon colour. Within a week the colour changes to purplish or brown and the lesions become nodular. Rarely there may be a single growth. The majority of patients develop multiple lesions.

Metastases to the nasal skin

The commonest internal malignancy to metastasize to the nose is probably lung carcinoma, which usually produces firm cutaneous nodule/s. Skin metastases are usually late events.

Sarcoidosis

Sarcoidosis is a chronic granulomatous disease of unknown aetiology. It is a 'multisystem' disorder but cutaneous disease may occur without systemic involvement. In one series of 188 patients with cutaneous sarcoid (Veien, Stahl and Brodthagen, 1987) 50 had no systemic involvement. Where cutaneous and systemic disease coexist, there is poor correlation between the extent of the cutaneous lesions and the severity or extent of systemic disease. However, nasal involvement in sarcoidosis, particularly the lesions of lupus pernio (Plate 4/2/III) and nasal rim papules have been associated with significant sarcoidosis of the upper respiratory tract, and these cutaneous lesions are markers of possible granulomatous infiltration of the nasal mucosa and upper airway.

Lupus pernio (Plate 4/2/III)

Lupus pernio was first described by Besnier (1889) and so called because of the resemblance of the lesion to perniosis or cold-induced injury. However, it is distinguished from true pernio by persistence in warm weather. The typical plaque of lupus pernio involves the nose and is a symmetrical bluish-red and dusky violaceous lesion which may feel soft, doughy or indurated. The surface is glistening and the epidermis stretched with large pilosebaceous follicles and maybe telangiectasia. Similar lesions may affect the cheeks, lips, fingers and ears ('turkey ears'). Pressing a glass slide against the skin at the edge of a plaque (diascopy) will sometimes reveal the typical yellowish-brown appearance of a granulomatous reaction. Lupus pernio of the skin rarely ulcerates.

When the nasal mucosa is involved in sarcoidosis, patients present with crusting, swelling, discharge, ulceration or difficulty breathing. The nasal bones may be affected. Nasal bone radiographs in a series of 26 patients with lupus pernio showed that 34% had bony porosis and destruction of the nasal bones (Spiteri *et al.*, 1985).

Lupus pernio portends a chronic course and, in addition to lesions of the upper respiratory tract, is associated with bone cysts, lacrimal gland and renal sarcoid, and hypercalcaemia.

Nasal rim papules and nodules

Sarcoidal papules and nodules involving the nasal rim may indicate involvement of the nasal mucosa and upper respiratory tract as mentioned above.

Papular sarcoidosis

Orange or yellowish papules, 2–6 mm in diameter, which later become violaceous are a common skin manifestation particularly in the black patient. The face, eyelids, nasolabial folds, nape and upper back are usually involved.

Nodular sarcoidosis

Individual lesions are larger and fewer than in the papular type.

Annular sarcoidosis

Annular lesions may affect the cheek adjacent to the nose.

Scar sarcoidosis

Scars at sites of trauma, nose piercing, operation, inoculation site or tattoo may become purple, swollen and tender at the time of presentation or during disease reactivation.

Sarcoid in Black Americans

The skin is especially affected and lesions may be exuberant and bizarre with atypical plaques, nodules and keloid-like forms. Psoriasiform, verrucous and lupus-erythematosus-like lesions may occur in addition to patches of hypopigmentation.

Diagnosis

Histological examination of biopsy samples of skin or nasal mucosa will show non-caseating granulomas. Multinucleate giant cells are usually present. The rim of lymphoid cells surrounding the granuloma is never well developed, hence the term 'naked tubercle'. A fine reticulin network encircles the granuloma and may penetrate it.

Blood tests may show hypercalcaemia, elevated serum angiotensin converting enzyme and abnormal liver enzymes in cases with liver involvement.

Course and prognosis

Cutaneous papules tend to resolve within months or years. Plaques persist and lupus pernio is particularly persistent. Its prognosis is modified by the extent of the accompanying systemic involvement.

Treatment

Small cutaneous lesions may be treated with potent topical corticosteroids or with intralesional triamcinolone injections. Caution should be exercised in excising any sarcoidal lesion because of the risk of scar sarcoidosis and of keloid formation. Systemic corticosteroids are indicated for disfiguring skin disease, and antimalarials (chloroquine) have been used with some success. Lupus pernio is a particularly difficult management problem, but it may respond to a combination of methotrexate and systemic corticosteroids.

Patients with lupus pernio and those who find their cutaneous lesions cosmetically embarrassing may benefit from cosmetic camouflage.

Connective tissue diseases
Lupus erythematosus

Lupus erythematosus may be systemic (systemic lupus erythematosus) or largely confined to the skin (chronic discoid lupus erythematosus).

Systemic lupus erythematosus

Systemic lupus erythematosus (SLE) is a generalized autoimmune disorder with a predilection for young females. It shows a spectrum of severity from a mild recurring illness to a fulminant rapidly fatal disease. Fortunately many patients with SLE have a disease that is intermediate in severity, with relapses and remissions spanning many years. Any organ system may be involved, but most commonly the joints (95%), kidneys (55%) and cardiopulmonary system (40%). Renal disease varies from mild focal lupus nephritis to diffuse proliferative glomerulonephritis.

Those with cardiopulmonary involvement present with pleuritic chest pain or have evidence of pleural effusion, pulmonary infiltrates, pericarditis, myocarditis, endocarditis or conduction abnormalities. Patients with active SLE are systemically unwell with malaise, fever (low grade or spiking), anorexia, weight loss and lymphadenopathy. Central nervous system involvement (psychosis, convulsions, neuropathy or paralysis) portends a poor prognosis.

Approximately 80% of patients with SLE have a rash at some stage and it is the presenting complaint in up to 25%. The characteristic eruption is the 'butterfly' rash which is intensely red on both cheeks, sharply demarcated at the nasolabial areas and extends across the bridge of the nose. There may be associated facial oedema and scale. Some patients have a more diffuse erythema involving the face and upper trunk and one-third of patients have increased sensitivity to light. Lesions resembling chronic discoid lupus (described below) occur in one-third of patients with SLE at some stage. Further lesions include diffuse alopecia, Raynaud's phenomenon, livedo reticularis, vasculitis, bullous lesions, pigmentary abnormalities and calcinosis cutis. Mucous membrane ulceration, particularly involving the buccal mucosa, occurs during active phases of the disease. Ulceration of the mucosa of the nasal septum occurs in approximately 5% of patients. Perforation of the nasal septum may occur during disease exacerbations and presents as epistaxis.

Chronic discoid lupus erythematosus

Chronic discoid lupus erythematosus (CDLE) is characterized by well-defined red scaly plaques which tend to heal by atrophy, scarring and pigmentary change. Removal of the adherent scale may reveal horny plugs in the undersurface which have occupied dilated pilosebaceous orifices ('carpet-tack' sign). There may be areas of follicular plugging and hyperkeratosis. The hyperkeratosis may be sufficiently marked to produce warty lesions which most commonly affect the nose, temples, ears and scalp. Lesions of CDLE vary in size from a few millimetres to several centimetres and may be localized with lesions occurring on the face and scalp or more generalized with lesions elsewhere on the body. Facial lesions most commonly affect the cheeks, bridge of the nose, tip of the nose and the ears. Examination of the scalp may show well-defined areas of scarring alopecia. A small proportion of patients have Raynaud's phenomenon or chilblains.

CDLE-type lesions may occur in patients with SLE, but less than 5% of patients with CDLE will progress to SLE. The overall prognosis for CDLE is good. However, there may be considerable psychological morbidity due to facial scarring.

Diagnosis

The cutaneous lesions of SLE and CDLE may be histologically indistinguishable. The histological features include hyperkeratosis, follicular plugging, epidermal atrophy, degeneration of the basal layer and a periappendageal lymphocytic inflammatory infiltrate.

Antinuclear antibodies are present in high titre in patients with active SLE and antibodies to double-stranded DNA are specific to SLE. Other abnormalities include elevated ESR, hypergammaglobulinaemia, hypocomplementaemia, anaemia, leukopenia, thrombocytopenia, positive rheumatoid factor, a false positive test for syphilis and urinary abnormalities.

Approximately 50% of patients with CDLE have haematological and serological abnormalities. Antinuclear antibody, when positive, is usually present in lower titre than in SLE and antibodies to double-stranded DNA are negative.

Treatment

The wide range of involvement and severity in SLE means that treatment must be tailored to the individual's needs. Choice of therapy is dictated by the extent of vital organ involvement. Corticosteroids in high dose are required in acute disease, and may be combined with azathioprine or cyclophosphamide. Lupus nephritis may respond to a combination of prednisolone and chlorambucil.

Patients must be advised to avoid strong sunlight which is well known to provoke exacerbations of SLE.

Lesions of CDLE will improve with potent topical corticosteroids. Active cutaneous lesions warrant topical corticosteroids under occlusion, intralesional triamcinolone or hydroxychloroquine. Patients with active facial CDLE or with residual scarring often gain considerable benefit from the use of cosmetic camouflage.

Wegener's granulomatosis

This is a rare granulomatous necrotizing condition of the upper and lower respiratory tract associated with generalized arteritis and focal or diffuse glomerulitis. Rhinological symptoms in Wegener's granulomatosis include nasal crusting, bloody rhinorrhoea, progressive nasal obstruction and vague pain and tenderness of the dorsum of the nose. Papular, plaque-like and ulcerative lesions are the most common of the cutaneous signs. Granulomatous involvement of the nasal septum with dissolution of the cartilage leads to the typical saddle nose deformity, and necrotizing granulomatous lesions may lead to complete destruction of the nose. The skin elsewhere may show the 'palpable purpura' of cutaneous vasculitis.

Diagnosis

Antineutrophil cytoplasmic antibody with cytoplasmic staining (C-ANCA) has a high sensitivity (96%) in patients with generalized active Wegener's granulomatosis. Positivity is seen less commonly in active localized disease.

Treatment

Treatment with systemic corticosteroids and cyclophosphamide improves the otherwise poor prognosis.

Scleroderma

Scleroderma or systemic sclerosis is a disorder of unknown aetiology which incorporates Raynaud's phenomenon, sclerotic skin lesions and vasculitis. In the well-developed case the facial appearance is characteristic with a smooth forehead, pinched or beaked nose and peri-oral furrowing (purse-string mouth). There may be varying degrees of mat telangiectasia. Patients with limited cutaneous involvement are anticentromere antibody positive and usually have a better prognosis than patients with diffuse cutaneous systemic sclerosis, who have the Scl 70 antibody.

Relapsing polychondritis

Relapsing polychondritis is a rare disease characterized by recurring episodes of inflammation in cartilaginous tissues. Patients usually present with auricular chondritis and arthritis. The chondritis manifests as acute onset of redness, heat, swelling and tenderness of the affected part, mimicking cellulitis. Eventually more than 50% of affected patients will have involvement of the nasal cartilage. With recurrent bouts of inflammation the cartilage is destroyed and replaced with fibrous tissue, resulting in 'cauliflower' ears and a deformed and obstructed nose. There may be collapse of the cartilages of the larynx and trachea. Other features include aortic aneurysm, mitral regurgitation and eye inflammation.

Systemic corticosteroids are used to control acute disease. The course of relapsing polychondritis is highly variable and spontaneous remission may occur.

Other diseases affecting the external nose
Centrofacial ulcerations

Destructive processes of the facial midline may signify any of a range of infective, malignant or autoimmune diseases. As the diagnosis is frequently elusive repeat biopsy samples may be necessary and samples should be submitted for routine histology, special stains, microbiology and immunofluorescence. The term 'lethal midline granuloma' is a clinical description which embraces Wegener's granulomatosis, polymorphic reticulosis (lymphoid granulomatosis) and idiopathic midline destructive disease. However, there is no agreement in the literature and some authors exclude Wegener's granulomatosis from the range of diseases included under the umberella of 'lethal midline granuloma'.

The majority of lymphoid granulomatosis are peripheral T-cell lymphomas and there are occasional reports of B-cell lymphomas causing ulceration and destruction of the nose and paranasal sinuses. Treatment is with radiotherapy and some authors (Senan, Symonds and Brown, 1992) have found initial treatment with oral alkylating agents and steroids useful in newly diagnosed cases.

Idiopathic midline destructive disease or malignant granuloma (Stewart, 1933) usually commences insidiously with oedema of the nose and nasal congestion. This is followed by perforation of the nasal septum, ulceration of the hard palate and extensive mutilation of the centre of the face. Histology of involved tissue shows a diffuse infiltrate of lymphocytes, leucocytes and histiocytic-type giant cells. It may be distinguished from Wegener's granulomatosis by the absence of necrotizing granulomas. The disease lasts from 3 to 20 months. Most authors feel that local high-dose radiation offers the best hope of amelioration.

Rosacea

Rosacea is a chronic disease of unknown aetiology with a predilection for those of Celtic origin. Affected patients tend to be 'flushers and blushers' who flush more intensely and more persistently than those who blush when embarrassed. With progression the erythema becomes more fixed and associated with crops of red papules and small pustules. There may also be telangiectasia and facial oedema. Comedones are not a feature of rosacea and this fact as well as the occurrence of rosacea in an older age group helps to differentiate rosacea from acne vulgaris. The centre of the face is predominantly affected in rosacea. In the most severely affected patients disfiguring enlargement of the nose, rhinophyma (Plate 4/2/IV), develops. Tissue overgrowth begins at the tip of the nose and progresses to involve the ala nasae and the columella. There is irregular suffusion and enlargement of the nose with prominent pilosebaceous orifices. The paranasal areas may be affected in some patients. The diagnosis of rosacea is a clinical one. Histopathology shows dermal oedema and dermal connective tissue disorganization. Most stages of rosacea will improve with oral tetracycline 1 g/day. Topical metronidazole is also beneficial. Telangiectasia and florid erythema are poorly responsive to treatment. Rhinophyma warrants referral to a dermatological surgeon or to a plastic surgeon as excellent cosmetic results may be achieved by 'paring', electrodesiccation or laser therapy.

Seborrhoeic dermatitis

Seborrhoeic dermatitis is a constitutional disorder which typically affects the sebaceous follicle rich areas of the face and trunk. Lesions classically involve the nasolabial folds as a red eruption with a greasy scale. More extensive lesions involve the eyebrows, beard area, forehead, ears and the centre of the chest. Scalp involvement presents as itchy scaling on a red background (dandruff). A role for the yeast *Pityrosporum ovale* in the pathogenesis of seborrhoeic dermatitis is supported by the response of the condition to oral and topical ketoconazole. There is a high prevalence of seborrhoeic dermatitis in patients with AIDS where the condition may be particularly severe and extensive.

Contact dermatitis

Dermatitis localized to the nose and paranasal skin may be 'allergic' due to contact with nose drops or plants or 'irritant' due to rubbing, e.g. during acute coryza.

Dermatitis artefacta

Patients with dermatitis artefacta are usually women who produce factitious disease to satisfy a psychological need. Lesions may be produced by cutting, scratching, picking, burning or damaging the skin with chemicals. A wide range of bizarre and chronic skin lesions are thus produced. Diagnosis and treatment are very difficult due to the underlying psychopathology.

References

BESNIER, E. (1889) Lupus pernio de la face: synovites fougueuses (scrofulotuberculeuses) symetriques des extremities superieures. *Annales de Dermatologie et de Syphiligraphie (Paris)*, 10, 333–396

CHUANG, T. Y., POPESCU, N. A., SU, W. P. D. and CHUTE, C. G. (1990) Squamous cell carcinoma. A population-based incidence study in Rochester, Minn. *Archives of Dermatology*, 126, 185–188

MARCOVAL, J., SERVITJE, O., MORENO, A., JUCGLA, A. and PEYRI, J. (1992) Lupus vulgaris. Clinical, histopathologic, and bacteriologic study of 10 cases. *Journal of the American Academy of Dermatology*, 26, 404–407

ROENIGK, R. K., RATZ, J. L., BAILIN, P. L. and WHEELAND, R. G. (1986) Trends in the presentation and treatment of basal cell carcinomas. *Journal of Dermatologic Surgery and Oncology*, 12, 860–865

SEHGAL, V. N. and WAGH, S. A. (1990) Cutaneous tuberculosis. Current concepts. *International Journal of Dermatology*, 29, 237–252

SENAN, S., SYMONDS, R. P. and BROWN, I. L. (1992) Nasal peripheral T cell lymphoma. a 20-year review of cases treated in Scotland. *Clinical Oncology*, 4, 96–100

SPITERI, M. A., MATTHEY, F., GORDON, T., CARSTAIRS. L. S. and GERAINT JAMES, D. (1985) Lupus pernio: a clinico-radiological study of thirty-five cases. *British Journal of Dermatology*, 112, 315–322

STEWART, J. P. (1933) Progressive lethal granulomatous ulceration of the nose. *Journal of Laryngology and Otology*, 48, 657–701

TEICHGRAEBER, J. F. and GOEPFERT, H. (1990) Rhinectomy: timing and reconstruction. *Otolaryngology – Head and Neck Surgery*, 102, 362–369

USTVEDT, H. J. and OSTENSEN, I. W. (1951) The relation between tuberculosis of the skin and primary infection. *Tubercle*, 32, 36–39

VEIEN, N. K., STAHL, D. and BRODTHAGEN, H. (1987) Cutaneous sarcoidosis in Caucasians. *Journal of the American Academy of Dermatology*, 16, 534–540

3

Radiology of the nose and paranasal sinuses

P. D. Phelps

Plain radiography of the nose

Views for the nose

Radiological examination of the nasal bones can best be made by placing a dental film in direct contact with the side of the nose and centring the incident beam horizontally through the nose. This lateral view may be supplemented by a craniocaudal projection obtained by inserting an occlusal film between the teeth and directing the vertical beam through the nasal bones onto the film. These views are usually requested following facial trauma, to show fractures of the nasal bones as well as lateral shifts and displacements (Figure 3.1).

Standard sinus views

A specialized skull unit should be used whenever possible to allow accurate positioning and unvarying focus film distances with a moving grid. Pathological processes affecting the paranasal sinuses encroach on the air in the sinuses and are seen on the radiographs as alterations in the translucency of the sinus. Examination in the erect position is desirable to reveal

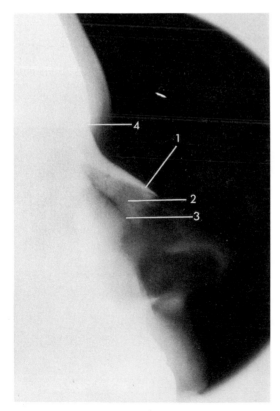

(a)

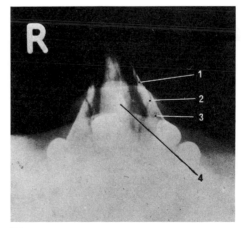

(b)

Figure 3.1 (a) Lateral view of nasal bones: 1. nasal bones. 2. Groove for anterior ethmoidal nerve. 3. Nasomaxillary suture. 4. Nasal process of frontal bone. (b) Superoinferior view of nasal bones: 1. nasal bones (lateral aspect). 2. Nasomaxillary suture. 3. Nasal process of maxilla. 4. Septum

fluid levels which may be present. It is possible to perform erect examinations on modern isocentric skull units, but without the advantages of fixed reference planes (see Volume 1, Chapter 17).

Asymmetry of the paired sinuses will usually result in the smaller sinus appearing more opaque because of its thicker bony walls. This should not be considered pathological. It is not uncommon for one frontal sinus to be much smaller than its fellow or even to be absent. Antra differ in size less often, though small differences are not uncommon. Rarely one maxillary antrum fails to develop and, in consequence, the maxilla looks dense on plain X-ray films. The smaller size of the affected antrum should alert the observer to this possibility (Figure 3.2).

The following projections allow a good all-round assessment of the paranasal sinuses; the occipitomental, the occipitofrontal, and either or both the lateral and the overshot axial views.

Occipitomental (or Waters') view (Figure 3.3)

The patient sits facing the Bucky support with the chin resting against it, the median sagittal plane aligned to the midline. The mouth is supported wide open with a transradiant perspex 'bite block' and the baseline is adjusted to make an angle of 45° with the film. In older patients it may be necessary to angle the central ray of the tube caudally to compensate for an inability to extend the head sufficiently, but if a skull table is used with the object table angled through 20° (or more) forwards towards the patient, the correct position will be consistently maintained, and will always allow the use of a horizontal X-ray beam. The tube is adjusted so that the central ray passes horizontally to the middle at the level of the inferior orbital margins and to the centre of the film.

Structures demonstrated

The antra are clearly visible, the frontal sinuses are projected obliquely, though their floors are clearly shown. The ethmoid cells are largely obscured, but a few cells may be seen within the nose and medial to the lamina papyracea on the inner wall of the orbit. The sphenoidal sinuses are visible through the open mouth. If, after examining the film, a fluid level is suspected, its presence or absence can be confirmed by repeating the view with the sagittal plane of the head tilted 20–40° to the side in question.

Occipitofrontal (or Caldwell) view (Figure 3.4)

The patient sits or lies prone with the forehead and part of the nose in contact with the Bucky support. The baseline is adjusted perpendicular to the film and the tube is angled 15° caudally. If a skull table is used the object table is angled 15–20° towards the patient, the central ray is directed horizontally to the nasion, and to the centre of the film.

Structures demonstrated

The frontal sinuses are clearly shown. The upper parts of the antra are obscured by the petrous bones but their lower parts are visible. The floor of the sella

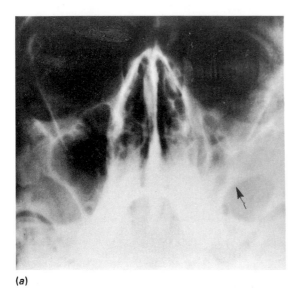

(a)

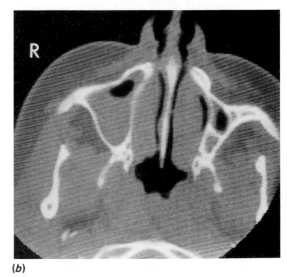

(b)

Figure 3.2 (*a*) Occipitomental view and (*b*) axial CT scan of the sinuses. Normal size antrum on the right, congenitally small and septate antrum on the left. There is mucosal thickening and fluid on both sides shown on the CT scan

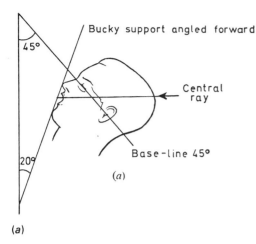

(a)

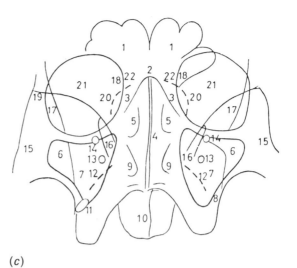

(c)

(b)

Figure 3.3 Occipitomental view of the sinuses: (a) technique, (b) radiograph, (c) line drawing of (b). 1. Frontal sinuses. 2. Nasal bones. 3. Nasal process of maxilla. 4. Nasal septum. 5. Middle turbinate. 6. Posterolateral wall of antrum. 7. Antrum. 8. Anterolateral wall of antrum. 9. Inferior turbinate. 10. Sphenoid sinus. 11. Foramen ovale overlying alveolar recess of antrum. 12. Soft tissue shadow cast by lips (dotted lines). 13. Foramen rotundum. 14. Infraorbital foramen. 15. Zygoma. 16. Superior orbital fissure. 17. Innominate line. 18. Lamina papyracea of ethmoid. 19. Frontozygomatic suture. 20. Soft tissue shadow cast by nares (dotted lines). 21. Orbit. 22. Ethmoid cells

turcica, the crista galli, the nasal septum and the middle and inferior turbinates can be seen. The ethmoidal and sphenoidal sinuses are superimposed.

Lateral (Figure 3.5)

The patient sits facing the Bucky table and the skull is then rotated into the lateral position. The central ray is directed horizontally to a point behind the outer canthus of the eye and to the centre of the film. When particular interest is directed to the nasopharynx, the patient sits sideways on with the head in the lateral position and the chin protruded. In children under 7 years of age the central ray is directed horizontally to a point immediately posterior to the angle of the mandible. In older children or adults the central ray is directed to a point 2.5 cm in front and 3.75 cm below the superimposed external auditory meatus and to the centre of the film. The focal film distance is increased from the standard 90 cm to reduce magnification.

Structures demonstrated

On the lateral projection the paired sinuses are superimposed on one another, but the extent of pneumatization of the frontal and sphenoidal sinuses can be gauged, especially in their vertical and horizontal directions. The thickness of the soft tissues in the nasopharynx, the uvula, and the extent of the nasopharyngeal airway can be asessed. Enlarged adenoids can be clearly shown.

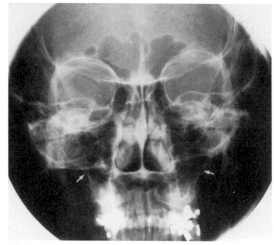

(a)

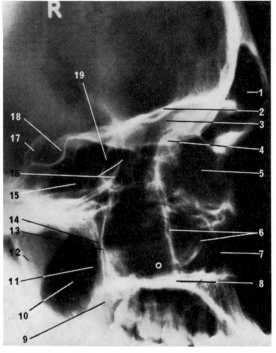

Figure 3.5 Lateral view of the sinuses: 1. Frontal sinuses, Vertical component; 2. Floor of anterior cranial fossa; 3. Frontal sinuses. Horizontal component; 4. Cribriform plate; 5. Orbit; 6. Zygoma; 7. Anterior wall of antrum; 8. Floor of antrum; 9. Uvula; 10. Air in nasopharynx; 11. Lateral pterygoid lamina; 12. Mandible; 13. Posterior wall of antrum; 14. Anterior wall of pterygoid process; 15. Sphenoid sinus; 16. Anterior wall of middle cranial fossa; 17. Dorsum sellae; 18. Anterior wall of pituitary fossa; 19. Anterior wall of sphenoid sinus.

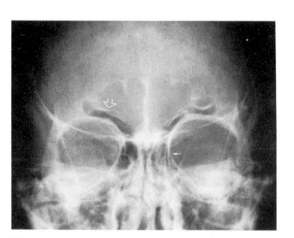

(b)

Figure 3.4 (*a*) Occipitofrontal views. Antra, ethmoid and frontal sinuses are shown. The white arrows point to the lateral walls of the antra, which should always be shown on this view. (*b*) The open arrow points to pneumatization of the orbital roof by ethmoid cells. The small arrow points to the lamina papyracea

This view is essential when opaque foreign bodies are being sought, or when surgery on the sphenoid bone or transnasal implantation of radioactive isotope seeds into the pituitary gland is contemplated. We use an alternative version of the lateral projection which better demonstrates the sinuses and postnasal space. This is a high kilovoltage lateral film using 150 kV or above and 3 mm of brass filtration (Figure 3.6).

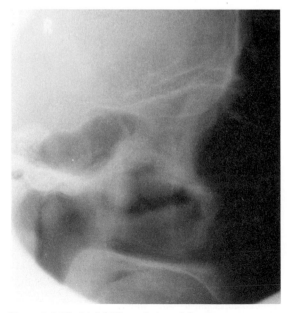

Figure 3.6 The high kV lateral view of the sinuses

Occipitomental views with varying angulation

Overangled or underangled occipitomental views may be used to give tangential views of the roof of the antrum in suspected injuries in that area. The patient is positioned as for a normal occipitomental view and the additional views are taken with the baseline at 60° and 30°, respectively. Increased angulation may be needed in patients in whom the petrous bones overlie the base of the antrum in the standard view.

Panoramic views (orthopantomography)

Panoral tomography in the plane of the dental arches is used for dental surveys (see Volume 1, Chapter 17) but, at the same time, the orthopantomograph gives a good display of the lower aspects of the antra which may be used to supplement the plain film demonstration of the sinuses.

Computerized tomography (CT)

The superiority of CT over other methods of imaging the sinuses can be summarized as follows:

1 The bony walls of the sinuses are demonstrated at least as well by CT in the high resolution mode as by conventional radiography and tomography
2 An excellent anatomical display of soft tissue densities, including fluid levels and polypoid masses, within the normally air-filled cavities of the sinuses, nasal cavity and postnasal space is provided
3 Most important of all, disease extending beyond the bony perimeters of the sinuses into the adjacent soft tissue of the orbit, brain and infratemporal fossa can be imaged.

These applications of CT have disappointed in only one way. While giving an excellent anatomical display, CT generally fails to predict the histological nature of the pathological process, unless there is characteristic calcification within a tumour such as a meningioma or chondroma.

'Tissue characterization' with or without contrast enhancement is almost always unsuccessful if measurement of attenuation values is used, and this was appreciated in the early days of CT (Forbes *et al.*, 1978). Contrast enhancement is required:

1 If intracranial extension of disease is suspected on clinical grounds or from the anatomical demonstration, particularly on the coronal CT sections
2 If a particularly vascular tumour such as a meningioma or juvenile nasopharyngeal angiofibroma is suspected; a contrast infusion to ensure that enhancement occurs in the vascular phase is required in such cases (see Volume 1, Chapter 17)
3 Occasionally if an inflammatory process is suspected.

Most American authorities, however, recommend routine use of contrast enhancement for the investigation of the facial area (Hasso, 1984). The present author does not advocate this approach, as intravenous contrast medium usually enhances all soft tissue structures around the sinuses, and is therefore unhelpful, besides adding to the length of the examination, increasing the not inconsiderable radiation dose to the patient, and adding the risk of a systemic reaction to the contrast agent. Soft tissue characterization is much better by magnetic resonance (MR).

The standard plane for CT scanning of the paranasal sinuses is parallel to the infraorbital meatal baseline. This plane is nearly parallel to the planes of the hard palate, the zygomatic arches and much of the orbital roof. The antra are seen in cross-section (Figure 3.7), the ethmoid and sphenoid sinuses are well demonstrated, as are the anterior and posterior walls of the frontal sinuses. These axial sections are also the best for demonstrating the orbital contents and the nasopharynx.

The axial scans are then reviewed to decide whether further sections are necessary in the coronal plane. Generally, evaluation of structures parallel to the infraorbital baseline or evidence of intracranial extension of the disease process necessitates coronal sections (Figure 3.8). For both axial and coronal scans, contiguous sections, 5 mm thick, are usual. Degradation of the images by metal fillings in the teeth, especially in the coronal plane, may require repositioning of the patient's head or the angle of the gantry.

The soft tissue structures of the face need to be assessed on a window setting of 400–800 Hounsfield units (HU), while bone detail is best shown at a setting of 1000–3000 Hounsfield units. Even at the wide window setting, thin plates of bone, especially the lamina papyracea forming part of the medial wall of the orbit, may appear to be dehiscent because of partial volume averaging. Erosion of a thin plate of bone should not be diagnosed on the CT scan unless an adjacent soft tissue mass can be demonstrated, and then the problem of soft tissue silhouetting is added to that of partial volume averaging (see Volume 1, Chapter 17).

Functional endoscopic sinus surgery (FESS)

Recent developments in nasal endoscopy have coincided with the development of improved high resolution CT to give a better demonstration of nasal and sinus anatomy. Greater attention is now paid to the ethmoid labyrinth and in particular the so-called ostiomeatal complex where the ostium of the antrum opens into the middle meatus. Obstruction to this and other major routes of mucociliary drainage such as the

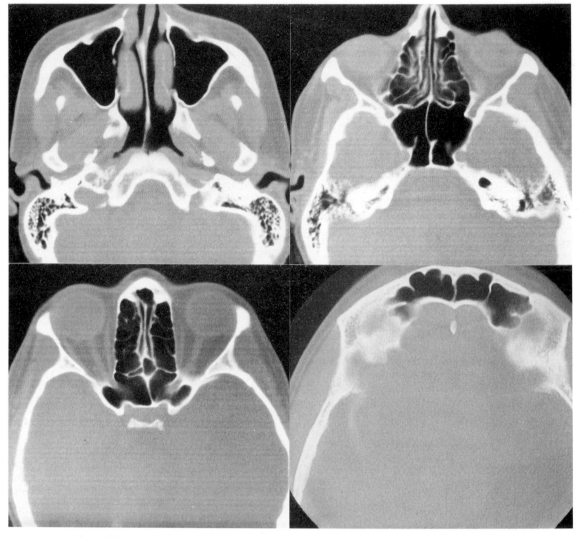

Figure 3.7 Axial CT of the sinuses showing antra, ethmoid and sphenoid sinuses, and frontal sinuses in successive sections

spheno-ethmoidal recess are thought to be the prime causes of sinus disease. Their accurate demonstration by imaging is of great importance for FESS and preoperative coronal CT sections (3 or 4 mm thick) are mandatory (Figure 3.9). The sections are imaged on a bone algorithm and wide window setting (4000 HU) to give maximum anatomical detail as well as outlining any soft tissue opacities. A common variant is the pneumatized middle turbinate or concha bullosa (Figure 3.10).

The maxillary antra are small at birth and expand progressively during the first decade of life. Occasionally they may remain infantile (Figure 3.11) and then it can be difficult, on plain films, to distinguish this cause of opacity from the more usual such as chronic infection or fibrous dysplasia. The antra are rarely asymmetrical but the absence of pathological features and presence of a normal ostium can be confirmed by axial CT (Figure 3.12). Sometimes a small sinus may be double (see Figure 3.2).

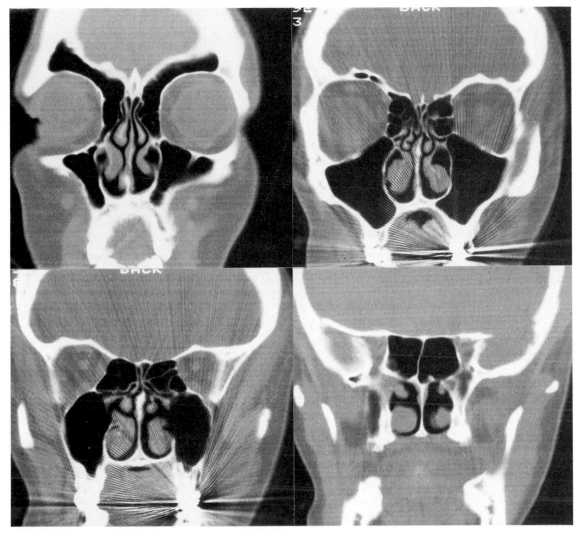

Figure 3.8 Coronal CT of the sinuses showing all the sinuses in successive sections

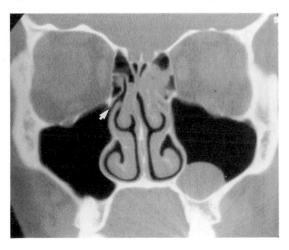

Figure 3.9 The ostiomeatal unit. The arrow points to the normal ostium while the other side shows mucosal obstruction

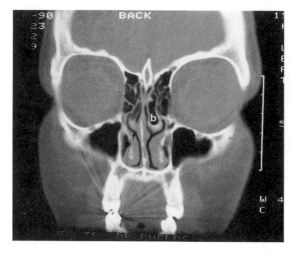

Figure 3.10 Concha bullosa (b) shown on this coronal CT section. The arrow shows apposition of the mucosal surfaces on the other side

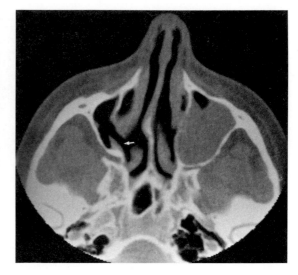

Figure 3.12 A small, but air-containing, antrum on the right. The section was taken at the level of the sinus ostium (arrow). Swollen mucosa fills the other antrum

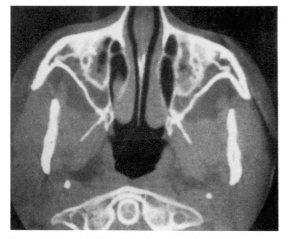

Figure 3.11 Axial CT section showing infantile antra having a double wall appearance. There is also some mucosal thickening within the antra

Magnetic resonance (MR) (Figure 3.13)

The bony margins of the sinuses appear as a plane of absent signal on MR scans and this limits the usefulness of the technique for examination of the sinuses. Moreover, the intense signal from the high fat content of bone marrow, as in the basisphenoid and petrous apices and around the frontal sinuses, can be very confusing for the radiologist interpreting the scans. This is particularly so as retained fluid within the sinuses gives a similar intense signal from the high water content.

It is difficult or impossible on a CT scan to differentiate tumour tissue from retained fluid in sinuses where the drainage of a sinus is blocked by obstruction from the tumour. Differentiation on an MR scan is simple and clear (Figure 3.14). Extension of sinus neoplasia into the cranial cavity is shown very well by MR and the ability to image in any plane is a considerable advantage.

Specific clinical situations

Trauma

Injuries to the face and sinuses are considered in Chapter 16. Fractures are usually demonstrated by conventional radiographic techniques, but CT is often necessary to show the fracture lines. Fluid levels in sinuses indicating a cerebrospinal fluid fistula are well shown by CT (Figure 3.15). The improved soft tissue imaging of CT and MR imaging can also be an advantage in trauma cases, especially for showing the state of the orbital contents (Figure 3.16) and CT is especially good for assessing 'blow out' fractures (Figure 3.17).

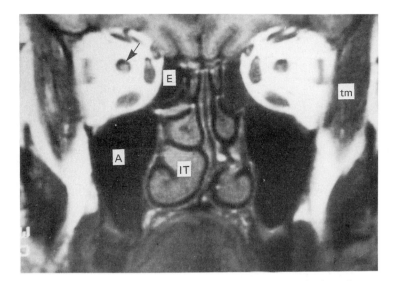

Figure 3.13 Normal MR scan. Coronal section through the antra (A), ethmoids (E) and orbits. The arrow points to the optic nerve. IT = inferior turbinate, tm = temporalis muscle

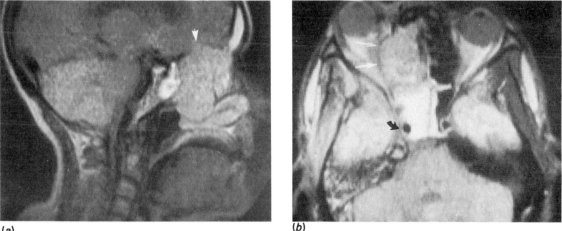

(a)　　　　　　　　　　　　　　　　**(b)**

Figure 3.14 MR scan. (*a*) Lateral view showing a mass in the nasal cavity extending up into the anterior cranial fossa (arrow). Note the high signal of retained fluid in both frontal and sphenoid sinuses on this T2-weighted image; (*b*) axial view shows the mass displacing the medial wall of the orbit which appears as a dark line (white arrows). The black arrow points to the internal carotid artery

Inflammatory disease

Mucosal thickening, a common finding on plain sinus views, is shown far more readily on CT scans. Normal mucosa is too thin to be demonstrated on the scan, but minor degrees of thickening in the absence of relevant symptoms may be dismissed as an incidental finding. If the sinus ostium becomes blocked, a completely opaque sinus will result. An air/fluid level may be observed at an intermediate stage before the obstructed sinus becomes totally opacified.

Chronic obstruction of the ostium or a septate portion of the sinus cavity gives rise to mucocoeles. Proptosis is often the presenting symptom. The diag-

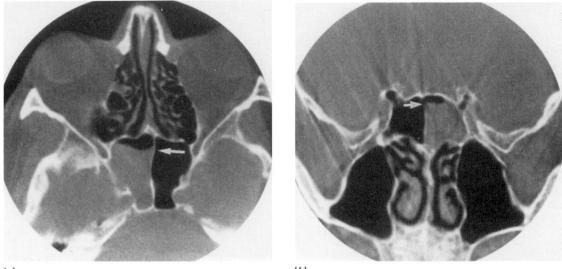

(a)   **(b)**

Figure 3.15 A patient with a spontaneous cerebrospinal fluid rhinorrhoea. (*a*) Axial CT section and (*b*) the coronal show the fluid level in the left sphenoid sinus only, indicating that this was the pathway of the leak. The arrow indicates the fluid level

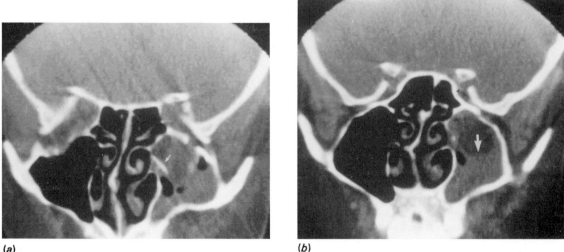
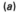

(a)   **(b)**

Figure 3.16 Coronal CT sections showing a fracture of the orbital floor ((*a*) small arrow). Note the clear distinction between orbital fat and blood in the antrum ((*b*) large arrow)

nosis is often suspected on plain skull radiographs, but CT confirms the benign nature of the lesion and gives an accurate display of its extent (Price and Danziger, 1980). Initially it was hoped that a low CT attenuation reading would help to confirm the diagnosis of mucocoele but such readings have proved extremely variable. Nevertheless, the diagnosis can usu-ally be made from the expansile appearance of the lesion (Figure 3.18).

The characteristic radiological features of benign nasal polyposis are familiar to otolaryngologists. How-ever, in a proportion of patients the changes are much greater and include widening of the ethmoid labyrinth and nasal cavity, bone thinning and expan-

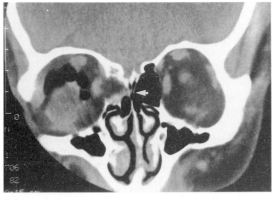

(a)

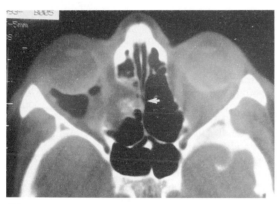

(b)

Figure 3.17 The less common medial blow out fracture (arrow) with air in the orbit. (*a*) Coronal CT section; (*b*) axial view

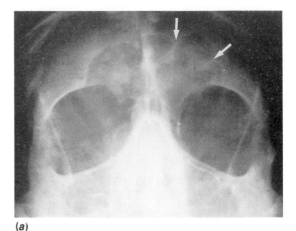

(a)

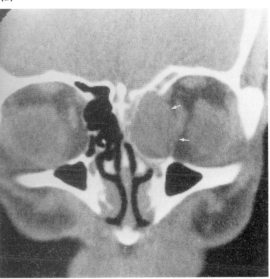

(b)

Figure 3.18 (*a*) Plain occipitofrontal view showing frontal sinus mucocoele. Note the loss of scalloping on the right, and the normal partitions (arrows) on the left. (*b*) The typical appearance of an ethmoid mucocoele. Note the expansile nature of the lesion extending into the orbit

sion, and mucocoele formation (Lund and Lloyd, 1983). The ethmoid widening and opacity can be shown by plain films or CT (Figure 3.19).

Most acute sinus infections are successfully treated by antibiotics, but sometimes the inflammatory process spreads beyond the confines of the sinus cavities. The close association with the orbit means that the most frequent complication of acute inflammatory sinus disease is orbital cellulitis with pain, oedema and proptosis. A subperiosteal or orbital abscess is a more serious complication which may require surgical exploration and drainage. The decision regarding surgical intervention is greatly helped by the CT demonstration of the site of the abscess (Figure 3.20). Patients with orbital cellulitis frequently require external drainage. Frontal ethmoidectomy may be required if resolution does not occur or chronic infection is present. Pus between bone and orbital periosteum is well shown by coronal CT (Figure 3.20). If the infection breaches the periosteum the normal muscle and fat planes rapidly become indistinct and vision deteriorates.

Postoperative state of the sinuses

Following surgery on the paranasal sinuses, radiological investigation may be required to determine the presence of recurrent disease. After the Caldwell-Luc operation, the postoperative appearance is opaque on plain sinus views, but CT has shown that this opacification is commonly due to bone thickening (Cable *et al.*, 1981). This would seem to be the result of peri-

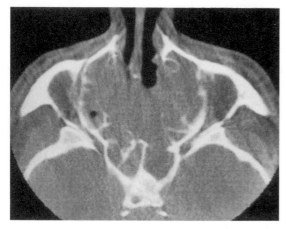

Figure 3.19 Axial CT section showing severe polyposis of nose and ethmoids, causing hypertelorism

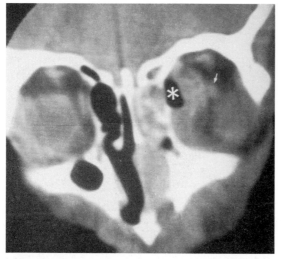

(a)

osteal stripping followed by the deposition of new bone (Figure 3.21). The postoperative antrum is often smaller than normal. Although CT differentiates well between bone and soft tissue, unfortunately it is not so satisfactory for excluding residual soft tissue disease such as loculated pus.

Tumours

The CT diagnosis of a tumour requires the presence of a soft-tissue tumour mass. Changes in the adjacent bones are secondary features. Categorizing the bone destruction seen on CT as either aggressive bone destruction or bone remodelling aids differential diagnosis. Bone remodelling or expansion reflects slow growth of the tumour. New bone is laid down on the outer surface of the sinus wall as erosion takes place from the inner wall adjacent to the tumour and differentiation from a mucocoele or expansion by benign simple polyposis (see Figure 3.19) may be difficult.

A mass in the middle meatus of the nasal cavity extending into the antrum is highly suggestive of an inverting papilloma (Lund and Lloyd, 1984). Other features of this tumour which have been shown by CT are small areas of calcification within the tumour mass and sclerosis of the sinus walls (Figure 3.22), although the latter is a non-specific change most frequently seen in chronic sinus infection. More obvious extensive and dense calcification within an expansile mass is a feature of chondroma or chondrosarcoma. This calcification is an important feature in the diagnosis, well demonstrated by CT (Figure 3.23) but not shown by MR, although enhancement of the periphery of the tumour with gadolinium is almost pathognomonic. Lloyd and Phelps (1986) have shown significant advantages in entirely different

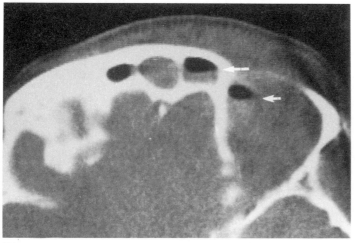

(b)

Figure 3.20 (*a*) Subperiosteal abscess (asterisk), displacing the orbital contents. The arrow points to the optic nerve. Note the opaque ethmoid sinuses on this side. (*b*) Axial CT section of another case with a subperiosteal abscess affecting the orbit. The arrow points to the fluid levels in the frontal sinus, and the abscess

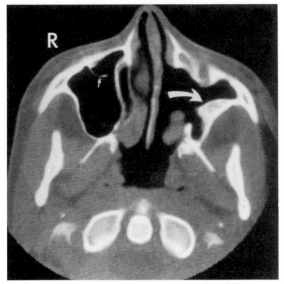

Figure 3.21 The typical appearance on axial CT following a previous Caldwell-Luc operation. Note the arrow in the wide antrostomy opening, indicating new bone formation on the posterolateral wall of the left antrum. There is a small septum in the right antrum (small arrow)

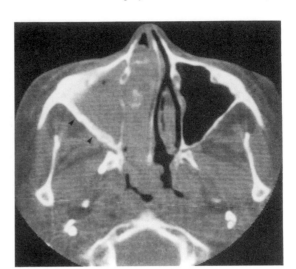

(a)

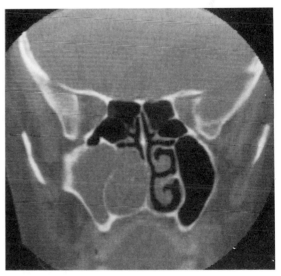

(b)

Figure 3.22 (*a*) Axial and (*b*) coronal CT sections showing the typical appearances of an inverting papilloma. The mass fills the antrum and extends out into the middle meatus of the nose. Note the thickening of the antral wall (arrow heads), and also some calcification within the mass

ways for both CT and MR in the diagnosis and assessment of one particular rare benign tumour, namely juvenile angiofibroma. Thirty cases were described, all of whom had bone destruction at the base of the pterygoid lamina. The distinctive radiological features of these tumours are discussed in Volume 6, Chapter 2, and the radiological anatomy and pathology of the infratemporal fossa and parapharyngeal region in volume 5, Chapter 2.

Malignant sinus neoplasms characteristically produce aggressive bone destruction: the bone is rapidly permeated and destroyed. Such destruction is seen primarily with squamous cell carcinoma which accounts for nearly 80% of all paranasal sinus malignancies (Som, 1985). Where plain sinus views are the usual primary means of imaging, it is most important for both radiologists and surgeons to look carefully for erosion of the bony margins of the sinuses, especially in the presence of suspicious clinical features.

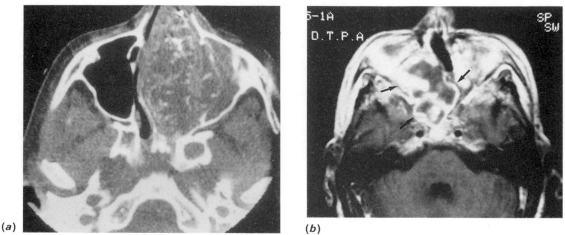

(a)   **(b)**

Figure 3.23 (*a*) Calcification in a chondrosarcoma in the ethmoid region. (*b*) The pathognomonic appearance of a chondrosarcoma is the intense enhancement around the periphery of the lesion after gadolinium

Obliteration of fascial planes beyond the sinus walls is the most characteristic CT sign for the identification of malignancy (Figure 3.24). Whenever a soft tissue mass extends beyond the bony confines of a sinus, neoplasia should be ruled out by biopsy. Extension of sinus neoplasia into the orbit or cranial cavity (Figure 3.25) affects the management of the disease. This extension is shown better by MR than CT, especially with gadolinium enhancement. Differentiation of tumour from mucosa and retained fluid is possible (Figure 3.26).

Bony tumours and bone dysplasias

Osteomas are common benign tumours which produce no symptoms unless they extend beyond the sinus, block the ostium, cause pressure on a nerve or displace other structures. They are commonest in the frontal sinuses and are readily demonstrated by plain radiographs (Figure 3.27).

Tomography or CT is sometimes required to show the point of attachment to the sinus wall and axial CT (Figure 3.28) gives a good demonstration of the

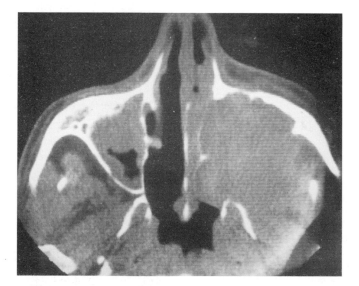

Figure 3.24 Axial CT section showing the typical appearances of an antral carcinoma. Note the destruction of the posterolateral wall of the antrum and extension backwards into the soft tissues. There is marked mucosal thickening of the other antrum

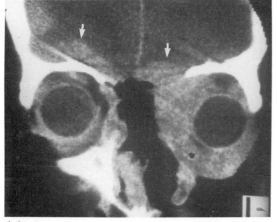

(a)

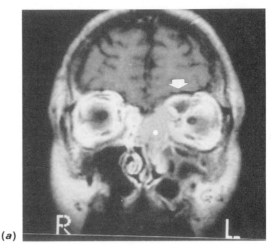

(a)

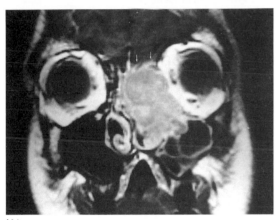

(b)

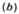

Figure 3.25 (above) (*a*) Extension of a carcinoma into the orbit and anterior cranial fossa shown by enhanced CT (arrows); (*b*) coronal GdMR section showing an ethmoid carcinoma extending back into the orbit and up and into the anterior cranial fossa (arrows)

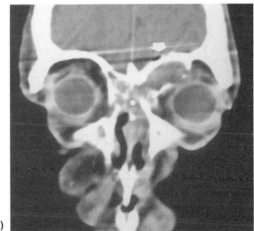

(b)

posterior extent. The density of the mass depends on the amount of ivory and cancellous bone present in the tumour. A benign bony tumour which fills the sinus, with no radiographic features to suggest an osseous lesion, may cause problems in assessment. A

Figure 3.26 (right) Adenocarcinoma of the ethmoids (asterisk) with a secondary mucocoele of the frontal sinus (arrow) shown on coronal section imaging by (*a*) CT; (*b*) unenhanced MR; and (*c*) MR after gadolinium. Note how the mucocoele becomes clearly apparent after Gd

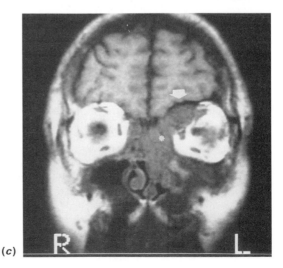

(c)

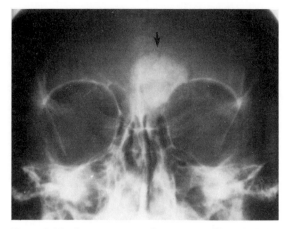

Figure 3.27 Plain sinus view of an osteoma filling the left frontal sinus

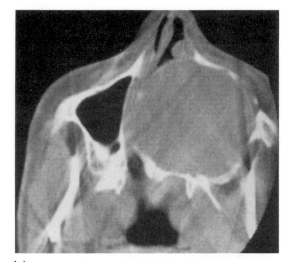

(a)

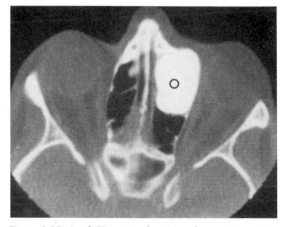

Figure 3.28 Axial CT section showing a dense osteoma in the ethmoids (O)

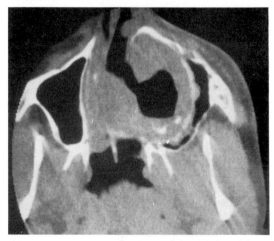

(b)

Figure 3.29 A giant-cell reparative granuloma arising from the alveolus fills the antrum (*a*), but after biopsy air can be seen between the mass and the antral wall (*b*)

large mass in the antrum (Figure 3.29) which appeared to have arisen from the alveolus was histologically diagnosed as a giant-cell reparative granuloma and its true relation to the antrum only revealed at surgery. Other benign tumours of the jaws can produce a similar appearance on CT with destruction of the alveolus and evidence of spread into the soft tissues. Meningiomas may very rarely arise in the sinuses but are more likely to affect the sinuses by extension from within the cranial cavity. CT is the imaging investigation of choice, not only to demonstrate calcification within a tumour mass, but also to show the osseous sclerosis that occurs with meningioma (Figure 3.30). Nevertheless, differentiation of meningioma en plaque from developmental diseases such as fibrous dysplasia may be difficult. Fibrous

dysplasia is either polyostotic or monostotic and usually develops early in life. The skull and facial bones may be affected singly or as part of a more generalized disease (Figure 3.31).

Characteristically there is thickening and expansion of bone but the density of the lesion depends on the amount of fibrous tissue present; when this is high, a 'ground glass' appearance is seen (Figure 3.32). In other cases dense bone predominates and, less commonly, a mixed type occurs with islands of dense bone in a fibrous matrix (Figure 3.33).

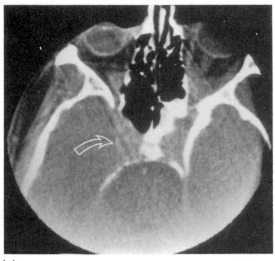

(a)

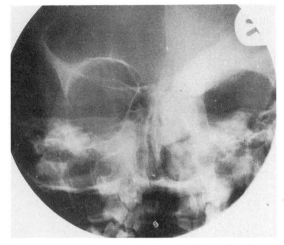

Figure 3.31 Albright's syndrome. Dense fibrous dysplasia affects the supraorbital ridge

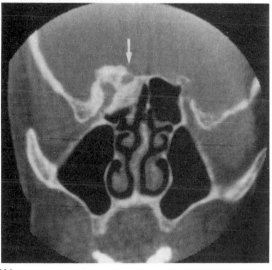

(b)

Figure 3.30 A sphenoid ridge meningioma producing bone sclerosis in the region of the superior oblique fissure. (*a*) Axial section showing extension of the soft tissue mass into the anterior cranial fossa (curved arrow), (*b*) coronal section showing bone sclerosis (white arrow) and extension into the sphenoid sinus

Figure 3.32 Fibrous dysplasia encroaching on the sphenoid sinus and the orbit showing the 'ground glass' appearance on this axial CT scan

The nasopharynx (postnasal space)

These alternative terms to describe the space behind the posterior choanae of the nose highlight the dilemma of whether the nasopharynx should be considered with the nose or the rest of the pharynx. Traditionally, radiological examination of the nasopharynx was by lateral and submentovertical views to show soft tissue masses distorting or obstructing the airway or eroding the base of the skull (Figure 3.34). CT is now the usual means of demonstrating the nasopharynx. Although an excellent demonstration of the air mucosal interface is obtained, it should be remembered that this is better assessed clinically with a

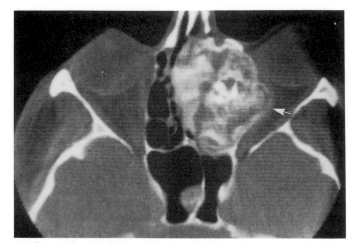

Figure 3.33 Axial CT section showing localized fibrous dysplasia displacing the optic nerve (arrow)

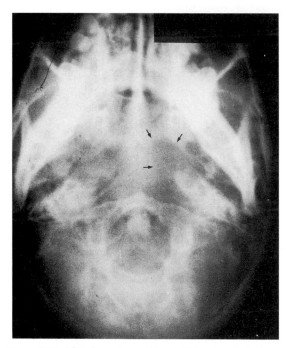

Figure 3.34 Plain base view of the skull showing typical erosion in the region of the foramen lacerum by a nasopharyngeal carcinoma

tissue planes which lie beneath the mucosa. The axial view of these planes complements the clinical examination because deep extension is the hallmark of malignancy in the nasopharynx. The pterygoid muscles attached to the lateral pterygoid plate and the deglutition muscles can be recognized as well as the fat in the paranasopharyngeal space between them. Further consideration of these parapharyngeal structures is given in Volume 5 on the pharynx. Diseases of the nasopharynx frequently obstruct the

mirror or endoscope. The characteristic shape of the nasopharynx on axial CT shows the torus tubaris as the most prominent landmark. In front is the opening of the eustachian tube and behind the lateral pharyngeal recess, or fossa of Rosenmüller (Figure 3.35). What is more important, and a great advance in imaging, is the ability of CT to demonstrate the deep

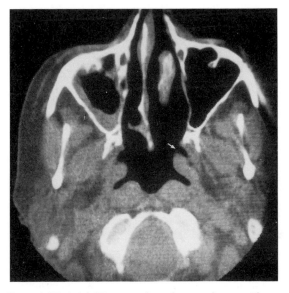

Figure 3.35 Axial CT scan to show the nasopharynx. The arrow points to the opening of the eustachian tube

eustachian tube, and the subsequent opacity of the middle ear cleft is easily demonstrated by CT or MR.

Magnetic resonance has several advantages over CT for imaging the nasopharynx. As well as the facility for three-plane imaging, the soft tissue structures in the paranasopharyngeal region are demonstrated better than by CT. The standard head coil is used. T1-weighted images, 5 mm thick, are obtained in the axial plane after an initial sagittal scout view. Further views in the coronal plane or using a T2-weighted protocol are then obtained if necessary but, more usually, depending on the pathology to be demonstrated, the initial T1 axial and coronal scans are repeated after the intravenous administration of gadolinium (Gd) DTPA. Lymphoid tissue is relatively hyperintense compared to the surrounding musculature and enhancement of the normal mucosa by Gd makes the mucosal lining more obvious.

Malignant tumours of the nasopharynx

Almost all deeply infiltrating lesions of the nasopharynx will prove to be primary neoplasms, usually squamous cell carcinoma. The most important feature on the CT scan is obliteration of the paranasopharyngeal soft tissue planes and in particular the fat in the paranasopharyngeal space (Figure 3.36). The deep soft-tissue structures are normally very symmetrical so comparison between the two sides is

useful. Such symmetry is not so constant in the normal outline of the mucosal surface.

Sometimes carcinomas of the upper aerodigestive tract are not apparent on examination of the mucosal surfaces because the tumour arises either submucosally or within a deep crypt and then extends into the deep tissue planes rather than the lumen. In one series (Mancuso and Hanafee, 1983) there were 19 mucosally inapparent carcinomas of the upper aerodigestive tract out of 160 cases examined. There may or may not be a mass bulging the wall of the nasopharynx, but diagnosis can only be made by CT or MR guided biopsy. Endoscopy and biopsy compromise the effectiveness of CT and therefore should be carried out after the CT examination.

Asymmetry of the muscle layers may be due to atrophy after radiotherapy or sometimes to neurogenic muscular atrophy from infiltration by a carcinoma (Figure 3.37). Occasionally nasopharyngeal

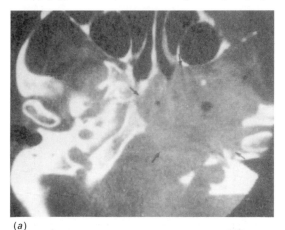

(a)

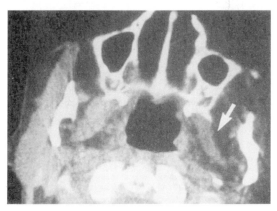

(b)

Figure 3.37 A carcinoma eroding the base of the skull ((a) small arrows), although the nasopharynx appeared normal. The patient complained of trigeminal pain for a long period and the large arrow (b) indicates the atrophic pterygoid muscles

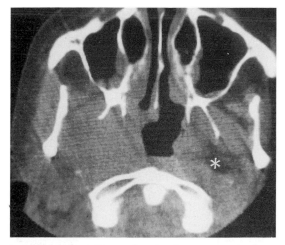

Figure 3.36 Axial CT scan showing the appearances of a typical deeply infiltrating carcinoma of the nasopharynx. Note the abnormal outlines of the nasopharynx, but more particularly the obliteration of the soft tissue planes. The asterisk indicates fat in the normal paranasopharyngeal space on the opposite side

carcinomas grow in a more exophytic manner into the lumen of the nasopharynx, but this is usually a feature of lymphomas.

Erosion of the skull base and extension of tumour into the cranial cavity along the carotid artery or through the foramen lacerum can be shown by enhanced CT, but much better by enhanced MR in the coronal plane, which is the optimum investigation for showing this upwards extension of malignant neoplasms of the nasopharynx through the floor of the middle cranial fossa into the cavernous sinus and parasellar region (Figure 3.38). This information

alters management, giving the lesion a grading of T4 requiring a larger field of radiation in a region containing several important structures (Phelps and Beale, 1992). Persistent pain in the face is often the presenting feature and, if severe, and if prolonged and unexplained, may warrant a Gd-enhanced MR examination in the coronal plane. Inflammatory disease of the mouth and paranasal sinuses may mimic neoplastic invasion, including upward spread into the middle cranial fossa. We have encountered cases of fungal disease, aspergillosis (Figure. 3.39) and mucormycosis, as well as actinomycosis which pen-

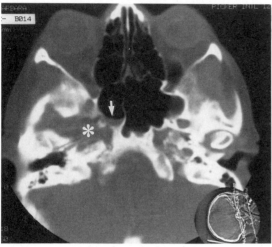

(a)

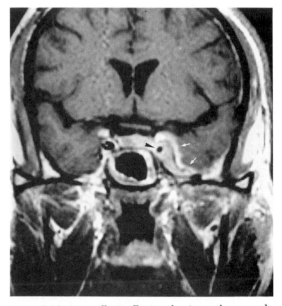

Figure 3.39 Aspergillosis affecting the sinuses has spread upwards into the left cavernous sinus, resulting in narrowing of the internal carotid artery (arrowhead). Note the inflammation of the dura (white arrow) shown on this coronal MR scan after gadolinium

etrated the skull base in the vicinity of the foramen lacerum and invaded the cranial cavity. They were indistinguishable by imaging from infiltrating neoplasms.

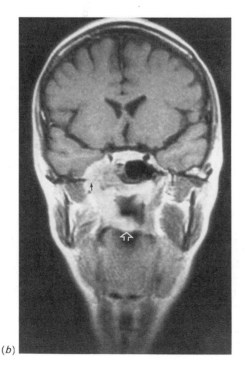

(b)

Figure 3.38 (a) Axial CT scan of the base of the skull showing some bone erosion as well as a fluid level in the right sphenoid sinus. (b) Coronal MR section with gadolinium enhancement showing tumour arising from the soft palate (open arrow) and extending upwards through the base of the skull (black arrow) into the right cavernous sinus and parasellar region

Chordoma

Chordomas are predominantly midline tumours. A large soft tissue mass in the postnasal space is associated with destruction of the basisphenoid and sometimes flecks of calcification best shown by CT (Figure 3.40). There is usually an associated intracranial mass and irregular destruction of adjacent bone depending on the site of origin. The tumour is best demonstrated by MR especially in the sagittal plane and typically there is a non-homogeneous appearance on T1-weighted protocols (Figure 3.41) and heterogeneous enhancement with gadolinium is usual (Meyers *et al.* 1992) (see also volume 6, Figure 2.31).

Summary

Conventional plain radiographs continue to have a role in the initial investigation of diseases of the paranasal sinuses, despite the limitations of this technique. Good radiographic method and positioning of the patient are important, as is the ability of the observer to detect early signs of disease such as erosion of the sinus walls. High resolution CT gives an excellent demonstration of both fine bone detail and soft tissue anatomy on the same sectional picture and is now the investigation of choice. CT can demonstrate a tumour early in the course of the disease and can be used to recognize the exact extent of the

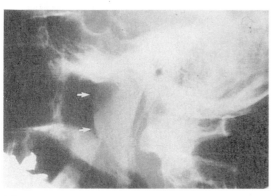
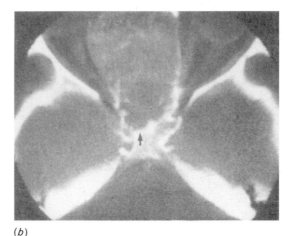

(*a*)   (*b*)

Figure 3.40 (*a*) Lateral plain film view showing a mass in the nasopharynx. (*b*) Axial CT scan shows erosion of the basisphenoid (black arrow) and calcification within this midline tumour, typical of a chordoma

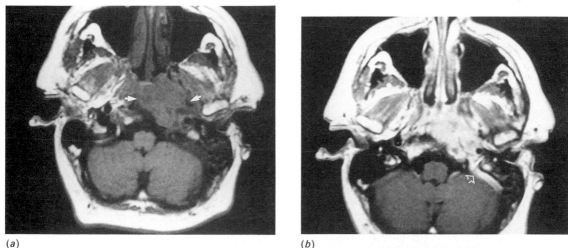

(*a*)   (*b*)

Figure 3.41 Axial MR scan before (*a*) and after (*b*) gadolinium showing a carcinoma of the nasopharynx (arrows). Note that on the enhanced scan the tumour appears to have extended into the posterior cranial fossa, although is probably still extradural (open arrow)

lesion for optimal staging prior to therapy. CT plays an important role in follow up and can be used to show residual or recurrent disease. MR gives better soft tissue imaging in three planes and appears to be better than CT for showing extension of disease into the cranial cavity. MR is now the investigation of choice for malignant disease of the nasopharynx, giving the best assessment of the radiation fields required (Figure 3.42).

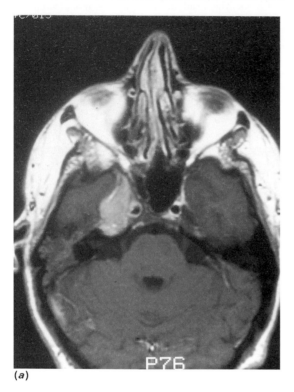

(a)

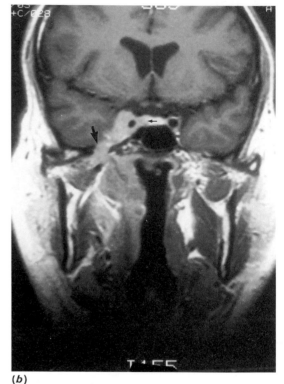

(b)

Figure 3.42 Gadolinium enhanced T1 MR scan in (*a*) axial and (*b*) coronal planes. A squamous cell carcinoma of the nasopharynx has extended up through the foramen ovale (large arrow) and into the cavernous sinus engulfing the carotid artery and almost reaching the midline (small arrow)

References

CABLE, H. R., JEANS, W. D., CULLEN, R. J., BULL, P. D. and MAW, A. R. (1981) Computerized tomography of the Caldwell-Luc cavity. *Journal of Laryngology and Otology*, **95**, 775–783

FORBES, W. ST. C., FAWCITT, R. A., ISHERWOOD, I., WEBB, R. and FARRINGTON, T. (1978) Computed tomography in the diagnosis of diseases of the paranasal sinuses. *Clinical Radiology*, **29**, 501–511

HASSO, A. N. (1984) CT of tumours and tumour-like conditions of the paranasal sinuses. *Radiologic Clinics of North America*, **22**, 119–130

LLOYD, G. A. S. and PHELPS, P. D. (1986) Juvenile angiofibroma: imaging of magnetic resonance, CT and conventional techniques. *Clinical Otolaryngology*, **11**, 247–259

LUND, V. J. and LLOYD, G. A. S. (1983) Radiological changes associated with benign nasal polyps. *Journal of Laryngology and Otology*, **97**, 503–510

LUND, V. J. and LLOYD, G. A. S. (1984) Radiological changes associated with inverted papilloma of the nose and paranasal sinuses. *British Journal of Radiology*, **57**, 455–461

MANCUSO, A. A. and HANAFEE, W. N. (1983) Elusive head and neck carcinomas beneath intact mucosa. *Laryngoscope*, **93**, 133–138

MEYERS, S. P., HIRSCH, W., JR, CURTIN, H. D., BARNES, L., LALIGAM, N. S. and SEN, C. (1992) Chordomas of the skull base: MR features. *American Journal of Neuroradiology*, **13**, 1627–1636

PHELPS, P. D. and BEALE, D. J. (1992) The foramen lacerum – a route of access to the cranial cavity for malignant tumours below the skull base. *Clinical Radiology*, **46**, 179–183

PRICE, H. I. and DANZIGER, A. (1980) Computerised tomographic findings in mucoceles of the frontal and ethmoid sinuses. *Clinical Radiology*, **31**, 169–174

SOM, P. M. (1985) CT of the paranasal sinuses. *Neuroradiology*, **27**, 189–201

4

Evaluation of the nasal airway and nasal challenge

Ronald Eccles

The nasal airway and factors influencing nasal resistance to airflow

Site of nasal resistance

In adults, the nose contributes two-thirds of the total airway resistance (Ferris, Mead and Opie, 1964; Speizer and Frank, 1964). This nasal resistance can be divided into three components: the nasal vestibule, the nasal valve and the turbinated nasal passage (Figure 4.1).

The nasal vestibule, because of its compliant walls, is liable to collapse in response to the negative pressure created during inspiration, and in this way the nasal vestibule can limit nasal airflow and act as a flow-limiting segment or Starling resistor. Bridger (1970) described this flow-limiting segment of the nose as lying in the nasal vestibule between the upper lateral cartilages and the septum. Collapse of the compliant lateral wall of the nasal vestibule has been shown to occur when ventilation through one nostril reaches around 30 l/min (Bridger and Proctor, 1970; Haight and Cole 1983a). The flow limiting effect of the compliant nasal vestibule only occurs on inspiration as expiratory airflow creates a positive dilating pressure within the nasal vestibule.

The narrowest point of the nasal passage determines the nasal resistance to airflow and this region is often referred to as the 'nasal valve' (Dishoeck, 1965; Bridger 1970; Haight and Cole 1983a). However, there is some dispute in the literature as to whether the nasal valve lies in the nasal vestibule or more posteriorly within the bony cavum of the nose. The anatomical and physiological evidence indicates that the nasal valve occurs at the entrance of the pyriform aperture with the major site of nasal resistance just anterior to the tip of the inferior turbinate (Bachman and Legler, 1972; Haight and Cole 1983a).

The change in airway resistance along the nasal passage can be determined by passing a pressure sensing cannula carefully along the passage and determining the pressure-flow relationships during quiet breathing (Bridger and Procter, 1970). Using this

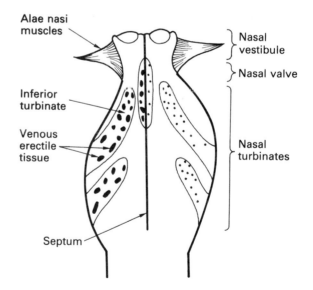

Figure 4.1 Diagram of the nose. The compliant wall of the nasal vestibule is supported by the alae nasi muscles. The nasal valve is at the level of the anterior tip of the inferior turbinate. The diagram illustrates the normal asymmetry of nasal congestion with one side of the nose congested due to swelling of the venous erectile tissue and the other side open and decongested due to constriction of the venous erectile tissue. The degree of congestion of the tip of the inferior turbinate and nasal septum determines the cross-sectional area of the nasal valve area and therefore regulates nasal airway resistance

technique. Haight and Cole (1983a) clearly demonstrated that the major site of nasal resistance lies at the anterior end of the inferior turbinate within the first few millimetres of the bony nasal cavity (Figures 4.1 and 4.2).

The nasal valve is the narrowest point of the airway and it is a dynamic valve as swelling of the venous erectile tissue of the inferior turbinate and nasal septum can cause complete obstruction of the nasal passage. The significance of the erectile properties of the inferior turbinate has been described by Haight and Cole (1983a) who found that the anterior end of the turbinate could advance by as much as 5 mm after application of histamine.

The anterior site of the major component of nasal resistance at the level of the tip of the inferior turbinate has important surgical implications as it follows that treatment aimed at reducing the swelling of the inferior turbinate will have major effects on nasal resistance, whereas minor corrective surgery such as trimming of septal spurs posterior to the nasal valve region will have little effect on nasal resistance.

The turbinated region of the nasal passage has a relatively large cross-sectional area compared to the nasal valve area. In the normal nose the turbinated area has only a minimal contribution to the airway resistance of a nasal passage as illustrated diagrammatically in Figure 4.1 and as demonstrated by Haight and Cole (1983a) in Figure 4.2.

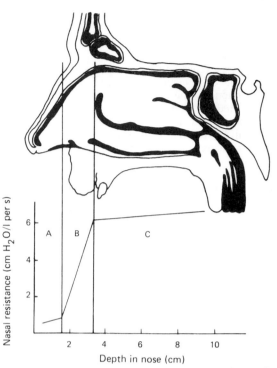

Figure 4.2 Changes in resistance to airflow along the nasal passage. Nasal resistance can be divided into the three components illustrated: (A) nasal vestibule, (B) nasal valve and (C) nasal turbinates. (Based on the results of the study by Haight and Cole, 1983a)

Control of nasal resistance

In the normal healthy subject nasal resistance is mainly determined by the degree of engorgement of venous erectile tissue and the activity of accessory respiratory muscles which maintain the patency of the nostril on inspiration. In allergic and infective rhinitis, it is congestion of venous erectile tissue which causes nasal obstruction as the airway can be readily opened by administration of a topical sympathomimetic decongestant.

The mechanism regulating the swelling of the erectile tissue is poorly understood; Cauna and Cauna (1975) described throttle or cushion veins which may control its filling. Wright (1895) and Burnham (1935) suggested that the close apposition of arteries and veins in the bony canals of the turbinates was significant, as arterial dilation would cause compression of the venous plexus draining the erectile tissue and this would lead to swelling of the erectile tissue.

The venous erectile tissue of the nasal mucosa has a dense adrenergic sympathetic innervation (Dahlstrom and Fuxe, 1965) and electrical stimulation of the sympathetic nerves to the nose causes a pronounced vasoconstriction and a marked decrease in the volume of blood held in the mucosa (Ang-

gard and Edwall, 1974; Eccles and Wilson, 1974; Malm, 1977; Eccles, 1982). Under normal conditions, there is a continuous sympathetic vasoconstrictor tone to the nasal venous erectile tissue and section or local anaesthesia of the cervical sympathetic nerves which supply the nasal mucosa causes ipsilateral nasal congestion and an increase in nasal resistance to air flow (Beickert, 1951; Stoksted and Thomsen, 1953; Eccles, 1978b, 1982). The sympathetic division of the autonomic nervous system has a major role to play as a final effector pathway in the reflex regulation of nasal resistance (Eccles, 1982).

The parasympathetic nerve supply to the nose controls nasal secretion but has little role in the control of nasal resistance to airflow (Eccles and Wilson, 1973, 1974). Parasympathetic nerve stimulation causes a watery nasal secretion which is rapidly cleared from the nasal passages without any effect on nasal resistance. Thick viscous mucus associated with upper respiratory tract infection can influence nasal resistance and complicate the measurement of nasal resistance. In order to eliminate any component of nasal resistance due to the accumulation of mucus in the nasal cavity, subjects should be asked to blow the nose gently prior to each measurement of nasal airway resistance.

The nasal vestibule is surrounded by cartilages which are attached to muscles controlled by the facial nerve. These muscles are important in facial expression as is apparent in facial palsy caused by interruption of the motor pathways in the facial nerve. Activity of the alae nasi muscles and the movement of the alar cartilage can be used as a test of facial nerve integrity in suspected cases of facial nerve damage or compression (Sasaki and Mann, 1976).

Contraction of the alae nasi muscles causes a dilation or flaring of the nostril but, according to Haight and Cole (1983a), this has little effect on nasal resistance to air flow as the major resistance lies at the tip of the inferior turbinate at the entrance of the pyriform aperture. However, Strohl, O'Cain and Slutsky (1982) reported that voluntary flaring of the nostril can cause a 20% reduction in nasal resistance and Rivron and Sanderson (1991) reported a 67% increase in resistance on voluntary constriction of the alar margins of the nose.

The function of the alae nasi muscles and other muscles around the nasal cartilages is probably to stabilize the nasal vestibule and prevent alar collapse during the high negative pressures developed during deep and rapid inspiration. Upper airway negative pressure in the anaesthetized rabbit has been shown to increase the activity of nasal muscles and this observation supports a stabilizing role for nasal muscles (Mathew, 1984). Nasal air flow has also been shown to enhance the activity of the alae nasi muscles in the cat and this finding suggests that nasal air flow is an important stimulus in the control of upper airway accessory respiratory muscles (Davies and Eccles, 1987). At peak inspiratory nasal air flow, the pressure within the nasal vestibule falls well below atmospheric pressure and, when this suction effect exceeds the supporting tension of the lateral nasal wall, nasal collapse occurs and flow is limited.

Factors influencing nasal resistance

In subjects free from signs of nasal disease mean total resistance has been reported to be 0.23 Pa/cm³/s with a range from 0.15 to 0.39 Pa/cm³/s as illustrated in Figure 4.3 (Morris, Jawad and Eccles, 1992). Cole (1988) reported that normal total nasal resistance lay in the range 0.15–0.30 Pa/cm³/s.

Nasal resistance is maximum in the infant at around 1.2 Pa/cm³/s and declines to the adult value at around 16–18 years of age and then shows only a slow decline with increasing age (Polgar and Kong, 1965; Saito and Nishihata, 1981; Syaballo *et al.*, 1986). Unlike other respiratory parameters such as vital capacity, etc. there is no correlation in the adult between total nasal resistance and age, sex or height

(Saito and Nishihata, 1981; Morris, Jawad and Eccles, 1992).

The airflow through the nasal passages is normally asymmetrical and most subjects show reciprocal changes in nasal resistance to airflow (Figure 4.4). The oscillations in nasal resistance are commonly referred to in the literature as the 'nasal cycle', but Gilbert (1989) stated that this term is confusing as there is little evidence for true cyclical changes in the majority of subjects who exhibit reciprocal changes

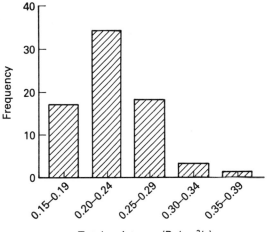

Figure 4.3 Frequency distribution of total nasal airway resistance in asymptomatic subjects. (Mean 0.23 Pa/cm³/s, medium 0.23 Pa/cm³/s, (Adapted from Morris, Jawad and Eccles, 1992)

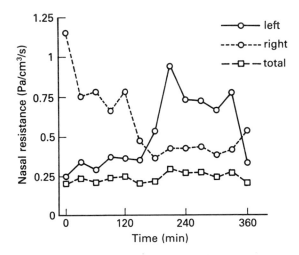

Figure 4.4 Nasal cycle in healthy subject. Spontaneous reciprocal changes in unilateral nasal airway resistance. Note that total nasal resistance remains relatively stable when compared with changes in unilateral resistance.

in unilateral nasal resistance. Because of the reciprocal changes in nasal resistance to airflow, one nasal passage usually has a higher resistance than the other. Therefore it is not very informative to quote mean unilateral resistances for right and left nasal passages. It is more useful to consider the nasal passages as high and low resistance sides and Williams and Eccles (1992) quoted a ratio between the high and low sides in healthy subjects as 1.7:1, with the high resistance side having a mean of 0.6 Pa/cm³/s (range 0.32–0.75 Pa/cm³/s) and the low resistance side a mean of 0.36 Pa/cm³/s (range 0.25–0.52 Pa/cm³/s).

Since the reciprocal changes in nasal airway resistance were first described by Kayser (1895), there have been many other studies extending our knowledge of this unusual asymmetry in nasal airflow (Heetderks, 1927; Stoksted, 1953; Eccles 1978a; Hasegawa and Kern, 1978b). However, the functional significance of the nasal cycle is still obscure, apart from the fact that the alternation of nasal airflow allows a rest period from the damaging effects of nasal airflow.

The reciprocal changes in nasal resistance are caused by changes in sympathetic nervous tone to the nasal venous erectile tissue, with the low resistance side having the greatest sympathetic vasoconstrictor tone (Stoksted and Thomsen, 1953; Eccles, 1978b). Animal experiments indicate that reciprocal changes in nasal resistance are controlled from the respiratory areas of the brain stem with control of nasal resistance closely integrated with respiratory activity (Bamford and Eccles, 1982; Eccles, 1983).

Other factors which influence nasal resistance to airflow are listed in Figure 4.5. Exercise causes a decrease in nasal airway resistance (Richerson and Seebohm, 1968; Dallimore and Eccles, 1977; Hasegawa and Kern, 1978a; Syaballo, Bundgaard and Widdicombe, 1985).

Exercise is more potent than a topically applied decongestant in reducing nasal airway resistance as it decongests those areas of the nose which may not be accessible to a nasal spray or drops. Since exercise can cause a decrease in nasal airway resistance it is important to rest subjects for up to 30 minutes prior to any measurement of nasal resistance. When measurements of nasal resistance are made over several hours there is a significant increase in nasal resistance and this may be due to a period of imposed rest and lack of exercise (Eccles, Jawad and Morris, 1990).

Changes in ventilation cause changes in nasal resistance to airflow probably by the effects of carbon dioxide on the arterial chemoreceptors. An increase in arterial carbon dioxide due to rebreathing or asphyxia causes nasal vasoconstriction and a reduction in nasal resistance; and a reduction in arterial carbon dioxide due to hyperventilation causes nasal vasodilation and an increase in nasal resistance to airflow (Tatum, 1923; Dallimore and Eccles, 1977; Hasegawa and Kern, 1978a; Babatola and Eccles, 1986).

Changes in posture can cause marked changes in nasal resistance due to changes in jugular venous pressure and reflex changes in sympathetic tone to the nose. The change from erect to supine posture causes an increase in total nasal resistance to air flow which may be explained by an increase in jugular venous pressure (Rundcrantz, 1969; Hasegawa, 1982).

On adoption of the lateral recumbent posture, reflex changes in nasal resistance occur so that the dependent nasal passage congests and the upper nasal passage decongests. This partitioning of nasal air flow ensures that the upper nasal passage is responsible for the major component of the nasal air flow. The changes in nasal air flow are caused by a pressure stimulus to the skin, with the axillary region being

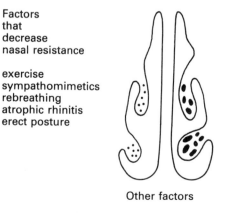

Factors
that
decrease
nasal resistance

exercise
sympathomimetics
rebreathing
atrophic rhinitis
erect posture

Factors
that
increase
nasal resistance

infective rhinitis
allergic rhinitis
vasomotor rhinitis
hyperventilation
supine posture
ingestion of alcohol
aspirin
sympathetic antagonists
cold air

Other factors

nasal cycle
nasal sensation

Figure 4.5 Factors which influence nasal airway resistance

the most sensitive area for the initiation of the reflex (Rao and Potdar, 1970; Haight and Cole, 1983b, 1984; Davies and Eccles, 1985a).

Warming or cooling of the skin surface can induce reflex changes in nasal mucosal blood flow and there are several detailed studies on this area which indicate that the nasal mucosa responds in the same way as the skin (Cole, 1954, 1982; Drettner, 1961). Although the effects of changes in skin temperature on nasal blood flow are well documented, those of changes in the temperature of inspired air on nasal blood flow have not been studied in as much detail and the results of these studies are inconclusive (Drettner, 1961; Cole, 1982). Cole, Forsyth and Haight (1983) demonstrated that inhalation of cold air caused nasal congestion but with a wide variation in response between subjects and, more recently, cold air blown into the nose has been used as a nasal challenge (Iliopoulos *et al.*, 1988.)

The subjective sensation of nasal air flow is very important as regards patient comfort, but it is a parameter which is often overlooked by clinicians treating nasal obstruction. In some patients the objective measurement of nasal resistance determined by rhinomanometry may indicate a normal airway, but the subjective impression of the patient is one of nasal obstruction. In these cases there may be some loss of nasal sensation of air flow, perhaps due to nasal pathology or damage to sensory pathways (Eccles, 1991).

Nasal air-flow sensory receptors have been proposed by several groups (McBride and Whitelaw, 1981; Burrow, Eccles and Jones, 1983), and there is evidence that anaesthesia of these air-flow receptors can lead to disturbances of respiration during sleep (White *et al.*, 1985). Experiments on anaesthetized animals indicate that nasal air-flow receptors are present in the nasal vestibule and that the sensory pathway is via branches of the infraorbital branch of the trigeminal nerve (Davies and Eccles, 1987).

The sensation of nasal air flow is markedly enhanced by aromatics, such as menthol, which are frequently incorporated in preparations used to treat nasal obstruction associated with the common cold; these have a marked effect on the subjective sensation of nasal air flow but do not have any decongestant action (Burrow, Eccles and Jones, 1983; Eccles, Jawad and Morris, 1990). The sensitization or stimulation of nasal air-flow receptors by menthol has been shown to enhance the activity of upper airway accessory respiratory muscles and this action may help to prevent upper airway collapse especially during sleep (Davies and Eccles, 1985b).

Evaluation of the nasal airway

Rhinomanometry is generally accepted as the standard technique of measuring nasal airway resistance and assessing the patency of the nose, but there are other useful methods of obtaining objective measurements of nasal function. This section will include details of rhinomanometry and compare the technique with newer techniques such as acoustic rhinometry.

Rhinomanometry

Nasal resistance to air flow is calculated from two measurements: nasal air flow and transnasal pressure as shown in Figure 4.6. Both these parameters are measured by means of differential pressure transducers and this is why the study of nasal pressure and flow is termed 'rhinomanometry', since manometry involves the measurement of pressure. Nasal air flow can be measured by means of a pneumotachograph which usually consists of a gauze resistance inside a cone-shaped tube. The pressure difference across the gauze generated by air flow through the tube is used to measure air flow. Transnasal pressure can be measured by relating the pressure at the posterior nares to that at the entrance of the nostril which will normally be atmospheric pressure or nasal mask pressure.

Nasal resistance to air flow may be calculated from the following equation:

$$R = \Delta P / \dot{V}$$

R = resistance to air flow, in cmH$_2$O/litre/s or Pa/cm^3/s
ΔP = transnasal pressure, in cmH$_2$O or Pa
$\dot{V}$ = nasal air flow, in litre/s or cm^3/s

This equation is a compromise which has been generally accepted by rhinologists and it does not take into consideration separate components of laminar and turbulent air flow (Clement, 1984).

Rohrer (1915) described an equation which allowed for both components of laminar and turbulent air flow in the respiratory tract, but his conclusions concerning the significance of laminar air flow in the airways have not been universally accepted (Williams, 1972; Hey and Price, 1982). For the greater part of the respiratory cycle, nasal air flow is turbulent

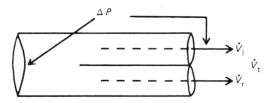

Figure 4.6 Model of the nose to illustrate parameters measured in the determination of nasal resistance to airflow. ΔP = pressure change across nose; $\dot{V}_l$ = left nasal airflow; $\dot{V}_r$ = right nasal airflow; $\dot{V}_t$ = total nasal airflow

and this turbulence aids in mixing the air and facilitates the exchange of heat and moisture. Nasal air flow shows evidence of turbulence when transnasal pressures exceed 40–80 Pa and therefore laminar air flow would only be found when dynamic pressure and flow values are close to zero (Hey and Price, 1982).

A plot of the dynamic relations of transnasal pressure and flow on an x/y plotter shows a curvilinear relationship (Figure 4.7). Nasal air flow rises with increase of transnasal pressure, but at the higher pressures there is a limitation of flow due to the increased frictional effects of turbulent air flow. The flow-limiting effect of nasal alar collapse is only apparent during rapid or close to maximum inspiratory manoeuvres.

The curvilinear relationship between transnasal pressure and flow means that one cannot simply determine nasal resistance from the slope of the graph, as would be the case with a straight line relationship. The slope of the $P/\dot{V}$ plot varies along its length and, therefore, it is not possible to describe the curve with a single numerical value for resistance. It is, however, possible to define the resistance at any given sample point along the curve and this has been the solution recommended for a standardized measurement of nasal resistance (Clement, 1984).

The positive or negative pressure at the posterior nares results in air flow through both nasal passages. The right and left nasal air flows are normally asymmetrical due to the nasal cycle and therefore a single pressure value may relate to two different air flows. It is, therefore, sensible to standardize nasal resistance by measuring both nasal air flows at the same sample pressure point rather than by measuring transnasal pressures at the same sample flow point.

Unilateral nasal air flow measured at a sample pressure point of 150 Pa and bilateral nasal air flow measured at 75 Pa have been recommended as universal standards (Clement, 1984). However, the Asian population cannot always achieve these pressures during normal quiet breathing and the lower sample pressures of 100 and 50 Pa, respectively, are generally accepted for nasal resistance measurements in Japan.

Total nasal resistance to air flow can be determined either directly using the posterior method of rhinomanometry (see below) or it can be calculated by combining the two separate values of nasal resistance for the two nasal passages as shown in the formula below:

$$\frac{1}{R(\text{total})} = \frac{1}{r(\text{left})} + \frac{1}{r(\text{right})}$$

where the reciprocal of total resistance is equal to the sum of the reciprocals of left and right resistance.

Total resistance in units of Pa/cm³/s can also be directly calculated from the separate nasal airflows obtained at a sample pressure, e.g. at 150 Pa:

$$R_t = \frac{\Delta P(150 \text{ Pa})}{\dot{V}_r + \dot{V}_l}$$

R_t = total nasal resistance (Pa/cm³/s)
ΔP = transnasal pressure at sample point (150 Pa in this example)
$\dot{V}_r$ = right nasal air flow (cm³/s)
$\dot{V}_l$ = left nasal air flow (cm³/s)

When quoting values for total nasal resistance it should be stated whether the value was obtained by measurement of total nasal air flow using posterior rhinomanometry, or whether the air flows of the nasal passages have been measured separately.

The use of a sample pressure point to determine nasal resistance is a compromise, as the single numerical value calculated as nasal resistance only describes one point on the $P/\dot{V}$ respiratory curve.

It is possible to sample the curve at numerous points and obtain an average resistance value with the aid of a microprocessor, and this technique has particular advantages when comparing the resistance values of different segments of the respiratory tract (Cole, Fastag and Niinima, 1980).

Another approach to defining the $P/\dot{V}$ curve has been described by Broms, Jonson and Lamm (1979) who found that curves from a large sample of subjects could be arranged in radial order and that the curves only rarely crossed each other. From this arrangement of the curves, it was possible to define nasal resistance in terms of a polar coordinate system. This particular system of determining nasal resistance is now commonly used in Sweden.

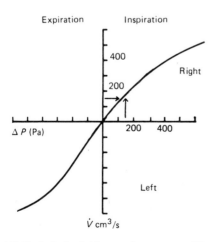

Figure 4.7 Typical x/y plot for nasal pressure and flow. In order to calculate nasal resistance the nasal airflow is measured at a sample pressure of 150 Pa. Note that nasal resistance varies with the slope of the curve. 1 mmH₂O = 10 Pa

Techniques of rhinomanometry

The determination of nasal resistance involves the measurement of nasal pressure and flow as described above. Active rhinomanometry involves the generation of nasal air flow and pressure with normal breathing. Passive rhinomanometry involves the generation of nasal air flow and pressure from an external source, such as a fan or pump, to drive air through the nose.

Active rhinomanometry can be divided into anterior and posterior methods according to the siting of the pressure-sensing tube.

In active anterior rhinomanometry, the pressure-sensing tube is normally taped to one nasal passage (Figure 4.8). The sealed nasal passage acts as an extension of the pressure-sensing tube to measure pressure in the posterior nares. With this method, nasal air flow is measured from one nostril at a time and the pressure-sensing tube is moved from one side to the other. The $P/\dot{V}$ curves and nasal resistance are determined separately for each nasal passage and the total resistance is then calculated by summing the values as shown in the formulae above.

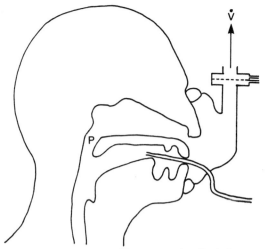

Figure 4.9 Active posterior rhinomanometry. Posterior nares pressure is measured by means of an oral cannula. Total nasal resistance may be measured by determining total nasal airflow; or by sealing one nostril at a time, the separate left and right nasal resistances may be measured

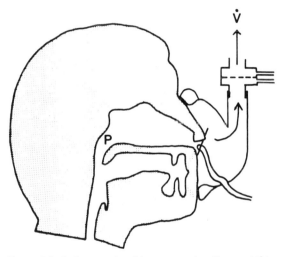

Figure 4.8 Active anterior rhinomanometry. One nostril is sealed with a pressure-sensing tube by means of surgical tape in order to measure posterior nares pressure. The sealed nasal passage has no airflow and acts as an extension of the pressure-sensing tube. The resistance to airflow of each nasal passage is measured separately by taping the pressure-sensing tube alternately from one nasal passage to the other

In active posterior rhinomanometry, the pressure-sensing tube is held in the mouth and detects the posterior nares pressure when the soft palate is relaxed allowing an airway to the mouth (Figure 4.9). Total nasal air flow can be measured from both nasal passages; or by taping off one nostril, the right and left nasal air flow can be measured separately. Total nasal resistance can be determined directly from the

total nasal air flow and transnasal pressure. A disadvantage of this method, when compared with the anterior method, is that not all subjects can relax the soft palate sufficiently. With some training of subjects using feedback from the $P/\dot{V}$ plot on an oscilloscope or monitor, it is possible to obtain satisfactory results from about 90% of subjects. The use of a $P/\dot{V}$ plot is necessary when performing posterior rhinomanometry as this method is more prone to artefacts than anterior rhinomanometry because of pressure changes in the mouth due to tongue movements.

Passive rhinomanometry involves the direction of an external flow of air through the nose and out of the mouth (Figure 4.10). The method may involve either measurement of a driving pressure at a constant flow or measurement of the flow at a constant pressure. Passive rhinomanometry is particularly useful if it is necessary to separate the upper and lower airways for experimental work (Syaballo, Bundgaard and Widdicombe, 1985).

Active anterior rhinomanometry, using surgical tape to seal a pressure-sensing tube into the nasal passage, is one of the most commonly used methods for clinical determination of nasal resistance (Solow and Greve, 1980).

The following precautions are recommended when determining nasal resistance to air flow:

1 The use of a face mask is recommended rather than nasal cannulae as the insertion of a cannula into the nostril is likely to cause distortion of the airway and irritation. The face mask should form a soft airtight seal and should not pull on the cheek as this can distort the nasal vestibule and disturb nasal resistance.

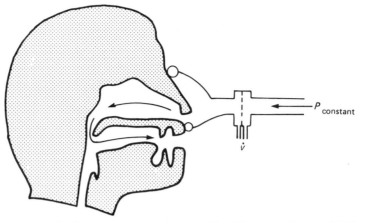

Figure 4.10 Passive rhinomanometry. Nasal resistance may be determined by either measuring nasal airflow at a constant driving pressure or by measuring the driving pressure required to maintain a constant air flow

2 Equipment should be routinely calibrated for pressure and flow measurement. A sloping manometer filled with light paraffin can be used to calibrate the pressure and a rotameter with an air pump or pressurized air cylinder to calibrate flow.

3 A single determination of nasal resistance is unreliable because of possible air leaks around the mask, etc. It is therefore important to take a series of readings with a change in mask position between sets (Eccles, Jawad and Morris, 1990; Morris, Jawad and Eccles, 1992).

Acoustic rhinometry

Acoustic rhinometry has been developed from methods previously used to measure lower respiratory tract resistance (Jackson *et al.*, 1977). The method consists of generating an acoustic pulse from a spark source or speaker which is transmitted along a tube and into the nose. The sound from the pulse wave is reflected back from inside the nose according to changes in the local acoustic impedance which are related to the cross-sectional area of the nasal cavity. The reflected sound is detected by a microphone that transmits the sound signal to an amplifier and computer system for processing into an area–distance graph.

The technique of acoustic rhinometry for evaluation of nasal geometry has been evaluated by Hilberg and colleagues who demonstrated that the cross-sectional area measurements correlated very well with measurements made by computed tomography scans, nasal volume and rhinomanometry (Hilberg *et al.*, 1989; Grymer *et al.*, 1991).

A major advantage of the technique of acoustic rhinometry is that it provides a measure of nasal cross-sectional area along the length of the nasal passage,

unlike rhinomanometry which is limited to measuring the narrowest point of the nasal airway. The plot of cross-sectional area against distance can also be expressed as nasal volume for given distances along the nasal passage. A typical graph obtained by acoustic rhinometry is illustrated in Figure 4.11. The normal value for minimum cross-sectional area for a nasal passage is quoted as 0.7 cm^2 with a range from 0.3 to 1.2 cm^2 and this increases on decongestion to 0.9 cm^2 with a range from 0.5 to 1.3 cm^2 (Grymer *et al.*, 1991).

The diagnostic value of acoustic rhinometry has been investigated by Lenders and Pirsig who could distinguish various deviations of nasal structure such as valve stenosis, septal deviation, turbinate hypertrophy and tumour masses (Lenders and Pirsig, 1990).

The technique of acoustic rhinometry is quicker and easier to perform than rhinomanometry but its accuracy, like rhinomanometry, is determined by the interface between the equipment and the nose. For example, the cross-sectional area of the nasal vestibule is susceptible to distortion if a tube is inserted into the nose. Malpositioning of the nasal tube and air leaks are just as likely to give spurious measurements with acoustic rhinometry as face mask leaks with rhinomanometry but, with care, the technique of acoustic rhinometry provides reproducible data.

Nasometry

During speech, sound is transmitted through both the oral and nasal passages. Nasal obstruction causes a reduction in the amount of sound transmitted through the nose and results in the type of hyponasal speech, which typifies the subject suffering from nasal congestion associated with the common cold.

Until recently there has been no objective measure of the nasal component of speech. Speech therapists

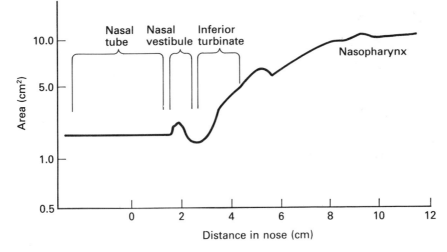

Figure 4.11 Acoustic rhinometry. Plot of nasal cross-sectional area by distance into nose. The curve illustrates a typical record obtained when a tube of constant diameter is inserted for approximately 1 cm into the nasal vestibule with the entrance of the nostril making a seal around the tube. In this record the cross-sectional area of the nasal vestibule at the end of the tube is greater than the cross-sectional area of the tube. This is not always the case as with a narrow nasal vestibule the curve may show a dip or notch at this point

have for many years used a purely subjective assessment of nasality. The level of nasality is a subjective impression of the sound contribution from the nose to the sound content of normal speech. Subjects with nasal obstruction have flat sounding hyponasal speech that is unaffected by occlusion of the nostrils. Phrases that contain nasal consonants such as 'n', 'm' and 'ng' highlight the nasality. The amount of sound transmitted via the nose is influenced by the position of the soft palate and hyponasal speech can be mimicked by closing off the nasopharynx from airflow generated during speech. Disorders of palatal function such as congenital cleft palate cause hypernasality because more of the sound during speech is directed through the nose. Speech therapists have developed several objective measurements of nasality by monitoring nasal pressure and nasal airflow during speech or measuring the relative sound energy directed through the nasal and oral passages.

Nasalance, which is the ratio of sound energy from the nasal and oral passages can be measured by means of two microphones placed close to the nose and mouth and separated by a steel plate. The instrument used to measure nasalance is often called a 'nasometer' (Kay Electronics, Pine Brooke, NJ, USA). With normal nasal and palatal function, the nasalance is dependent on the phonetic content of speech and is normally around 40% of the total sound energy during a typical English sentence. Using a standard sentence with a lot of nasal consonants the nasalance value is increased to 60%.

The measurement of nasalance has been proposed as a useful method of selecting children for adenoidectomy (Parker, Maw and Szallasi, 1989). Nasalance has also been shown to correlate directly with total nasal airway resistance measured by rhinomanometry (Williams, Eccles and Hutchings 1990; Parker *et al.*, 1990). In a study in which nasal airway resistance and nasalance were measured before and after administration of a topical decongestant, there were highly significant changes in both parameters and the changes in resistance and nasalance were significantly correlated (Williams, Eccles and Hutchings 1990).

Nasalance is a relatively new measurement for assessing nasal function and the simplicity of the method and ease of use in children makes it very attractive to the clinician. Nasalance is particularly useful when used as a measure of nasal obstruction in severely obstructed patients because nasalance is then a much more stable parameter than nasal resistance (Williams, Eccles and Hutchings 1990). However, since the nasalance measurement can be influenced by palatal function some caution must be used in the interpretation of results to ensure that changes in nasalance are related to changes in nasal airway resistance.

Peak nasal airflow

Peak expiratory flow is used as a clinical measure of lung function and the small portable peak flow meter provides a simple, quick and inexpensive way of assessing the degree of airway obstruction in conditions such as asthma.

Peak expiratory nasal airflow can be measured by adapting the standard peak flow meter with a nasal mask, but this is not a very satisfactory method due to expulsion of nasal secretions, which then contaminate the instrument (Taylor, MacNeil and Freed, 1973).

Peak inspiratory nasal airflow is a more suitable measure of nasal function because it avoids contamination of the instrument with secretions. The measurement of inspiratory airflow is influenced by any tendency of the airway to collapse in response to the subatmospheric pressures generated on deep inspiration and therefore this measurement will detect any tendency to alar collapse. Therefore, peak inspiratory airflow is affected by both nasal obstruction and the stability of the airway, whereas peak expiratory nasal airflow is determined solely by the degree of nasal obstruction to airflow. Peak inspiratory nasal airflow using a modified peak flow meter has been used to assess changes in nasal resistance associated with the use of nasal decongestants, exercise and histamine challenge (Benson, 1971; Gleeson *et al*, 1986). In healthy subjects the peak inspiratory nasal airflow is reported to be a mean value of 200 l/min (range 9–300 l/min) (Gleeson *et al*. 1986).

Peak nasal airflow can also be measured by means of a nose mask and spirometer during forced vital capacity manoeuvres and Pertuze, Watson and Pride (1991) reported that peak inspiratory nasal airflow in healthy subjects was around 3 l/s and peak expiratory airflow around 4 l/s.

The measurement of peak inspiratory airflow is a useful technique for obtaining a quick measure of nasal obstruction and it is particularly useful when looking for large changes in nasal resistance as, for example, in allergen challenge studies and for studying the effects of topical nasal decongestants on nasal obstruction. However, it is important that the subjects are carefully trained in the method of measurement as the peak nasal airflow is effort dependent. Leaks around the nasal mask are also a common source of error and a soft, close-fitting nasal mask is essential.

Head-out body plethysmograph

A common problem in measuring nasal resistance to airflow is ensuring a leak-free seal around any nasal mask but this problem can be eliminated if nasal airflow is measured via a head-out body plethysmograph. The head-out body plethysmograph was developed from the body plethysmograph used to measure the airway resistance of the lungs. The subject sits in an airtight box and air is displaced from the box through a nylon mesh filter fixed in the side wall, as the subject breathes in and out. The mesh filter acts as a large flow head and because airflow is not measured by means of a face mask, the nose is free for inspection and available for observation and investigations such as nasal electromyographic recording (Niinima *et al*., 1979; Cole *et al*., 1985). Transnasal pressure measurements that are required for the calculation of nasal

resistance are made via an 8 F gauge infant feeding tube passed along the floor of the nasal passage. The passage and presence of the feeding tube do not appear to influence the nasal resistance and many subjects have tolerated the tube in situ for several hours. The per nasal technique of measuring transnasal pressure does not require much cooperation from the patient and is less time consuming than rhinomanometry. The head-out body plethysmograph may appear rather cumbersome compared to the standard methods of rhinomanometry, but it is a reliable and stable apparatus that is not as prone to air leaks as a face mask.

The technique of head-out body plethysmography has been used by Cole and associates in Toronto to assess nasal airway resistance in thousands of patients but it has not been developed as a method in other centres because the head-out body box is not commercially available.

Nasal challenge

Nasal challenge, or nasal provocation as it is sometimes termed, involves the administration of substances directly into the nose. In a narrow definition this would only include suspected allergens, as a diagnostic test, but a broad definition of nasal challenge would include a large number of substances, and some examples of challenge substances are listed in Table 4.1. Nasal challenge with allergens or substances such as histamine, bradykinin, etc. can be used to investigate the pathophysiology of nasal disease and a great deal of new knowledge is being generated in this area, especially in studies where nasal lavage and biochemical analysis are combined with nasal challenge.

Nasal challenge with suspected allergens can be used as a diagnostic procedure in cases where there is some doubt over the results of skin and blood tests (Mygind, 1978; Weeke, Davies and Okuda, 1985;

Table 4.1 Examples of substances used in nasal challenge

Nasal challenge	Authors
Histamine	Mullins, Olson and Sutherland (1989)
Cold air	Iliopoulos *et al*. (1988)
Serotonin	Tonnesen, Demuckadell and Mygind (1987)
Ozone	Koren, Hatch and Graham (1990)
Capsaicin	Rajakulasingam *et al*. (1992)
Bradykinin	Rajakulasingam *et al*. (1992)
Metacholine	Borum (1978)
Hyperosmolar saline	Krayenbuhl *et al*. (1989)
Diesel exhaust particulates	Takafuji *et al*. (1987)
Aspirin	Schapowal and Schmitzschumann (1992)

Druce and Schumacher, 1990; Small, Biskin and Barrett, 1992). However, the clinical usefulness of nasal challenge as a diagnostic procedure is debatable. In 1986, Mygind *et al.*, stated that 'to do nasal provocation testing is to ask for trouble', and the authors doubted that nasal challenge would find a place in clinical practice. Although skin testing is recognized as a useful indicator of IgE-mediated disease it does not necessarily predict the presence or severity of clinical symptoms and that is why nasal challenge has been investigated as a means of diagnosing and monitoring allergic rhinitis. However, nasal challenge studies on patients with ragweed allergic rhinitis did not show any relationship between the response to nasal challenge and the seasonal symptoms (Small, Biskin and Barrett, 1992). A more positive report by Clarke (1988) found that nasal challenge was a useful tool in selecting patients for immunotherapy and that the response to nasal challenge with allergen was a reliable means of monitoring the effectiveness of immunotherapy treatment. The clinical usefulness of nasal challenge is therefore still controversial and there has been little progress over the last decade except for the use of nasal challenge as a research tool in studies on mediators of nasal inflammation.

Mygind and Lowenstein (1982) stated that nasal challenge in patients with negative skin tests has no place in clinical practice, except perhaps for diagnosis of occupational allergy. The usefulness of nasal challenge in studying occupational rhinitis is supported by the results of researchers who have found the procedure useful in identifying occupational allergens (Okuda *et al.*, 1982; Gervais, Ghaem and Eloit, 1985).

Local and reflex effects

The tickling sensation, sneezing and hypersecretion caused by allergen challenge are due to stimulation of sensory nerve endings in the nasal mucosa. There is evidence that histamine is the mediator responsible for these responses as they can be reduced by H_1 antagonists, such as chlorpheniramine. From this evidence it has been proposed that there are histamine H_1-receptors on the sensory nerves supplying the nasal mucosa (Kirkegaard, Secher and Mygind, 1983).

The nasal congestion and increase in nasal resistance caused by allergen challenge is due mainly to the local effects of mediators released from mast cells acting directly on nasal blood vessels. Unilateral antigen challenge causes unilateral nasal congestion without any contralateral congestion (Konno, Togawa and Nishihiara, 1982; Haight and Cole, 1983a). Thus, the vascular response to mediators can be explained by their local actions, whereas the secretory response depends on a reflex activation of parasympathetic nerves to nasal glands (Figure 4.12).

Histamine, when administered into the circulation or applied topically, causes nasal vasodilatation and an increase in nasal resistance and there is evidence for both histamine H_1- and H_2-receptors on nasal blood vessels (Hiley, Wilson and Yates, 1978).

Nasal challenge with histamine induces symptoms which are very similar to those caused by allergen challenge in the sensitive subject, and this, together with the presence of histamine in the basophilic cells of the nasal mucosa, has implicated histamine as an important mediator of nasal allergy (Mygind, 1982). However, there are important differences between nasal challenges with histamine or allergen which indicate that histamine is not the sole mediator of nasal allergy. First, nasal challenge with allergen, but not histamine, gives rise to local eosinophilia, which can be demonstrated in a nasal smear from 1–3 hours to 1–3 days after allergen challenge, and secondly allergen challenge, but not histamine challenge, increases nasal reactivity (Connel, 1968).

The allergic response is dependent on a complex soup of mediators whose time course of release and activation varies widely; however, the time course of response can often be divided into early and late phases. The response to allergen challenge in the lungs is often divided into an immediate response occurring in a matter of minutes and a late response occurring after several hours; however, this separation of early and late responses has not been conclusively shown in the nose (Richardson, Rajtora and Pennick, 1979; Davies *et al.*, 1985).

Standardization of nasal challenge

At the time of writing, there is no generally accepted procedure for nasal challenge and, before any progress can be made in this field, several variables in the procedure need to be standardized.

The actual allergen preparation itself can be a source of much variability. Purification of pollen extracts may give a more consistent product, but many active substances may be removed. The initial material itself can vary according to how, when and from where it is collected. The final concentration of allergen applied to the nasal mucosa and the area of mucosa over which it is spread can also determine the level of allergic response (Mygind, 1978).

The method of administering the allergen varies from one centre to another with nasal drops, nebulized droplets, powders and allergen-soaked filter paper discs all being used (Wihl and Mygind, 1977; Konno, Togawa and Nishihiara, 1982; Weeke, Davies and Okuda, 1985). It is difficult to compare responses when such different methods are used.

The severity of the allergic response to nasal challenge may be measured in terms of sneezes, secretion weight, changes in nasal resistance and the levels of mediators in nasal secretion or nasal lavage fluid.

Measurement of nasal resistance to air flow alone

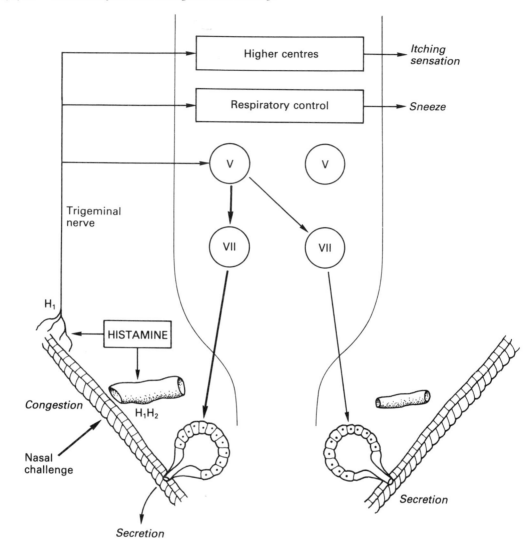

Figure 4.12 Diagrammatic representation of events of unilateral nasal challenge with allergen. The allergen challenge triggers the release of histamine from mucosal basophils. Histamine causes ipsilateral nasal congestion by a direct local action on H_1- and H_2-receptors on nasal blood vessels. Histamine also stimulates H_1-receptors on trigeminal sensory nerve endings in the nasal mucosa to initiate a bilateral reflex nasal secretion and a sensation of itching and sneezing

does not always provide a comprehensive measure of the allergic response and patient symptom scores often give a better measure of the response to challenge.

Once there is some generally agreed standardization of nasal challenge, then the procedure may provide useful diagnostic information in the clinic, but at present it is still very much a laboratory-based procedure with specific uses in basic research on rhinitis.

References

ANGGARD, A. and EDWALL, L. (1974) The effects of sympathetic nerve stimulation on the tracer disappearance rate and local blood content in the nasal mucosa of the cat. *Acta Otolaryngologica,* **77,** 131–139

BABATOLA, F. D. O. and ECCLES, R. (1986) Nasal vasomotor responses in man to breath-holding and hyperventilation recorded by means of intranasal balloons. *Rhinology,* **24,** 271–276

BACHMANN, W. and LEGLER, U. (1972) Studies on the structure and function of the anterior section of the nose by means of luminal impressions. *Acta Otolaryngologica*, **73**, 433–442

BAMFORD, O. S. and ECCLES, R. (1982) The central reciprocal control of nasal vasomotor oscillations. *Pfluegers Archiv European Journal of Physiology*, **394**, 139–143

BEICKERT, P. (1951) Halsbeitenrhythmus der vegativen Innervation. *Archiv für Klinische und Experimentelle Ohren-, Nasen- und Kehlkopfheilkunde*, **157**, 404–411

BENSON, M. K. (1971) Maximal nasal inspiratory flow rate. Its use in assessing the effect of pseudoephedrine in vasomotor rhinitis. *European Journal of Clinical Pharmacology*, **3**, 182–184

BORUM, P. (1978) Intranasal ipatropium. Inhibition of metacholine-induced hypersecretion. *Rhinology*, **16**, 225–233

BRIDGER, G. P. (1970) Physiology of the nasal valve. *Archives of Otolaryngology*, **92**, 543–553

BRIDGER, G. P. and PROCTOR, D. F. (1970) Maximum nasal inspiratory flow and nasal resistance. *Annals of Otology, Rhinology and Laryngology*, **79**, 481–488

BROMS, P., JONSON, B. and LAMM, C. J. (1979) A universal way to evaluate the curve in rhinometry. *Acta Otolaryngologica*, **360**, 22–23

BURNHAM, H. (1935) An anatomical investigation of blood vessels of the lateral nasal wall and their relation to turbinates and sinuses. *Journal of Laryngology and Otology*, **50**, 569–593

BURROW, A., ECCLES, R. and JONES, A. S. (1983) The effects of camphor, eucalyptus and menthol vapour on nasal resistance to airflow and nasal sensation. *Acta Otolaryngologica*, **96**, 156–161

CAUNA, N. and CAUNA, D. (1975) The fine structure and innervation of the cushion veins of the human nasal respiratory mucosa. *Anatomical Record*, **181**, 1–16

CLARKE, P. S. (1988) Improved diagnosis and treatment of allergic rhinitis by the use of nasal provocation tests. *Annals of Allergy*, **60**, 57–60

CLEMENT, P. A. R. (1984) Committee report on the standardisation of rhinomanometry. *Rhinology*, **22**, 151–155

COLE, P. (1954) Respiratory mucosal vascular responses, air conditioning and thermo regulation. *Journal of Laryngology and Otology*, **68**, 613–622

COLE, P. (1982) Modification of inspired air. In: *The Nose Upper Airway Physiology and the Atmospheric Environment*, edited by D. F. Proctor and I. Andersen. Amsterdam: Elsevier Biomedical, pp. 351–375

COLE, P. (1988) Nasal airflow resistance. In: *Respiratory Function of the Upper Airway. Lung Biology in Health and Disease vol. 35*, edited by O. P. Mathew and G. Sant' Ambrogio. New York: Marcell Dekker. pp. 391–414

COLE, P., FASTAG, O. and NIINIMA, V. (1980) Computer-aided rhinometry. *Acta Otolaryngologica*, **90**, 139–142

COLE, P., FORSYTH, R. and HAIGHT, J. S. J. (1983) Effects of cold air and exercise on nasal patency. *Annals of Otology, Rhinology and Laryngology*, **92**, 196–198

COLE, P., HAIGHT, J. S. J., LOVE, L. and OPRYSK, D. (1985) Dynamic components of nasal resistance. *American Review of Respiratory Disease*, **132**, 1229–1232

CONNEL, J. T. (1968) Quantitative intranasal pollen challenge. *Journal of Allergy*, **41**, 123–139

DAHLSTROM, A. and FUXE, K. (1965) The adrenergic innervation of the nasal mucosa of certain mammals. *Acta Otolaryngologica*, **59**, 65–72

DALLIMORE, N. S. and ECCLES, R. (1977) Changes in human nasal resistance associated with exercise, hyperventilation and rebreathing. *Acta Otolaryngologica*, **84**, 416–421

DAVIES, A. M. and ECCLES, R. (1985a) Reciprocal changes in nasal resistance to airflow caused by pressure applied to the axilla. *Acta Otolaryngologica*, **99**, 154–159

DAVIES, A. M. and ECCLES, R. (1985b) The effects of nasal airflow and menthol on the nasal electromyographic activity of the anaesthetized cat. *British Journal of Pharmacology*, **85**, 254

DAVIES, A. M. and ECCLES, R. (1987) Electromyographic responses of a nasal muscle to stimulation of the nasal vestibule in the cat. *Journal of Physiology*, **391**, 25–38

DAVIES, R. J., ANGGARD, A., CORRADO, O. J. and BORUM, P. (1985) Rhinitis and asthma. In: *Allergic and Vasomotor Rhinitis: Clinical Aspects*, edited by N. Mygind and B. Weeke. Copenhagen: Munksgaard. pp. 65–79

DISHOECK, VAN H. A. E. (1965) The part of the valve and turbinates in total nasal resistance. *International Rhinology*, **3**, 19–26

DRETTNER, B. (1961) Vascular reactions of the human nasal mucosa on exposure to cold. *Acta Otolaryngologica Supplementum*, **166**, 1–105

DRUCE, H. M. and SCHUMACHER, M. J. (1990) Nasal provocation challenge. *Journal of Allergy and Clinical Immunology*, **86**, 261–264

ECCLES, R. (1978a) The central rhythm of the nasal cycle. *Acta Otolaryngologica*, **86**, 464–468

ECCLES, R. (1978b) The domestic pig as an experimental animal for studies on the nasal cycle. *Acta Otolaryngologica*, **85**, 431–436

ECCLES, R. (1982) Neurological and pharmacological considerations. In: *The Nose Upper Airway Physiology and the Atmospheric Environment*, edited by D. F. Proctor and I. Andersen. Amsterdam: Elsevier Biomedical. pp. 191–214

ECCLES, R. (1983) Sympathetic control of nasal erectile tissue. *European Journal of Respiratory Disease*, **64**, (Suppl. 128), 150–154

ECCLES, R. (1991) Relationship between measured nasal airway resistance and the sensation of nasal airflow. *Facial Plastic Surgery*, **7**, 278–282

ECCLES, R. and WILSON, H. (1973) The parasympathetic secretory nerves of the nose of the cat. *Journal of Physiology*, **230**, 213–233

ECCLES, R. and WILSON, H. (1974) The autonomic innervation of the nasal blood vessels of the cat. *Journal of Physiology*, **238**, 549–560

ECCLES, R., JAWAD, M. S. and MORRIS, S. (1990) The effects of oral administration of (-)-menthol on nasal resistance to airflow and nasal sensation of airflow in subjects suffering from nasal congestion associated with the common cold. *Journal of Pharmacy and Pharmacology*, **42**, 652–654

FERRIS, B. G., MEAD, J. and OPIE, L. H. (1964) Partitioning of respiratory flow resistance in man. *Journal of Applied Physiology*, **19**, 653–658

GERVAIS, P. GHAEM, A. and ELOIT, C., (1985) Occupational allergic rhinitis. *Rhinology*, **23**, 92–98

GILBERT, A. N. (1989) Reciprocity versus rhythmicity in spontaneous alternations of nasal airflow. *Chronobiology International*, **6**, 251–257

GLEESON, M. J., YOULTEN, L. J. F., SHELTON, D. M., SIODLAK, M. Z., EISER, N. M. and WENGRAF, C. L. (1986) Assessment of nasal airway patency: a comparison of four methods. *Clinical Otolaryngology*, **11**, 99–107

GRYMER, L. F., HILBERG, P., PEDERSEN, O. F. and RAMUSSEN, T.

R. (1991) Acoustic rhinometry: values from adults with subjective normal nasal patency. *Rhinology*, **29**, 35–47

HAIGHT J. S. J. and COLE, P. (1983a) The site and function of the nasal valve. *Laryngoscope*, **93**, 49–55

HAIGHT, J. S. J. and COLE, P. (1983b) Nasal responses to local unilateral stimuli in man. *Rhinology*, **21**, 67–72

HAIGHT, J. S. J. and COLE, P. (1984) Reciprocating nasal airflow resistances. *Acta Otolaryngologica*, **97**, 93–98

HASEGAWA, M. (1982) Nasal cycle and postural variations in nasal resistance. *Annals of Otology, Rhinology and Laryngology*, **91**, 112–114

HASEGAWA, M. and KERN, E. B. (1978a) The effects of breath holding, hyperventilation and exercise on nasal resistance. *Rhinology*, **16**, 243–249

HASEGAWA, M. and KERN, E. B. (1978b) Variations in nasal resistance in man: a rhinomanometric study of the nasal cycle in 50 human subjects. *Rhinology*, **16**, 19–29

HEETDERKS, D. L. (1927) Observations on the reaction of normal nasal mucous membrane. *American Journal of Medical Science*, **174**, 231–244

HEY, E. N. and PRICE, J. F. (1982) Nasal conductance and effective airway diameter. *Journal of Physiology*, **330**, 429–437

HILBERG, O., JACKSON, A. C., SWIFT, D. L. and PEDERSEN, O. F. (1989) Evaluation of nasal cavity geometry by acoustic reflection. *Journal of Applied Physiology*, **62**, 295–303

HILEY, C. R., WILSON, H. and YATES, M. S. (1978) Identification of beta-adrenoceptors and histamine receptors in the cat nasal vasculature. *Acta Otolaryngologica*, **85**, 444–448

ILIOPOULOS, O., PROUD, D., NORMAN, P. S., LICHENSTEIN, L. M., KAGEYSOBOTKA, A. and NACLERIO, R. M. (1988) Nasal challenge with cold, dry air induces a late-phase reaction. *American Review of Respiratory Disease*, **138**, 400–405

JACKSON, A. C., BUTLER, J. P., MILLET, E. J., HOPPIN, F. G. and DAWSON, S. V. (1977) Airway geometry by analysis of acoustic pulse response measurements. *Journal of Applied Physiology*, **43**, 523–536

KAYSER, R. (1895) Die exacte Messiung der Luftdurchgangikeit der Nase. *Archiv für Laryngologie und Rhinologie*, **3**, 101–120

KIRKEGAARD, J., SECHER, C. and MYGIND, N. (1983) Inhibition of histamine induced nasal sumptoms by the H_1 antihistamine chlorpheniramine maleate. Demonstration of topical effects. *British Journal of Diseases of the Chest*, **77**, 113–122

KONNO, A., TOGAWA, K. and NISHIHIARA, S. (1982) Participation of vascular reflex in swelling in nasal allergy. *Acta Otolaryngologica*, **94**, 131–140

KOREN, H. S., HATCH, G. E. and GRAHAM, D. E. (1990) Nasal lavage as a tool in assessing acute inflammation in response to inhaled pollutants. *Toxicology*, **60**, 15–25

KRAYENBUHL, M. C., HUDSPITH, B. N., BROSTOFF, J., SCADDING, G. K., GUESDON, J. L. and LATCHMAN, Y. (1989) Nasal histamine release following hyperosmolar and allergen challenge. *Allergy*, **44**, 25–29

LENDERS, H. and PIRSIG, W. (1990) Diagnostic value of acoustic rhinometry: patients with allergic and vasomotor rhinitis compared with normal controls. *American Review of Respiratory Disease*, **25**, 5–16

MCBRIDE, B. and WHITELAW, W. A. (1981) A physiological stimulus to upper airway receptors in humans. *Journal of Applied Physiology*, **51**, 1189–1197

MALM, L. (1977) Sympathetic influence on the nasal mucosa. *Acta Otolaryngologica*, **83**, 20–21

MATHEW, O. P. (1984) Upper airway negative-pressure effects on respiratory activity of upper airway muscles. *Journal of Applied Physiology*, **56**, 500–505

MORRIS, S., JAWAD, M. S. M. and ECCLES, R. (1992) Relationships between vital capacity, height and nasal airway resistance in asymptomatic volunteers. *Rhinology*, **30**, 259–264

MULLINS, R. J., OLSON, L. G. and SUTHERLAND, D. C. (1989) Nasal histamine challenges in symptomatic allergic rhinitis. *Journal of Allergy and Clinical Immunology*, **83**, 955–959

MYGIND, N. (1978) *Nasal Allergy*. Oxford: Blackwell

MYGIND, N. (1982) Mediators of nasal allergy. *Journal of Allergy and Clinical Immunology*, **70**, 149–159

MYGIND, N. and LOWENSTEIN, H. (1982) Allergy and other environmental factors. In: *The Nose Upper Airway Physiology and the Atmospheric Environment*, edited by D. F. Proctor and I. Andersen. Amsterdam: Elsevier Biomedical. pp. 377–397

MYGIND, N., BORUM, P. SECHER, C., and KIRKEGAARD, J. (1986) Nasal challenge. *European Journal of Respiratory Disease*, **68** (Suppl. 143), 31–34

NIINIMA, V., COLE, P., MINTZ, S. and SHEPHARD, R. J. (1979) A head-out exercise body plethysmograph. *Journal of Applied Physiology*, **47**, 1336–1339

OKUDA, M., OHTSUKA, K., SAKAGUCHI, S., TOMIYAMA, M., OHNISHI, M. and USIAMI, A. (1982) Diagnostic standards for occupational nasal allergy. *Rhinology*, **20**, 13–19

PARKER, A. J. CLARKE, P. M., DAWES, P. J. D. and MAW, A. R. (1990) A comparison of active anterior rhinomanometry and nasometry in the objective assessment of nasal obstruction. *Rhinology*, **28**, 47–53

PARKER, A. J., MAW, A. R. and SZALLASI, F. (1989) An objective method of assessing nasality: a possible aid in the selection of patients for adenoidectomy. *Clinical Otolaryngology*, **14**, 161–166

PERTUZE, J., WATSON, A. and PRIDE, N. B. (1991) Maximum airflow through the nose in humans. *Journal of Applied Physiology*, **70**, 1369–1376

POLGAR, G. and KONG, P. G. (1965) The nasal resistance of newborn infants. *Journal of Pediatrics*, **67**, 557–567

RAJAKULASINGAM, K., POLASA, R., LAU, L. C. K., CHURCH, M. K., HOLGATE, S. T. and HOWARTH, P. H. (1992) Nasal effects of bradykinin and capsaicin: influence on plasma protein leakage and role of sensory neurons. *Journal of Applied Physiology*, **72**, 1418–1424

RAO, S. and POTDAR, A. (1970) Nasal airflow with body in various positions. *Journal of Applied Physiology*, **28**, 162–165

RICHERSON, H. and SEEBOHM, M. (1968) Nasal airway response to exercise. *Journal of Allergy*, **41**, 269–284

RICHARDSON, H. B., RAJTORA, J. W. and PENNICK, G. D. (1979) Cutaneous and nasal allergic responses in ragweed hay fever: lack of clinical and histopathological correlation with late phase reactions. *Journal of Allergy and Clinical Immunology*, **64**, 67

RIVRON, R. P. and SANDERSON, R. J. (1991) The voluntary control of nasal airway resistance. *Rhinology*, **29**, 181–184.

ROHRER, F. (1915) Der Stromungswiderstand in den menschlichen Atemwegen und der Einfluss der ungregelmassigen Verzwigung des Bronchialsystems auf den Atmungsverlaufin verschiedenen Lungenbezirken. *Pfluegers Archiv für gestalte Physiologie*, **162**, 225–299

RUNDCRANDTZ, H. (1969) Postural variations of nasal patency. *Acta Otolaryngologica*, **68**, 435–443

SAITO, A. and NISHIHATA, S. (1981) Nasal airway resistance in children. *Rhinology*, **19**, 149–154

SASAKI, C. T. and MANN, D. G. (1976) Dilator naris function. A useful test of facial nerve integrity. *Archives of Otolaryngology*, **102**, 365–367

SCHAPOWAL, A. and SCHMITZSCHUMANN, M. (1992) Provocation test for the diagnosis of aspirin-sensitive asthma and aspirin-sensitive rhinosinusitus. *Allergologie*, **15**, 158–164

SMALL, P., BISKIN, N. and BARRETT, D. (1992) Does nasal provocation play a role in the diagnosis and management of ragweed-induced allergic rhinitis. *Annals of Allergy*, **68**, 274–278

SOLOW, B. and GREVE, E. (1980) Rhinomanometric recording in children. *Rhinology*, **18**, 31–42

SPEIZER, F. E. and FRANK, R. (1964) A technique for measuring nasal and pulmonary flow resistance simultaneously. *Journal of Applied Physiology*, **19**, 176–178

STOKSTED, P. (1953) Rhinometric measurements for determination of the nasal cycle. *Acta Otolaryngologica Supplementum*, **109**, 176–181

STOKSTED, P. and THOMSEN, K. (1953) Changes in the nasal cycle under stellate ganglion blockade. *Acta Otolaryngologica Supplementum*, **109**, 176–181

STROHL, K. P., O'CAIN, C. F. and SLUTSKY, A. S. (1982) Alae nasi activation and nasal resistance in healthy subjects. *Journal of Applied Physiology*, **52**, 1432–1437

SYABALLO, N. C., BUNDGAARD, A. and WIDDICOMBE, J. G. (1985) Effects of exercise on nasal airflow resistance in healthy subjects and in patients with asthma and rhinitis. *Bulletin Europeen de Physiopathologie Respiratoire*, **21**, 507–513

SYABALLO, N. C., BUNDGAARD, A., ENTHOLM, P., SCHMIDT, A. and WIDDICOMBE, J. G. (1986) Measurement and regulation of nasal airflow resistance in man. *Rhinology*, **24**, 87–101

TAKAFUJI, S., SUZUKI, S., KOIZUMI, K., TADAKORO, K., MIYAMOTO, T. and IKEMORI, R. (1987) Diesel-exhaust particulates inoculated by the intranasal route have an adjuvant activity for IgE production in mice. *Journal of Allergy and Clinical Immunology*, **79**, 639–645

TAYLOR, G., MACNEIL, A. R. and FREED, D. L. J. (1973) Assessing degree of nasal patency by measuring peak expiratory flow rate through the nose. *Journal of Allergy and Clinical Immunology*, **52**, 193–198

TATUM, A. L. (1923) The effects of deficient and excessive pulmonary ventilation on nasal volume. *American Journal of Physiology*, **65**, 229–233

TONNESEN, P., DEMUCKADELL, O. B. S. and MYGIND, N. (1987) Nasal challenge with serotonin in asymptomatic hayfever patients. *Allergy*, **42**, 447–450

WEEKE, B., DAVIES, R. J. and OKUDA, M. (1985) Allergy diagnosis in vivo. In: *Allergic and Vasomotor Rhinitis: Clinical Aspects*, edited by N. Mygind and B. Weeke. Copenhagen: Munksgaard pp. 97–107

WHITE, D. P., CADIEUX, R. J., LOMBARD, R. M., BIXLER, E. O., KALES, A. and ZWILLICH, C. W. (1985) The effects of nasal anaesthesia on breathing during sleep. *American Review of Respiratory Disease*, **132**, 972–975

WIHL, J. A. and MYGIND, N. (1977) Studies on the allergen-challenged human nasal mucosa. *Acta Otolaryngologica*, **84**, 281–286

WILLIAMS, H. L. (1972) A reconsideration of the relation of the mechanics of nasal airflow to the function of the nose in respiration. *Rhinology*, **10**, 145–161

WILLIAMS, R. G. and ECCLES, R. (1992) Nasal airflow asymmetry and the effects of a topical nasal decongestant. *Rhinology*, **30**, 277–282

WILLIAMS, R. G., ECCLES, R. and HUTCHINGS, H. (1990) The relationship between nasalance and nasal resistance to airflow. *Acta Otolaryngologica*, **110**, 443–449

WRIGHT, J. (1895) A consideration of the vascular mechanisms of the nasal mucous membrane and its relation to certain pathological processes. *American Journal of Medical Science*, **109**, 516–523

5

Abnormalities of smell

Victoria L. Moore-Gillon

The extent to which an individual's daily life is disrupted by a reduced or absent sense of smell is much less apparent to others than where there is impairment or loss of sight or hearing. There is also a widespread belief that the association of smell with social and sexual behaviour, so obvious in the animal world, is not applicable in man. It is perhaps for these reasons that complaints of olfactory dysfunction have in the past been relatively ignored by clinicians. Like animals lower in the evolutionary scale, however, humans are warned of environmental dangers by odours. We tend to experience such odours as unpleasant, although much of this is likely to be social conditioning rather than an innate aversion to the stimulus, such as occurs with pain sensation. Odours perceived as pleasant can have erogenous qualities in social interaction, and although much of this is again conditioning, some human odours may have direct effects on sexual interest (Engen, 1983). Studies also suggest that like many other mammals, humans have the potential for communicating basic biological information via the sense of smell (Doty, 1981). With increasing recognition of the distress felt with an absent or impaired sense of smell, and a growing understanding of its relevance to everyday interaction with others, there is developing a greater awareness of the importance of smell and its disorders.

For the sufferer there are problems over and above the obvious one of the loss of enjoyment of pleasant odours. Many affected individuals express anxiety about inability to detect spoiled food, offensive body odours in themselves, leaking gas, or fire. Their anxiety may be intensified by fears that the loss is indicative of a serious underlying disorder as, indeed, it occasionally is. Mood change may accompany olfactory loss, and there is an increased incidence of depression in individuals who develop anosmia. Some authorities have reported a link between olfactory impairment and sexual dysfunction, although this is disputed by others. The sensation of taste is complex and is linked to odour perception. In many individuals whose presenting complaint is of taste disturbance or loss, true taste function is itself normal but there is unrecognized loss of smell.

The investigative and therapeutic nihilism which has been the approach of most doctors to olfactory problems has not been due exclusively to lack of recognition of the importance of such loss. Our understanding of the physiological mechanisms of the sense of smell has been poor. There have been no accurate and simple objective ways of assessing olfaction. Finally, there has been the widespread perception, only partly justified, that there is no treatment. There have been, however, major advances in understanding of basic olfactory physiology and in the clinical methods of testing the sense of smell. Furthermore, it is now appreciated that rhinitis is a major cause of loss of smell, opening up the possibility of treatment, both medical and surgical, for many patients who present with olfactory disturbance.

Mechanisms of olfaction
The experience of odour

The everyday experience of 'smell' is made up of much more than the detection and analysis of impulses from the olfactory nerves. There is also cerebral input from trigeminal, glossopharyngeal and vagus nerves, which can create problems both in the interpretation of symptoms and in practical testing. A patient who detects the 'smell' of substances such as ammonia or bleach may have no true olfactory function at all, but is detecting the presence of the vapour via stimulation of trigeminal irritant receptors. To these varied peripheral inputs from no fewer than four cranial nerves must be added the cortical influences upon odour perception that may be produced by association and past exposure. The term 'total odour experience' may be more accurate and informative than 'smell' but is, fortunately, unlikely to become acceptable.

Development of the olfactory system in humans

The olfactory neuroepithelium is well developed in the human fetus and by 11 weeks' gestation there is complete differentiation of olfactory cells. As in other mammals, the human fetus also possesses a well-developed vomeronasal organ, with a cellular configuration similar to olfactory epithelium, on each side of the nasal septum. In common with other primates, however, the vomeronasal organ in man regresses in late fetal life and only remnants are found in the adult (Nakashima *et al.*, 1985). The human olfactory system is operative at birth and neonates respond preferentially to maternal odour.

Anatomy and physiology of olfaction in the adult

The olfactory epithelium occupies about 1 cm² on each side of the nose, over the cribriform plate and on the upper septum and superior turbinate. Figure 5.1 shows in diagrammatic form the highly specialized nature of the olfactory epithelium. The long cilia projecting from the bipolar olfactory neurons (Figure 5.2) are unlike those elsewhere in the nose and respiratory tract in being immotile. Instead, they are involved in odour reception and transduction. The axons of the primary olfactory neurons pass through the cribriform plate to synapse in the olfactory bulb with the second order neurons, called mitral and tufted cells. The intracerebral pathway of the olfactory impulse is not fully understood, but involves the lateral olfactory tract, anterior olfactory nucleus, olfactory tubercle, the nucleus of the lateral olfactory tract, and the corticomedial nucleus of the amygdala. The cortical representation of olfactory processing in man appears to be bilateral in the pyriform cortex, and there is also evidence for functional lateralization with additional cortical activity in the right, but not the left, orbitofrontal cortex (Zatorre *et al.*, 1992). With these complex intracerebral pathways, it is not surprising that olfactory dysfunction can result from other than purely nasal conditions, as will be discussed.

During normal tidal breathing, only 5–10% of

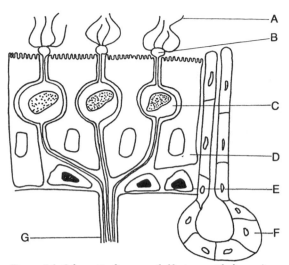

Figure 5.1 Schematic diagram of olfactory epithelium. A, Cilia; B, dendritic knob; C, bipolar receptor neuron; D, supporting cell; E, basal cell; F, Bowman's gland; G, olfactory axon. (Reproduced by kind permission of the Royal Society of Medicine Services Ltd. from Moore-Gillon, V. Olfactometry. In: *Rhinitis – Mechanisms and Management*, edited by I. Mackay)

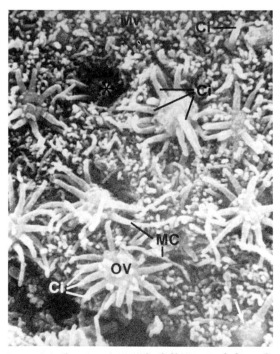

Figure 5.2 Electron micrograph of olfactory epithelium. Ci, Cilia; Ov, olfactory vesicle; Mc, modified cilia; Mv, microvilli on sustentacular cell; *, partially projected olfactory vesicle. (Reproduced from Kessel and Kardon *Tissues and Organs*, Fig. 2, p. 132. By kind permission of W. H. Freeman and Co.)

nasal inspired air reaches the region of the olfactory mucosa. Sniffing not only increases flow rate but also alters flow pattern so that during this manoeuvre 20% of the increased total flow reaches the olfactory epithelium. Odour molecules entering the olfactory region are absorbed into the nasal mucus and carried on a binding globulin to receptors on the cilia. The mechanism of odour 'transduction', by which odorant binding to the cilia initiates membrane depolarization, and the processes involved in odour recognition are at last becoming clear (Ronnett and Snyder, 1992; Anholt, 1993; Scott *et al.*, 1993). Odour molecule binding produces allosteric changes in the receptor which activates a stimulatory GTP-binding protein. In turn, the enzyme adenyl cyclase is activated, and cyclic AMP synthesized. This opens a cation channel in the ciliary plasma membrane, leading to depolarization and the subsequent generation of an action potential. Odour molecule binding also leads to the activation of a separate second messenger system, involving inositol triphosphate which opens a calcium channel in the membrane. Calcium entering through both this and the cyclic-AMP gated channel binds to calmodulin and modulates odorant response by amplifying the generation of cyclic AMP.

It is currently believed that odour *recognition* can occur because cells in the olfactory epithelium are broadly 'tuned': each neuron will respond to many odours, but different neurons do not respond to exactly the same odours. Odours are accordingly recognized by the *combination* of olfactory neurons in which they produce membrane depolarization. For any given odour, a unique pattern of neuronal depolarization is stimulated, and it is this which, after central processing and analysis, gives rise to the characteristic olfactory sensation associated with that odour. Support for this concept comes from the demonstration by Buck and Axel (1991) of proteins in the membranes of olfactory neuronal cilia which, in common with many protein receptor molecules, have a characteristic seven transmembrane domain (7TD) structure. Using an oligonucleotide primer specific for the 7TD protein superfamily, amplification by the polymerase chain reaction, and restriction fragment analysis of the amplified DNA, they showed that in the olfactory mucosa there are large numbers – probably hundreds – of broadly similar but subtly different 7TD receptor proteins. This particular receptor family is apparently unique to olfactory neurons, and it seems there may be 15–20 different members of the family present on the surface of each olfactory neuron. Any one cell may thus react to some, but not all odours, and a pattern of excitation is built up across the olfactory mucosa. There is thus now support at the molecular level for the physiological theories about the basis of an individual's ability to distinguish between thousands of different odours.

Olfactory disturbance and olfactory testing

Definitions and principles

Complete loss of the sense of smell is called *anosmia*. Individuals with a diminished sense of smell are said to be *hyposmic*, but an apparent residual smell sense may represent stimulation of irritant receptors in a person who is, in fact, anosmic. A hyperacute sense of smell, which sometimes is only for a few odours, is much less common but is called *hyperosmia*. Some hyposmic individuals may experience a distorted perception of odours, *dysosmia*.

Olfactory testing involves two processes: first, the preparation and delivery of an odour stimulus and, second, the assessment of the response of the olfactory system. This assessment may be by some form of objective measurement of the physiological events produced by the olfactory stimulus; in the past, olfacto-pupillary and olfactorespiratory responses have been investigated but they are imprecise and unreliable. The value of attempting to investigate olfactory evoked cortical potentials, analogous to visual evoked responses, is disputed. Despite current renewed interest in the technique, there are problems in separating the true olfactory component of the response from the potentials associated with tactile and irritant stimulation, and those associated with the muscular concomitants of smelling or sniffing (Hummel and Kobal, 1992; Auffermann *et al.*, 1993). Newer methods assessing cortical activity, such as positron emission tomographic scanning (Zatorre *et al.*, 1992) are finding applications in the investigation of olfaction, but the complexity and cost of the technique makes it likely to remain of use in research rather than clinically.

Assessments of olfactory function which involve at least some element of subjective response on the part of the patient are potentially simpler than attempts at purely objective methods. Such assessments may involve the patient detecting the presence of an odour or series of odours, or identifying an odour or series of odours. The *detection threshold* is the lowest concentration of an odour that can be detected as being present. At a higher concentration for any given odour is the *recognition threshold*, the minimum concentration for recognition of the odour. In practice, the term *olfactory threshold* is applied to the detection threshold. Techniques which investigate minimum detectable concentrations are thus usually known as *threshold techniques*, and those which involve odour recognition as *suprathreshold techniques*. Threshold techniques give quantitative information, while suprathreshold ones give qualitative information. It must be remembered, however, that the task of actually naming odours, even apparently familiar ones, is a challenge quite independent of any impairment of smell itself. Sumner (1962), using four well-known smells in conventional smell-testing bottles, found that only two-thirds of his subjects could correctly name three or more of the four smells. It is likely that in many individuals, no more information is gained by using conventional smell bottles than simply by asking them if they have noticed any impairment or change of their sense of smell. The accuracy of subjective assessement of olfactory impairment may be improved by eliminating the free-recall component of the test using a multiple choice procedure. The subject is given a number of possible alternative identifications for each bottle and chooses the one which is thought to be correct.

Historical development of methods of olfactory assessment

Strictly speaking, any technique used in threshold (quantitative) testing is olfactometry. The use of the word *olfactometer* is, however, usually confined to a piece of equipment designed to prepare and deliver varying concentrations of an olfactory stimulus. In 1848, Valentin produced the first such device. Measured amounts of odorant were introduced into a large open vessel into which subjects put their noses and immediately took a sniff. The same principle has been applied to a whole room (an olfactorium) in which the subject sits. Proetz (1924) and Elsberg (1935) moved towards modern concepts of olfactometry by introducing, respectively, a bank of serial dilutions of odorant and the idea that air in a closed bottle above the level of odorant-containing fluid becomes saturated with odorant.

The most accurate olfactometers in use today use the air dilution principle illustrated in Figure 5.3. A warmed, filtered and humidified air stream is split into two. One of these streams passes through an odorant saturator, and is then diluted in various proportions with the unsaturated stream, producing highly accurate and known dilutions of the odour. A 10-fold concentration increase may, however, produce only a twofold odour intensity change as perceived by the subject, so olfactometers must be able

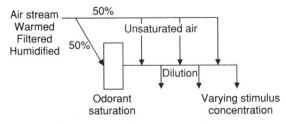

Figure 5.3 The principle of the air dilution olfactometer. (Reproduced by kind permission of the Royal Society of Medicine Services Ltd. from Moore-Gillon, V. Olfactometry. In *Rhinitis – Mechanisms and Management*, edited by I. Mackay)

to change the stimulus concentration over several orders of magnitude. Olfactometers of this kind (Figure 5.4) are invaluable for basic research in specialized centres, but are extremely expensive to build and maintain, and are not mobile. Developments over the past decade or so have accordingly concentrated on producing reliable methods of olfactory assessment which are cheap and convenient enough to be used in clinical assessment.

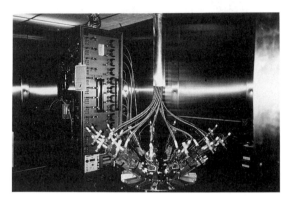

Figure 5.4 Air dilution olfactometer at the Smell and Taste Research Center, University of Pennsylvania, USA

Olfactory assessment in the clinical setting

Olfactory threshold determinations are most easily carried out using one of the several commercially available 'squeeze bottle' techniques (Amoore and Ollman, 1983; Amoore and O'Neill, 1986) (Figure 5.5). These tests use a series of paired bottles, one of which contains a known dilution of odorant and the other diluent only. The series of pairs represents serial dilutions of the odorant stimulus. A puff of air is squirted into the nose, and the subject asked to say which of the pair contains an odour (but is not asked to name it). A correct choice between the odour-containing bottle and that containing diluent only has to be made on three separate presentations for that concentration to be taken as the detection threshold. The threshold is compared with reference values determined empirically from population studies, and the test subject is then placed into the normal, hyposmic, and hyperosmic ranges.

Threshold evaluation may not, in some patients, correlate closely with impairment of olfactory performance in everyday life. There may be an apparently normal threshold, but problems with odour recognition at low concentrations, which may be to a few specific odours only. The subject may also be unable to perceive changes in smell intensity in the suprathreshold range. The substitution of suprathreshold

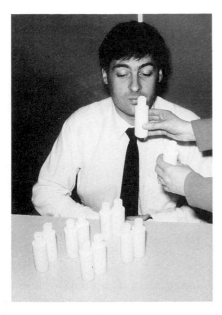

Figure 5.5 Olfactory threshold testing using PM Carbinol delivered by squeeze bottles. (Olfacto-Labs, 1414 Fourth Street, Berkeley, CA 94710, USA)

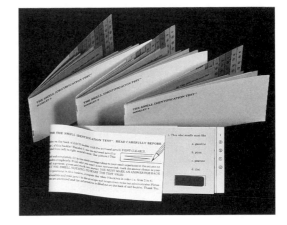

Figure 5.6 UPSIT – University of Pennsylvania Smell Identification Test. (Sensonics, 15 Haddon Street, Philadelphia, USA)

studies for measurements of olfactory threshold, or their addition to threshold techniques, is thus obviously of potential value. In view of the drawbacks of conventional smell identification bottles mentioned above, however, alternative methods of suprathreshold testing have been devised.

Doty, Shaman and Dann (1984) have developed the UPSIT (University of Pennsylvania Smell Identification Test), using odours microencapsulated in 10–50 μm crystals mounted on a series of cards in booklets (Figure 5.6). When scratched by a fingernail or pencil, the smell is released and is sniffed by the subject, who attempts to identify it with the help of four proffered alternative identifications, one of which must be chosen even if the subject believes that nothing can be smelt. Population studies show that when presented with a series of 40 different odour-impregnated cards, normal subjects give 32–40 correct responses, hyposmic individuals 20–30, and total anosmics score 7–14 correct answers (by chance alone).

The patient with olfactory impairment

Odour perception depends upon the anatomical state of the nose, the functional state of the olfactory epithelium and its connections with the second-order olfactory neurons, and the state of the central olfactory pathways and the olfactory cortex. There is a decline in olfactory function with age (Doty *et al.*,

1984; Doty and Snow, 1988), but it is uncommon for elderly individuals to present with complaints of olfactory loss alone and alternative explanations should be sought before attributing such complaints to ageing. As noted above, smell is such an important determinant of taste that the presenting symptom is frequently of apparent taste impairment, rather than olfactory loss.

Most patients complaining of olfactory disturbance will fall into one of three groups: after a head injury, after a viral infection, or as a result of poor odorant access to the olfactory mucosa. Other causes are uncommon, but are of importance for two reasons. First, they include individuals in whom the olfactory loss is due to a serious but potentially treatable condition, such as sphenoidal ridge meningiomas, frontal gliomas, and the occasional pituitary tumour. Olfactory groove meningiomas almost always cause anosmia several years before the development of visual disability, which is likely to be irreversible. Second, olfactory impairment may indicate the presence of other disorders. Alzheimer's disease, Parkinson's disease, Huntington's chorea and Korsakoff's psychosis may be asociated with olfactory disturbance and, indeed, olfactory loss may be a very early manifestation of some of these conditions. Anosmia or hyposmia has also been reported in association with hypogonadotrophic hypogonadism (Kallman's syndrome), Turner's syndrome, schizophrenia, diabetes mellitus, and in those with migraine or a history of alcoholism (Doty *et al.*, 1991, 1992; Hirsch, 1992; Kopala, Clark and Hurwitz, 1993; Shear *et al.*, 1992; Wu *et al.*, 1993; Weinstock, Wright and Smith, 1993).

Where olfactory loss occurs after a head injury, it is usually complete and olfactory testing shows the patient to be anosmic. It is believed that the anosmia results from shearing of the olfactory neurons as they pass through the cribriform plate. Contrary to some previous teaching, the responsible head injury is not always severe, there is frequently no skull fracture, and there is not always a history of unconsciousness. It should also be remembered that many individuals with a head injury may also have a nasal injury. In such cases, there may be nasal obstruction due to structural changes and clinical experience suggests that even where there is no deformity, nasal obstruction may be present due to the development of vasomotor instability. Identification of this group of individuals who become apparently anosmic following head injury is important because anosmia due to problems of odorant access to the olfactory mucosa is potentially remediable, while that due to olfactory neuronal damage is not. A clue is often given by the finding, on careful testing, that the individual has marked hyposmia rather than complete anosmia.

Olfactory disturbance following viral infections may be due to damage to the olfactory neurons by the virus itself, in which case loss is usually complete and permanent, but there may also be dysosmias which can be extremely distressing. As sometimes occurs with nasal injuries, however, a post-viral vasomotor rhinitis may lead to hyposmia or complete anosmia. Treatment of the rhinitis may restore the sense of smell and such individuals, along with others where olfactory disturbance is due to impaired odorant access to the olfactory mucosa, constitute the only group who may be cured. The fact that they constitute about 30% of those presenting with olfactory complaints, however, highlights the importance of the investigation of all cases of smell loss. Since, as noted above, so little of normal tidal respiration reaches the olfactory epithelium the absence of a subjective sensation of nasal obstruction is not an indication that odorant access is satisfactory. Figure 5.7 shows a CT scan of an individual with complete anosmia, but with no complaints of nasal obstruction. Surgical removal of the multiple small polyps led to the return of a normal sense of smell.

Investigation and management of the patient presenting with olfactory impairment

The investigation of a patient with a smell problem must start with a careful history. General medical health and mental state may point to a possible aetiology. The olfactory history itself should include details of the onset of symptoms and the events surrounding the loss, with particular attention to viral infections and head or nasal trauma. Congenital smell loss is rare but is often unrecognized by the patient or family until the teenage years. Both complete and partial congenital smell loss have been described (Amoore and Steinle, 1991). In acquired smell loss, the exact nature of the deficit (complete,

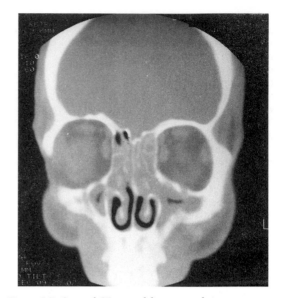

Figure 5.7 Coronal CT scan of the nose and sinuses showing ethmoid opacity and obstruction to the olfactory area by nasal polyps

partial, constant, variable) is important. Symptoms suggestive of rhinitis or sinus disease should be carefully elicited, although it should be stressed yet again that the lack of a sensation of nasal obstruction does not mean that odorant access to the olfactory mucosa is necessarily unimpaired.

Physical examination of the internal anatomy of the nose and the postnasal space is of obvious importance and a neurological examination will indicate whether the olfactory loss is an isolated problem, is due to a focal lesion, or is part of a more generalized disorder. If focal neurological signs are present or if the history and examination do not suggest a clear cause for the olfactory loss, a CT or MRI scan should be performed. Unless there is a definite history of immediate and total olfactory loss after a head injury or of symptoms suggesting nasal obstruction, a CT scan of the nose, sinuses and cribriform plate area should be carried out.

Olfactory testing is helpful as a means of establishing whether smell loss is partial or complete and of providing a baseline for assessment of response after treatment. Both threshold (using commercially available squeeze-bottles) and suprathreshold (using the UPSIT technique) measurements should be included. More complex olfactory testing is rarely required except for research.

Treatment

The contribution that poor odorant access plays in cases of hyposmia and anosmia has in the past been inadequately appreciated by clinicians. In the 30% of cases attributable to such problems some improvement in smell function may be obtained. Even small amounts of mucosal oedema around the middle turbinates or upper nasal septum may prevent odour access to the olfactory tract. In such cases, treatment with topical nasal steroids or even a short course of systemic steroids may improve odorant access. The CT scan may indicate those individuals who may benefit from surgical intervention.

Many claims have been made for the efficacy of zinc and this matter is discussed by Price (1986). Similarly, vitamin supplements and theophylline treatment has been recommended in cases of idiopathic smell loss. Results have not stood up to critical scientific analysis apart from those cases in which there is a clearly documented zinc or vitamin deficiency.

Conclusions

After decades of relatively slow progress, dramatic advances in unravelling the complexities of the mechanisms of odour detection and recognition are now taking place. The development of reliable and relatively simple clinical methods of olfactory testing, along with the availability of modern imaging techniques, means that individuals with olfactory complaints may now be investigated with greater ease and accuracy than in the past.

Loss or impairment of the sense of smell leads to distress, anxiety, and significant impairment of the quality of life. The widespread trivialization of olfactory symptoms by clinicians is inappropriate, but has probably been perpetuated by the widely held but misplaced belief that all cases of smell loss are untreatable. Even if the condition is found to be irremediable after careful investigation, many patients express relief that no serious underlying cause has been found, and many also find it much easier to accept their disability and adjust to life ahead knowing that all avenues have been explored.

References

AMOORE, J. E. and OLLMAN, B. G. (1983) Practical test kits for quantitatively evaluating the sense of smell. *Rhinology*, 21, 49–54

AMOORE, J. E. and O'NEILL, R. S. (1986) Clinical olfactometry: improved convenience in squeeze-bottle kits, and a portable olfactometer. *Chemical Senses*, 11, 576–577

AMOORE, J. E. and STEINLE, S. (1991) A graphic history of specific anosmia. In: *Chemical Senses: Vol. 3 Genetics of Perception and Communication*, edited by C. J. Wysocki and M. R. Kare. New York: Marcel Dekker Inc. pp. 331–350

ANHOLT, R. R. (1993) Molecular neurobiology of olfaction. *Critical Reviews in Neurobiology*, 7, 1–22

AUFFERMANN, H., GERULL, G., MATHE, F. and MROWINSKI, D. (1993) Olfactory evoked potentials and contingent nega-tive variation simultaneously recorded for diagnosis of smell disorders. *Annals of Otology, Rhinology and Laryngology*, 102, 6–10

BUCK, L and AXEL, R. (1991) A novel multigene family may encode odorant receptors: a molecular basis for odor recognition. *Cell*, 65, 175–187

DOTY, R. L. (1981) Olfactory communication in humans. *Chemical Senses*, 6, 351–376

DOTY, R. L. and SNOW, J. B. (1988) Age-related alterations in olfactory structure and function. In: *Molecular Neurobiology of the Olfactory System*, edited by F. Margolis and T. Getchell. New York: Plenum Press. pp. 355–374

DOTY, R. L., SHAMAN, P. and DANN, M. (1984) Development of the UPSIT: a standardised microencapsulated test of olfactory function. *Physiology and Behavior*, 32, 489–502

DOTY, R. L., STERN, M. B., PFEIFFER, C., GOLLOMP, S. M. and HURTIG, H. I. (1992) Bilateral olfactory dysfunction in early stage treated and untreated idiopathic Parkinson's disease. *Journal of Neurology, Neurosurgery and Psychiatry*, 55, 138–142

DOTY, R. L., SHAMAN, P., and APPLEBAUM, S. L., GIBERTSON, R., SIKSORSKI, L. and ROSENBERG, L. (1984) Smell identification ability: changes with age. *Science*, 226, 1441–1443

DOTY, R. L., PERL, D. P., STEELE, J. C., CHEN, K. M., PIERCE, J. D. REYES, P. *et al.* (1991) Olfactory dysfunction in three neurodegenerative diseases. *Geriatrics*, 46, 47–51

ELSBERG, C. A. (1935) The sense of smell: Introduction. *Bulletin of the Neurological Institute of New York*, 4, 1–19

ENGEN, T. (1983) The human uses of olfaction. *American Journal of Otolaryngology*, 4, 250–252

HIRSCH, A. R. (1992) Olfaction in migraneurs. *Headache*, 32, 233–236

HUMMEL, T. and KOBAL, G. (1992) Differences in human evoked potentials related to olfactory or trigeminal chemosensory activation. *Electroencephalography and Clinical Neurophysiology*, 84, 84–89

KOPALA, L. C., CLARK, C. and HURWITZ, T. (1993) Olfactory deficits in neuroleptic naive patients with schizophrenia. *Schizophrenia Research*, 8, 245–250

MOORE-GILLON, V. (1989) Olfactometry In: *Rhinitis – Mechanisms and Management*, edited by I. Mackay. London: Royal Society of Medicine Services Ltd. pp. 69–79

NAKASHIMA, T., CHARLES, P., KIMMELMAN, P. and SNOW, J. B. (1985) Vomeronasal organs and nerves of Jacobsen in the human fetus. *Acta Otolaryngologica*, 99, 266–271

PRICE, S. (1986) The role of zinc in taste and smell. In: *Clinical Measurement of Taste and Smell*, edited by H. L. Meiselman and R. S. Rivlin. New York: Macmillan Publishing Co. Inc. pp. 443–445

PROETZ, A. W. (1924) A system of exact olfactometry. *Annals of Otology*, 33, 746–763

RONNETT, G. V. and SNYDER, S. H. (1992) Molecular messengers of olfaction. *Trends in Neurosciences*, 15, 508–513

SCOTT, J. W., WELLIS, D. P., RIGGOTT, M. J. and BUONVISO, N. (1993) Functional organisation of the main olfactory bulb. *Microscopy Research and Technique*, 24, 142–156

SHEAR, P. K., BUTTERS, N., JERNIGAN, T. L., DITRAGLIA, G. M., IRWIN, M., SCHUCKIT, M. A. and CERMAK, L. S. (1992) Olfactory loss in alcoholics: correlations with cortical and subcortical MRI indices. *Alcohol*, 9, 247–255

SUMNER, D. (1962) On testing the sense of smell. *Lancet*, ii, 895–897

VALENTIN, G. G. (1848) *Lehrbuch der Physiologie*, 2nd edn. Braunschweig: F Vieweg

WEINSTOCK, R. S., WRIGHT, H. N. and SMITH, D. U. (1993)

Olfactory dysfunction in diabetes mellitus. *Physiology and Behavior*, **53**, 17–21

WU, J., BUCHSBAUM, M. S., MOY, K., DENLEA, N., KESSLAR, P., TSENG, H. *et al.* (1993) Olfactory memory in unmedicated schizophrenics. *Schizophrenia Research*, **9**, 41–47

ZATORRE, R. J., JONES-GOTMAN, M., EVANS, A. C. and MEYER, E. (1992) Functional localization and lateralisation of human olfactory cortex. *Nature*, **360**, 339–340

6

Mechanisms and treatment of allergic rhinitis

S. R. Durham

Allergic rhinitis is an IgE-mediated hypersensitivity disease of the mucous membranes of the nasal airways characterized by sneezing, itching, watery nasal discharge and a sensation of nasal obstruction. The lining of the nose is continuous with the paranasal sinuses which may also be involved. Associated allergic conjunctivitis and bronchial asthma may occur. Allergic rhinitis occurs in atopic individuals who are exposed to common aeroallergens. Allergic rhinitis is either seasonal (e.g. summer hayfever) or perennial. Perennial rhinitis, at least in the UK, is most commonly due to sensitivity to the house dust mite, *Dermatophagoides pteronysinnus*, and/or allergy to domestic pets, although sensitivity to an agent inhaled in the workplace should always be sought (occupational rhinitis). Perennial rhinitis with seasonal exacerbations may occur.

Although frequently trivialized by patients and doctors (particularly non-sufferers!) allergic rhinitis remains a common cause of morbidity, social embarrassment and impaired performance either at school or in the workplace. The disease is extremely common, although prevalence depends critically upon the age, gender and geographical locations of populations studied and, more importantly criteria for definition of rhinitis (Fleming and Crombie, 1987). Estimates vary from 10% to 20% with a male predominance and peak age distribution in young adulthood (Table 6.1). Recent evidence suggests the prevalance of hayfever in western developed countries has increased in recent years. For example in the UK, over the past 30 years there has been a fourfold increase in the prevalence of general practitioner consultations for summer hayfever (Fleming and Crombie, 1987). The reasons for this increase in prevalence are unknown and it cannot be explained by changes in diagnostic fashion or a greater awareness of the condition alone (Table 6.2).

Table 6.1 Age distribution of hayfever consultation (per 1000 population)

Age (years)	Distribution
0–4	12.6
5–14	48.0
15–24	47.2
25–44	29.8
45–64	12.6
65–74	8.9
75 +	4.0

Data from the Office of Population Census and Surveys (1982). Royal College of General Practitioners

Table 6.2 Consultation per 1000 population for hayfever (male and female) in the UK

Consultations (per 1000)	Years
5.1	1955–1956
10.6	1970–1971
19.8	1981–1982

Reproduced from Fleming D. M., Crombie D. L. (1987), *British Medical Journal*, **294**, 279–283, with permission

In this chapter the aetiology of allergic rhinitis is discussed in terms of genetic predisposition, nature of the provoking allergens and the possible role of pollution. There follows a section on pathogenesis which evaluates the role of immunoglobulin E, mediators of hypersensitivity, cellular interactions and recent data on the role of cytokines. Clinical features are presented including differential diagnosis and an approach to differential diagnosis and management. Finally treatment is discussed with emphasis on recent advances and prospects for novel treatments in the future.

Aetiology

Atopy

Atopy refers to the tendency to develop an exaggerated IgE antibody response as reflected by a positive skin prick test response to one or more common aeroallergens. It follows that atopy represents a *predisposition* to develop allergic disease. Allergy represents the clinical expression of atopic disease. The common allergic disorders include rhinitis, asthma and eczema. The prevalence of atopy when defined in this way is extremely common, affecting up to one-third of the general population. It follows that not all atopic individuals develop symptoms.

Atopy is genetically inherited as confirmed by family studies and, in particular, twin studies (Hanson *et al.*, 1991). The mode of inheritance is controversial (Marsh, Meyers and Bias, 1981). Suggestions have included autosomal recessive, autosomal dominant, mixed and multifactorial genetic influences. Interpretation is confounded by criteria used to define atopy, methods of genetic analysis (e.g. segregation analysis or sib pair analysis) and the population studied.

A recent study from Oxford (Cookson and Hopkin, 1988) defined atopy in terms of either an elevated total IgE or a positive skin prick test (greater or equal to 2 mm greater than a negative control prick test) or elevated allergen specific IgE concentrations. Several large families were initially studied and the investigation was then extended to include multiple small families. Segregation analysis (and more recently sib pair analysis) suggested autosomal dominant inheritence with a strong maternal influence. Genetic analysis of DNA from family members implicated genetic linkage with a gene (or genes) on chromosome 11q (Cookson *et al.*, 1989). An exciting recent development is the colocalization on chromosome 11q of the gene for the high affinity IgE receptor, disorders of which, at least in part, may contribute to the atopic trait (Sandford *et al.*, 1993). These findings have been confirmed by some but not all investigators (Amelung *et al.*, 1992) and clearly further studies are required. The role of chromosome 11, and in particular the high affinity IgE receptor gene will depend upon comparison of the precise sequence data of the IgE receptor gene between atopic and non-atopic individuals.

It seems likely that genetic influences in atopy will turn out to be multifactorial. The development of allergy, in addition to genetic predisposition, depends upon exposure to environmental allergens.

Allergens

Seasonal rhinitis

Seasonal allergic rhinitis in the UK (Varney, 1991) is most commonly due to allergy to grass pollen with seasonal symptoms in June or July corresponding to peak grass pollen counts. The commonest grass in the UK is perennial rye (*Lolium perenne*), the large leafed Timothy-grass (*Phleum pratense*) and cocksfoot (*Dactylis glomerata*). Other varieties include meadow fescue (*Festuca pratensis*) and Yorkshire fog (*Holcus lanatus*). Grasses are flowering plants whose pollens are dispersed by the wind. The timing of the peak pollen season varies with ambient temperatures and tends to occur 2–4 weeks later in the North of England and Scotland compared with South and South-East England. The majority of grasses flower in the early morning when pollen grains become airborne, rise on hot air currents, only to fall in the evening and at night when pollen counts at ground level are at their highest, corresponding to exacerbation of hayfever symptoms. Pollen counts are increased by warm, dry clear conditions and fall during unseasonal cold or wet periods. Pollen counts above $50/m^3$ are considered the level at which most, but not all, hayfever sufferers may develop symptoms. Patients with high sensitivity may suffer for 10–12 weeks during the summer. Owing to 'priming' of the nasal mucosa, exposure to even low counts late in the season may provoke symptoms.

Seasonal allergic rhinitis occurring during the spring time may occur following exposure to tree pollens including birch, hazel, plane tree, ash and pine. Weed pollens, including nettle, dock and mugwort flower in late summer. Fungi spore in late summer and autumn. Common species include *Cladosporium*, *Alternaria*, *Aspergillus* and *Basidiospores*. The number of outdoor air spores averages on a daily basis $10\,000–20\,000/m^3$ with peak concentrations up to $200\,000$ or higher for short periods. Paradoxically, rain fall may provoke an initial increase in spore numbers. For example epidemics of asthma and rhinitis which occur following thunderstorms have been attributed to a rapid increase in *Didymella* spores. The characteristics of common allergenic fungi including aerobiology and identification is covered in detail elsewhere (Salkin and Haines, 1984).

The dominant seasonal allergens vary widely throughout the world. In Scandinavia tree pollen allergy is far more prominent than in the UK. In southern Europe the grass pollen season occurs much earlier and dominant seasonal allergens include weeds (e.g. *Parietaria*) and olive tree pollen. In the USA ragweed pollen is a major seasonal allergen whereas in Japan the Japanese cedar tree has been identified as a major cause of seasonal allergy over the past 30 years.

Perennial allergic rhinitis

Worldwide the commonest cause of perennial allergic rhinitis is allergy to house dust mite species including *D. pteronysinnus*, *D. farinae* and *Euroglyphus maynei* (Colloff *et al.*, 1992). In the UK *D. pteronysinnus* is most common. In rural homes and those with damp, the storage mites of *Euroglyphus maynei* and *Lepidoglyphus destructor* may be very abundant. House dust mites are the dominant allergens in house dust. The optimal conditions for mite growth are approximately 15–20°C, relative humidity 60–70%. Mites are more abundant in humid homes. In temperate climates, the number of house dust mites increases during the humid late summer months. In houses the bedroom is the preferential breeding ground, particularly the mattress where abundant food, in the form of human skin scales, is present. Mites also flourish in the pillow, bed clothes, carpets, curtains and soft furnishings. The major allergens of house dust mite have been identified as digestive enzymes (cysteine proteases, group 1 allergens, e.g. Der p1) present in the digestive tract and excreted in mite faeces. Mite faecal pellets are relatively large (20 μm). Although mite faecal particles become airborne when room air is disturbed, faecal particles rapidly settle within 20 minutes.

The precise chemical structure and nucleotide sequence of the major mite allergens have now been reported (reviewed in Colloff *et al.*, 1992). The advent of specific monoclonal antibodies directed against major mite allergens has enabled the development of highly specific and sensitive radioimmunoassays which enable more precise environmental measurements of mite allergen levels. This should allow a more scientific evaluation of environmental control/allergen avoidance measures (Colloff *et al.*, 1992). In children, significant associations have been found between the presence of airborne mite allergen and mite sensitivity and between high mite allergen exposure by the age of 1 year and development of asthma at the age 11 years (Sporik *et al.*, 1990).

Other major perennial allergens include domestic pets (cats, dogs, rabbits, guinea pigs, gerbils, hamsters and horses) (Colloff *et al.*, 1992). Cat allergens are well characterized. The major cat allergen Fel d1, is a salivary protein which is preened on to the fur where it dries and becomes airborne on minute particles (less than 5 μm). Fel d1 may remain airborne on the surface of respirable small particles for prolonged periods and may provoke immediate symptoms of allergic rhinitis or asthma many hours later. Cockroach is a recently identified cause of rhinitis and asthma in inner city areas within the USA.

Occupational allergens

Rhinitis may occur as a consequence of exposure to allergens inhaled in the workplace. Occupational rhinitis is far less well characterized as a disease entity than occupational asthma. Frequently, asthma and rhinitis due to occupational allergen exposure may coexist in the same patient. The presence of work-related symptoms with improvement during periods away from work provide the essential clue to diagnosis. Common biological causes include flour (in bakers, grain workers), laboratory animals including guinea-pigs, rats and mice (in laboratory workers) and wood dusts (Western red cedar, oreoko in saw mill workers and carpenters), biological washing-powders (enzymes e.g. *Bacillus subtilis*, in soap powder manufacturers) and colophony (due to the emanations of solder flux in electronics workers).

A further recently identified allergen is latex. Latex allergy may provoke rhinitis, asthma, urticaria and, occasionally, life threatening anaphylaxis. Susceptible workers include surgeons, nurses, dental nurses, other health workers and patients with indwelling latex urinary catheters (e.g. spina bifida patients). Latex in surgical gloves may also provoke unsuspected intraoperative anaphylaxis in latex-sensitive subjects. Chemical causes include two part paint systems and resins (catalysts include di-isocyanates, acid anhydrides and polyamines in paint manufacturers and painters, particularly spray painters). Other chemical causes include platinum salts (in platinum refiners) and drugs (antibiotics, in pharmaceutical workers and nurses).

Food and drug-induced rhinitis (see Chapter 7)

Food may occasionally provoke IgE-mediated allergic rhinitis (Bindslev-Jensen, 1993). Typically patients with rhinitis due to food allergy are atopic with sensitivity to common aeroallergens and develop immediate nasal symptoms, *as well as* symptoms in other organs including the mouth, tongue, skin and digestive tract. In addition to IgE-mediated mechanisms, food-induced rhinitis may be due to sensitivity to preservatives such as sulphites, benzoates and tartrazine. Histamine-containing foods such as cheese, poorly kept fish and certain wines may also provoke 'pseudo-allergic' reactions including flushing, headache and rhinitis. Alcohol may provoke nasal congestion in anyone although this may be exaggerated in allergic rhinitis sufferers. Food-induced allergic rhinitis is more common in children. Particular triggers include milk, eggs and cheese. In adults nuts, fish, shellfish and citrus fruits may provoke immediate symptoms in sensitive subjects.

The mechanism of drug-induced rhinitis is largely unknown. Aspirin sensitivity is an important cause of rhinitis which may be severe and prolonged (Christie *et al.*, 1991). Aspirin-induced rhinitis is frequently associated with nasal polyposis and late onset (intrinsic) asthma. Aspirin sensitivity is frequently, although not always, associated with sensitivity to other non-steroidal anti-inflammatory drugs. The mechanism is unknown. Antihypertensive drugs (propranolol, other beta blockers, adrenergic neuron blocking drugs and ACE inhibitors) may provoke rhinitis with predominantly nasal congestion and rhinorrhoea.

Rhinitis medicamentosa refers to rebound hyperaemia, nasal congestion and obstruction with tachyphylaxis that occurs following prolonged and repeated use of topical vasoconstrictors. Although isolated cases undoubtedly occur, the risk of this complication has probably been overstated in the past and there is a paucity of reliable data. In general patients should be advised not to use topical vasoconstrictors for more than 2 weeks at a time.

Role of pollution

Nasal hyperreactivity refers to a heightened sensitivity of the nasal mucosa to a range of non-specific irritants. This may occur in so-called idiopathic rhinitis (cause unknown) or, more commonly, in association with prolonged allergen exposure in sufferers of allergic rhinitis. Typical irritants include perfumes, tobacco smoke, traffic fumes, domestic sprays and bleach. Watery rhinorrhoea following changes in temperature is also extremely common, and almost diagnostic of the presence of nasal hyperreactivity.

From the above it can be seen that irritants in high concentrations may provoke acute nasal symptoms in everyone, whereas lower levels of exposure may provoke symptoms in patients with 'idiopathic' rhinitis and nasal hyperreactivity or in patients with nasal hyperreactivity associated with allergic rhinitis. It has also been suggested that urban pollution particularly from motor exhaust fumes may be one factor responsible for increasing the prevalence of hayfever. Support for this concept comes from Japan where hayfever due to Japanese cedar pollen, first reported in the early 1960s, has shown a rapid increase in prevalence over the past 30 years which has coincided with a dramatic increase in motor vehicle exhaust pollution (Muranaka *et al.*, 1986). This increase in Japanese cedar pollen allergy in Japan is largely confined to urban rather than rural areas. Exhaust fumes include nitrogen dioxide, ozone and (from diesel engines) diesel particulates. Diesel particulates have been shown to be adjuvant for antibody production *in vivo* in animal models. Very recent data suggest that pre-exposure to a combination of nitrogen dioxide and ozone may amplify subsequent pollen-induced immediate symptoms of rhinitis (Rusznak *et al.*, 1994).

In contrast, a recent study compared the prevalence of hayfever in heavily polluted districts in Leipzig compared with the relatively pollution free area of Munich. In contrast to the Japanese findings, hayfever was more common in Munich where pollution

did not appear to be a major provoking factor (Von Mutius *et al.*, 1992). In summary, the role of pollution in hayfever remains controversial. Undoubtedly pollutants may irritate or exacerbate symptoms of nasal hyperreactivity in hayfever sufferers, although the role of specific pollutants in the development of pollen sensitivity and the persistence of hayfever symptoms remains controversial.

Pathogenesis

Immunoglobulin E

Immunologbulin E (IgE) (reviewed in Vercelli and Geha, 1993) has the unique property of binding reversibly to high affinity receptors on mast cells and basophils. The interaction of allergen with IgE initiates secretion of pharmacologically active mediators that cause clinical manifestations of immediate hypersensitivity.

IgE is composed of two heavy chains (*epsilon*) and two light chains (*kappa or lambda*). The intact molecule has a molecular weight of 188 000. IgE is heat labile. Heating for 2 hours at 56°C destroys its capacity to interact with heavy chain receptor (FcR) but not its allergen binding capacity. High affinity IgE receptors (Fc *epsilon* R1) are present on mast cells and basophils and have recently been described on Langerhans cells (dendritic cells present in the skin and at mucosal surfaces) and eosinophils. Antigenically distinct low affinity IgE receptors (Fc *epsilon* R2) have been demonstrated on subpopulations of T and B lymphocytes, monocytes and macrophages, eosinophils and platelets. However the biological significance of these low affinity receptors has yet to be determined.

As mentioned above, the characteristic feature of atopy is the preferential production of IgE antibodies by human B lymphocytes in response to antigenic stimulation by common aeroallergens. Allergen is captured by allergen specific B cells via their surface immunoglobulin receptors, internalized, processed into peptides and then expressed on the B cell surface in association with MHC class II molecules. CD4 + T lymphocytes are essential for IgE production by B cells. The production of interleukin 4 (IL-4) by activated CD4 + T lymphocytes follows cognate interaction between the T-cell receptor and processed allergen expressed along with the appropriate MHC class II restriction molecule on the surface of allergen specific B lymphocyte. IL-4 is the first signal necessary for preferential IgE production by B cells (Del Prete *et al.*, 1988). The precise molecular mechanism is unknown at the present time. However IL-4 promotes the production of *epsilon* heavy chain germ line transcripts (Vercelli and Geha, 1993). The production of mature C *epsilon* mRNA by allergen specific B lymphocytes requires a second signal. This may be provided by T cell contact. Recent studies have confirmed that this contact dependent signal may be delivered by engagement of a B cell specific antigen, CD40, with its ligand expressed on T lymphocytes (Jabara *et al.*, 1990). The role of CD40 has been further established by showing that anti-CD40 monoclonal antibodies may induce IgE synthesis by B lymphocytes. Alternative second signals which may substitute T cell contact include presence of Epstein-Barr virus (EBV) or hydrocortisone (Vercelli and Geha, 1993). The biological significance of these alternate MHC-unrestricted non-cognate T–B cell interactions in providing a second signal for IgE synthesis is unknown. Paradoxically topical corticosteroids, *in vivo*, are known to inhibit IL-4 messenger RNA by human T lymphocytes (Masuyama *et al.*, 1994; Sun Ying *et al.*, 1994).

Recently, CD40 antigen has been demonstrated on the surface of human mast cells and basophils (Gauchat *et al.*, 1993) (as well as T lymphocytes). Human mast cells may also express IL-4 (Bradding *et al.*, 1993). These interesting observations raise the possibility that mast cells may themselves promote an increase in B cell IgE production independent of T lymphocytes. Recent studies have shown that interleukin 6 (IL-6) may enhance IL-4-induced IgE production by B cells (Vercilli and Geha, 1993). Furthermore the recently described interleukin 13 (IL-13) may substitute for IL-4 whereas interleukin 12 (IL-12), a potent inducer of Th1-type T lymphocytes may enhance *interferon* gamma production, a potent inhibitor of IL-4-induced IgE production by B lymphocytes (Kiniwa *et al.*, 1992). Rapidly advancing knowledge of the factors involved in IgE regulation should identify novel therapeutic interventions in the future.

Mediators of hypersensitivity

Allergen-IgE dependent activation of mast cells and basophils results in the production of a whole range of pharmacologically active mediators. Translocation of cytosolic granules to the cell surface occurs where membrane exposes the granular matrix to the extracellular environment. Granule-associated mediators are thereby released from the partially solubilized granule matrix.

In parallel with events leading to granule secretion, stimulation of membrane phospholipases (C and A2) generate increased membrane levels of phospholipids including arachidonic acid. Subsequent metabolism of arachidonic acid by the cyclo-oxygenase pathway generates predominantly prostaglandin D2 (PGD$_2$) while the lipoxygenase pathway generates leukotriene B4, a chemotactic factor, and leukotrienes C4 and D4 which constitute the biological activity previously recognized as slow releasing substance of anaphylaxis (SRS-A).

Granule-associated mediators include histamine and tryptase. Bradykinin is also generated following mast cell activation, possibly via conversion of plasma protein precursors by products of mast cell activation.

The biological properties of these mediators include vasodilatation, an increase in vascular permeability and plasma exudation. Leukotriene B4 and platelet-activating factor (a further potent lipid-derived mediator) are potent chemoattractants for eosinophils and neutrophils. Leukotriene C4 is a potent mucus secretogogue. Histamine, acting directly or via neuronal reflexes, promotes itch, sneezing and mucus secretion.

In addition to preformed mediators and lipid mediators, mast cells have recently been demonstrated to produce cytokines, including IL-4 (Bradding *et al.*, 1993), interleukin 5 (IL-5) and tumour necrosis factor alpha (TNF-alpha) and thus represent an alternative source of cytokines to T lymphocytes. Unlike T lymphocytes, mast cells have the capacity to store cytokines within their cytoplasmic granules. However, the biological role of cytokines produced by mast cells (as well as T lymphocytes) has yet to be determined.

Mast cells (Irani and Schwartz, 1989) are located within the epithelium and submucosa of the upper and lower respiratory tract and gut and within the skin. Although largest numbers are located within the submucosa, mucosal type (tryptase only) mast cells migrate through the human nasal epithelium during natural seasonal grass pollen exposure (Bentley *et al.*, 1992). Connective tissue type mast cells (tryptase and chymase positive cells) are more prominent within the nasal submucosa and do not migrate in response to allergenic stimulation. Basophils are also found in blown secretions of patients with rhinitis. Thus water soluble allergens are free to interact with IgE-sensitized mast cells (and basophils) superficially within the nasal epithelium and in nasal secretions. The resulting rapid release of mediators from cells located in the epithelium or free on the nasal mucosa are responsible for immediate allergen-induced symptoms of itch, sneeze, watery rhinorrhoea, nasal congestion and blockage. Pharmacological mediators, including histamine, prostaglandin D2, bradykinin and TAME-esterase have been demonstrated in nasal lavage fluid during both early and late nasal responses (Naclerio *et al.*, 1985) following allergen provocation and are inhibited by topical corticosteroids (Pipkorn *et al.*, 1987). It is of interest that, in contrast to histamine, prostaglandin D2 is only identified during early responses which implies that late histamine release (6–12 hours after allergen provocation) may be derived from basophils rather than mast cells (Naclerio *et al.*, 1985). (Prostaglandin D2 is specific for mast cells.) Basophils have also been identified in nasal washes during late phase responses and are inhibited by corticosteroids (Naclerio *et al.*, 1985).

The biological importance of various mediators released following mast cell/basophil activation must ultimately depend upon the role of specific mediator antagonists, *in vivo*, during experimental or naturally occurring disease. The role of histamine is confirmed by the beneficial effect of antihistamines. Lipoxygenase inhibitors and leukotriene C4 receptor antagonists have been shown to have a beneficial effect in allergic rhinitis. Bradykinin antagonists are only recently available and the results of human studies are awaited. However, it is clear that a single mediator is not responsible for all rhinitis symptoms and specific receptor antagonists are therefore unlikely to control all symptoms of the disease.

Cellular recruitment and activation

A characteristic feature of allergic inflammation is the local accumulation of inflamatory cells including CD4 + T lymphocytes, mast cells, eosinophils, basophils and neutrophils (Bascom *et al.*, 1988; Varney *et al.*, 1992). Cellular recruitment and activation has been measured in nasal lavage fluid and in biopsies of the nasal mucosa obtained following both local allergen provocation and during natural seasonal allergen exposure. For example, following allergen challenge, immediate symptoms of itching, sneezing and rhinorrhoea occur within minutes. Depending upon the allergen dose and the allergen sensitivity of the subject a proportion of subjects develop late phase responses at 6–12 hours, resolving in 24 hours. When repeated nasal provocations are performed the number of pollen grains required to elicit a positive response may be reduced. This 'priming effect' disappears when the interval between challenges is increased. This priming is thought to be due to influx of inflammatory cells following the initial challenge (Bentley *et al.*, 1992). The clinical importance of this phenomenon is that patients allergic to tree pollens may be 'primed' during the spring time and develop exaggerated grass pollen-induced symptoms following exposure to even low pollen counts. This emphasizes the importance of early intervention with anti-inflammatory treatment before exposure begins. Chronic perennial rhinitis is characterized by chronic inflammation of the nasal epithelium and mucosa as a consequence of prolonged exposure to perennial allergens such as house dust mite, domestic pets and cockroach. Nasal biopsies from patients with perennial rhinitis have confirmed an intense inflammatory infiltration (Bradding *et al.*, 1993).

Mast cells/basophils

Mucosal (tryptase only) and connective tissue (tryptase and chymase positive cells) mast cells are distributed throughout the nasal mucosa in approximately equal proportions (Irani and Schwartz, 1989; Bentley *et al.*, 1992). Mast cell degranulation has been demonstrated histologically following allergen provocation

(Gomez *et al.*, 1986). Mast cell numbers increase within the epithelium during the pollen season (Viegas *et al.*, 1987). This epithelial migration involves tryptase only (mucosal type) cells (Bentley *et al.*, 1992). Allergic rhinitis sufferers have increased circulating numbers of mast cells/basophil progenitors which decrease during the pollen season, possibly due to recruitment to the nose. Seasonal epithelial mast cell migration (Gomez *et al.*, 1988) and the basophil influx (Bascom *et al.*, 1988), which is identifiable in nasal washings during late responses, are inhibited by corticosteroids.

Eosinophils

Eosinophils are prominent in nasal washings, smears and biopsies of the nasal mucosa of patients with both seasonal and perennial allergic rhinitis. Eosinophil numbers increase during the pollen season (Bentley *et al.*, 1992) and following allergen provocation (Varney *et al.*, 1992). Eosinophils are a major source of leukotriene C4 (a potent mucous secretogogue) and platelet-activating factor. Platelet-activating factor promotes vasodilatation, increased permeability and is a potent chemotactic factor for both eosinophils and neutrophils. Eosinophils produce a number of potent, highly positively charged proteins which are toxic to human respiratory epithelium (Frigas *et al.*, 1981). These include major basic protein, eosinophil cationic protein, eosinophil peroxidase and eosinophil-derived neurotoxin. Major basic protein is present in sputum from patients with asthma in concentrations which are toxic *in vitro* to human bronchial epithelial cultures. Parodoxically, unlike bronchial asthma, epithelial desquamation and damage is not a characteristic feature of allergic rhinitis (at least not following challenge or during seasonal exposure). Eosinophil recruitment and activation after challenge and during the pollen season is inhibited by treatment with corticosteroids (Sun Ying *et al.*, 1994).

T lymphocytes

Previous studies have focused mainly on the role of mediators and, as stated above, effector cells including mast cells, basophils and eosinophils. However, recent evidence suggests that IgE-dependent activation and cellular recruitment, particularly tissue eosinophilia, are under the local regulation of distinct cytokines (Mosmann *et al.*, 1986). Cytokines, originally described as products of T lymphocytes are peptide messengers which are also produced by alternative cells including mast cells (Bradding *et al.*, 1993), eosinophils (Gounni *et al.*, 1994) and the respiratory epithelium (Calderon *et al.*, 1994). However the principal cellular source of cytokines is the T lymphocyte. *In vitro* studies in murine models have identified two distinct classes of T helper lymphocytes distinguished on the basis of their profile of cytokine release (Mossman *et al.*, 1986; Robinson *et al.*, 1993). Th1 cells produce IL-2 and interferon (IFN-) gamma whereas 'Th2' cells elaborate principally IL-4 and IL-5. Both subsets produce IL-3 and granulocyte/macrophage colony stimulating factor (GM-CSF). IL-3 is a mast cell growth factor (Otsuka *et al.*, 1988) and IL-3, IL-5 and GM-CSF promote differentiation and maturation of eosinophils from bone marrow precursors (Owen *et al.*, 1987; Clutterback, Hirst and Sanderson, 1988; Lopez *et al.*, 1988; Rothenberg *et al.*, 1988). IL-5 has selective effects on eosinophils which include an increase in eosinophil adhesion to vascular endothelium (Walsh *et al.*, 1990) and activation and persistence of eosinophils in culture and, presumably in tissues. IL-4, in addition to its essential role in B lymphocyte switching in favour of IgE production (Del Prete *et al.*, 1988), may also selectively influence eosinophil recruitment by stimulating increased expression of vascular cell adhesion molecule 1 (VCAM-1) on vascular endothelium (Schleimer *et al.*, 1992). VCAM-1 selectively promotes eosinophil but not neutrophil adhesion. In contrast IFN-gamma inhibits IL-4-induced IgE production by B cells and inhibits proliferation of Th2-type lymphocytes (Mosmann *et al.*, 1986). Nasal biopsies performed during late nasal responses have shown increases in CD4 + T lymphocytes and CD25 + (IL-2R bearing) cells, presumed T lymphocytes, in addition to tissue neutrophilia and eosinophilia (Varney *et al.*, 1992). Double immunostaining has recently confirmed that the majority of IL-2R bearing cells during late responses are indeed T cells (Hamid *et al.*, 1992). *In situ* hybridization studies demonstrated allergen-induced increases in Th2 type cytokines, particularly IL-4 and IL-5 (Durham *et al.*, 1992). There was a close correlation between numbers of IL-4 and IL-5 + cells and the number of activated eosinophils. Double *in situ* immunostaining experiments revealed that the majority of cells expressing mRNA for IL-4 and IL-5 were indeed T cells with a contribution from mast cells and (for IL-5) a small contribution from eosinophils (Masuyama *et al.*, 1994; Sun Ying *et al.*, 1994). Studies of patients with perennial allergic rhinitis involving specific immunostaining for cytokines have also demonstrated the mast cell as an alternative source of cytokines (Bradding *et al.*, 1993). Thus both T lymphocytes and mast cells represent sources of IL-4 and IL-5. These results support the hypothesis that cytokines from T lymphocytes and mast cells may be responsible for local IgE production and tissue eosinophilia during human allergic rhinitis.

Influence of treatment on cells and cytokines

A hypothesis regarding pathogenic mechanisms of allergic rhinitis is summarized in Figure 6.1. Therapeutic intervention may be directed at the level of allergen exposure through appropriate avoidance measures or, occasionally and in defined circumstances by use of specific immunotherapy. Alternatively specific mediator antagonists may be of value and the role of antihistamines is clearly defined. Topical corticosteroids, as mentioned above, are extremely effective in prevention and treatment of allergic rhinitis. Likely mechanisms include reduction of mast cell epithelial migration and tissue eosinophilia. However, rather than a direct effect on mast cells and eosinophils, it seems likely that corticosteroids

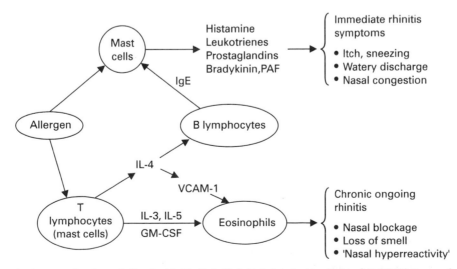

Figure 6.1 Hypothesis on mechanisms of allergic rhinitis. IL-3, IL-4, IL-5, interleukins 3, 4 and 5; VCAM-1, vascular cell adhesion molecule 1; GM-CSF, granulocyte/macrophage colony stimulating factor; PAF, platelet activating factor

may be effective by suppressing cytokine release, particularly release of IL-4 and IL-5 from T lymphocytes and, possibly mast cells. A recent study involving allergen provocation demonstrated that corticosteroids inhibited the late response, as well as the early response following allergen provocation. This was accompanied by a decrease in CD4 + T lymphocytes, mast cells and eosinophils and inhibition of cells mRNA + for IL-4 (Masuyama *et al.*, 1994). Specific immunotherapy may act in a different manner by promoting preferential Th1 responses with an increase in local production of IFN-gamma with inhibition of Th2 cells and antagonism of the effects of Th2 type cytokines (Durham *et al.*, 1994).

Clinical features

Effective treatment of rhinitis symptoms depends upon accurate clinical diagnosis and assessment of the patient's dominant symptoms. In general, the diagnosis of allergic rhinitis is straightforward and dependent upon the clinical history. However, the aetiology of rhinitis symptoms is frequently multifactorial. A careful history, local examination of the nose and performance of skin prick tests should be performed in all patients presenting with rhinitis symptoms. Additional tests including flexible and rigid endoscopy, mucociliary clearance studies and immunological tests may be required in certain circumstances. It should be remembered that the nose represents a 'window' to the respiratory tract and may also reflect systemic disease elsewhere (Durham, 1993).

History

A simple, arbitrary clinical definition of rhinitis is symptoms of nasal discharge, sneezing or nasal congestion/obstruction (two out of three) occurring for more than one hour on most days either seasonally or throughout the year. Rhinitis covers a spectrum of symptoms from a minor trivial inconvenience to profuse symptoms which adversely affect the quality and enjoyment of life and work or school performance. Certain individuals may be incapacitated for several days. It is important to establish the patient's *dominant* symptom and the impact of rhinitis symptoms on daily life.

Seasonal rhinitis

The first symptom of the hayfever season is usually sneezing. In severe cases paroxysms of sneezing occur at frequent intervals throughout the day. Sneezing is probably largely due to histamine release acting through reflexes. Excessive fluid and mucus secretion

(rhinorrhoea) is believed to be the response of seromucus glands to mast cell/basophil derived mediators. Nasal obstruction or blockage is the result of vascular engorgement, with resulting vasodilatation and oedema formation. Itchiness of the nose, eyes and palate are common features resulting from histamine and/or neural reflexes. Tearing, itching and redness of the eyes together with some degree of periorbital oedema is usual in hayfever. Other symptoms may include a burning or raw sensation in the throat and development of asthma symptoms such as wheezing and chest tightness.

Perennial rhinitis

The symptoms of perennial rhinitis differ from seasonal rhinitis largely as a result of long-standing nasal mucosal inflammation. Rhinorrhoea may be more viscous or purulent depending on the degree of cellular recruitment. Conjunctivitis is far less frequent in perennial rhinitis. Perennial rhinitis may also be accompanied by secondary symptoms including loss of smell, loss of taste and associated sinusitis or eustachian tube dysfunction. In general, sneezing is less common and prolonged continuous symptoms of nasal congestion and postnasal drip are more common.

In taking a history the seasonality, frequency and severity of symptoms and the patient's dominant symptom should be identified. A history of potential allergic triggers including occupational causes should be sought. A personal or family history of atopic disease is frequently obtained. It should be remembered that rhinitis is frequently multifactorial. A previous history of trauma may be relevant to a structural problem such as a deflected septum contributing to symptoms. A history of mucopurulent rhinorrhoea, facial pain and systemic symptoms of fever and malaise may point to associated infective sinusitis. A careful drug history and history of food-provoking factors should also be taken. Food allergy is almost invariably accompanied by other manifestations of allergy such as oral and gastrointestinal symptoms, rash or occasionally anaphylaxis.

Examination

In patients *with current symptoms* the allergic nasal mucosa appears pale or bluish, boggy with swelling and watery discharge. Frequently, if the patient is seen when asymptomatic the nasal mucosa appears entirely normal. The presence of polyps, septal deflection or prominent nasal turbinates should also be recorded. Further endoscopic otolaryngological examination, examination of the chest and general examination may be relevant if the diagnosis is not clear-cut.

Laboratory tests

In the diagnosis of allergic rhinitis, helpful supportive information for the clinical history may simply be achieved with skin prick testing. Skin prick testing is inexpensive, accurate, rapid and can be undertaken with a wide variety of allergens at a single skin prick testing session. Skin prick tests are preferred to scratch or intradermal tests which are less reproducible, more dangerous and may give false-positive responses. The usefulness and limitations of skin prick testing are summarized in Table 6.3. Skin prick tests should be performed with standardized commercially available extracts. Extracts of foods are, in general, less reliable with a higher rate of both false-positive and false-negative responses when compared to aeroallergens. Immediate sensitivity to raw fruit and vegetables and other fresh foods may simply be tested directly using a 25 gauge orange needle applied repeatedly through the surface of the fruit before skin prick testing.

Table 6.3 Use of skin prick tests

They diagnose (or exclude) 'atopy' – the predisposition to develop allergic disorders

They provide helpful supportive evidence (positive or negative) for the clinical history

Skin prick tests are essential when potentially expensive time-consuming allergen avoidance measures or the removal of a pet are involved

Skin prick tests have educational value and provide an illustration to the patient which may reinforce verbal information

Practice points. Skin prick tests may be invalid in patients on antihistamines, patients with severe eczema or patients with dermatographism. Always include a positive control (histamine 10 mg/ml) and a negative control test (allergen diluent). Check storage of extracts used for skin prick tests

Where skin prick testing is not possible owing to lack of availability of extracts, associated skin disease or in patients taking antihistamines, serum IgE measurements may be performed. The principle of the radioallergosorbent test (RAST) is summarized in Figure 6.2. More modern automated methods employ enzyme-linked immunoabsorbent assays (ELISA) which depend upon the development of a colour reaction which is measured by optical densitometry.

Nasal cytology is helpful in differential diagnosis of nasal complaints. Samples may be obtained either by blown secretions or by gentle scraping of the lateral nasal wall. The material is smeared on to a glass slide fixed in ethanol and stained with May Grünwald or Giemsa. The presence of eosinophils, neutrophils, basophils, mast cells, epithelial cells and bacteria should be recorded. Nasal swabs for bacteriology or viral studies may also be taken.

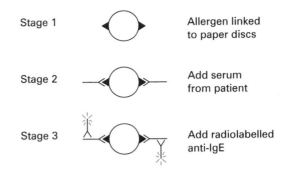

Figure 6.2 Principle of radioallergosorbent test (RAST)

Approach to differential diagnosis and management

Rhinitis is defined in terms of the presence and duration of common nasal symptoms. The need for taking a history, examining the nose and performing skin prick tests on every patient is emphasized. This should enable identification of significant allergy, infection or structural problems contributing to the development of nasal symptoms. A logical and simple strategy for management of these conditions is given in Figure 6.3. The differential diagnosis including rare causes of nasal symptoms is mentioned. The need for re-evaluation and appropriate referral upon failure of treatment to an allergist and/or otolaryngologist is emphasized. The scheme highlights that a simple approach in a general practice setting may be effective in diagnosing and treating the majority of patients with rhinitis, whereas difficult diagnostic problems, in patients with persistent symptoms and treatment failure should be referred to a combined medical/surgical rhinology clinic for specialist investigation and treatment. Detailed discussion of differential diagnosis of rhinitis is covered elsewhere in this volume.

Complications

It has been suggested that allergy may contribute to serous otitis media. However, the evidence is conflicting; some studies have not demonstrated a greater prevalence of atopy and allergy in otitis media patients compared with normal control subjects. It is possible that pathological changes associated with rhinitis may lead to obstruction of the eustachian tube with dysfunction and middle ear effusion. It seems more likely that serous otitis is not an allergic disease *per se* but a frequent complication of nasal allergy, particularly in children (Van Cauwenberge and Ingels, 1993).

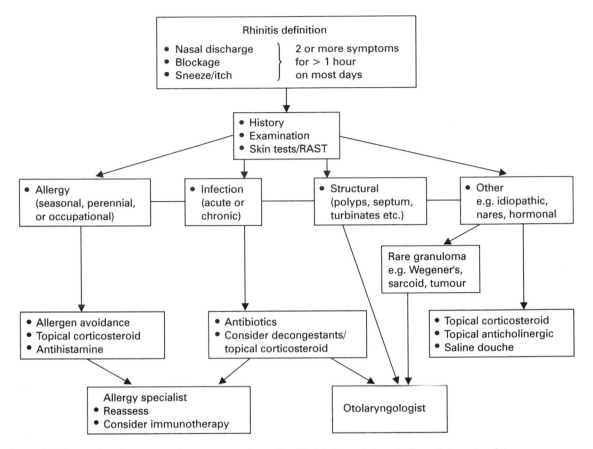

Figure 6.3 Approach to diagnosis and management (reproduced by kind permission of *Allergy*. International Consensus Report on Rhinitis Management, *Allergy* (1994; **49** suppl. 19, 1–34). RAST, radioallergosorbent test

The association between allergy and sinusitis is essentially twofold. First, allergy may contribute to obstruction of the sinus ostia and, in this sense, represents a predisposing factor. Second, perennial allergic rhinitis has some of the features of chronic sinusitis particularly nasal discharge and obstruction (Slaviu, 1988).

Allergic rhinitis and bronchial asthma frequently coexist (Slaviu, 1988). For example, patients with severe seasonal rhinitis commonly develop symptoms of peak seasonal wheezing and chest tightness. It is important to recognize and treat associated asthma. Furthermore, treatment of rhinitis with improvement in the nasal airway may also improve symptoms of bronchial asthma.

Treatment

The mainstay of treatment of allergic rhinitis involves identification and avoidance of provoking allergens (where possible) and the use of topical corticosteroid nasal sprays and oral antihistamines. Immunotherapy retains a place in treatment in patients with severe isolated grass pollen allergy. Surgery should not be considered 'a last resort' but rather complementary to medical treatment of allergic rhinitis when this is complicated by structural problems such as deflected septum, nasal polyps or enlarged turbinates (Zinreich *et al.*, 1987; Mackay, 1992).

Allergen avoidance

Management of patients with rhinitis symptoms should always include identification and, where possible, avoidance of causal factors. Although the concept of allergen avoidance seems straightforward and obvious, in practice it is often difficult to undertake. However, it is now possible to document environmental allergen exposures with a great degree of precision. Allergen avoidance measures which have been shown effectively to eliminate the allergen load have also been shown to be clinically efficacious.

House dust mite avoidance measures

The major sources of house dust mite are the mattress, pillow and bed covers (Colloff *et al.*, 1992). Other sources include carpets (particularly wool carpets) and soft furnishings throughout the home. Optimal conditions for mite growth are 15°C and 60–70% relative humidity (approximating to the average modern centrally heated home!). Theoretical approaches to house dust mite avoidance/reduction are listed in Table 6.4. Mattress/bedding barrier intervention has been shown to reduce mite allergen levels and improve clinical symptoms of both asthma and rhinitis. Acaracides kill mites although do not eliminate the allergen. The allergen may be modified by protein denaturing agents (tannic acid). Although theoretically useful, careful prospective controlled trials are required before these additional methods can be routinely recommended. The recent position paper by the British Society of Allergy and Clinical Immunology recommends use of bedding barrier intervention, regular vacuuming of carpets and soft furnishings and, where possible, use of alternative cork, vinyl or hard wood floors (Colloff *et al.*, 1992).

Table 6.4 Theoretical approaches to house dust mite avoidance/reduction

Mattress covers
Covers for pillows and bedding
Vacuuming
Liquid nitrogen
Acaricides
Protein denaturing agents
Regulation of ventilation, humidity of the home

Animal allergens

The major cat allergen (Fel D1) is present in minute (less than 2.5 μm) particles which may remain airborne for many hours and are very respirable (Colloff *et al.*, 1992). Families with atopic members should be advised against having furred animals in the home (cats, dogs, gerbils, hamsters, guinea pigs and rabbits). However, psychosocial factors may render dogmatic statements about removal of a family pet unwise. In such circumstances advice may be ignored and the doctor–patient relationship embarrassed. Where removal of a pet is not possible advice can be given to confine the animal outside or to the kitchen. Families may be advised that an animal should not be replaced. Recent studies have suggested that washing the cat (once weekly) when combined with other cleaning measures may be effective. The assumption is that this will reduce symptoms of cat allergy although this remains, at the present time, unproven. Cat allergen may remain in the home for many months after the removal of a pet. Patients should be advised that vigorous prolonged cleaning measures are required in order to reduce satisfactorily cat allergen levels.

Pollens

Avoidance of pollens is often not practicable (Varney, 1991). However, simple advice includes keeping windows shut in cars and buildings. Wearing sunglasses may reduce eye symptoms. Certain modern cars have pollen filters. Patients should be advised against walking in open grassy spaces particularly during the evening and at night. If affordable, a holiday by the sea or abroad during the peak pollen season may be recommended.

As mentioned above the availability of monoclonal antibodies to the major allergens of house dust mite and cat allergens should enable more precise identification of threshold levels for sensitization and threshold levels at which attacks of acute rhinitis/asthma may occur. Accurate quantification of environmental levels should also enable the development of more effective environmental control measures. Previous pessimism regarding the potential value of allergen avoidance measures is unfounded. However, as for any new treatment, the same stringent criteria should be used to assess efficacy of allergen avoidance methods, particularly when expensive and time-consuming measures are involved. There are exciting prospects for improving environmental caution measures which should be considered as complementary to pharmacotherapy in the management of allergic rhinitis.

Pharmacotherapy

Treatment of rhinitis, not surprisingly, has similarities to generally accepted guidelines for treating bronchial asthma (Naclerio, 1991; International Consensus Report on Management of Rhinitis, 1994). With the exception of patients with mild occasional symptoms, treatment is required with 'relievers', drugs which control symptoms and relieve acute attacks, and 'preventors' or anti-inflammatory, anti-allergic drugs which suppress the underlying disease process. Where appropriate, allergen avoidance measures should be employed.

Topical corticosteroids

Topical corticosteroid nasal sprays are extremely effective in controlling nasal symptoms of allergic rhinitis in the majority of patients (Juniper *et al.*, 1989; Naclerio, 1991; Naclerio and Mygind, 1993). Topical corticosteroids, in recent years, have become the mainstay of treatment based on their efficacy and lack of side effects. Topical corticosteroids are highly effective against *all* nasal symptoms, including nasal congestion and blockage. Beclomethasone (Beconase) and budesonide (Rhinocort) are available as metered dose freon propellant inhalers and as aqueous nasal sprays. The latter are more pleasant to take, are better tolerated and have the advantage of a better local distribution within the nasal cavity. Side effects are minimal. Local irritation generally settles when the underlying inflammation responds to treatment. If local irritation is a problem, a short course of oral corticosteroids may be justified in the first instance. Slight bleeding may occur in 5–10% of patients. A recent alternative is fluticasone propionate (Flixonase) which is potent, effective once daily and may have even less potential for systemic effects. However, this drug is more expensive and should be reserved at present for patients not responding to the above medications.

The commonest reason for treatment failure with corticosteroid nasal sprays is that the medication has not been taken regularly or because of faulty inhaler technique. In seasonal allergic rhinitis the drug should ideally be commenced early in the season before onset of symptoms. Systemic effects of nasal corticosteroids are virtually absent in usual recommended therapeutic doses. Nonetheless, care should be taken in children, particularly when other topical corticosteroid preparations for either eczema or asthma are being taken.

Short courses of oral corticosteroids (e.g. prednisolone 20 mg for 5 days) are very effective for severe peak pollen seasonal symptoms or when complete nasal blockage prevents effective penetration of corticosteroid nasal sprays. Depot intramuscular corticosteroids are not recommended. Although effective, the dose is high, irretrievable and may be associated with an increased risk of both local side effects such as atrophy at the injection site and systemic side effects.

Betamethasone (Betnesol) nasal drops, when used in the head down and forward position, may also be effective. However, this drug is usually reserved for patients with ostiomeatal complex disease, sinusitis and nasal polyps. In general, allergic rhinitis is better treated with corticosteroid nasal sprays rather than drops.

Sodium cromoglycate is an alternative prophylactic treatment for both seasonal (Orgel *et al.*, 1991) and perennial (Cohen *et al.*, 1976; Druce *et al.*, 1990) allergic rhinitis and remains the treatment of first choice in young children. Sodium cromoglycate is less effective than topical corticosteroids, although is effective in placebo controlled trials when taken four times daily. Sodium cromoglycate eye drops are very effective in controlling allergic conjunctivitis symptoms. Cromoglycate is safe and non-toxic although may occasionally provoke local irritation.

Antihistamines

Antihistamines are particularly effective for symptoms of sneezing, itching and watery rhinorrhoea although, unlike topical corticosteroids have little effect on nasal congestion and blockage (Anon., 1990; Simons, 1993). However, antihistamines are additionally effective for eye, palate and throat symptoms. Some patients prefer the convenience of a once or twice daily oral tablet to use of nasal sprays. Many patients with mild disease find the older antihistamines such as chlorpheniramine (Piriton) satisfactory, especially when taken at night. However, although inexpensive, major disadvantages of the old antihistamines include sedative effects and anticholinergic side effects. For these reasons the first generation antihistamines have been virtually superseded by newer H1-specific histamine receptor antagonists which have minimal side effects.

Terfenadine has virtually no sedative properties, little interaction with alcohol and is an effective, relatively inexpensive antihistamine. A rare but important complication is QT prolongation on the ECG which, on extremely rare occasions, has resulted in development of ventricular arrhythmias (torsades de pointes) (Warin, 1991). However this risk is *only* present when the drug is taken in overdosage, in the presence of impaired liver function or when ketoconazole or erythromycin are taken concurrently. QT prolongation has not been reported when terfenadine is used in recommended doses as indicated in the package insert. QT prolongation and arrhythmias have also been reported with astemizole (Hismanal, Pollon-eze) (Craft, 1986). It is not clear whether this rare complication is specific for these two drugs or represents a class effect involving other antihistamines.

Astemizole is an alternative effective second generation antihistamine with a low sedative profile. A disadvantage is a very prolonged half life (skin prick tests should not be performed within 6 weeks of taking astemizole). Weight gain has been occasionally reported with this drug.

Newer alternatives include acrivastine (Semprex). Acrivastine is an effective drug with a rapid onset of action and short half-life. This is of value in patients with occasional intermittent symptoms who do not wish to take regular long-acting oral antihistamines or nasal sprays. Loratadine (Clarityn) is effective when used once daily and has the advantage of a very rapid onset of action. Cetirizine (Zirtek) is extremely effective although may occasionally cause sedation. Cetirizine, in addition to its antihistamine properties, has been shown both *in vitro* and *in vivo* to inhibit eosinophil migration. However, it is not clear whether these additional anti-allergic properties contribute to its efficacy over and above its potent antihistaminic effects. Unfortunately there is a paucity of clinical trials comparing these newer antihistamines which are more expensive than terfenadine and astemizole and should probably be reserved for patients who fail to respond to these drugs.

A novel topical antihistamine, azelastine (Rhinolast) is now available. This approach seems logical. However, further clinical trials to evaluate efficacy are required and patients may find its taste unpleasant.

Other treatments

Topical vasoconstrictors (Anggard and Malm, 1984; Bende and Loth, 1986) are effective against nasal blockage and safe when used for short periods only. They are particularly helpful to open up a blocked nose prior to for example, commencing topical nasal corticosteroid treatment. They may provide relief from the common cold and may be useful as prophylaxis against barotrauma. Topical anticholinergics (ipratropium bromide) are only effective against watery nasal rhinorrhoea (Knight, Kazim and Salvatori, 1986; Dolovich et al., 1987). Ipratropium may be added to topical corticosteroids and antihistamines for the treatment of allergic rhinitis when watery rhinorrhoea remains the dominant persistent symptom. Over-use may provoke excessive nasal dryness and crusting.

In summary, pharmacotherapy should always be combined with allergen avoidance where possible. It is essential to elicit the patient's dominant symptom and match the drug profile (doses and dose intervals) to the patient's symptoms (Table 6.5).

The importance of inhaler technique and regular prophylactic treatment should be emphasized, particularly the advantages of introducing topical corticosteroid early in the pollen season. Treatment failure should always prompt re-evaluation of the diagnosis and management.

Immunotherapy

Immunotherapy should be considered in pollen sensitive patients who fail to respond to conventional treatment (Position Paper, 1993; Varney et al.,

1991). Immunotherapy was initiated in the UK in the early 20th century. The efficacy of immunotherapy in seasonal allergic rhinitis (grass pollen, ragweed and birch) has been confirmed in a number of double-blind placebo-controlled clinical trials. Although immunotherapy may also be effective in patients with perennial allergy due to house dust mite (Ewan et al., 1988; Corrado et al., 1989) and animal danders (Ohman, Findlay and Leitermann, 1984), at the present time, at least in the UK it is not recommended outside the context of controlled clinical trials.

Allergen injection immunotherapy is widely used in Europe and the USA. Although effective when compared with placebo, the place of immunotherapy will ultimately depend upon comparative studies with the best available pharmacotherapy and 'add on' trials where the addition of immunotherapy to existing pharmacotherapy is assessed. Allergen immunotherapy represents a specific treatment for allergic disease and, unlike conventional pharmacological treatment, has at least the theoretical potential to alter the course of allergic disease with, for example, prevention of progression of allergic rhinitis to asthma. However, this hypothesis requires testing in long-term prospective controlled trials which employ biologically standardized extracts.

Allergen injection immunotherapy may also be criticized on grounds for safety. Following a Committee on the Safety of Medicines Report, in 1986, allergen immunotherapy in the UK largely ceased. Concern was expressed at occasional deaths from severe bronchospasm and anaphylaxis which were almost exclusively confined to patients with asthma. Quite rightly, the Committee recommended that immunotherapy should only be given by trained personnel where facilities for resuscitation are available and that patients should be kept under medical observation following injections. However, the recommendation of a postinjection observation period of 2 hours (unlike 30 minutes recommended in USA and Europe) has made immunotherapy impracticable for both physicians and patients in the UK.

Indications and contraindications for immuno-

Table 6.5 Treatment of allergic rhinitis in adults*. (Reproduced from *Allergy*, 1994; **49** (suppl. 19), p. 20. International Consensus Report on the diagnosis and management of rhinitis)

	Itch/sneezing	Discharge	Blockage	Impaired smell
Sodium cromoglycate	+	+	±	—
Oral antihistamines	+ + +	+ +	±	—
Ipratropium bromide	—	+ + +	—	—
Topical decongestants**	—	—	+ + +	—
Topical corticosteroids	+ + +	+ + +	+ +	+
Oral corticosteroids	+ + +	+ + +	+ + +	+ +

*   Match drug profile to patients' symptoms and always include allergen avoidance advice where appropriate.
** Restrict use of topical decongestants to 7 days. In USA, (oral) decongestants may be an alternative.

therapy are summarized in Table 6.6. Careful patient selection is crucial for the success of immunotherapy. In the UK immunotherapy is confined to patients with seasonal grass pollen allergy confirmed on skin prick testing and/or RAST determination. Patients with multiple allergies or chronic asthma are specifically excluded. Future studies should include further assessment of the efficacy and safety of immunotherapy for perennial mite-induced rhinitis and 'add on' studies and long-term preventative studies. A review of immunotherapy has recently been published by the British Society of Allergy and Clinical Immunology (Position Paper, 1993). Practical guidelines for immunotherapy are more comprehensively covered in the European Academy of Allergy and Immunology Position Paper on immunotherapy (Malling and Weeke, 1993).

Table 6.6 Indications and contraindications for allergen injection immunotherapy for use in allergic rhinitis

Indications
1 Evidence of IgE-mediated disease in which allergens are considered to be the major triggers
2 Inability to avoid allergens
3 Inadequacy of drug therapy or intolerable side effects of such treatment
4 Limited spectrum of allergen sensitivities (in general one, or at most, two allergens)
5 Compliance

Contraindications
1 Non-availability of suitable allergen extracts
2 Significant medical or immunological disease
3 Multiple allergies
4 Concurrent treatment with drugs likely to impair possible treatment for anaphylaxis (beta-blockers or other adrenergic blocking drugs)

Adapted from WHO/IUIS Report (WHO/IUIS working group. Current status of allergen immunotherapy. Shortened version of WHO/IUIS working group report. Lancet, i, 259–261, 1989).

Conclusions

The mainstay of modern management of allergic rhinitis involves topical corticosteroids and oral antihistamines combined with effective allergen avoidance measures. In resistant cases it seems logical to use a combined approach involving allergen avoidance and topical corticosteriods and immunotherapy, the effects of which may be complementary, and possibly synergistic. Future strategies may include the use of specific antagonists directed against Th2-type cytokines, e.g. anti-IL-4 or IL-5, or possibly soluble IL-2R which may antagonize effects of these cytokines. It might be predicted that IFN-gamma may be effective in allergic rhinitis. Although initial reports of systemic IFN-gamma were disappointing, a trial of topical IFN-gamma would be of interest.

References

AMELUNG, P. J., PANHUYSEN, C. I. M., POSTMA, D. S., LEVITT, R. C., KOETER, G. H., FRANCOMANO, G. A. et al. (1992) Atopy and bronchial hyperresponsiveness: exclusion of linkage to markers on chromosome 11q and 6p. *Clinical Experimental Allergy*, **22**, 1077–1084

ANGGARD, A. and MALM, L. (1984) Orally administered decongestant drugs in disorders of the upper respiratory passages: a survey of clinical results. *Clinical Otolaryngology*, **9**, 43–49

ANON (1990) Three new 'non-sedative' antihistamines. Worth staying awake for? *Drugs and Therapy Bulletin*, **28**, 38–40

BASCOM, R., WACHS, M., NACLERIO, R. M., PIPKORN, U., GALLI, S. J. and LICHTENSTEIN, L. M. (1988) Basophil influx occurs after nasal antigen challenge: effects of topical corticosteroid pretreatment. *Journal of Allergy and Clinical Immunology*, **81**, 580

BENDE, M. and LOTH, S. (1986) Vascular effects of topical oxymetazoline on human nasal mucosa. *Journal of Laryngology and Otology*, **100**, 285–288

BENTLEY, A. M., JACOBSON, M. R., CUMBERWORTH, V., BARKANS, J. A., MOQBEL, R., SCHWARTZ, L. B. et al. (1992) Immunohistology of the nasal mucosa in seasonal allergic rhinitis: increases in activated eosinophils and epithelial mast cells. *Journal of Allergy and Clinical Immunology*, **89**, 821–829

BINDSLEV-JENSEN, C. (1993) Food allergy and intolerance. In: *Allergic and Non-Allergic Rhinitis: Clinical Aspects*, edited by N. Mygind and R. M. Naclerio. Copenhagen: Munksgaard. pp. 46–50

BRADDING, P., FEATHER, I. H., WILSON, S., BARDIN, P. G., HEUSSER, C. H., HOLGATE, S. T. et al. (1993) Immunolocalization of cytokines in the nasal mucosa of normal and perennial rhinitis subjects. *Journal of Immunology*, **151**, 3853–3865

CALDERON, M. A., DEVALIA, J. L., RUSZNAK, C., EVANS, K. and DAVIES, R. J. (1994) The effect of ozone (oz) on epithelial permeability and synthesis of IL-8 and GM-CSF by cultured nasal epithelial cells from non-atopic non-rhinitic subjects. *Clinical and Experimental Allergy*, **9**, 166

CHRISTIE, P. E., TAGARI, P., FORD HUTCHINSON, A. W. et al. (1991) Urinary leukotriene E4 concentrations increase after aspirin challenge in aspirin-sensitive asthmatic subjects. *American Review of Respiration Disease*, **143**, 1025–1029

CLUTTERBACK, E. J., HIRST, E. M. A. and SANDERSON, C. J. (1988) Human interleukin-5 (IL-5) regulates the production of eosinophils in human bone marrow cultures: comparison and interaction with IL-1, IL-3, IL-6 and GM-CSF. *Blood*, **73**, 1504

COHEN, R. H., BLOOM, R. L., RHWADES, R. B., WITTIG, H. L. and HAUGH, L. D. (1976) Treatment of perennial allergic rhinitis with cromolyn sodium. *Journal of Allergy and Clinical Immunology*, **58**, 121–128

COLLOFF, M. J., AYRES, J., CARSWELL, F., HOWARTH, P. H., MERRETT, T. G., MITCHELL, E. B. et al. (1992) The control of allergens of dust mites and domestic pets: a position paper. *Clinical and Experimental Allergy*, **22**, (suppl. 2), 1–28

COMMITTEE ON THE SAFETY OF MEDICINES (1986) CSM update: Desensitizing vaccines. *British Medical Journal*, **293**, 948

COOKSON, W. O. C. M. and HOPKIN, J. M. (1988) Dominant inheritance of atopic immunoglobulin-E responsiveness. *Lancet*, i, 86–88

COOKSON, W. O. C. M., SHARP, P. A., FAUX, J. A. and HOPKIN, J. M. (1989) Linkage between immunoglobulin-E responses underlying asthma and rhinitis and chromosone 11q. *Lancet*, i, 1292–1295

CORRADO, O. J., PASTORELLO, E., OLLIER, S., CRESWELL, L., ZANUSSI, C., ORTOLANI, C. et al. (1989) A double-blind study of hyposensitisation with an alginate conjugated extract of *D. pteronyssinus* 'Conjuvac' in patients with perennial rhinitis. *Allergy*, 44, 108–115

CRAFT, T. M. (1986) Torsades de pointes after astemizole overdose. *British Medical Journal*, 292, 660

DEL PRETE, G. F., MAGGI, E., PARRAONCHI, P., CHRETIEN, I., TIRI, A., MACCHIA, D. et al. (1988) IL-4 is an essential factor for the IgE synthesis induced *in vitro* by human T cell clones and their supernatants. *Journal Immunology*, 140, 4193

DOLOVICH, J., KENNEDY, L., VICKERSON, R. and KAZIM, F. (1987) Control of the hypersecretion of vasomotor rhinitis by topical ipratropium bromide. *Journal of Allergy and Clinical Immunology*, 80, 274–278

DRUCE, H. M., GOLDSTEIN, S., MELAMED, J., GROSSMAN, J., MOSS, B. A. and TOWNLEY, R. G. (1990) Multicentre placebo-controlled study of nedocromil sodium 1% nasal solution in ragweed seasonal allergic rhinitis. *Annals of Allergy*, 65, 212–216

DURHAM, S. R. (1993) Medical approach to rhinitis. *British Journal of Hospital Medicine*, 50, 458–462

DURHAM, S. R., SUN YING, VARNEY, V. A., JACOBSON, M. R., SUDDERICK, R. M., MACKAY, I. S. et al. (1992) Cytokine messenger RNA expression for IL-3, IL-4, IL-5, and granulocyte/macrophage-colony-stimulating factor in the nasal mucosa after local allergen provocation: relationship to tissue eosinophilia. *Journal of Immunology*, 148, 2390

DURHAM, S. R., VARNEY, V. A., SUN YING, JACOBSON, M. R., SUDDERICK, R. M., MACKAY, I. S. et al. (1994) Effect of grass pollen immunotherapy on cell infiltration and cytokine mRNA expression during allergen-induced late nasal responses. *Journal of Allergy and Clinical Immunology*, 93, 230

EWAN, P. W., ALEXANDER, M. M., SNAPE, C., IND, P. W. and AGRELL, B. (1988) Effective hyposensitization in allergic rhinitis using a potent partially purified extract of house dust mite. *Clinical Allergy*, 18, 501–508

FLEMING, D. M. and CROMBIE, D. L. (1987) Prevalance of asthma and hayfever in England and Wales. *British Medical Journal*, 294, 279–283

FRIGAS, E., LOEGERING, D., SOLLEY, G., FARROW, G. and GLEICH, G. J. (1981) Elevated levels of the eosinophil major basic protein in the sputum of patients with bronchial asthma. *Mayo Clinic Proceedings*, 56, 345–353

GAUCHAT, J. F., HENCHOZ, S., MAZZEI, G., AUBRY, J. P., and BRUNNER, T. (1993) Induction of human IgE synthesis in B cells by mast cells and basophils. *Nature*, 365, 340–343

GOMEZ, E., CORRADO, O. J., BALDWIN, D. L., SWANTON, A. R. and DAVIES, R. J. (1986) Direct in vivo evidence for mast cell degranulation during allergen-induced reactions in man. *Journal Allergy and Clinical Immunology*, 78, 637–645

GOMEZ, E., CLAGUE, J. E., GATLAND, D. and DAVIES, R. J. (1988) Effect of topical corticosteroids on seasonally induced increases in nasal mast cells. *British Medical Journal*, 296, 1572–1573

GOUNNI, A. S., LAMKHIOUED, B., OCHIAL, K., TANAKA, Y., DELAPORTE, E. and CAPRON, A., (1994) High-affinity IgE receptor on eosinophils is involved in defence against parasites, *Nature*, 367, 183–186

HAMID, Q., BARKANS, J., ROBINSON, D. S., DURHAM, S. R. and KAY, A. B. (1992) Co-expression of CD25 and CD3 in atopic allergy and asthma. *Immunology*, 75, 659

HANSON, B., MCGRUE, M., ROITMAN-JOHNSON, B., SEGAL, N. L., BOUCHARD, T. J. and BLUMENTHAL, M. N. (1991) Atopic disease and immunoglobulin E in twins reared apart and together. *American Journal of Human Genetics*, 48, 514–521

INTERNATIONAL CONSENSUS REPORT ON THE DIAGNOSIS AND MANAGEMENT OF RHINITIS. (1994) *Allergy*, 49 (suppl. 19), 1–34

IRANI, A.-M.A. and SCHWARTZ, L. B. (1989) Mast cell hetrogeneity. *Clinical and Experimental Allergy*, 19, 143–155

JABARA, H. H., FU, S. M., GEHA, R. S. and VERCELLI, D. (1990) CD40 and IgE: synergism between anti-CD40 mAb and IL-4 in the induction of IgE synthesis by highly purified human B cells. *Journal of Experimental Medicine*, 172, 1861

JUNIPER, E. F., KLINE, P. A., HARGREAVE, F. E. and DOLOVICH, J. (1989) Comparison of beclomethasone diproprionate aqueous nasal spray, astemizole, and the combination in the prophylactic treatment of ragweed pollen-induced rhinoconjunctivitis. *Journal of Allergy and Clinical Immunology*, 83, 627–633

KINIWA, M., GATELY, M., GUBLER, V., CHIZZONITE, R., FARGEAS, C. and DELESPESSE, G. (1992) Recombinant interleukin-12 suppresses the synthesis of immunoglobulin E by interleukin-4 stimulated human lymphocytes. *Journal of Clinical Investigation*, 90, 262–266

KNIGHT, A., KAZIM, F. and SALVATORI, A. V. (1986) A trial of intranasal Atrovent versus placebo in the treatment of vasomotor rhinitis. *Annals of Allergy*, 57, 348–354

LOPEZ, A. F., SANDERSON, C. J., GAMBLE, J. R., CAMPBELL, H. D., YOUNG, I. G. and VADAS, M. A. (1988) Recombinant human interleukin-5 is a selective activator of human eosinophil function. *Journal of Experimental Medicine*, 167, 219

MACKAY, I. S. (1992) Functional endoscopic sinus surgery. *Clinical Otolaryngology*, 17, 1–2

MALLING, H. J. and WEEKE, B. (1993) Revised EAACI position paper on immunotherapy. *Allergy*, 48, S14

MARSH, D. G., MEYERS, D. A. and BIAS, W. B. (1981) The epidemiology and genetics of atopic allergy. *New England Journal Medicine*, 305, 1551–1559

MASUYAMA, K., JACOBSON, M. R., RAK, S., MENG, Q., SUDDERICK, R. M., KAY, A. B. et al. (1994) Topical glucocorticosteroid (fluticasone propionate) inhibits cells expressing cytokine mRNA for interleukin-4 (IL-4) in the nasal mucosa in allergen-induced rhinitis. *Immunology*, 82, 192–199

MOSMANN, T. R., CHERWINSKI, H., BOND, M. W., GIELDIN, M. A. and COFFMAN, R. L. (1986) Two types of murine helper T cell clone. *Journal of Immunology*, 136, 2348–2357

MURANAKA, M., SUZUKI, S., KOIZUMI, K., TAKAFUJI, S., MIYAMOTO, T., IKEMORI, R. et al. (1986) Adjuvant activity of diesel exhaust particulates for the production of IgE antibodies in mice. *Journal of Allergy and Clinical Immunology*, 77, 616–623

NACLERIO, R. M. (1991) Allergic rhinitis. *New England Journal of Medicine*, 325, 860–869

NACLERIO, R. M. and MYGIND, N. (eds) (1993) Intranasal corticosteroids. In: *Allergic and Non-Allergic Rhinitis: Clinical Aspects*. Copenhagen: Munksgaard. pp. 114–122

NACLERIO, R. M., PROUD, D., TOGIAS, A. G., ADKINSON, N. F., MEYERS, D. A., KAGEY-SOBOTKA, A. et al. (1985) Inflammatory mediators in late antigen-induced rhinitis. *New England Journal of Medicine* 313, 65–70

OHMAN, J. L., FINDLAY, S. R. and LEITERMANN, K. M. (1984)

Immunotherapy in cat-induced asthma. Double-blind trial with evaluation of in vivo and in vitro responses. *Journal of Allergy and Clinical Immunology*, **74**, 230–239

ORGEL, H. A., MELTZER, E. O., KEMP, J. P., OSBORN, N. K. and WELCH, M. J. (1991) Comparison of intranasal cromolyn sodium, 4%, and oral terfenadine for allergic rhinitis: symptoms, nasal cytology, nasal ciliary clearance and rhinomanometry. *Annals of Allergy*, **66**, 237–244

OTSUKA, T. A., MIYAJIMA, N., BROWN, K., OTSU, J., ABRAMS, S., SEALAND, C. et al. (1988) Isolation and characterization of an expressible cDNA encoding human IL-3. *Journal of Immunology*, **140**, 2288

OWEN, W. R. Jr, ROTHENBERG, M. E., SILBERSTEIN, D. S., GASSON, J. C., STEVENS, R. L., AUSTEN, K. F. et al. (1987) Regulation of human eosinophil viability, density and function by granulocyte macrophage colony-stimulating factor in the presence of 3T3 fibroblasts. *Journal of Experimental Medicine*, **166**, 129

PIPKORN, U., PROUD, D., LICHTENSTEIN, L. M. et al. (1987) Effect of short term systemic glucocorticosteroid treatment on human nasal mediator release after antigen challenge. *Journal of Clinical Investigation*, **80**, 957–961

POSITION PAPER ON ALLERGEN IMMUNOTHERAPY (1993) Report of a BSACI working party. *Clinical Experimental Allergy*, **23** (suppl. 13), 1–44

ROBINSON, D. S., HAMID, Q., JACOBSON, M. R., SUN YING, KAY, A. B. and DURHAM, S. R. (1993) Evidence of TH2-type T helper cell control of allergic disease in vivo. *Springer Seminars in Immunopathology*, **15**, 17–27

ROTHENBERG, M. E., OWEN, W. F., SILBERSTEIN, D. S., WOODS, J., SOBERMAN, R. J., AUSTEN, K. F. et al. (1988) Human eosinophils have prolonged survival, enhanced functional properties and become hypodense when exposed to human interleukin-3. *Journal of Clinical Investigation*, **81**, 1986

RUSZNAK, C., DEVALIA, J. L., HERDMAN, M. J. and DAVIES, R. J. (1994) Effect of six hours exposure to 400PPB nitrogen dioxide (NO_2) and/or 200PPB sulphur dioxide (SO_2) on inhaled allergen response in mild asthmatic subjects. *Clinical and Experimental Allergy*, (abstract), **4**, 186

SALKIN, I. F. and HAINES, J. H. (1984) The biology and identification of fungi. In: *Rhinitis*, edited by G. A. Seltipane. Providence, Rhode Island: The New England and Regional Allergy Proceedings. pp. 45–51

SANDFORD, A. J., SHIRAKAWA, T., MOFFAT, M. F., DANIELS, S. E., RA, C., FANX, J. A. et al. (1993) Localisation of atopy and βsubunit of high-affinity IgE receptor (FCΣRI) on chromosone 11q. *Lancet*, i, 332–334

SCHLEIMER, R. P., STERBINSKY, S. A., KAISER, J., BICKEL, C. A., KLUNK, D. A., TOMIOKA, M. et al. (1992) IL-4 induces adherence of human eosinophils and basophils but not neutrophils to endothelium: association with expression of VCAM-1. *Journal of Immunology*, **148**, 1086

SIMONS, F. E. R. (1993) Antihistamines. In *Allergic and Non-*

allergic Rhinitis: Clinical Aspects, edited by N. Mygind and R. M. Naclerio. Copenhagen: Munksgaard. pp. 123–135

SLAVIU, R. G. (1988) Sinusitis in adults and its relation to allergic rhinitis asthma and nasal polyps. *Journal of Allergy and Clinical Immunology*, **82**, 950–956

SPORIK, R., HOLGATE, S., PLATTS MILLS, T. A. E. and COGSWELL, J. (1990) Exposure to house-dust mite allergen (Der P1) and the development of asthma in childhood. *New England Journal of Medicine*, **323**, 502–507

VAN CAUWENBERGE, P. and INGELS, K. (1993) Rhinitis and otitis. In: *Allergic and Non-Allergic Rhinitis: Clinical Aspects*, edited by N. Mygind and R. M. Naclerio. Copenhagen: Munksgaard. pp. 189–193

VARNEY, V. A. (1991) Hayfever in the United Kingdom. *Clinical and Experimental Allergy*, **21**, 757–762

VARNEY, V. A., GAGA, M., FREW, A. J., ABER, V. R., KAY, A. B. and DURHAM, S. R. (1991) Usefulness of immunotherapy in patients with severe summer hayfever uncontrolled by anti-allergic drugs. *British Medical Journal*, **302**, 265–269

VARNEY, V. A., JACOBSON, M. R., SUDDERICK, R. M., ROBINSON, D. S., IRANI, A.-M. A., SCHWARTZ, L. B. et al. (1992) Immunohistology of the nasal mucosa following allergen-induced rhinitis: identification of activated T lymphocytes, eosinophils and neutrophils. *American Review of Respiratory Diseases*, **146**, 170

VERCELLI, D. and GEHA, R. S. (1993) Regulation of IgE synthesis: from the membrane to the genes. *Springer Seminars in Immunopathology*, **15**, 5–16

VIEGAS, M., GOMEZ, E., BROOKS, J., GATLAND, D. and DAVIES, R. J. (1987) Effect of the pollen season on nasal mast cells. *British Medical Journal*, **294**, 414

VON MUTIUS, E., FRITZSCH, C., WEILAND, S. K., ROELL, G. and MAGNUSSEN, H. (1992) Prevalence of asthma and allergic disorders among children in united Germany: a descriptive comparison. *British Medical Journal*, **305**, 1395–1399

WALSH, G. M., HARTNELL, A., WARDLAW, A. J., KURIHARA, K., SANDERSON, C. J. and KAY, A. B. (1990) IL-5 enhances the in vitro adhesion of human eosinophils, but not neutrophils, in a leucocyte integrin (CD11/18)-dependent manner. *Immunology*, **71**, 258–265

WARIN, R. P. (1991) Torsades de pointes complicating treatment with terfenadine. *British Medical Journal*, **303**, 58

WHO/IUIS WORKING GROUP (1989) Current status of allergen immunotherapy. Shortened version of WHO/IUIS working group report. *Lancet*, i, 259–261

YING, S., DURHAM, S. R., JACOBSON, M. R., RAK, S., MASUYAMA, K., LOWHAGEN, O. et al. (1994) T lymphocytes and mast cells express messenger RNA for interleukin-4 in the nasal mucosa in allergen-induced rhinitis. *Immunology*, **82**, 200–206

ZINREICH, S. J., KENNEDY, D. W., ROSENBAUM, A. E., GAGLER, B. W., KUMAN, A. J. and STAMMBERGER, H. (1987) Paranasal sinuses: CT imaging requirements for endoscopic surgery. *Radiology*, **163**, 769–775

7

Food allergy and intolerance

Carsten Bindslev-Jensen

The term 'adverse reactions to foods and food additives' describes a clinically abnormal response to an ingested food or food additive. Adverse reactions to foods are divided into hypersensitivity reactions and non-hypersensitivity reactions. The incidence of true food hypersensitivity is rare occurring immediately after ingestion of even a small amount of the substance. The reaction is unrelated to any physiological effect of the food or additive. In contrast, non-hypersensitivity reactions may occur in any individual due to contamination, poisoning, pharmacological reactions or metabolic phenomena.

Examples of non-hypersensitivity reactions are salmonella enteritis due to ingestion of contaminated hen's eggs, botulism due to ingestion of food contaminated with toxins from *Clostridium botulinum*, flushing due to tyramine, e.g. from bananas, or diarrhoea due to lack of the lactase enzyme in adults.

Food hypersensitivity is subdivided into *food allergy*, characterized by a proven involvement of the immune system, and *food intolerance*, which has not been proven to be immunological. Most authors include *coeliac disease* in food hypersensitivity reactions, although a firm *causal* relationship between the clinical symptoms and the presence of antibodies directed against the gliadin fraction of wheat or rye for example has not been established.

The characteristics of the various adverse reactions are summarized in Table 7.1. The term food intolerance has been widely misused, mainly due to uncontrolled reports in the literature claiming a relationship between ingestion of a food item and occurrence of symptoms. Since most humans eat every day, a connection between daily occurring symptoms, e.g. joint complaints and intake of food often seems reasonable to the patient, although no causal relationship has been demonstrated.

Adverse reactions to food can only be verified by the use of double-blind, placebo-controlled food challenge (DBPCFC) (Metcalfe and Sampson, 1990) and by using this procedure, only the classical symptoms and signs listed in Table 7.1 have convincingly been demonstrated to be true food hypersensitivity.

Sensitization

At least three routes of sensitization exist. The classical route, by ingestion, is by far the most common in infants and may apparently occur in close relation to childbirth. In a cohort study on 1749 newborns, only the infants who were fed cow's milk formula in the maternity ward and thereafter breastfed for a period of weeks to months developed cow's milk allergy, whereas this was not the case in either the group who were exclusively breastfed or in the group who were fed cow's milk formula in the maternity ward and thereafter continued on formula (Host and Halken, 1990). Intrauterine sensitization occurs rarely as does sensitization to cow's milk protein present in undigested forms in human milk (Husby, 1988). The exact mode of sensitization is at present unknown, as is the exact place in the human body (mouth, intestine, respiratory tract ?), where the sensitization takes place.

Sensitization by inhalation can occur in two different ways. First, inhaled allergens sensitize the body in the same classical way as any other inhalant allergen, in the nose or in the lungs. This is most typically seen in baker's asthma, where inhaled proteins from flour will result in asthma (and rhinitis) in up to 20% of bakers after 15–20 years of exposure (Anderson, 1991). Sensitization by inhalation also occurs in the very common oral allergy syndrome (OAS), where the food allergy is due to allergenic cross-reaction between epitopes in pollen (to which

Table 7.1 Characteristics of the various forms of adverse reactions to food

Disease	Symptoms and signs	Diagnosis
Food allergy	Anaphylaxis, diarrhoea, vomitus, urticaria, contact urticaria, angioedema, dermatitis herpetiformis, atopic dermatitis, contact eczema, asthma, rhinitis, conjunctivitis, Schoenlein Henoch's purpura, eosinophil gastroenteritis, Heiner's syndrome, the oral allergy syndrome (OAS)	Double blind placebo-controlled food challenge (DBPCFC), except in infants, where open, controlled challenges are sufficient Positive skin prick test (SPT), specific IgE (RAST), basophil histamine release (HR) or patch test (PT) indicative but not sufficient
Food intolerance	Symptoms as above	As above, except SPT, HR, RAST or PT always negative
Coeliac disease	Diarrhoea, fatigue, anaemia, dermatitis herpetiformis, deficiency diseases	Intestinal biopsies. Demonstration of gliadin antibodies (IgG or IgA) indicative
Microbial	Depending on the microorganism. Most often several cases at the same time	Demonstration of the relevant microorganism or toxin
Toxic	Depending on toxin	Demonstration of toxic concentrations of the compound in tissue, organ or food item
Lactase deficiency	Diarrhoea after ingestion of larger amounts of lactose in cow's milk	Determination of lactose threshold value
Other disaccharidase deficiencies	Diarrhoea after ingestion of larger amounts of disaccharide	Determination of disaccharide threshold value
Pharmacological	Depending on agent	Demonstration of agent in relevant tissue, organ or food item

the patient is sensitized by inhalation) and various fruits and vegetables (Amlot *et al.*, 1987; Ortolani *et al.*, 1989).

The third route of sensitization is via the skin, where younger women especially develop a type IV sensitivity to nickel and in some cases thereafter also react with exacerbation of their eczema after oral intake of higher amounts of nickel containing foods (Veien, 1987).

Allergens

The allergens which most often give rise to an IgE-mediated reaction are milk, egg, cod fish, wheat, soy and in the USA peanut (American Academy of Allergy and Immunology Committee on Adverse Reactions to Foods, 1984). This reflects both the fact that these are foods commonly eaten in high quantities by adults and infants and that they contain allergenic glycoproteins, characterized by being heat- and acid-stable and thus not degraded in the stomach.

Pollen cross-reacting foods contain proteins sharing epitopes with the pollen. In contrast to what was previously believed, where the oral allergy syndrome was thought to be elicited by lectins in the food cross-binding IgE-molecules on the surface of mast cells in the mouth and throat, it has now been demonstrated in several of the cross-reacting food items, including hazelnut, apple and kiwi, that these reactions are due to common epitopes of approximately 18 kD in size in the pollen allergen and for example in hazelnut (Hirschwehr, Valenta and Ebner, 1992). The pollen cross-reacting proteins are seldom heat- and acid-stable, and are therefore usually destroyed by heat or by stomach acid, thus in the majority of cases only giving rise to symptoms when eaten raw and fresh. Examples of cross-reacting food items are shown in Table 7.2.

The most common allergens giving rise to type IV reactions are nickel and cobalt (Veien, 1987). Sensitization to nickel requires binding of the hapten to a carrier protein prior to presentation to the Langerhans' cell in the skin; the events giving rise to reactivation of the eczema following the ingestion of nickel are unknown.

The mode of action of food additives (preservatives and colourants) is also unknown. A clinically significant cross-sensitization between aspirin (which is not found in nature) and the preservative salicylate, which may also occur naturally in high quantities in certain foods has still not been demonstrated convincingly. The same is true for the alleged connection between aspirin and the colourant tartrazine. Stevenson *et al.* (1986) challenged 80 aspirin-sensitive asthmatics with large quantities of tartrazine without any positive reactions. Also, in a survey of respiratory reactions to monosodium glutamate, Schwartzstein

Table 7.2 **Cross-reacting foods**

Birch pollen	Grass pollen	Mugwort pollen	Cow's milk	Hen's egg	Cod fish	Peanut
Hazelnut, apple, kiwi, avocado, tomato, almond, potato, walnut, cashew nut, plum, carrot, cherry	Bean, lentil, pea, wheat, rye	Celery, parsley, chive, banana, melon, parsnip	Milk from goat mare sheep	Egg from turkey duck goose seagull Meat	Plaice, herring, mackerel	Soy, pea, limabean, bean, garbanzo

(1992) was unable to find more than one report of a positive reaction in double-blind, placebo controlled food challenge in the medical literature from 1966 to 1991. Contrary to these findings, a proportion of patients with bronchial asthma will experience dyspnoea upon oral intake of sulphite (Dahl, Henriksen and Harving, 1986) – data on rhinitis provoked by sulphite have not been published. Food additives are generally believed to be harmful by the public; a fact that has not been supported in trials using double-blind, placebo-controlled food challenges. As an example the artificial sweetener aspartame (Nutrasweet) was investigated for a period of several years in the USA without finding a single patient whose symptoms could be attributed to aspartame (Metcalfe, 1991), although the product was banned by ecological organizations in many countries because of its alleged allergic potential.

It is important to discriminate between immunological and clinical cross-reactivity. In the first case, the cross-reactivity is demonstrated in the laboratory by sophisticated immunochemical techniques. However, such a cross-reactivity does not imply clinical cross-reactivity as demonstrated by the fact that up to 65% of grass-pollen allergic patients with specific IgE to grass pollen epitopes will demonstrate specific IgE to wheat in one or more of the new and very sensitive tests for specific IgE (radioallergosorbent tests, 'RASTs') without ever having reacted upon ingestion of white bread (Poulsen, L.K. and Bindslev-Jensen, C., unpublished results). Another example applies to immunological cross-reactivity between peanut and various other vegetables (see Table 7.2), where Bernhisel-Broadbent could elicit a clinical response to the other vegetables in only two of 41 children allergic to peanut, verified by double-blind, placebo-controlled food challenge (Bernhisel Broadbent and Sampson, 1989). Thus, the clinical significance of cross-reactivity must be evaluated for each and every allergen in every patient if the management is to be correct. As a rule, probability of a clinical reaction reflects the heat- and acid-stability of the food, but also normal preparation of a given food is important, for example those allergic to grass pollen would probably react clinically to wheat if they ingested raw, fresh and unprocessed wheat.

Prevalence

The prevalence or incidence of adverse reactions to food or food additives vary immensely depending on the method used. By using a questionnaire, the prevalence of cow's milk allergy in infants exceeds 25%, whereas if a double-blind, placebo-controlled food challenge is used in the same population, a prevalence of 2.2% is obtained (Host and Halken, 1990). In a prospective study by Bock (1987), the cumulative prevalence of adverse reactions to food during the first 3 years of life was found to be 5.2% using open and double-blind challenges. Interestingly, in Bock's study a large proportion of the children (11.7%) reacted to the sugars in fruit or juices (enzyme deficiency). Such reactions are not hypersensitivity reactions, and should not be included in prevalence studies.

The incidence of adverse reactions to food additives has been widely overestimated. By using double-blind, placebo-controlled food challenges, Fuglsang et al. (1994) estimated the prevalence of reactions in school children to a maximum value of less than 2%. Although the validity of that study is hampered by the lack of data on the frequency of reactions to placebo in the food challenges, the results are supported by Rosenhall's (1982) results in 504 patients with a history of asthma or rhinitis elicited by food additives. At present, no data exist on the prevalence of nickel-sensitive patients reacting to nickel in food, but Veien (1987) has estimated the number to be 10% of the severe cases at the most.

Depending on the allergen, many patients will develop tolerance to the food in question. In Host and Hallken's study (1990), more than 90% of the children who had a confirmed allergy to cow's milk in the first year of life had outgrown their clinical allergy by the age of 3 years. Skin tests and RASTs may be positive for a period of time after clinical tolerance has evolved, it is therefore important regularly to rechallenge the patients with an established diagnosis of cow's milk

Table 7.3 Duration of clinical disease

	Milk	Egg	Fish	Soy	Wheat	Additives
Duration	90% < 3 years	50% < 5 years	20% < 5 years	90% < 5 years	Not known	Not known

Kjellman *et al.*, 1988; Host and Halken, 1990

allergy. Patients with other food allergies especially cod fish will develop tolerance less frequently (Table 7.3).

Symptoms and signs

Patients with food hypersensitivity present with classical allergic symptoms and signs. Although a vast variety of other symptoms has been ascribed to the intake of food or additives, none of these (with the exception of the excacerbation of frequency and severity in selected migraine patients (Pradalier and Bindslev-Jenen, 1993) has been proven in trials using double-blind, placebo-controlled food challenges (Pearson, 1988; Parker *et al.*, 1990). Verified symptoms and signs are listed in Table 7.1. Oral intake of a specific food item will elicit a characteristic series of events in a sensitive individual: the initial symptoms usually experienced by the patient are oral and pharyngeal itching and swelling, *the oral allergy syndrome*, followed by objective signs with further ingestion of the offending food item (Amlot *et al.*, 1987).

The majority of patients with food hypersensitivity will present *concomitant symptoms and signs from two or more organ systems* (respiratory, skin, gastrointestinal) upon intake of the offending food. Thus, an isolated reaction such as asthma, urticaria or diarrhoea is rarely due to food hypersensitivity, whereas a history of concomitant development of all three signs upon food intake is suggestive. Gastrointestinal symptoms and signs are most frequent, followed by skin symptoms. Symptoms of asthma or rhinitis/conjunctivitis are the least frequent (Sampson and Mc-Caskill, 1985; Bindslev-Jensen, 1992a; Bock, 1992).

Food hypersensitivity reactions are usually immediate reactions, where symptoms and signs develop within the first hour after ingestion. Whether isolated late reactions, developing hours to days after challenge exist is debated – a dual response consisting of an immediate reaction followed hours later by a late phase reaction has been described, whereas the isolated late reactions in the nose in children allergic to cow's milk are mainly due to a confusion in definition (Hill, Ball and Hosking, 1988). Hill, Ball and Hosking defined reaction time as the time between the first challenge dose and clinical reaction, and since some of their patients did not react until the second day of challenge, where the cumulated dose was sufficient to elicit a response, these patients were classified as 'late reactors', although the last challenge dose was administered 30 minutes before clinical symptoms evolved.

The diagnosis of food allergy and intolerance

At present, double-blind, placebo-controlled food challenge is the only reliable test for the diagnosis of adverse reactions to foods. No other diagnostic procedure can exclude the need for double-blind, placebo-controlled food challenge (Table 7.4) (Atkins, Steinberg and Metcalfe, 1985; Sampson, Buckley and Metcalfe, 1987; Bock *et al.*, 1988; Metcalfe and Sampson, 1990; Hansen and Bindslev-Jensen, 1992; Norgaard and Bindslev-Jensen, 1992).

Skin prick test, tests for specific IgE, histamine release

It must be emphasized that the outcome of a diagnostic test should be compared to the outcome of double-blind, placebo-controlled food challenge and not a comparison with other tests or with the patient's case history. Only by comparison with a double-blind, placebo-controlled food challenge is it possible to validate any given test (Metcalfe and Sampson, 1990).

As a result of the variable quality of the food extract used for *in vivo* or *in vitro* tests, caution should be taken when transferring results obtained with one type of food to other foods. Most investigators have obtained a high sensitivity and specificity for skin prick test or RAST with cod allergen, whereas in most cases sensitivity and specificity with extracts of fruits and vegetables have resulted in poor correlation.

The basic problem concerning the other diagnostic tests is that unlike inhaled allergens, no commercially available *standardized* extracts exist (Norgaard, Skov and Bindslev-Jensen, 1992). It is therefore often not possible to distinguish the real value of a test in the diagnosis of food allergy because of the unreliability to the allergen extract. This is probably the reason for the great variability in diagnostic sensitivity and specificity reported in the literature (Bindslev-Jensen *et al.*, 1994). Another problem which must be borne in mind when interpreting the diagnostic values of a

Table 7.4 Diagnostic tests

Accepted tests	Not fully validated tests
Double-blind, placebo-controlled food challenge	Case history
	Skin prick test (SPT)
Open food challenge (OFC) in infants	Measurement of specific IgE (RAST)
	Histamine release from basophils (HR)
	Patch test (type IV hypersensitivity)

test is the different time course of sensitization and clinical disease. In many cases the diagnostic tests remain positive for a period after the patient has developed clinical tolerance, thus further hampering the specificity of the test. Moreover, in some cases, especially in young children, clinical disease precedes positive results in the diagnostic tests, impairing the sensitivity of the test applied. On the other hand, in some cases the opposite picture is seen, i.e. the test is positive prior to clinical disease. In this case, the specificity of the test will be hampered.

A detailed knowledge of the single allergen in question and the performance of the chosen test (skin prick test, RAST, histamine release) with the particular allergen is therefore important when interpreting the outcome of the test in correlation to patient's symptoms and case history.

Food allergy versus food intolerance

When using the double blind, placebo controlled food challenge, the clinical features of food allergy and food intolerance are identical, i.e. concomitant symptoms and signs from two or more organ systems. The distinction therefore depends on whether the involvement of the immune system can be verified. Since the methods for determining a possible involvement of the immune system are not standardized, many cases of low sensitivity will be misdiagnosed as food intolerance, which would be diagnosed as allergic when tests with a high sensitivity are applied (Norgaard, Skov and Bindslev-Jensen, 1992; Bindslev-Jensen *et al.*, 1994). Since the clinical pictures are identical, the term *food hypersensitivity* may be used to describe both food allergy *and* food intolerance to proteins, whereas the term food intolerance would still seem more appropriate for reactions to food additives (Bindslev-Jensen *et al.*, 1994).

Controlled programme for diagnosing food hypersensitivity

The central phase in the diagnosis of food hypersensitivity (type I and type IV reactions, food intolerance) is the *provocation programme*, concluding with a

double-blind, placebo-controlled food challenge. A flow chart for a controlled programme is presented in Figure 7.1. Before initiating the controlled programme, other causes for the patient's symptoms should be excluded.

The *history* is of paramount importance. Atopic diseases are frequent in siblings and parents of children with food hypersensitivity, and therefore a detailed history of allergic disposition is important. Careful recording of food intake and its relation to the disease often provides useful information. A record of food intake particularly in small children provides useful information, whereas in older children and adults, problems with the interpretation of such a 'food intake history' often emerge. A 'run-in' diary of symptom scores determines the nature and severity of the patient's complaint. In this period the patient eats a normal diet. Patients at risk of a severe systemic reaction should be observed during this phase. The *diet period* serves to obtain freedom from symptoms or at least a significant reduction in symptom severity. Several 'elimination diets' exist, all based on the exclusion of the food items most frequently causing food hypersensitivity. If no reduction in symptom score is obtained, (even on a very restricted diet) the controlled programme should be abandoned. Reduction in symptom severity enables the specific diagnosis to be established by a double-blind, placebo-controlled food challenge. The initial *allergy testing* may comprise a skin prick test, RAST, histamine release test and/or patch test. Patients with allergy to pollen and concomitant pollen cross-reactivity should not be diagnosed according to Figure 7.1. These patients should be informed of the possible cross-reacting fruits and vegetables and in avoidance measures. Several procedures for performing double-blind, placebo-controlled food challenges have been developed (Table 7.5). The use of any of these methods in normal clinical practice is hampered by the high demand of resources and time.

In many cases, it may be convenient to apply open food challenges (OFC) prior to verification of the positive results by double-blind, placebo-controlled food challenge. It is important, however, to emphasize that double-blind, placebo-controlled food challenges have not yet been fully validated. Several hazards exist, as reviewed by David (1989):

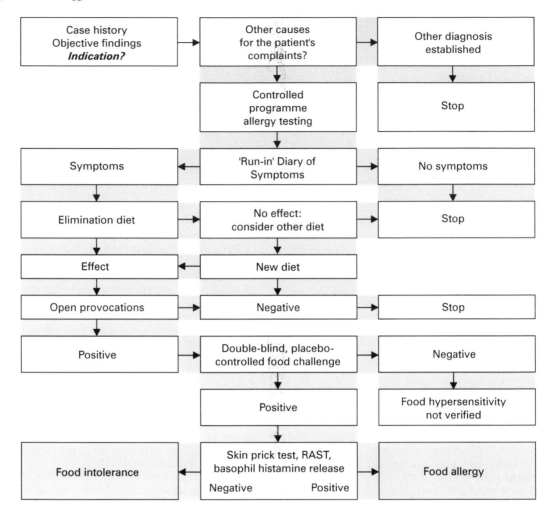

Figure 7.1 Flow chart for controlled diagnosis of food hypersensitivity. (Adapted from Bindslev-Jensen, 1992b)

1 The nature of food being tested – should raw, freeze-dried or cooked food be used?
2 Double-blind, placebo-controlled food challenges may bypass important sites, as is the case when using capsules
3 Failure to employ double-blind methodology is a potential hazard
4 Failure to employ double-blind placebo control
5 The state of disease in question – is the sensitivity of the test altered by changes in activity of the disease?
6 Development of tolerance
7 Additive effect of multiple hypersensitivities, e.g. concomitant sensitization to pets or mites
8 Disease may be suppressed by pharmacological treatment.

Furthermore, problems may arise in patients with late reactions.

When applying proper double-blind, placebo-controlled food challenges, only a portion of patients suspected of food hypersensitivity will be diagnosed as true positive; this has been reviewed by Bock (1986) and Atkins (1986), reporting a percentage of positive results ranging from 0 to 50% of the patients, mainly depending of the age of the patient.

The number of single provocations in a provocation programme depends on the nature of the patient's complaints. In a patient reporting objective signs (asthma, urticaria, rhinitis, diarrhoea, vomiting) upon ingestion of a food item, administration of one active and one placebo provocation is usually sufficient to verify or exclude the diagnosis. This recommendation is based on the low frequency (1–2%) of reactions to placebo provocations in these patients (Hansen and Bindslev-Jensen, 1992); Norgaard and Bindslev-Jensen, 1992).

Table 7.5 Challenge models

Method	Characteristics	Advantages	Disadvantages
DBPCFC with capsules or tablets	Dehydrated food. Can be titrated. Commercially available	Known quantity. Convenient for additives	Many capsules. Reactions in mouth and throat not diagnosed. Food quality unknown.
DBPCFC with foods	Fresh food in relevant amount. Can be titrated, given via tube or masked in a vehicle	Quality of allergen. Reactions in mouth diagnosed. Normal route of administration	Resource-demanding Not standardized
Open challenge with a food (OFC)	Fresh food in relevant amount. Can be titrated	Easily performed. Negative test makes DBPCFC superfluous	Risk of false-positive results
Open provocation with a meal	Mixture of fresh or processed foods in relevant amount	Easily performed. Negative test makes DBPCFC superfluous	Risk of false-positive results. Difficulties in interpretation

DBPCFC: double-blind, placebo-controlled food challenge

On the other hand, when patients only present with subjective symptoms, which cannot be objectively verified (abdominal pain, the oral allergy syndrome, itching, headache), the number of provocations must be increased to three active and three placebo provocations in order to avoid false-positive reactions and in order to obtain statistical significance (Hansen and Bindslev-Jensen, 1992). In patients who have experienced severe reactions upon intake of a food item and especially in patients having experienced anaphylaxis upon ingestion, double-blind, placebo-controlled food challenges should be performed in hospital, if at all, where resuscitation equipment is available.

Negative results should be followed by an open-meal provocation with the food processed in the normal way in order to exclude false-negative reactions due to epitope loss in the material used for double-blind, placebo-controlled food challenges.

Food hypersensitivity and rhinitis

Although less frequent than gastrointestinal or skin symptoms, respiratory symptoms may be elicited during a double-blind, placebo-controlled food challenge or experienced by the patient following accidental intake of a non-tolerated food (Bindslev-Jensen 1992a; Bock, 1992).

Although the value of the study by Amlot *et al.* (1987) is impeded by the lack of blind challenges, the careful demonstration of the oral allergy syndrome in all patients within less than 10 minutes followed by objective signs within 30 minutes (urticaria in 22%, conjunctivitis in 25%, asthma in 28%, vomiting and nausea in 28%) is valuable. Rhinitis (8%) and anaphy-

laxis (8%) were rarely reported. In most other studies on adults (Bindslev-Jensen, 1992a), rhinitis symptoms are less frequent and most often in combination with symptoms of asthma. In children, rhinitis symptoms in combination with symptoms and signs from other organ systems appear more frequent. Sampson and James (1992) reported respiratory symptoms elicited by double-blind placebo-controlled food challenges in 59% of selected patients with atopic dermatitis, of these, 66% were rhinitis symptoms, 13% were laryngeal and only 24% were asthma symptoms. Interestingly, in this study, 20 of 70 patients developing rhinitis upon challenge had no previous history of allergic rhinitis, whereas only three of 34 developing wheezing had no previous history of asthma.

Thus in conclusion, rhinitis symptoms in food hypersensitivity mostly develop in combination with other symptoms and signs, except in obvious cases such as gustatory rhinitis due to intake of hot and spicy foods (Raphael, Raphael and Kaliner, 1989).

Therapy

The specific therapy of food hypersensitivity is avoidance. The patient and family should be educated in how to avoid the offending food. Prompt administration of adrenalin in cases of anaphylaxis is mandatory and life-saving (Sampson, Mendelson and Rosen, 1992). Corticosteroids are only of value as adjuvants in the treatment of anaphylaxis and in eosinophil gastroenteritis.

The place of sodium cromoglycate in therapy is disputed since most double-blind studies have failed to demonstrate any value, whereas several open or single-blind trials have reported benefit (Shapiro and Konig, 1985; Sogn, 1986). Antihistamines (H_1-antagonists) abolish the itching in the oral allergy syndrome, but will not protect against a systemic reaction (Bindslev-Jensen *et al.*, 1991; Bindslev-Jensen, 1992c). Antihistamines may thus be potentially dangerous because the initial warning sign preceding the more serious systemic reaction is eliminated.

References

American Academy of Allergy and Immunology Committee on Adverse Reactions to Foods (1984) Adverse Reactions to Food. Bethesda: National Institutes of Health. 84–2442

AMLOT, P. L., KEMENY, D. M., ZACHARY, C., PARKES, P. and LESSOF, M. H. (1987). Oral allergy syndrome (OAS): symptoms of IgE-mediated hypersensitivity to foods. *Clinical Allergy*, **17**, 33–42

ANDERSON, J. A. (1991) The clinical spectrum of food allergy in adults. *Clinical and Experimental Allergy*, **21** (suppl. 1), 304–315

ATKINS, F. M. (1986) A critical evaluation of clinical trials in adverse reactions to foods in adults. *Journal of Allergy and Clinical Immunology*, **78**, 174–182

ATKINS, F. M., STEINBERG, S. S. and METCALFE, D. D. (1985) Evaluation of immediate adverse reactions to foods in adult patients. II. A detailed analysis of reaction patterns during oral food challenge. *Journal of Allergy and Clinical Immunology*, **75**, 356–363

BERNHISEL BROADBENT, J. and SAMPSON, H. A. (1989) Cross-allergenicity in the legume botanical family in children with food hypersensitivity. *Journal of Allergy and Clinical Immunology*, **83**, 435–440

BINDSLEV-JENSEN, C. (1992a) Respiratory reactions induced by food challenges in adults. *Pediatric Allergy and Immunology*, **3**, 201–206

BINDSLEV-JENSEN, C. (1992b) Rhinitis and food allergy. In: *Allergic Rhinitis – Clinical Aspects*, 2nd edn, edited by R. Naclerio and N. Mygind. Copenhagen: Munksgaard. pp. 34–37

BINDSLEV-JENSEN, C. (1992c) Double-blind, placebo-controlled food challenge (DBPCFC) in food allergy – effect of Astemizole. *Journal of Allergy and Clinical Immunology*, **89**, 161

BINDSLEV-JENSEN, C., SKOV, P., MADSEN, F. and POULSEN, L. K. (1994) Food allergy and food intolerance – what is the difference? *Annals of Allergy*, **72**, 317–320

BINDSLEV-JENSEN, C., VIBITS, A., SKOV, P. and WEEKE, B. (1991) Oral allergy syndrome: the effect of astemizole. *Allergy*, **46**, 610–613

BOCK, S. A. (1986) A critical evaluation of clinical trials in adverse reactions in children. *Journal of Allergy and Clinical Immunology*, **78**, 165–174

BOCK, S. A. (1987) Prospective appraisal of complaints of adverse reactions to foods in children during the first 3 years of life. *Pediatrics*, **79**, 683–688

BOCK, S. A. (1992) Respiratory reactions induced by food challenges in children with pulmonary disease. *Pediatric Allergy and Immunology*, **3**, 188–195

BOCK, S. A., SAMPSON, H. A., ATKINS, F. M., ZEIGER, R. S., LEHRER, S., SACHS, M. *et al.* (1988) Double-blind, placebo-controlled food challenge (DBPCFC) as an office procedure:

a manual. *Journal of Allergy and Clinical Immunology*, **82**, 986–997

DAHL, R., HENRIKSEN, J. M. and HARVING, H. (1986) Red wine asthma: a controlled challenge study. *Journal of Allergy and Clinical Immunology*, **78**, 1126–1129

DAVID, T. J. (1989) Hazards of challenge tests in atopic dermatitis. *Allergy*, **44** (suppl 9), 101–107

FUGLSANG, G., MADSEN, C., HALKEN, S., JORGENSEN, M., OSTER-GÅRD, P.A. and OSTERBALLE, D. (1994) Adverse reactions to food additives in children with atopic symptoms. *Allergy*, **49**, 31–38

HANSEN, T. K. and BINDSLEV-JENSEN, C. (1992) Codfish allergy in adults. Identification and diagnosis. *Allergy*, **47** 610–617

HILL, D., BALL, G. and HOSKING, C. S. (1988) Clinical manifestations of cows' milk allergy in childhood. I. Associations with in-vitro cellular immune responses. *Clinical Allergy*, **18**, 469–479

HIRSCHWEHR, R., VALENTA, R. and EBNER, C. (1992) Identification of common allergenic structures in hazel pollen and hazelnuts: a possible explanation for sensivity to hazelnuts in patients allergic to tree pollen. *Journal of Allergy and Clinical Immunology*, **90**, 927–936

HOST, A. and HALKEN, S. (1990) A prospective study of cow milk allergy in Danish infants during the first 3 years of life. Clinical course in relation to clinical and immunological type of hypersensitivity reaction. *Allergy*, **45**, 587–596

HUSBY, S. (1988) Dietary antigens: uptake and humoral immunity in man. *APMIS*, Suppl. 1, 1–40

KJELLMAN, N. I., BJORKSTEN, B., HATTEVIG, G. and FALTH MAG-NUSSON, K. (1988) Natural history of food allergy. *Annals of Allergy*, **61**, 83–87

METCALFE, D. D. (1991) Food allergy. *Current Opinions in Immunology*, **31**, 881–886

METCALFE, D. D. and SAMPSON, H. A. E. (1990) Workshop on experimental methodology for clinical studies of adverse reactions to foods and food additives. *Journal of Allergy and Clinical Immunology*, **861**, 421–442

NORGAARD, A. and BINDSLEV-JENSEN, C. (1992) Egg and milk allergy in adults. Diagnosis and characterization. *Allergy*, **47**, 503–509

NORGAARD, A., SKOV, P. S. and BINDSLEV-JENSEN, C. (1992) Egg and milk allergy in adults: comparison between fresh foods and commercial allergen extracts in skin prick test and histamine release from basophils. *Clinical and Experimental Allergy*, **22**, 940–947

ORTOLANI, C., ISPANO, M., PASTORELLO, E. A., ANSALONI, R. and MAGRI, G. C. (1989) Comparison of results of skin prick tests (with fresh foods and commercial food extracts) and RAST in 100 patients with oral allergy syndrome. *Journal of Allergy and Clinical Immunology*, **83**, 683–690

PARKER, S. L., LEZNOFF, A., SUSSMAN, G. L., TARLO, S. M. and KRONDL, M. (1990) Characteristics of patients with food-related complaints. *Journal of Allergy and Clinical Immunology*, **86**, 503–511

PEARSON, D. J. (1988) Psychologic and somatic interrelationships in allergy and pseudoallergy. *Journal of Allergy and Clinical Immunology*, **81**, 351–360

PRADALIER, A. and BINDSLEV-JENSEN, C. (1993) Immunological aspects of migraine. In: *The Headaches* edited by J. Olesen, P. Tfelt-Hansen and K. M. A. Welch. New York: Raven Press. pp. 719–740

RAPHAEL, G., RAPHAEL, M. H. and KALINER, M. (1989) Gustatory rhinitis: a syndrome of food-induced rhinorrhea. *Journal of Allergy and Clinical Immunology*, **83**, 110–115

ROSENHALL, L. (1982) Evaluation of intolerance to analgesics, preservatives and food colourants with challenge tests. *European Journal of Respiratory Diseases*, **63**, 410–419

SAMPSON, H. A. and JAMES, J. M. (1992) Respiratory reactions by food challenges in children with atopic dermatitis. *Journal of Allergy and Clinical Immunology*, **3**, 195–201

SAMPSON, H. A. and MCCASKILL, C. C. (1985) Food hypersensitivity and atopic dermatitis: evaluation of 113 patients. *Journal of Pediatrics*, **107**, 669–675

SAMPSON, H. A., BUCKLEY, R. H. and METCALFE, D. D. (1987) Food allergy. *Journal of the American Medical Association*, **258**, 2886–2890

SAMPSON, H. A., MENDELSON, L. and ROSEN, J. P. (1992) Fatal and near-fatal anaphylactic reactions to food in children and adolescents. *New England Journal of Medicine*, **327**, 380–384

SCHWARTZSTEIN, R. M. (1992) Pulmonary reactions to monosodium glutamate. *Pediatric Allergy and Immunology*, **3**, 228–232

SHAPIRO, G. G. and KONIG, P. (1985) Cromolyn sodium: a review. *Pharmacotherapy*, **5**, 156–170

SOGN, D. (1986) Medications and their use in the treatment of adverse reactions to foods. *Journal of Allergy and Clinical Immunology*, **78**, 238–243

STEVENSON, D. D., SIMON, R. A., LUMRY, W. R. and MATHISON, D. A. (1986) Adverse reactions to tartrazine. *Journal of Allergy and Clinical Immunology*, **78**, 182–191

VEIEN, N. K. (1987) Systemically induced eczema in adults. *Acta Dermatologica et Venereologica*, Suppl. 147, 1–49

8

Infective rhinitis and sinusitis

N. Weir and D. G. Golding-Wood

As the lining of the nose and paranasal sinuses is continuous, inflammatory processes tend to involve both areas to a greater or lesser extent. Rather than distinguish rhinitis and sinusitis separately rhinosinusitis has become a suitable descriptive term. The aim of this chapter is to consider the aetiology, differential diagnosis and medical treatment of rhinosinusitis and detail the specific inflammatory conditions of the nose and paranasal sinuses.

Classification

There remains no universally accepted classification of rhinosinusitis. Division into allergic and non-allergic, the latter being infective and non-infective has the advantage of simplicity, but disguises the fact that rhinosinusitis is often of multifactorial aetiology with considerable overlap of clinical manifestations. The underlying cause is rarely apparent from different symptom complexes, e.g. swelling of the lining of the nose and paranasal sinuses may occur from underlying atopy, leading to stasis and subsequent infection, but the presenting symptoms of mucopurulent rhinorrhoea, nasal obstruction and facial pain would not necessarily suggest an underlying allergic aetiology. Conversely, not all patients presenting with purulent mucus in the nasal fossae have infection; a smear may reveal the presence of eosinophils, and the patient will often respond dramatically to topical or systemic corticosteroids. The classification is summarized in Table 8.1.

Allergy

While allergy is a common cause of rhinitis, it is not the exclusive cause as sometimes perceived by many practitioners. Allergic rhinitis, strictly speaking, relates to the immediate immunoglobulin (IgE) antibody-mediated hypersensitivity reaction to specific allergens, a type I hypersensitivity reaction. Most allergens are proteins with a molecular weight between 10 000 and 50 000. In practice, many allergens causing rhinitis are complex compounds often consisting of a number

Table 8.1 Aetiology of rhinosinusitis

Allergy
Seasonal
Perennial
Occupational

Infection
Acute
Chronic
   specific, e.g. fungal
   non-specific
      host defence deficiency
         local
         systemic

Structural
e.g. Ostiomeatal complex, deviated nasal septum, hypertrophic turbinates

Other
Idiopathic
Nares
Occupational
Hormonal
Drug-induced
Irritants
Food
Emotional
Atrophic

After International Consensus Report on the Diagnosis and Management of Rhinitis. *Allergy Suppl. 19*, **49**, 1994

of immunogenic molecules called antigens. The term 'allergen extract' is thus used, e.g. pollen, house dust mite, etc., each of which contains many antigens, all or only a few of which may induce the IgE response, leading to symptoms. IgE antibodies evoked by exposure to antigens become attached to the surface of tissue mast cells and basophil leucocytes as cytophilic antibodies. Interaction between the cell-bound IgE antibodies and the respective allergens results in the release of histamine and other mediators from these cells, causing the signs and symptoms of rhinitis. The mechanism and treatment of allergy, particularly allergen avoidance measures, are covered in Chapter 6.

A complex array of inflammatory mediators may be released by other mechanisms, e.g. non-specific irritants (cold air, fumes and dust), as well as ingested acetylsalicylic acid and certain food preservatives and dyes. These latter responses are not necessarily IgE mediated, the terms hyperreactivity or hyperresponsiveness are therefore often used to encompass these forms of provocation.

Itching and sneezing with profuse watery nasal discharge are characteristic symptoms of allergic rhinitis. There may be redness and excoriation of the skin of the nose following excessive nose blowing and wiping. The eyes may be red and watery in the typical seasonal rhinoconjunctivitis due to pollen allergy. Concomitant coughing and wheezing characteristic of asthma may be present.

The nasal mucous membranes are usually pale, boggy, hypertrophic and wet. Classically the inferior turbinates are bluish in colour sometimes with posterior lobulated ends, referred to as mulberry turbinates. It can at times be difficult to differentiate between hypertrophic, pale, swollen, polypoidal turbinates and polyps. Although the latter are insensitive when lightly probed and can be displaced, the turbinates remain fixed.

Nasal secretions with a very high eosinophil count associated with allergic rhinitis may appear yellow or green and the patients may be diagnosed as having infective rhinosinusitis. Conversely, nasal secretions accompanying acute coryza may be clear and mistakenly assumed to be non-purulent, allergic rhinitis.

The distinction between allergic rhinitis and infective rhinitis may not always be clear cut. The two may, and often do, occur at the same time, with allergy leading to swelling and inflammation of the nasal mucous membranes causing mechanical obstruction which impedes drainage and clearance from the sinuses and allows 'secondary' bacterial infection. In such cases, it will be necessary to treat the inflammatory process first with antibiotics and anti-inflammatory drugs (and possibly surgery) to restore the normal patency to the sinuses. Once this has been achieved, the underlying allergic problem will require maintenance therapy.

The treatment of allergic rhinitis has been revolutionized over the last few years by the introduction of first, topical corticosteroids (beclomethasone, flunisolide, budesonide and fluticasone) and second, non-sedating H_1-antagonist antihistamines (e.g. acrivastine, astemizole, cetirizine, loratadine and terfenadine). The latter rarely sedate or potentiate the action of alcohol. Terfenadine must be taken twice daily and is rapidly effective although remains so for a relatively short period (6–12 hours). Astemizole has the advantage of once daily dosage although its maximum effectiveness may not be obtained for a week or more. Skin tests may remain negative for up to 4 weeks from the last dosage. Both are contraindicated in pregnancy. Serious cardiac side effects have been observed with some antihistamines. Terfenadine and astemizole should not be given in conjunction with macrolide antibiotics (e.g. erythromycin) and some oral antifungal agents (e.g. ketoconazole and itraconazole) or in the presence of liver disease. Occasional dryness and bleeding may occur with topical steroids but no irreversible damage to the mucosa has been reported and, provided they are used in the recommended dosage, they have no systemic side effects.

Systemic corticosteroids are probably underused in the management of this condition. Because of their well-recognized side effects, they are not suitable for long-term maintenance therapy but are very useful as a short course to bring the symptoms under control with a view to maintaining any improvement using topical corticosteroids, antihistamines or sodium cromoglycate. The latter is less effective than topical corticosteroids but is an entirely safe medication, is only effective as a prophylactic agent and is more likely to be effective in atopic patients.

The prospect of long-term maintenance therapy does not appeal to some patients and hyposensitization or surgery may be requested. Hyposensitization, more effective in children than adults, is only of proven value in the treatment of single allergen (pollen or house dust mite) disease.

While allergy cannot be 'cured' by surgery, surgical reduction of the turbinates, correction of deviation of the nose or septum and surgery to improve sinus patency may all play an important role, particularly where nasal obstruction is the patient's main symptom. Some patients may be able to contend with sneezing and rhinorrhoea provided they have an adequate airway. For many, however, surgery is indicated to restore function followed by long-term medication to maintain it.

Infection

Infective rhinitis may be acute or chronic and the latter may arise as the result of an infection with a specific chronic infective agent, as considered later in this chapter, or may be the consequence of a local or systemic host defence deficiency.

Local defence mechanisms

The two cardinal factors in the maintenance of normal physiology of the paranasal sinuses and their mucous membranes are drainage and ventilation. Normal drainage of the paranasal sinuses depends on effective mucociliary clearance. This is largely dependent upon the amount of mucus produced, its composition, the effectiveness of ciliary action, mucosal reabsorption and the condition of the sinus ostia.

The nose and paranasal sinuses are lined with respiratory epithelium that is essentially a pseudostratified ciliated columnar epithelium with interspersed goblet cells. Non-ciliated and basal cells are also present. The cilia are approximately 6 μm long, 0.25 μm in diameter and number about 100–200 per cell. In cross-section, each cilium can be seen to have two central microtubules surrounded by a ring of nine doublet microtubules, protruding from one side of which are inner and outer dynein arms composed of ATPase protein responsible for the energy production required for the beating of the cilium. On each ciliated and non-ciliated cell there are 200–400 microvilli, the number increasing towards the nasopharynx. These microvilli are approximately one-third of the size of the cilia and have a central core of actin filaments. Microvilli are non-motile and their function is probably to promote ion and fluid transport between the cells and the periciliary fluid regulating the composition of the latter and overlying mucus (Petruson, Hansson and Karlsson, 1984).

The goblet cells are unicellular mucus-secreting glands found above the basement membrane. They possess well-developed Golgi apparatus and endoplasmic reticulum of mainly granular type, consistent with high synthetic activity. The distribution and density of goblet cells have been extensively studied by Tos (1982) who found the highest density in the inferior turbinate (11 000 cells/mm²) and lowest in the septum (5700/mm²), the density in the sinuses being in the mid-range but highest in the maxillary sinuses. Generally, there is a higher density of goblet cells posteriorly near the nasopharynx. In addition to goblet cells within the epithelium there are multicellular glands deep to the basement membrane in the lamina propria. The anterior serous nasal glands are not thought to play an important role in man. Small seromucous glands are evenly distributed in the mucosa of the respiratory region (8–9/mm²) although in the paranasal sinuses the density is very much lower (0.06–0.47/mm²) (Tos, 1982).

Nasal secretion is a complex mixture containing material secreted by the goblet cells, seromucous glands and lacrimal glands, material transported across the membrane of epithelial cells equipped with microvilli, together with microorganisms and condensed water from expired air. These secretions comprise a 'mucus blanket'. This mucus film has two layers for effective mucociliary transport; a superficial viscid sheet, the *gel layer*, moving over underlying serous fluid, the *sol layer*, which bathes the cilia and microvilli (Lucas and Douglas, 1934). The cilia beat in a synchronized (transversally) and metachronized (longitudinally) manner, although the mechanism of this synchronization is not fully understood. The cilia move in the low-viscosity periciliary layer at a frequency of 12–15 Hz with a rapid 'stiff-armed' effective stroke during which claw-like projections from the tips of the cilia (Jeffery and Reid, 1975) engage the thick, viscous gel layer to propel this towards the nasopharynx. During the recovery phase, the cilia bend to return entirely within the thin sol layer in a plane at right angles to the effective beat and sweeping across the surface of the cell (Figure 8.1).

In health, the mucus layer is steadily transported. Endoscopic studies indicate that a healthy maxillary sinus renews its mucus layer every 20–30 minutes. Normally the secretion covers the underlying mucosa with a homogeneous layer of consistent thickness. The viscous layer appears somewhat thicker near the ostia of the larger sinuses probably because of convergence of the secretion of the entire sinus. The cohesive nature of the mucus allows the mucus to be transported across small mucosal defects or lesions. Bony crests are usually traversed without difficulty unless the secretion becomes unduly viscous when secretions may be retained and drain by gravity.

In addition to ciliary action movements of the mucosa, pulsation associated with inflammation or movements of the fontanelles, may assist the transportation of secretions out of the maxillary sinus. Mucus transport from the sinuses into the nose is greatly enhanced by unimpeded nasal airflow creating negative pressure within the nasal cavity during inspiration.

Pathways of secretion transport

One of Messerklinger's most important observations is that the secretions of various sinuses do not reach their respective ostia randomly but by definite pathways which seem genetically determined (Messerklinger, 1966, 1967). Even when these pathways may be pathologically impeded or blocked, their direction is not significantly altered.

Within the maxillary sinus, secretion transport starts from the sinus floor in a stellate pattern. The mucus is transported along the sinus walls to converge at the natural sinus ostium and from there is transported through the infundibulum to the middle meatus and over the medial wall of the inferior turbinate to the nasopharynx (Figure 8.2). Secretion is always directed to the natural ostium even when one or more accessory ostia are present. A surgically created inferior meatal antrostomy may allow drain-

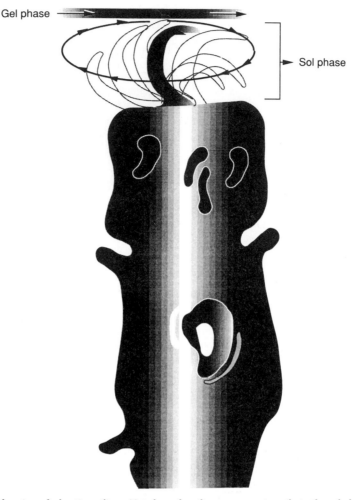

Figure 8.1 A schematic drawing of a beating cilium. Note how the cilium moves primarily in the sol phase and touches the gel phase only briefly during its fast active beat thus pushing the gel and the blanket in the direction of the active beat. (After Stammberger, 1991)

age of a fluid sump and provide ventilation but it will not actively aid outward transport.

The frontal sinus is unique in having active inwardly directed mucus transport. Mucus is transported along the interfrontal septum, then laterally along its roof and back medially via the floor and inferior walls of the sinus. The secretion then encounters a whorl-like ciliary pattern just above the frontal ostium together with the inwardly directed transport route. Mucus may therefore recycle through the sinus several times before it exits through the lateral aspect of the ostium (Figure 8.3). Once through the ostium, the secretion is transported through the frontal recess eventually to merge with secretions from the maxillary sinus.

Within the ethmoidal cells, drainage will occur to a dependent ostium or by a spiral transport pattern toward the ostium. All anterior ethmoidal cells, anterior to the ground lamella, will drain into the middle meatus, whereas posterior air cells will drain into the superior meatus and sphenoethmoidal recess. Similarly the sphenoid sinus exhibits a spiral pattern of drainage towards the ostium and into the sphenoethmoidal recess.

Secretion transport pathology

In cases of hypersecretion, mucus flows toward the dependent part of the respective sinus under the influence of gravity. Provided that the mucus composition remains balanced, a gel layer persists on the surface. This leaves only those 'non-drowned' cilia to remove the fluid, but the transport of mucus in different directions is hindered by the cohesion of the

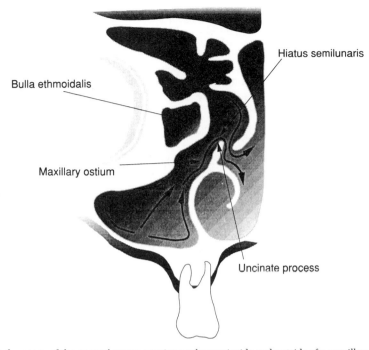

Figure 8.2 Schematic drawings of the normal transportation pathways inside and outside of a maxillary sinus. (After Stammberger, 1991)

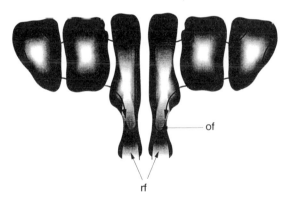

Figure 8.3 Schematic drawing of secretion transport inside and out of the frontal sinus. of, frontal sinus ostium; rf, frontal recess. (After Stammberger, 1991)

surface gel layer because of the limited power of the intact ciliary activity (Figure 8.4). Secretion transport ceases completely despite a normally functioning ciliated mucosa. If the sump of mucus is aspirated, normal transport will recommence almost immediately.

A change in the viscosity of the mucus, by an alteration in the composition of the secretion will

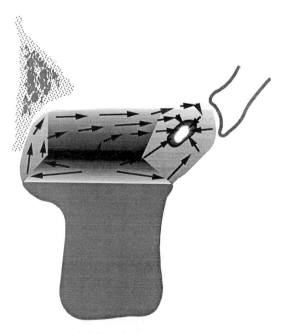

Figure 8.4 In this schematic drawing of a maxillary sinus half-filled with secretions, the transportation of the mucus layer is held back by the cohesional forces of the gel layer on the surface. The cilia of the still intact mucosal areas are not powerful enough to tear off the gel layer from the surface. (After Stammberger, 1991)

tend to produce a thicker gel layer impeding its passage through sinus ostia. This will encourage mucus retention. Conversely, a reduction in the amount of secretion or a loss of humidity at the mucosal surface, will tend to reduce the sol layer bringing the gel layer into close contact with the cilia thus impeding their action. The addition of a few drops of saline may rehydrate the mucus and restore normal mucociliary transport.

When inflamed the mucosa of the sinuses may swell considerably and rapidly. When bacterial or viral infection is present, not only are the mucosal glands affected but the entire mucosal surface may be partially destroyed or paralysed and thus unable to provide its mucociliary clearance function. Optimal function of the mucociliary clearance system requires normal ventilation, humidification, metabolism, osmotic pressure and pH as much as protection from external noxious stimuli. General factors that also affect ciliary function include long-standing dehydration, medication such as atropine and antihistamines, chemical substances or cigarette smoke and foreign bodies. A reduced oxygen supply slows ciliary movement and enriched oxygenation may increase ciliary beat frequency by 30–50%.

The two largest sinuses, the frontal and maxillary communicate with the middle meatus via narrow and delicate prechambers. The maxillary sinus ostium opens into the ethmoidal infundibulum. The frontal sinus ostium opens into an hourglass-shaped cleft, the frontal recess. In each of these prechambers, the mucosal surfaces are closely apposed such that mucus can be more readily cleared by an effective ciliary action on two or more sides (Figure 8.5). If the opposing mucosal surfaces become closely apposed as the result of mucosal swelling, the ciliary action is immobilized (Figure 8.6). Small contact areas like these in key sites such as the infundibulum or frontal recess may impair ventilation and drainage of the larger dependent sinus and lead to retention of secretions. If the area of blockage extends or infection occurs, the retained mucus provides an excellent culture medium for both viral and bacterial growth thus producing a vicious circle.

The concept of such limited disease producing extensive changes is central to our understanding and appropriate treatment of rhinosinusitis. The 'key region' for these changes is that part of the lateral

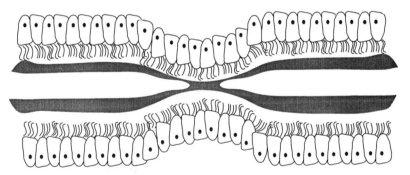

Figure 8.5 A schematic drawing of an ethmoidal 'bottle neck' in a healthy individual. In this instance the ciliary beat can work on secretion from two sides and thus promote mucus transportation. (After Stammberger, 1991)

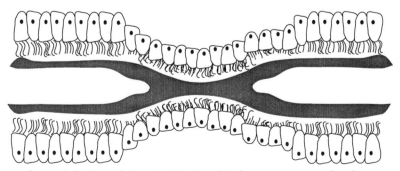

Figure 8.6 A schematic drawing of a diseased ethmoidal 'bottle neck'. The opposing mucosal surfaces are in intimate contact, with the pressure stopping the coordinated ciliary beat. The mucus between the apposed surfaces is thus no longer transported away. (After Stammberger 1991)

nasal wall that encloses the sinus ostia and their adjacent mucosa and prechambers. This region escapes precise anatomical description but is referred to as the ostiomeatal complex. The anterior ethmoid is the principal central component of the ostiomeatal complex and as such has a central role in the physiology of the normal and diseased paranasal sinuses.

It follows that our understanding and therapeutic efforts should be focused on those conditions which might further narrow the delicate system of clefts and air cells of the ostiomeatal complex. These include the anatomical variations that may interfere with normal nasal function and predispose to recurrent sinusitis. Specific targeted therapy towards the area of obstruction may allow the resolution of even massive mucosal pathology in the dependent sinuses without direct intervention upon them.

A guide to these features both in physiological and anatomical terms, is found within the excellent monograph, *Functional Endoscopic Sinus Surgery*, by Stammberger (1991).

Abnormal mucociliary clearance

The transport rate of mucus averages about 6 mm/minute but a wide range is found in normal subjects. Slow clearance rates of less than 1 mm/minute have not been adequately explained but would appear to be related in most cases to variations in physicochemical properties of secretions rather than in the rate of ciliary beating. Systemic dehydration and certain air pollutants may also reduce mucus clearance rates (Proctor, 1982) and there is evidence for bacterial products reducing mucus clearance by slowing ciliary beating. In a few cases, however, deficient clearance may be attributable to genetically determined abnormalities in ciliary morphology and function.

In 1933, Kartagener described a syndrome consisting of bronchiectasis, sinusitis and *situs inversus*. More recently this was associated with a genetically inherited autosomal recessive abnormality of the respiratory tract cilia, usually partial or complete dynein arm deficiency (Figure 8.7) (Afzelius, 1976; Pedersen and Mygind, 1976; Eliasson *et al.*, 1977). In this condition, which was initially termed 'immotile cilia syndrome', there is severe disturbance of the normal pattern of ciliary beating with a very variable degree of immotility (Rossman *et al.*, 1980) so that the preferred term is now 'primary ciliary dyskinesia'. Mucociliary clearance is profoundly impaired resulting in chronic or recurrent infection. Males are infertile because of the basically similar structure of cilia and the sperm tail, rendering the latter dyskinetic also (Pedersen and Rebbe, 1975). The relationship between primary ciliary dyskinesia and dextrocardia is postulated to be due to random rotation of the archenteron when cilia on embryonic cells are not

functioning (Afzelius, 1976). The important implication of this is that only half of the patients with this condition will be detected by dextrocardia found on chest X-ray or at examination. Therefore, the possibility of primary ciliary dyskinesia should not be excluded simply because dextrocardia is not found. These patients may simply present with a life-long history of rhinorrhoea and cough.

While slow clearance may result from dyskinesia of the cilia, it is equally likely to occur with abnormalities of the mucus. Patients with Young's syndrome (obstructive azoospermia, sinusitis and bronchiectasis or bronchitis) present with infertility, chronic sinusitis and often cough with purulent sputum, reminiscent of primary ciliary dyskinesia but examination of their cilia reveals that these are normal in structure and function. Examination of the semen reveals azoospermia and exploratory scrototomy reveals normal spermatogenesis, but a hold-up of sperm transport down the genital apparatus at the level of the caput epididymis where the sperm are found in a viscous, lipid-rich fluid, thought possibly to be due to a metabolic abnormality of the cells lining the tract (Young, 1970; Hendry, Parslow and Stendronska, 1983). Similar affection of respiratory mucus may account for the viscid sinus and respiratory secretions in this syndrome.

Kartagener's and Young's syndromes are excellent examples of primarily ciliary and primarily mucus abnormalities respectively.

Far more common, however, are secondary mucociliary transport abnormalities from such insults as upper respiratory tract infections. The nasal secretions become thick and mucopurulent and are not cleared in the normal manner. Viral infections of the upper respiratory tract damage the ciliated epithelium thereby reducing mucociliary clearance (Wilson *et al.*, 1987a). Certain bacteria associated with chronic sinus and bronchial sepsis (*Haemophilus influenzae*, *Streptococcus pneumoniae* and *Pseudomonas aeruginosa*) have been shown to release factors slowing and disrupting cilia (Wilson, Roberts and Cole, 1985) and, in the case of *P. aeruginosa*, these factors have been characterized as the low-molecular-weight pigments pyocyanin and 1-hydroxyphenazine (Wilson *et al.*, 1987b). Such molecules slow mucus transport in animal models and are found in human respiratory secretions during chronic sepsis in amounts sufficient to have a ciliary dyskinetic effect *in vivo* (Sykes *et al.*, 1987).

Examination of the nose in patients with primary ciliary dyskinesia usually reveals mucopurulent secretions on the floor of the nasal cavity and in the postnasal space. Polyps are occasionally seen (Greenstone *et al.*, 1985; Pedersen and Mygind, 1982; Levison *et al.*, 1983). If these do not respond to topical corticosteroids, their removal is indicated. The ears should be examined as a high proportion of these patients will be found to have glue ear. Persistent

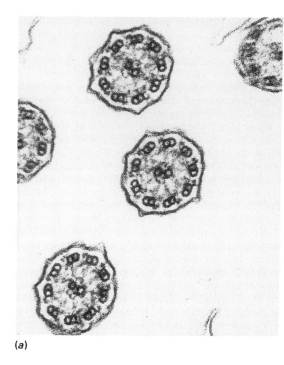

(a)

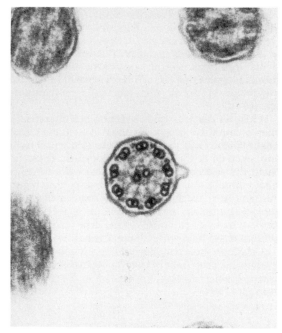

(b)

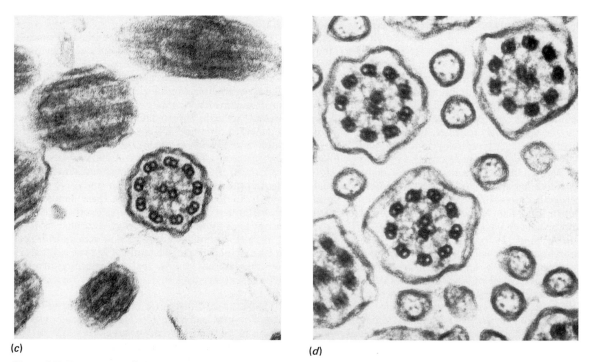

(c)

(d)

Figure 8.7 Transmission electron micrographs of representative cross-sections of cilia from samples of nasal epithelium showing: (*a*) normal ultrastructure (93% outer, 69% inner dynein arms present); (*b*) deficiency of inner dynein arms (89% outer, 17% inner dynein arms present); (*c*) deficiency of outer dynein arms (10% outer, 65% inner dynein arms present); (*d*) deficiency of outer and inner dynein arms (3% outer, 7% inner dynein arms present). (Magnification × 110 000; prepared by Andrew Rutman)

discharge through inserted ventilation tubes until they are either removed or extruded is a common experience (Greenstone *et al.*, 1985). Since there is no likelihood of primary ciliary dyskinesia resolving, it would seem unhelpful to advocate insertion of ventilation tubes. There is little reported evidence to suggest progression towards chronic ear disease despite these difficulties.

While primary syndromes remain 'incurable' secondary abnormalities (due to changes in mucus viscoelasticity induced by bacterial infection, e.g. after a viral infection of the upper respiratory tract or due to bacterial product or neutrophil elastase inhibition of ciliary function) can be treated in the expectation that in a reasonable proportion of patients the underlying condition will resolve and allow mucus and/or cilia to return to normal. In many cases, the chest is also involved in such disease and requires corresponding treatment (Stanley *et al.*, 1985). Cigarette smoking reduces mucociliary clearance and ciliary beat frequency in the nose as well as the bronchial tree, such habits may adversely affect treatment for secondary clearance abnormalities (Stanley *et al.*, 1986).

Symptomatic treatment can be helpful. Experience suggests that these patients can obtain symptomatic relief with topical mucolytics such as alkaline nasal douche which is sniffed through the nose two or three times daily followed by the application of topical corticosteroids. Antral washout will not give lasting relief as it will do nothing to improve the underlying primary problem. Endoscopic sinus surgery to improve drainage and ventilation in the region of the ostiomeatal complex may be useful in some patients.

For many patients with primary nasal mucociliary clearance problems, their otolaryngological symptoms present little more than an inconvenience possibly because their symptoms have been present for most of their life and they accept them as normal. For many, a simple medical regimen will be helpful; in some, surgical procedures to improve sinus drainage may be indicated. The most important aspect, however, should be an awareness of the condition in the hope that early diagnosis and referral for appropriate chest management may prevent or delay the onset of serious chest disease such as bronchiectasis.

Patients with Young's syndrome tend to have a similar clinical picture to those with primary ciliary dyskinesia, although it is interesting that in both groups, the nasal symptoms seldom cause more than mild inconvenience to the patient, and in primary ciliary dyskinesia have been present since birth.

Test for nasal mucociliary clearance

Quinlan *et al.* (1969) developed a method for measuring nasal mucociliary clearance in humans; this involved placing a radioisotopically labelled particle on the anterior nasal mucosa and tracing its clearance with a gamma camera. This method, while having research potential, is not practical in the routine clinical situation. Andersen *et al.* (1974) described a technique in which they replaced the labelled particle by saccharin and this has become the standard method for measuring nasal mucociliary clearance. A 0.5 mm particle of saccharin is placed approximately 1 cm behind the anterior border of the inferior turbinate. It is important not to place it too far anteriorly as clearance here is forwards rather than backwards. The time elapsing until the first experience of a sweet taste at the posterior nasopharynx is recorded as the nasal mucociliary clearance time in minutes. If carefully performed, the test is reproducible (Stanley *et al.*, 1984). Patients should be tested in standard environmental conditions and must be instructed not to sniff, eat or drink and to avoid coughing and sneezing if possible. They should be tested in the sitting position with the head flexed about 10° to avoid the particle falling backwards into any postnasal stream, and should not be told the nature of the particle. The particle should be inserted under direct vision to ensure there is no gross mechanical obstruction to the test. If a patient is unable to perceive the correct (sweet) taste after 60 minutes, it is important to test his ability to taste saccharin placed directly on the tongue as, rarely, persons may lack this ability.

The rate of clearance has a wide range in normal persons. Proctor (1982), using the radioisotopically labelled particle method, found that in apparently healthy adult subjects under optimal environmental conditions, the result ranged from 1 to over 20 mm/minute. Nevertheless, the saccharin clearance method is simple, inexpensive and useful as a routine investigation to screen gross mucus transport abnormality. In children, dyeing the particle of saccharin can assist in verifying when the child tastes, the dye appearing from the postnasal space on oral examination. In one study, all but two of 30 healthy controls tasted saccharin within 20 minutes while 28 out of 158 patients presenting with mucopurulent rhinitis did not perceive a sweet taste after 60 minutes or more (Mackay *et al.*, 1983). It is wise to repeat the test if it is abnormal, using the opposite nostril. There was a good correlation between the results of tests in normal volunteers performed 2 weeks apart and in opposite nostrils (Stanley *et al.*, 1984) and, in most, the transport time was 30 minutes or less.

If a patient, in the absence of mechanical obstruction, is found consistently to be unable to perceive the taste of saccharin 60 minutes after the test is commenced (innate inability to taste it having been ruled out by testing the taste of it directly on the tongue), mucus transport is grossly abnormal and further tests are required to indicate whether the ciliary or mucus component of transport is responsible.

Ciliary beat frequency

When the saccharin test reveals a grossly prolonged mucus transport time, it is simplest first to ask whether the cilia are capable of beating normally. A qualitative judgement can be gained simply by microscopic examination of strips of ciliated epithelium harvested from the lateral aspect of the inferior turbinate using a fibreoptic bronchoscopy cytology brush (Figure 8.8). This procedure requires no anaesthesia and can be safely employed at all ages, if necessary serially. The specimens are transferred to buffered saline by agitating the brush in the solution, and mounted on a coverslip-slide preparation sealed with silicone grease. This assessment can be quantified using a photometric method (Rutland and Cole, 1980) to measure the beat frequency of cilia which are kept at body temperature on the warm stage of a phase-contrast microscope; light is 'gated' and shone through a small area of cilia from below, the effective 'straight arm' beat of the cilium interrupting the light beam which is detected by a photometer. The electrical signal generated is processed by a ciliary beat frequency analyser (Greenstone, Logan–Sinclair and Cole, 1984) and the beating expressed in Hertz (beats/second). The normal range in humans for nasal cilia is 12–15 Hz, there being a gradient with slower beating more peripherally in the bronchial tree (Rutland, Griffin and Cole, 1982).

Simultaneous with this measurement of ciliary beat frequency, the percentage of cilia which are immotile can be determined by direct vision as, occasionally ciliary beat frequency may be only at the lower limit of the normal range but the number of cilia beating is low.

Patients with 'primary ciliary dyskinesia' initially present to paediatricians and otolaryngologists and can be diagnosed with this technique. However, recently, it has been recognized that cilia obtained from sites of purulent infection beat slower than normal (Wilson *et al.*, 1986). Therefore as this slowing is a secondary effect due to elastase 'leaked' from neutrophils (Smallman, Hill and Stockley, 1984) and toxins released by bacteria (Wilson, Roberts and Cole, 1985; Sykes *et al.*, 1987), it is important to be sure that primary ciliary dyskinesia is only diagnosed from specimens taken from areas which are not grossly purulent. If necessary, infection may need to be treated and the test repeated.

The definitive investigation to prove primary ciliary dyskinesia is electron microscopy. Care must be taken in the assessment of cilial structure as the occasional absence of dynein arms may occur in normal subjects. Equally the absence of dynein arms is not a universal finding in all cilia in patients with primary ciliary dyskinesia.

Immunity deficiency

A variety of defence mechanisms exists to eliminate inhaled foreign material. These can be considered either as those 'resident' in the respiratory tract or those attracted from the systemic circulation when the local mechanisms fail. In each case, such defences

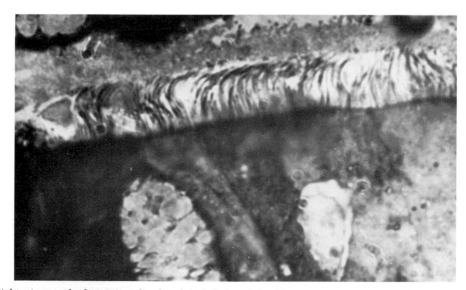

Figure 8.8 Light micrograph of a portion of a ciliated epithelial strip obtained by brushing the inferior nasal turbinate and used for determining the ciliary beat frequency. It shows a thick mucus layer overlying cilia lying in thin periciliary fluid above the epithelial cells (magnification × 2000, prepared by Andrew Rutman)

can be divided into those which are non-specific and those which are immunologically specific (Table 8.2). These divisions are perhaps artificial because of considerable interactions between these different mechanisms. In turn, this makes the identification of an isolated defect, as the sole cause of respiratory tract infections, sometimes very difficult.

Table 8.2 System of defences of the respiratory tract

Local ('resident') mechanisms
1 Non-specific
   reflexes (cough, sneeze)
   mucociliary system
   epithelial integrity and lining fluid (anatomical barrier)
   antimicrobial substances in lining fluid (e.g. lysozyme)
   pulmonary macrophage

2 Specific
   immunoglobulin (secretory IgA, IgE)
   lymphocytes

Systemic ('recruited') mechanisms
1 Non-specific
   serum factors (e.g. opsonins, complement components)
   granulocyte phagocytes, mononuclear phagocytes

2 Specific
   serum immunoglobulins (IgG, IgA, IgM, IgE)
   lymphocytes

Deficiencies in the defence mechanisms of the respiratory tract may occasion infective episodes. As both upper and lower respiratory tracts are similarly affected, it is important to recognize immune deficiency (especially that which is treatable) as an underlying cause of infection, to prevent untoward damage to the delicate architecture of the lung. Chronic disease, respiratory insufficiency and predisposition to further infection can occur, because distorted anatomy may disrupt front line defences such as mucociliary clearance.

Three categories of presentation for upper and lower respiratory symptoms exist to suggest immune deficiencies. First, the acute overwhelming infection usually due to profound immunity deficiency (e.g. panhypogammaglobulinaemia; acquired immune deficiency syndrome, AIDS). Second, recurrent acute episodes of infection with apparently normal periods intervening. Here, there is a prevalence of immunological abnormality (notably selective IgA deficiency) of between 40 and 70% in the lower respiratory tract (higher in recurrent pneumonia than bronchial infections). Third, the patient with chronic purulent bronchial disease associated with upper respiratory symptoms and chronic purulent sinusitis in over one-third of cases. Here, paradoxically, immunity deficiency is uncommon but a 'vicious circle' of chronic mucosal damage occurs (see below)

which demands a particular attitude to treatment (Cole, 1981). Any of these three types of presentation should alert the otolaryngologist to the possibility of immunity deficiency or progressive disease requiring appropriate treatment if irreparable damage is not to occur and fatally affect the lower respiratory tract.

Systemic immunity deficiency

Patients with systemic immunity deficiency (e.g. lack of antibodies, panhypogammaglobulinaemia) frequently present with respiratory symptoms because the nose and paranasal sinuses are in the 'front line' of the respiratory tract they encounter greater attack from environmental agents. It is not surprising that rhinosinusitis is frequently the first presentation of such systemic immunity deficiency. Mackay *et al.* (1983) found nine patients with significant immunoglobulin deficiency in a series of 250 patients presenting with upper respiratory tract symptoms. Five of these patients with severe panhypogammaglobulinaemia, who had been referred from chest physicians, gave a history of having initially presented to otolaryngologists with infective upper respiratory tract symptoms before developing irreversible lung disease.

The protective role of IgA in the respiratory tract is far from clear. It has been estimated from blood transfusion screening, that selective IgA deficiency occurs in one in 500–700 healthy individuals (Bachmann, 1965). However, there is no doubt that some patients with severe, recurrent symptoms in the upper and lower respiratory tracts lack serum and secretory IgA and that there is a significant prevalence of this abnormality in patients presenting with infective rhinosinusitis and bronchial sepsis. This deficiency may not necessarily be causal but a marker of other associated deficiencies of defences. Oxelius *et al.* (1981) have shown an association of IgA deficiency with deficiency of certain subclasses of IgG (notably IgG2) in children and it may be that the subclass deficiency is causal, since IgG2 is a particularly important antibody against polysaccharide capsular antigens such as those of the microorganisms *H. influenzae* and *Pneumococcus*. It is important that this is confirmed also for adult infective respiratory disease because, although IgA deficiency is not routinely replaceable, normal human immunoglobulin replacement therapy can reconstitute IgG2 deficiency. Also, IgG2 subclass deficiency will be not diagnosed by routine quantitation of the total major immunoglobulin classes IgG, IgA and IgM, and requires separate estimation of IgG subclasses.

Despite the great advances in this field over the last few decades, it is still by no means rare to find patients who are unusually susceptible to upper respiratory tract infections and to be unable to identify any defect in defences, systemic disease or environmental exposure likely to offer a reasonable explanation (Andersen and Proctor, 1982).

Chronic infection without classical immunity deficiency (the vicious circle)

Most patients with chronic bronchial sepsis suffer upper respiratory symptoms and over one-third have frank chronic purulent rhinosinusitis. Yet, less than one-tenth of these patients have classical immunity deficiency. It is suggested that the colonization of the upper and lower respiratory tracts by predominantly non-invasive microorganisms (e.g. uncapsulated *H. influenzae*), leads to an exuberant immunological response. Progressive disease with gross scarring of the respiratory lining and sometimes death from ultimate respiratory failure may occur. These facts can be explained by a normal short-lived useful host response to eliminate invading microorganisms becoming subverted into a tissue-damaging chronic inflammatory response.

When the front-line clearance mechanisms are less than perfect either from a predisposing damaging insult (e.g. infection) or underlying disease (cystic fibrosis) microorganisms may loiter in the respiratory tract. Microbial persistence encourages a host response directed at their elimination. The host response is chronic and inflammatory which, unfortunately, is relatively unselective and damages 'bystander' normal mucosal surfaces and tissues leading to progressive tissue damaging disease (Figure 8.9). This process, termed a 'vicious circle' (Cole, 1984), is the antithesis of acute invasive infection such as acute sinusitis or pneumonia since the microorganism (which is actively invasive in the latter) is relatively passive and the tissue damage is mediated largely by host rather than microbe. This distinction is important for treatment as will be seen later.

Patients with systemic immunity deficiency often present with the signs of (recurrent) acute or acute on chronic infection with mucopurulent rhinorrhoea, hyperaemic and swollen mucous membranes and purulent postnasal drip. Infection may also be present at other sites such as ears, chest and skin.

Acquired immune deficiency syndrome (AIDS) may present with otolaryngological symptoms. There are frequently signs of rhinitis with 'granular' mucosa and purulent discharge not unlike the appearance of sarcoid, although with less bleeding and crusting. Infective rhinosinusitis is not unusual either with common or opportunistic organisms. Sinusitis in HIV-infected patients is common, severe and difficult to treat. Patients with CD4 counts less than 200/mm^3 are prone to pansinusitis that responds incompletely to antibiotic therapy, often resulting in chronic sinusitis. Unlike the immunocompetent host, the majority of HIV-infected patients with advanced immunodeficiency develop posterior sinus disease (Godofsky *et al.*, 1992). Patients frequently develop oral candidiasis and often otitis externa with occasional otitis media. Kaposi's sarcoma skin lesions can develop at any site but should be sought within the mouth and pharynx.

While several immunity deficiency states may present initially to otolaryngologists or paediatricians, it is particularly important to recognize and treat panhypogammaglobulinaemia (very low IgG, IgA and IgM) as irreparable lung damage may be avoided by appropriate immunoglobulin replacement.

The standard therapy has been the painful intramuscular injection of human immunoglobulin given weekly in a dose of approximately 25 mg/kg body weight. The dose in such patients was regulated according to clinical control of frequency and severity of infections rather than monitoring immunoglobulin serum levels. The addition of fresh frozen plasma infusions at intervals to the regimen was sometimes required in the more seriously affected patient. Untoward effects, such as anaphylaxis or rashes were common and unpredictable. The advent of intravenous immunoglobulin preparations has substantially lessened the morbidity of treatment. Such preparations are given by infusion at less frequent intervals (usually 2–4 weekly) and have the advantage that the dose can be increased without increasing discomfort as occurred with intramuscular preparations. However, the preparations are very expensive and the efficacy of some is not fully known because of their relatively recent introduction. Opsonization of bacteria for phagocytosis is one important function of immunoglobulin and this can be used as the basis

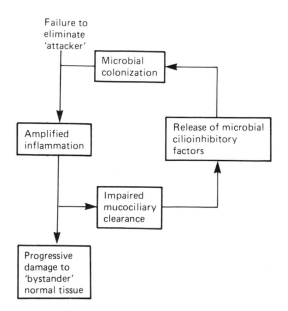

Figure 8.9 The vicious circle of chronic inflammation of the respiratory tract

of a laboratory test to compare the efficacy of various intravenous preparations *in vitro* (Munro, Stanley and Cole, 1985).

Selective immunoglobulin A deficiency is not treatable at present (and, as mentioned before, it is debatable whether reconstitution of IgA would affect bacterial infections). However, IgA deficiency seems to be a marker for IgG subclass deficiencies in some cases and the latter are probably treatable by replacement immunoglobulin. At present, the situation is much clearer in children (Oxelius *et al.*, 1981) than in adults.

The complexity of the immunological deficiencies which may be associated with chronic or recurrent rhinosinusitis make it mandatory to refer affected patients to a specialist centre.

The common cold (coryza)

Incidence

The common cold is probably the commonest viral infection in man. The incidence is variable but it is estimated that the average young adult has two to three colds a year. Children and young adults are particularly susceptible to rhinovirus infections and women may experience more infections than men perhaps because they are in closer contact with young children.

Predisposing factors

Climate

Colds occur all the year round but in temperate climates they are more common in winter than in summer. Rhinovirus infections are more prevalent in autumn and spring and coronavirus infections seem to occur mostly from December to March.

Environment, temperature, chills and humidity

Kerr and Lagen (1933–34) exposed groups of susceptible men in the same room, under perfect conditions of humidity, temperature and ventilation, with subjects in the early stages of a cold, and in some they even inoculated cold filtrates into the conjunctival sac without obtaining a single transfer, suggesting that an ideal environment increases resistance.

Van Cauwenberge (1985) in a study of 2065 healthy children between the ages of 2.5 and 6 years showed that there was a positive history of upper respiratory tract infections in the parents and the annual incidence of the common cold in the child. The higher the weight of the child, the lower was the incidence of common cold and the fewer pathological rhinoscopic findings. Children with a head circumference below the 2.5 centile had the highest incidence of infectious rhinitis as did children who lived in humid houses.

There is widespread belief that chilling may precipitate a cold in an individual; however, attempts to demonstrate such an effect experimentally have given negative results (Andrewes, 1950). Chill may act in two ways; by lowering the general resistance to infection and by causing reflex vasoconstriction of the nasal mucous membrane. The normal temperature of the mucous membrane of the nose has been shown to vary between 28 and 33°C. Chilling of the body surface may reduce the temperature of the nasal mucosa by as much as 6°C. The optimum relative humidity of the atmosphere is 45%. A lowering of relative humidity of 15%, as may easily occur when the relatively dry cold outside air in winter is heated indoors by radiators, withdraws more water than the nasal mucosa can supply, and causes drying of the mucous blanket. Excessive humidity is also harmful, as it reduces the evaporation of sweat from the skin and, owing to the high conductivity of water vapour, a slight lowering of temperature produces severe chilling, with the effects described above.

Hope Simpson (1958a,b) demonstrated a striking correlation between increase in the frequency of colds in a group of families and falls in the temperature of the soil. Humidity also affects the survival of viruses (Tyrrell and Bynde, 1961). Common cold viruses prefer high humidity whereas influenza viruses survive better in dry air.

Immune status

Local immunity in the nose is primarily the result of concentrations of IgA and IgG3, which are normally present in nasal secretions in the ratio of 3:1 compared with 1:5 in serum. IgA is produced in response to local antigen stimulation but does not combine with complement and therefore is unable to lyse bacteria; it is, however, effective as a viral neutralizing substance. IgA is a relatively short-lived antibody the half-life of which has been estimated to be 13 days but in practice, is more likely to be measured in minutes because, although there are very large numbers of IgA-producing plasma cells in submucosal tissues, it is soon carried away in mucus secretions. It is thus not uncommon to find reinfection with the same virus serotype in consecutive years. Total IgG analysis may be deceptive as the IgG1 component may mask low levels of IgG2 and IgG4 may mask IgG3 thus rendering the total IgG titre within normal range, albeit at the lower end. Subclass analysis is often worthwhile.

Failure to produce secretory IgA occurs in approximately one in 800 persons who live without ill effects. Patients with generalized hypogammaglobulinaemia, however, have frequent infections of the upper respiratory tract. A small group of patients lack IgA in the saliva and nasal mucus, despite normal serum levels. This situation should be considered in patients with recurrent infections who have not responded to multiple surgery.

Nutrition and vitamin deficiency

The lowering of resistance by hunger and under-nutrition was shown by Cruickshank (1942), who found that the death rate in measles, pertussis, influenza and bronchopneumonia among poor children was five times greater than among those better off. Deficiencies in vitamins A, C and D are said to increase susceptibility to infection but the claim that vitamin C is effective in preventing colds is not supported by controlled trials (Andrewes and Tyrrell, 1965).

Fatigue, fitness and exercise

Locke (1937) assessed the fitness of subjects by their oxygen consumption under standard exercise, and found that 64% of those with fitness above 0.6 had only one cold a year, while 80% of those below 0.5 had four colds a year. However, colds very often hit the man who is feeling very fit on his return from holiday (Andrewes and Tyrrell, 1965).

Nasal obstruction

Deviation of the nasal septum, hypertrophy of the turbinates, enlarged adenoids, polyps, scars and adhesions all interfere with ventilation and the free passage of air through the nasal chambers, and with the secretion and movement of the mucous blanket, and thus predispose to infection.

Foci of chronic infection

Foci of infection in the sinuses, nasopharynx or pharynx, by decreasing tissue resistance, favour infection. The most important of these in children are chronic adenoiditis, tonsillitis and sinusitis and, in adults, chronic sinusitis and tonsillitis.

The pH of nasal secretion

A drift to the acid side is associated with few bacteria, while an alkaline drift is associated with many bacteria in the nasal secretion. Rhinoviruses are destroyed by an acid pH (Ketler, Hamparian and Hilleman, 1962). Cilia prefer a pH of 7.0 but will function between pH 6.4 and pH 8.5.

General diseases

Any general disease, but particularly renal, hepatic and blood disorders, diabetes mellitus and tuberculosis, may lower general resistance to colds.

Causative agents

Viruses

In general it may be said that, in communities, the causative agent of the common cold is ubiquitous, but that infection occurs only when an individual's resistance is lowered, or when he is subjected to an overwhelming concentration and virulence of the causative agent. It is generally accepted that the common cold is due to infection with filterable viruses, followed by secondary infection with bacteria.

In spite of the rapid advances in virology and the isolation, identification and even culture of many viruses, it is still uncertain what proportion of respiratory illnesses is caused by them. The viruses responsible for colds are listed in Table 8.3 (Reed, 1981).

Table 8.3 Viruses causing the common cold

Virus	Serotypes	Proportion of colds (%)
Rhinovirus	89 different types, probably more	50
Coronaviruses	3 or more types, and possibly subtypes	15–20
Influenza	A and B and their subtypes; C	Together about 15–20
Parainfluenza	Types 1, 2, 3, 4	
Respiratory syncytial	One type	
Adenovirus	36 types, but only about half of them causing respiratory tract infection	
Other viruses	Includes some enteroviruses, other known viruses, and perhaps some unknown	10–20

Each of these viruses can be said to be associated with its own 'typical' clinical effect which, for rhinoviruses and coronaviruses, is the common cold syndrome. Influenza viruses, respiratory syncytial viruses are, however, known to cause more serious infections.

Rhinoviruses

These are members of the picornavirus group and are thus biologically related to polioviruses and other enteroviruses, and to foot and mouth disease virus. They are about 25 nm in diameter and incorporate protein subunits in which the antigenic specificity of each of 89 or more types is incorporated. They have an optimal growth temperature of 33°C. Nasal swabs and nasal washings produce the best specimens for culture on human embryonic fibroblasts such as WI-38. Identification of the serotype of a rhinovirus is difficult because of the large range of types. However antisera can be used against 89 types. A group-reactive serological test for rhinoviruses is not available and therefore retrospective diagnosis of rhinovirus infection cannot easily be established using paired sera collected in the acute and convalescent stages of the illness.

Coronaviruses

Coronaviruses were first classified as a distinct group in 1968 but are still not fully understood because of the technical difficulties in isolating them from clinicial specimens. They are RNA-containing viruses about 100–120 nm in diameter. Two early isolates were named 229E and OC_{43}. The former can be grown in tissue culture, but the latter needs organ cultures of human embryonic nasal epithelium or trachea. Serological tests available include complement fixation and neutralization tests for 229E, and complement fixation and haemagglutination inhibition for OC_{43}. Coronaviruses cause typical colds. The incubation period is slightly longer than for rhinovirus colds.

Mode of transmission

Droplet and dust

In talking, sneezing and coughing innumerable infected droplets are sprayed out which fall to the ground at distances of 0.9–1.8 m. A sneeze may generate as many as 20 000 droplets from the nose and mouth. Bedmaking, house dust and the manipulation of handkerchiefs also contribute large numbers of airborne particles.

Droplet nuclei

Droplet nuclei are small droplets which evaporate as they fall, and shrink to less than 0.1 mm in diameter.

In this form they remain suspended in the air as mist, and drift on the air currents for as long as 2 days, and thus have a much wider range than that of droplets. These will transport viruses, but are too small to carry the larger bacteria.

Contact

The causative organism may be transmitted by kissing, food, fingers and fomites.

Pathology

In the earliest stage of invasion there is transient vasoconstriction. This is followed by vasodilatation, oedema and increased activity of the seromucinous glands and goblet cells (Figure 8.10). Leucocytic infiltration of the tissues follows, with swelling and desquamation of the epithelial cells. The secretion is at first clear, watery and sterile, with a few epithelial and pus cells, but later it becomes coloured and viscid, stiffens on a handkerchief and contains many pus cells and bacteria.

Åkerlund *et al.* (1993) have shown that mucosal plasma exudation, as assessed by fibrinogen in lavage fluids, increased 100-fold following common cold virus inoculation. This exudate reflects the degree of subepithelial inflammation and suggests that fibrinogen, along with other potent protein systems may contribute to the resolution of common cold infections. The toxins produced in the mucous membrane are swiftly taken up by the lymphatics, and passing through the cervical lymph glands and ducts reach the blood stream. Resolution takes place by a reversal of these processes, and by proliferation of the remaining tissue cells to replace those that have been destroyed.

The lysozyme content is reduced in the early stages. The average pH of the nasal mucus lies between 5.5 and 6.5. During an acute rhinitis the reaction becomes alkaline, and during resolution it returns to neutral.

Bacteriology

Cultures from the normal mucous membrane of the posterior areas of the nose are usually sterile, provided that they are not contaminated from the vestibule and anterior areas. Cultures from the anterior nares show staphylococci in 43% of normal individuals.

In the first 3 days of a common cold the cultures from the posterior areas may be sterile, but after the third day pure or mixed cultures of streptococci, pneumococci, *Haemophilus influenzae*, or staphylococci are often shown.

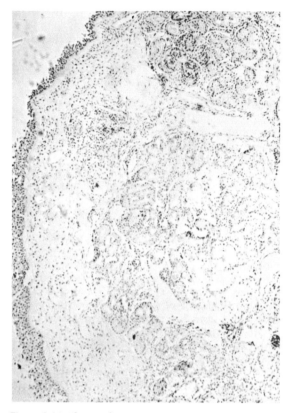

Figure 8.10 The nasal mucous membrane in acute rhinitis showing general oedema and hyperaemia with swelling of the seromucinous glands, desquamation of the epithelium, and cellular infiltration (× 100)

Clinical picture

The course of a cold may be described in four stages:

1 Prodromal or ischaemic stage. This lasts for a few hours, and represents the stage of local invasion and general nasal ischaemia. The familiar hot, dry or tickling spot is felt at the site of the invasion, while the general nasal airway seems unusually patent.
2 Early reaction and irritation. The infection, which is at first localized, spreads to the adjacent mucous membranes over the surface and by way of the lymphatics. This process may take a few hours or days. The site of invasion is often the first to recover, while the disease is still active in those areas which have been affected later. The throat is dry and sore on swallowing, and there is sneezing, watery nasal discharge and obstruction. The mucous membrane is red and swollen. General symptoms of mild toxaemia and fever now appear.

3 Stage of venous stasis and secondary infection. After the second day, the colour of the mucosa becomes dusky, with a bluish tinge, the discharge thickens, diminishes and becomes mucopurulent. The obstruction and toxaemia are at their maximum.
4 Resolution. The symptoms and signs gradually diminish, and after 5–10 days recovery takes place.

Complications

Nasopharyngitis and pharyngitis

The nasopharynx and pharynx are invariably infected to some extent in every cold.

Sinusitis

Sinusitis is one of the most common complications, but the sinuses are not invaded during the course of an uncomplicated cold.

Pharyngotympanic salpingitis, otitis media and mastoiditis

The infection ascends from the nasopharynx, invading the pharyngotympanic tube, middle ear and mastoid cells in sequence. It may be arrested at any point of the ascent.

Lymphadenitis

This is usually transient, and affects the retropharyngeal and deep cervical group.

Tonsillitis

A mild inflammation usually accompanies a cold, but parenchymatous or follicular tonsillitis is considered a complication.

Lower respiratory complications

Laryngotracheitis, bronchitis, pneumonia and asthma constitute the group of lower respiratory complications.

Gastroenteritis

This complication is rare except in infants.

Other complications

Nephritis and rheumatism are allergic and toxaemic manifestations.

Diagnosis

Other causes of rhinitis should be excluded.

Laboratory diagnosis may be made retrospectively by taking acute and convalescent sera and comparing the antibody levels. However, more rapid diagnostic techniques such as immunofluorescence are now available. In the course of an infection large numbers of infected cells are sloughed off into the respiratory secretions. These cells will carry markers or antigens specific for the virus involved and can be recovered by nasal swabs or washings, stained using specific antiviral antisera labelled with a fluorescent dye, and seen by fluorescence microscopy. This technique can now be applied to a range of common respiratory viruses including influenza viruses A and B, parainfluenza viruses 1–3, adenovirus and respiratory syncytial virus.

Prophylaxis and vaccines

Based on the observation that rhinovirus infections may possibly be spread by the manual route, thorough hand washing with soap and water will remove the virus from contaminated hands. Avoidance of fingering the nostrils and conjunctiva could reduce the chance of self-inoculation.

Because of the antigenic diversity of respiratory viruses with the exception of vaccines for influenza virus A and B infections, there are no suitable vaccines against the other respiratory viruses. No specific antirhinovirus compound has yet shown sufficient activity in man to merit further development but, nevertheless, work continues in this field.

Wide spectrum antiviral prophylaxis or therapy would have considerable theoretical advantages and the natural antiviral substance, interferon and its inducers, would seem to be an ideal solution. Double-blind placebo-controlled studies using interferon in rhinovirus-infected volunteers have given encouraging results. It is important though to ensure that any form of antiviral therapy should be of very low toxicity before its use in common colds can be justified.

Treatment

There is no known specific treatment for the common cold, but general and local supportive and palliative treatment can mitigate the severity and complications. There are so many different varieties of colds, so many different individual reactions to them, and so many different individual responses to treatment, that no hard and fast therapeutic rules can be laid down.

General treatment is directed to providing the best conditions for rest, both general and local, and at the same time supplying heat and the maximum blood flow to the infected tissues. Unfortunately, the majority of patients are not willing to submit to full-scale treatment for a cold of moderate severity, and modifications must be made, according to the circumstances.

Complete rest, both general and for the upper respiratory tract, necessitates confinement to bed in an even temperature of 18–20 °C, with a humidity of 45%.

Heat, both local and general, is provided at first by a hot bath. Inhalations of menthol or tincture of benzoin (BP) (one teaspoonful in a pint (0.57 l) of steaming water), may be soothing and will apply heat directly to the mucous membrane of the nose.

Analgesics and antipyretics, such as acetylsalicylic acid, may be valuable for the general malaise, aching and feverishness of the cold. Codeine compounds are more effective as sedatives. Both should be combined with a copious fluid intake.

Antihistamines have not been shown to reduce fully or abolish the symptoms of colds, but they can be particularly effective in the allergic patient who is often unduly susceptible to colds. Antihistamines can be usefully combined with an analgesic.

Alcohol is a sedative which is the chief justification for the faith placed in whisky as a treatment in the early stages of a cold. It is also a vasodilator and counteracts the discomfort of the peripheral vasoconstriction at that stage.

Local vasoconstrictors should be used sparingly as the excessive use of any vasoconstrictor agent should be avoided on the grounds of interference with ciliary activity, mucosal blood flow and local tissue resistance. Temporary relief may be achieved by using ephedrine 0.5% in isotonic saline. This is particularly helpful in enabling a child to sleep or a baby to suckle.

Antibiotics do not appear to influence the course of a cold and therefore should only be used, and then in full doses, if complications develop such as middle-ear infection, sinusitis, tonsillitis, bronchitis or pneumonia.

Influenzal rhinitis

Influenzal rhinitis occurs in association with an infection by one of the influenza viruses which are classified into three main unrelated antigenic groups (A, B and C).

The first isolation of a virus causing human influenza was made during the 1932/33 epidemic by Smith, Andrewes and Laidlaw. It was thought to have been the causative agent of the 1918 influenza pandemic in which an estimated 20 million people died worldwide. Influenza A infections (originally called H0N1) and its different strains lead to the greatest morbidity and are responsible for world-wide pandemics such as 1946 (strain H_1N_1), 1957 ('Asian' flu, strain H_2N_2), 1968 ('Hong Kong' flu, H_3N_2) and 1977 ('Red' flu, H_1N_1). Between pandemics the causative

break the immunoglobulin into its Fab and Fc fragments, thus masking the antigenic determinants and preventing more effective antibody attack. Indeed, the pathogenicity of the organism may be related to its ability to produce IgA protease (McNabb and Tomasi, 1981). *Bacteroides* produces IgG proteases, which prevent opsonization and phagocytosis of the facultative anaerobes. Ingham *et al.* (1977) and Kilian (1981) have suggested that facultative and obligate anaerobes may work synergistically to cause persistence of infection. While this is an attractive idea and helps explain the prevalence of mixed infection there is little evidence for synergistic action between aerobes and anaerobes as a factor in persistent inflammation of the ethmoid sinus (Frederich and Braude, 1974).

Often culture studies yield no growth unless strict anaerobic techniques are employed, but the Gram stain shows mixed flora. *Pseudomonas aeruginosa* is a prevalent pathogen in patients with extensive polyp formation, such as those with aspirin triad syndrome or cystic fibrosis.

An exacerbation of chronic sinusitis may be due to the pathogens of acute sinusitis. In quiescent stages, however, the organisms are often quite different (Frederich and Braude, 1974). Chronic sinusitis (if of nondental origin) is due to inadequate mucociliary function or to obstructed drainage; the infecting organisms are various opportunistic ones including a preponderance of anaerobes. Sinusitis of dental origin is invariably caused by anaerobic organisms and it is often of mixed flora.

Immunocompromised patients, including those with HIV infection, may develop sinusitis with common or opportunistic organisms including *Pseudomonas* species and fungi. The treatment depends on the causative agent.

Fungal infection is relatively rare by comparison with viral and bacterial infection. In many ways, it is surprising that fungal infection is not seen more often, particularly in view of the large number of patients now treated with topical corticosteroids. It is known to occur in cases of trauma to the face, poorly controlled diabetes, severely debilitated patients such as those with carcinomatosis and patients who have been treated with immunosuppressive drugs (Berlinger, 1985). It may, however, occur in otherwise healthy patients (Meikle, Yarington and Winterbauer, 1985). The commonest fungus involved is *Aspergillus*.

Investigations

Nasal endoscopy

An endoscopic examination of the nose is central to the appropriate management of any patient with nasal symptoms, particularly in cases resistant to treatment, to exclude aetiological factors and obtain accurate material for bacteriological examination. It must be emphasized that any nasal examination must be incomplete without endoscopic assessment which is fully described in Chapter 1. This will guide therapy more than any other investigation.

The endoscope allows the recognition of changes that are concealed from anterior rhinoscopy or even from inspection with the microscope. Topical vasoconstriction may be required. If this is necessary, it should be postponed until nasal mucociliary clearance tests and rhinomanometry have been performed, if it is intended that these should be done at the same visit.

Radiology

Sinus X-ray

The technique and overall interpretation of radiology of the nose and paranasal sinuses is covered in Chapter 3.

Plain X-rays are more appropriate in assessing the patient with acute rather than chronic inflammatory disease. They may show no abnormality, mucosal thickening, fluid levels (in which case, a tilted view will be helpful) or total opacity. However, it is important to remember that these X-rays are not infallible. The shadow of the lip may sometimes appear as mucosal thickening, totally clear X-rays will occasionally be taken of sinuses found to contain pus on wash-out. Equally up to half of sinuses showing a fluid level or opacity may yield no return on wash-out (Pfleiderer, Drake–Lee and Lowe, 1984). An opaque antrum on X-ray may on occasions be due to thickening of the bony wall (Proops, 1983), while previous Caldwell–Luc surgery results in scarring of the lining which, in most cases, will lead to great difficulty in interpreting the radiological appearance.

Sinus X-rays will frequently be requested by practitioners other than otolaryngologists and a report of mucosal thickening of the maxillary antra is then usually interpreted as 'sinusitis'. It is important to appreciate that the lining of the sinuses and nose is continuous and that many conditions producing swelling of the nasal mucosa will be associated with mucosal swelling in the antra without it necessarily being attributed to 'infection'. Hayfever, for example, with profuse watery rhinorrhoea may even be associated with fluid levels in the sinuses at times.

It should be stressed here that all patients with persistent nasal symptoms, particularly those resistant to treatment, should undergo sinus X-rays. At times these will result in unexpected information, such as bony erosion at the base of the skull, suggesting a postnasal space carcinoma, or opacity of the antrum with bony erosion from tumours of the sinuses presenting with symptoms of rhinosinusitis, although bony changes may be seen even with benign nasal polyps (Lund and Lloyd, 1983).

Computerized tomography

This examination is the optimum imaging technique to demonstrate the extent and distribution of mucosal disease together with any anatomical variant that may be relevant to the diagnosis of recurrent acute or chronic rhinosinusitis (Zinreich, 1993). Coronal views centred on the ostiomeatal complex are essential to fulfill these objectives. The addition of axial views is essential to define the relationship of the optic nerve to the posterior ethmoidal cells when operative treatment is contemplated. These issues are fully discussed in Chapter 3.

The value of CT scanning may be enhanced when taken together with clinical examination for the purposes of staging of rhinosinusitis. The staging of the extent of disease must rely heavily upon the assessment of the CT scan but contributions from symptom scores and endoscopic appearances can be added. While there is no uniform agreement on a staging system for rhinosinusitis, this is clearly an evolving concept which may yet become a useful guide to prognosis and therapeutic choice (Lund and Mackay, 1993).

While CT scanning is the optimal imaging technique for paranasal sinus disease, the radiation dose to the orbit and the lens in particular is not insignificant. Strategies for low dose assessment and thin sections away from the eye all help reduce the risk of cataract formation but this long-term complication demands that CT only be used when its results will make a positive impact on the patient's management.

Ultrasound

A transmitter emits soundwaves of high power and short duration which are reflected back to a receiver from the interface between objects of varying acoustic impedance. A probe, coated with electrode gel, is moved over the antrum and the 'echo' of the ultrasonic wave is recorded on an oscilloscope which can be photographed with a polaroid camera to produce a permanent record.

In an air-filled sinus, most of the ultrasound will be reflected from the interface between the anterior wall of the sinus and the air filling that sinus, leading to an early peak followed by a flat graph. Variations in this pattern will occur with fluid filling the sinus which will produce a 'back wall echo', a double peak will suggest a cyst and multiple peaks may be seen with mucosal thickening. The main advantages of using this technique to aid diagnosis are the freedom from the hazards of radiation to the orbit and the ability to use ultrasound repeatedly. The main disadvantage is the relatively low sensitivity in diagnosing sinus disease compared to plain radiography.

The diagnosis of maxillary sinusitis by plain X-ray or ultrasound is not wholly accurate when compared with proof puncture (Jensen and Sydow, 1987). However good correlation of up to 95% between plain X-ray and ultrasound can be achieved (Böckmann *et al.*, 1982). A-mode ultrasonography of the maxillary and frontal sinuses appears useful for initial examination and follow up of maxillary sinusitis (Jensen and Sydow, 1987). The improved imaging quality of B-mode ultrasonography allows greater confidence in diagnosis of lesions in the main sinuses as well as accurate assessment of the ethmoid sinuses. Giancoli, Mann and Miller (1992) compared the findings of B-mode ultrasonography with that of CT scanning. Excluding isolated mucous retention cysts and focal minimal mucosal thickening, they found a sensitivity of 100% for lesions within the major sinuses by ultrasound and specificities of 98%, 100% and 94% for the maxillary, frontal and ethmoid sinuses respectively. The discrepency between this and other studies may be related to the use of B-mode scanning and transglobe assessment of the ethmoid sinuses, that allows evaluation of both the anterior and posterior ethmoid. Clearly these assessments are heavily dependent on the equipment and reliant upon skilled performance and interpretation.

Swabs and antral lavage

The difficulty of interpreting nasal swabs as opposed to antral washings is the distinction of a causative pathogen from a commensal organism. This is shown by a review of 12 studies reporting the frequency of bacteria cultured from the nose in normal individuals (Gwaltney and Hayden, 1982). From the nasal vestibule they found 40–100% incidence of *Staphylococcus epidermidis* and *Micrococcus*, 25–40% *Staphylococcus aureus*, 90–100% diphtheroids and 1% Gram-negative bacteria. From the posterior nares, *Streptococcus pneumoniae* was isolated in 15–25%, *Haemophilus influenzae* in 6–40%, *Streptococcus pyogenes* in 6%, *Staphylococcus aureus* in 12%, *Neisseria meningitidis* in 4–27% and Gram-negative bacteria in 13%. If these are regarded as normal commensal flora, one is left in serious doubt as to the usefulness of nasal swab for bacteriology in the treatment of infective rhinosinusitis.

It must be appropriate that any swabs taken from the actively infected nose are carefully taken from the middle meatus to increase the chance that any cultured organism is responsible for the infection and not merely a contaminant. The optimal material for microbiological examination is pus aspirated from the infected sinuses. In acute sinusitis, the results of nasal cultures correlated poorly with those obtained by proof puncture (Axelsson and Brorson, 1973). This information is helpful in directing further antimicrobial therapy particularly in those cases resistant to treatment. The presence of anaerobic organisms is frequently obvious because of the putrid smell of any aspirated pus.

Branhamella catarrhalis is also a common pathogen

especially in children. While *Staphylococcus aureus* is commonly isolated from nasal swabs it is less commonly isolated from the acutely infected sinus. This suggests that *Staphylococcus aureus* is more usually a contaminant rather than a true pathogen. Once the probable causative organisms are identified and their patterns of antibiotic sensitivity are recognized, appropriate antibiotic treatment follows.

Those cases in which no significant growth is found may relate to failure to culture the responsible organism or they may be accounted for by Messerklinger's suggestion that mucosal apposition can lead to ciliary stasis and persistent inflammation (Messerklinger, 1978).

Sinoscopy

Sinoscopy provides the only certain method of providing accurate information about the nature of mucosal changes, the presence of secretions and the state of the natural ostium. Draf (1983), reviewing over 1000 cases in which sinoscopy of the paranasal sinuses was undertaken, concluded that in 20% of cases, it was not possible to ascertain the presence of suppurative maxillary sinusitis by means of X-rays and proof puncture alone. There appears surprisingly poor correlation between X-ray and endoscopic investigation (Draf, 1983; Pfleiderer, Croft and Lloyd, 1986).

As radiological investigations and even proof puncture can be misleading, sinoscopy is advocated as a technique that ensures accurate diagnosis upon which appropriate primary treatment can be recommended. One tangible benefit is the potential for the early detection of antral malignancies. Like proof puncture, however, sinoscopy is unpleasant whether undertaken via the canine fossa or the inferior meatus and is not without hazard. It is unlikely that it will ever be undertaken on a routine basis on all patients presenting with nasal symptoms.

A full history and examination, combined with radiological investigation and careful follow up to monitor response to treatment would appear to give sufficient information in the majority of cases, reserving endoscopy of the sinuses for those cases which are either refractory to treatment or where the former investigations indicate it.

Blood tests

Besides routine investigations such as full blood count with differential white cell count, erythrocyte sedimentation rate, urea and electrolytes, and liver function tests to detect underlying disease predisposing to infection, it is crucial to test immunological host defences (Cole, 1985). This can be done by testing serum for deficiency of IgG, IgA and IgM. In this way, panhypogammaglobulinaemia and selective antibody deficiency (e.g. IgA) will be diagnosed. Rarely, total Ig classes may be normal but subclasses of IgG may be deficient and require treatment (Stanley, Corbo and Cole, 1984).

The role of IgA in the respiratory tract is still much in doubt, although most books tend dogmatically to state its primary role in bacterial disease. Certainly, it has an important antiviral role but its antibacterial effect is not well worked out. Patients with local secretory IgA deficiency can usually be detected by their concomitant deficiency of serum IgA, but it is important to remember that local and systemic systems are distinct and a normal serum IgA does not exclude deficiency or absence of secretory IgA. The latter can be directly tested for in special centres (Stanley and Cole, 1985).

Treatment of acute rhinosinusitis

The treatment of acute sinusitis is primarily medical. Analgesics, antibiotics and decongestant medication reduce oedema and increase clearance and drainage from the sinuses. The appropriate use of these agents in combination will aid the rapid resolution of infection in most patients.

Analgesics

The pain of sinusitis can usually be relieved by aspirin and codeine preparations; it is unusual to have to resort to opiates. Special caution should be taken to ensure that the patient is not allergic to aspirin in view of the association between aspirin intolerance and rhinitis.

It is interesting to note that Mann *et al.* (1981) reported a 79% spontaneous cure after 2 weeks in patients treated with analgesics alone. Indeed, it may be that an accurate choice of antibiotic or selection of adjuvant treatment is relatively unimportant as the majority of maxillary sinusitis will resolve irrespective of treatment (Sydow, Axelsson and Jensen, 1982). Their conclusion was that the therapeutic outcome differs very little among the groups, although those patients treated with nasal decongestants alone (both topical and systemic) appeared to do least well.

Antibiotics

In general, treatment with an appropriate antibiotic for 10 days should suffice for the treatment of acute purulent sinusitis. More commonly the cases referred for specialist opinion are of either a recurrent or chronic nature, in these cases most authorities agree that antibiotic therapy should be given for a minimum of 2 weeks and treatment for 6 weeks or more is sometimes necessary. The predictability of culture studies in acute sinusitis indicates that a routine case of acute sinusitis can be managed without cultures. Treatment failure is uncommon provided the antibiotic chosen is effective against *Streptococcus pneumoniae*, *Haemophilus influenzae* and *Branhamella catarrhalis*. Oral amoxycillin (or if parenteral treatment is given, the less well orally absorbed but cheaper drug ampicillin) should be considered the drug of choice in treating acute sinusitis. It will be effective against *Streptococcus pneumoniae* and the majority of *Haemophilus* species, which are the commonest organisms involved. It will not, however, be effective against *Staphylococcus aureus*, beta-lactamase-producing *Haemophilus influenzae*, some anaerobes and some aerobic Gram-negative rods. Co-amoxiclav (Augmentin) provides the most suitable spectrum for any of the responsible organisms as a single agent. Cephalosporins also achieve good blood levels with an appropriate spectrum, cefuroxime (Zinnat) or cefixime (Suprax), which have efficacy against Gram-negative pathogens are frequently effective. In patients known to be allergic to penicillin, co-trimoxazole (trimethoprim 8 mg plus sulphamethoxazole 400 mg) two tablets, twice daily has been shown to be effective (Hamory et al., 1979). Although tetracyclines have been used in the past, pneumococci and *H. influenzae* are not always sensitive. Azithromycin (Zithromax) is reportedly effective against the three main pathogens of acute sinusitis. Any of these agents is a suitable choice for initial treatment. If the patient fails to respond, antral lavage should be undertaken and the washings sent for aerobic and anaerobic culture.

Sinusitis of dental origin is invariably caused by anaerobic organisms and it is often of mixed flora. The optimum treatment is the combination of amoxycillin (Amoxil) and metronidazole (Flagyl). Appropriate anaerobic activity is also achieved with single agent treatment with co-amoxiclav or clindamycin (Dalacin C).

In addition to the common pathogens, immunocompromised patients are often infected with *Pseudomonas* species and opportunistic organisms. Treatment depends on the causative organism. A narrow spectrum antibiotic chosen on the basis of known sensitivity is to be preferred, as recurrent sepsis is likely. Otherwise opportunistic or resistant organisms will emerge to cause further problems.

Decongestants

Decongestants induce vasoconstriction through alpha adrenergic receptors. The aim is to shrink the mucosa, improve the airway and assist sinus drainage. While there is symptomatic benefit the defence mechanisms are all dependent upon mucosal blood flow, if this is reduced the speed of resolution is unlikely to be helped (Falck, Svanholm and Aust, 1990). Most clinicians favour long-acting preparations such as oxymetazoline and xylometazoline hydrochloride which appear to be effective and have less 'rebound effect' than other topical decongestants. They should not be used for more than a few weeks, lest the patient develop rhinitis medicamentosa. Systemic decongestants do not appear to be as effective as topical preparations (Ånggård and Malm, 1984).

Potential systemic effects of decongestants include urinary retention, elevated blood and ocular pressure, tachycardia and dysrhythmias. They are best avoided in patients with hyperthyroidism, symptomatic prostatic hypertrophy, narrow angle glaucoma, hypertension and ischaemic heart disease. Patients taking monoamine oxidase inhibitors may have an enhanced response to decongestants.

A failure to respond to medical treatment, the presence of severe pain or incipient complications may require operative treatment when lavage is indicated to remove pus, restore ciliary activity and ventilate the sinus. Effective lavage will give the sinus mucosa the opportunity to restore its normal clearance mechanisms. The presence of pus under pressure requires more effective drainage and the appropriate surgical steps are covered in Chapter 12. On occasion repeated sinus lavage using the placement of an indwelling tube is of benefit allowing repeated and frequent irrigation without new punctures (Drettner, 1983).

Treatment of chronic rhinosinusitis

The principles involved in the the management of recurrent or chronic rhinosinusitis are first to attempt to identify and treat the underlying cause and second, if possible, to restore the functional integrity of the inflamed mucosal lining. Restoration of sinus ventilation and correction of mucosal apposition will allow restoration of the mucociliary clearance system. Anatomical obstruction requires operative treatment whereas medical treatment is most appropriate for obstruction resultant upon physiological abnormality.

Therapeutic entities include antibiotics, mucolytics, nasal irrigation, corticosteroids, and anti-allergic therapies when appropriate either individually or in combination. The treatment of underlying factors such as allergy, 'vasomotor instability', immune deficiency and mucociliary dysfunction have been covered under their separate headings and may be usefully combined with the more general strategies below.

Antibiotics

Chronic purulent sinusitis is associated with a much higher frequency of anaerobic organisms. An empirical trial of metronidazole, co-amoxiclav or even clindamycin is warranted by clinical suspicion if previous therapy has not been directed at anaerobic organisms. Persistent symptoms in the presence of infection require culture from nasal swabs or antral washings to direct further treatment. A failure to recognize the responsible organism(s) and treat them appropriately based on antibiotic sensitivity will naturally yield chronic infection. Persistent symptoms in the absence of overt infection may suggest ostial obstruction from other causes than sepsis as indicated above. Recurrent courses of antibiotics alone are certainly unhelpful in treating any primary cause and aiding long-term resolution.

Mucolytics

Characteristically, chronic sinusitis forms thick viscid secretions. Any assistance in reducing viscosity of secretion is helpful aiding sinus drainage and patient comfort. Mucolytic therapy is generally of limited efficacy for rhinosinusitis in common with home remedies such as increased fluid intake, horseradish and chicken soup (Ziment, 1991). Iodides given as drops (saturated solution of potassium iodide or SSKI) or as organic iodides have been documented as effective mucolytics and expectorants in patients with bronchitis. The use of SSKI was based upon anecdotal evidence from its benefit in treating thick pulmonary secretions. Similarly, acetylcysteine and carbocysteine have been used with some symptomatic benefit. Perhaps the most effective mucolytic for sinusitis is guaiphenesin which is a primary expectorant in many cough syrups and is available in liquid and tablet form (Druce, 1990). However, it must be administered in doses that are only just subemetic to be effective.

Nasal toilet

Cleansing of thick nasal and sinus secretions is achieved by saline sprays or irrigations. Specific commercial nasal irrigators are available but the use of a cannula together with a Higginson's syringe is as effective and certainly cheaper. Some symptomatic relief follows the use of moist heat to the face and the inhalation of steam. Commercially marketed facial saunas confer little additional benefit over steam inhalation, a hot shower or the application of a hot towel.

Corticosteroids

Anti-inflammatory drugs are particularly effective at reducing the mucosal swelling associated with the inflammatory response of infection. Systemic corticosteroids may yield undesirable sequelae and their use has been supplanted by topical preparations. It must be emphasized that topical steroids must reach the desired area to be effective. The preliminary use of a decongestant may improve the penetrance of the chosen agent. A topical spray (Dexarhinaspray) containing dexamethasone, neomycin and tramazoline (a decongestant) can be used but caution in its long-term application must be exercised because of the decongestant. Sprays, however, are poorly distributed to the majority of the nasal mucosa and this is

particularly true in the blocked nose where the best distribution is obtained from a pipette (Mygind, 1979). In addition to this, if there is any remaining activity of the mucociliary system, the effect will be to transport the preparations away from the sinuses. Logically, therefore, drops instilled into the nose in the head downwards position would appear to be the most effective way of decongesting the ostia of the sinuses. The head down and backwards position has been advocated by Mygind, but radiological studies and clinical evidence supports the head down and forwards position as shown in Figure 8.11 as the most effective (Charlton *et al.*, 1985; Wilson *et al.*, 1987c). Patients are instructed to instil two drops of betamethasone (Betnesol) into each nostril and remain in the head down and forwards position for 2 minutes, two or three times daily. Interestingly, betamethasone is absorbed and a systemic effect can be expected which may aid its topical effect. The steroid dose is low and when used as two drops each side twice daily, this is estimated as equivalent to 1.15 mg of prednisolone daily (Mackay, 1989). It is important that nasal steroids are continued at recommended doses for at least 2 weeks until a maximum effect is noted. It must be emphasized to the patient that they are not effective when used on an 'as-needed' basis. The duration of therapy depends on

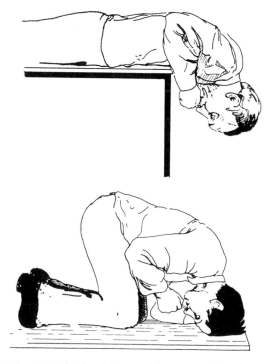

Figure 8.11 The 'head down and forwards position' for instilling intranasal drop medication. (Reproduced from *British Medical Journal*, 1985, **291**, p. 788, with permission)

therapeutic response, other treatments used and the nature of the underlying problem.

All the current nasal steroid preparations share the potential but uncommon side effects of nasal irritation, crusting and bleeding. These may be reduced to a large extent by aqueous propellants. Significant systemic absorption and undesirable side effects may be associated with the prolonged use of topical agents, especially at higher than recommended doses. The margin of safety varies with the agent chosen.

When maximal treatment over a period of 3–4 weeks fails, surgical treatment must be considered. Sinus washout may be helpful in the treatment of acute sinusitis before the mucosa has become too inflamed, but it is unlikely that a single washout will benefit a patient with chronic mucosal changes. The disadvantage of weekly washouts can be overcome by using an indwelling tube which can be used for daily lavage, instillation of medication and aeration. If simple medical treatment fails, it is likely that the problem will be recurrent and it appears more logical to attempt to provide more permanent drainage by surgical means together with any necessary correction of anatomical predisposing factors or the removal of any primary inflammatory focus within the ethmoid sinuses. These issues are described in Chapter 12.

Acute specific infective rhinitis
Acute nasal diphtheria

Definition

An acute infective rhinitis caused by *Corynebacterium diphtheriae*.

Clinical picture

Nasal diphtheria may be primary or secondary to the faucial form. In the latter case it indicates a severe attack. There is often a transient simple rhinitis in the early stage of faucial diphtheria, but no membrane forms and it passes off in a few days.

The acute form differs from the chronic form described later in the short duration, pyrexia and general toxaemia, adenitis and subsequent paralysis. In the UK immunization has practically eliminated diphtheria but the occasional case might arise from immigrants who have not been immunized (see Chronic diphtheritic rhinitis).

Treatment

C. diphtheriae is sensitive to penicillin, and a course of 4 or 5 days' intramuscular and local penicillin should be given in addition to the full doses of the antitoxin intravenously. Antitoxin neutralizes the toxins, while penicillin shortens the disease but does not neutralize the toxins.

There is a tendency for *C. diphtheriae* to persist in the nose for weeks after such an attack. Isolation should be continued until the cultures from three successive daily swabs have been negative.

Acute syphilis

The condition of acute syphilis is discussed under the heading of nasal syphilis.

Erysipelas

In erysipelas of the external nose, the nasal mucous membrane may become secondarily infected by the streptococci from the skin. The infection responds rapidly to penicillin.

Glanders

Acute glanders differs from the chronic form, described below, only in the rapidity of onset and the severity of both local and general manifestations. There is marked fever and prostration, and a pustular rash develops resembling smallpox. The nasal mucosa is greatly swollen, and later ulcers form and may destroy the septum and turbinates. The lymph glands are swollen and inflamed, and may suppurate. Death usually follows within a few weeks.

Diagnosis

Glanders is most likely to be confused with smallpox, typhus fever, erysipelas, impetigo or syphilis.

Anthrax

Primary anthrax of the nose with malignant pustule formation has been described.

Candidiasis (moniliasis)

This subject is discussed below.

Gonorrhoea

Rhinitis caused by infection with *Neisseria gonorrhoeae* is certainly rare. Unlike the conjunctivae the nasal mucous membrane has a high resistance to this infection. One or two doubtful cases of purulent rhinitis in infants have been said to be caused by gonorrhoea, but their authenticity has been doubted. The infection responds to penicillin or to co-trimoxazole (Septrin).

Chronic specific infective rhinitis

There are many forms of chronic rhinitis and not a little confusion has arisen from the fact that the term has been taken by different authorities to include different conditions. In the present section the accent has been laid on 'infection', and the conditions referred to are either the result of, or associated with, the latter.

Atrophic rhinitis

Atrophic rhinitis is a chronic nasal disease characterized by progressive atrophy of the mucosa and underlying bone of the turbinates and the presence of a viscid secretion which rapidly dries and forms crusts which emit a characteristic foul odour sometimes called ozaena (a stench). There is an abnormal patency of the nasal passages.

Aetiology

The aetiology of atrophic rhinitis is still unknown. In the past numerous organisms have been cited as the cause, among which are *Coccobacillus* (Loewenberg, 1894), *Bacillus mucosus* (Abel, 1895), *Coccobacillus foetidus ozaena*, diphtheroid bacilli, and *Klebsiella ozaenae* (Henriksen and Gundersen, 1959). It is true that these organisms may be found in cultures but there is little evidence that they cause the disease.

Other factors which have been regarded as possible causes are chronic sinusitis, excessive surgical destruction of the nasal mucous membrane and syphilis.

Atrophic rhinitis usually commences at puberty and is much more common in females than males; thus it is generally accepted that endocrine imbalance may play a part. Heredity is an important factor and there appears to be a racial influence in that the yellow races, Latin races and American Negroes are relatively susceptible, whereas the incidence is low in natives of equatorial Africa. Poor nutrition is undoubtedly a factor in the development of the condition and Bernat (1965) considered atrophic rhinitis to be an iron-deficiency disease. Recently, immunologists have considered atrophic rhinitis to be an autoimmune disease. Fouad *et al.* (1980) studied cellular immunity in patients with atrophic rhinitis using the leucocyte migration and spontaneous rosette tests *in vitro* and confirmed that there was an altered cellular reactivity or loss of tolerance to nasal tissues, which they considered might be precipitated primarily by virus infection, malnutrition and/or immunodeficiency which trigger a destructive autoimmune process with the release of antigen(s) of nasal mucosa into the circulation.

Pathology

Most authors agree that there are patches of metaplasia from columnar ciliated to squamous epithelium (Figure 8.12), that there is a decrease in the number and size of the compound alveolar glands, and that there are dilated capillaries; but some (Taylor and Young, 1961) were unable to demonstrate endarteritis and periarteritis of the terminal arterioles. It is possible, therefore, that there are two types of atrophic rhinitis:

1 Type 1, characterized by endarteritis and periarteritis of the terminal arterioles, which is the result of chronic infection and which might benefit from the vasodilator effect of oestrogen therapy
2 Type 2, in which there is vasodilatation of the capillaries, which might be made worse with oestrogen therapy.

It seems likely that in the past the majority of cases were of type 1.

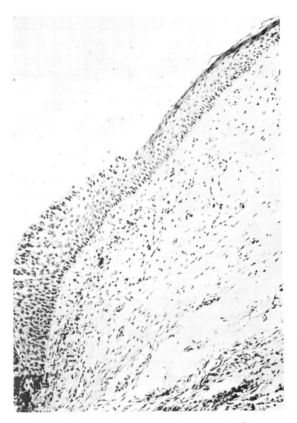

Figure 8.12 The nasal mucous membrane in atrophic rhinitis, showing metaplasia of the epithelium from columnar ciliated to squamous type, and fibrosis of the tunica propria

Taylor and Young (1961) also found that the endothelial cells lining the dilated capillaries had more cytoplasm than normal capillaries and showed a positive reaction for alkaline phosphatase which suggested the presence of active absorption of bone which is a feature of atrophic rhinitis.

Clinical picture

The presenting symptoms are most commonly nasal obstruction and epistaxis. Anosmia may be present and the patients are often only made aware of the loathsome effluvium surrounding them by the reluctance of others to come within their vicinity. Sometimes the symptoms are mainly pharyngeal and are caused by the pharyngitis sicca which often accompanies the condition or by choking when detached crusts slip from the nasopharynx into the oropharynx.

Clinical examination of the morose and dejected patient confirms the presence of fetor in all but the earliest cases and the nasal cavities are found to be lined with green, yellow and black crusts. Even before the removal of the latter the enormous capacity of the nasal passages is apparent and their detachment reveals a bleeding and ulcerated mucosa and shrivelled turbinates.

Investigations

Before embarking on treatment it is advisable to exclude the presence of sepsis in the paranasal sinuses by radiology, and if necessary by proof puncture. Swabs from the nasal secretions may be cultured, but while of interest, the results are unlikely to be of great value in the management of the case. Serological tests to exclude syphilis are essential as syphilis is certainly the most likely condition to be confused with atrophic rhinitis. The blood picture, serum proteins and iron should also be checked.

Treatment

Conservative

In the first place the patient should be instructed to douche the nose twice daily with an alkaline solution prepared by dissolving in 280 ml ($\frac{1}{2}$ pint) warm water a teaspoonful of the following powder: sodium bicarbonate 28.4 g, sodium diborate 28.4 g, sodium chloride 56.7 g.

Regular nasal cleansing is the basis of the conservative treatment in atrophic rhinitis and it may be of some consolation that, if the patient is prepared to carry out this simple treatment with unfailing regularity, freedom from offensive effluvia may almost always be achieved.

Following the removal of crusts by forceps or suction it is customary to apply either 25% glucose in glycerin, which inhibits the proteolytic organs, oestradiol in arachis oil 10 000 units/ml or Kemicetine antiozaena solution (each millilitre containing chloramphenicol 90 mg, oestradiol dipropionate 0.64 mg, vitamin D2 900 IU, propylene glycol). The use of potassium iodide by mouth with the object of increasing nasal secretion has been suggested. Autogenous vaccines may be given. Sinha, Sardana and Rjvanshi, (1977) have reported promising results using tissue therapy with systemic human placental extracts, which gave an 80% improvement in 2 years, and submucosal intranasal injection of human placental extracts which produced 93.3% relief over the same period of time. Qizilbash and Daif (1992) have reported good results in a small trial of treatment with rifampicin 600 mg orally once daily for 12 weeks.

Surgical

Numerous attempts to relieve the condition surgically have been made in the past. These include submucous injections of paraffin, and operations aimed at displacing the lateral nasal walls medially (Lautenslager's operation). More recently Teflon strips, polythene and cartilage have been inserted after flaps of mucoperichondrium were raised from the septum or mucoperiosteum from the floor or lateral walls. Wilson (1964) reported good results from the submucosal injection of a suspension of powdered Teflon in 50% glycerin paste. Chatterji (1980) reported successful results using autogenous medullary (cancellous) bone graft as a single long piece of bone.

Repeated stellate ganglion blocks have been employed with some success by Sharma and Sardana (1966) who advocated cervical sympathectomy or blockade as a possible first line of treatment. Previously, however, autonomic surgery for atrophic rhinitis had proved disappointing.

Encouraging results have been obtained following the closure of one or both nostrils by plastic surgery (Young, 1967). Young's method is to raise folds of skin inside the nostril and suture the folds together with the object of complete interruption of the air flow. After periods varying from months to several years the nostrils have been reopened revealing absence of crusting and normal mucosa. Sinha, Sardana and Rjvanshi (1977) found that bilateral closure was not tolerated by some patients who disliked mouth-breathing and a nasal voice. However, partial nostril closure leaving a 3 mm hole was well tolerated and gave similar results with no recurrence of disease over a 2-year period. Any further increase in size of the hole rapidly decreased their success rate.

Rhinitis sicca

Rhinitis sicca is the term often reserved for a dry, mildly atrophic anterior rhinitis which does not progress to the full clinical picture of atrophic rhinitis described above. The causes are not well defined but it is generally recognized that the condition occurs in alcoholism, anaemia, nutritional and constitutional diseases and in those engaged in dry, hot and dusty occupations.

The pathology resembles that of early atrophic rhinitis; indeed some authorities would not distinguish the two as separate entities. There is deficiency and inactivity of the seromucinous glands, metaplasia of the columnar ciliated epithelium to cuboidal or squamous epithelium and deficiency of the mucous blanket. A penetrating ulcer of the anterior part of the cartilaginous septum may be present.

The patient complains of discomfort, irritation and sometimes epistaxis and crusting but the crusts are thin and dry and do not as a rule extend to the posterior part of the nasal cavities as do the crusts of atrophic rhinitis; neither do they emit a characteristic fetor.

Clinical examination reveals a dry, whitish or glazed mucous membrane sometimes accompanied by crusting or complicated by a septal perforation.

As in atrophic rhinitis the patient should be investigated with a view to excluding nutritional deficiencies or local infection.

In treating the disorder all possible causes should be removed and if necessary iron and vitamins administered. Locally, douching with the solution advocated for the treatment of atrophic rhinitis is undoubtedly of value, but the time-honoured treatment with oily drops and sprays is to be deprecated owing to the danger of inhalation lipoid pneumonia and paraffin granuloma. These sinister conditions have been recognized for a number of years and their pathology is clearly described by Spencer (1985).

Rhinitis caseosa

Rhinitis caseosa (nasal cholesteatoma) is a chronic inflammation of the nose associated with the formation of granulation tissue and an accumulation of offensive cheesy material resembling cholesteatoma.

The condition is rare and is usually unilateral although bilateral involvement has been reported. It is slightly more common in males and can occur at any age. The cause of rhinitis caseosa is unknown but numerous theories have been advanced including those of tubercle, syphilis, cholesteatoma and polyp degeneration. The most widely accepted explanation is the theory of suppurative rhinitis complicated by obstruction where rhinitis caseosa is a secondary condition symptomatic of an underlying primary nasal abnormality (e.g. rhinoliths, deviated nasal septum, inflamed turbinates or polyps) which tends to interfere with the egress of discharge from the nose. There may be coexisting sinus infection.

Microscopical examination of the caseous debris shows keratinous material, numerous organisms and sometimes cholesterol crystals. The lining mucous membrane shows chronic inflammatory changes.

Clinical examination in the early stages merely reveals that one side of the nose is filled with whitish debris but later the bone is invaded, the soft tissues of the face are inflamed and abscesses may form and burst through the skin.

Careful investigation by means of radiology and histological examination is necessary to exclude the presence of coexistent conditions such as sinus infection or malignant disease, and treatment consists of thorough removal of the debris by scooping it out followed by repeated irrigation to ensure its complete removal. Any obstructive lesions should be corrected surgically. Surprisingly perhaps, the prognosis is extremely good provided that care is taken to follow up the patient and deal with any signs of stagnating discharge.

Gangosa

Gangosa (rhinopharyngitis mutilans; gangreangosa; kaninloma) is a slowly progressive ulceration and necrosis of the palate, nose and pharynx. As a disease it appears to be a separate entity but it may be clinically indistinguishable from tertiary yaws (see Yaws); thus there may arise a certain amount of confusion.

The geographical incidence of the specific form is limited to the Pacific Islands, Sri Lanka and equatorial Africa. Gangosa affects males and females of all ages and is associated with dirty and insanitary conditions. It is extremely rare in the white races but has been reported. The cause and mode of spread are unknown; no specific organisms have been found in the tissues or in the discharge.

The disease commences as a small painless nodule in the middle of the palate. This perforates into the nose and spreads intermittently destroying all structures including the nose, palate, orbit and its contents and even the entire face. Pain is absent. The disease may be steadily progressive, or may be arrested at any stage, the resulting scars resembling those of burns. Most cases survive (Arrowsmith, 1921; Myerson, 1933). Serological tests for syphilis are negative and there is no response to antisyphilitic treatment.

Nasal syphilis

Nasal disease secondary to infection with *Treponema pallidum* can occur in every age group from the neonate to the elderly. The disease is no longer common and the signs and symptoms in the early stages may be difficult to elicit, particularly if antibiotics have already been given.

The histological appearances of the syphilitic lesion

are characterized by oedema, and infiltration of the stroma with lymphocytes, plasma cells and endothelial cells. The perivascular cuffing by these cells and the endarteritis reduce the lumen of the blood vessels, and result in necrosis and ulceration.

Primary syphilis

The lesion of primary syphilis (chancre) can appear on the external nose or inside the vestibule. It presents as a hard, non-painful ulcerated papule that is often associated with an enlarged rubbery non-tender node some 3–4 weeks after contact. There may be malaise with a pyrexia. The lesion usually disappears spontaneously in 6–10 weeks. It has to be differentiated from malignant neoplasms and furunculosis. Malignant neoplasms are progressive, and occur in the later age groups. Furunculosis is painful and suppuration follows.

The following will be useful in establishing a diagnosis:

1 Cultures from the surface of the lesion will be negative
2 Smears examined by dark-ground illumination or after staining should show the spirochaete, *Treponema pallidum*
3 Serological tests for syphilis may be positive, except in the earliest cases, or in those cases already having antibiotics; serological tests in current use include: (a) Venereal Disease Reference Laboratory (VDRL) titres; (b) *Treponema pallidum* haemagglutination test (TPHA); (c) fluorescent treponemal antibody test (FTA-ABS)
4 A biopsy may be performed in doubtful cases; the microscopical appearances are characteristic.

Owing to its rarity and the fact that the chancre does not present a typical appearance, the diagnosis is often overlooked and may not be suggested until secondary manifestations are seen. The hardness and painless nature of the nodule, with early and great enlargement of the lymphatic glands, should suggest the diagnosis.

General antisyphilitic treatment with intramuscular penicillin, should be given at once, and the chancre may be cleansed with 1:2000 solution of perchloride of mercury and the surface smeared with 2% yellow mercuric oxide ointment.

Secondary syphilis

The secondary stage of syphilis is the most infectious and symptoms appear 6–10 weeks after inoculation. The most common manifestation is a simple catarrhal rhinitis. Clinically this does not show any special characteristic, except in its persistence. There may be crusting and fissuring of the nasal vestibule.

Secondary syphilis is rarely recognized in the nose, as mucous patches hardly ever occur on such a thin attenuated mucous membrane. The diagnosis is usually suggested by the appearance of other secondary lesions, particularly the development of mucous patches in the pharynx, roseolar or papular rashes, pyrexia and the shotty enlargement of many lymph nodes. The scar of the primary lesion may be visible. Serological tests for syphilis are positive. The response to antisyphilitic treatment is so rapid as to be of diagnostic value.

The condition responds to general antisyphilitic treatment.

Tertiary syphilis

This is the stage most commonly encountered in the nose. The pathological lesion is the gumma, invading mucous membrane, periosteum or bone. The bony portion of the septum is the site most commonly attacked. More rarely the lateral nasal wall, frontal sinus, nasal bones or floor of the nose are invaded. Pain and headache (which is always worse at night), swelling and obstruction are the early symptoms. The swelling may be diffuse or localized, and offensive discharge, bleeding and crusting follow, but the pain is then relieved. The olfactory acuity diminishes. In neglected cases perforation of the affected nasal wall, and collapse of the bony support of the nose may occur. Ultimately there may be severe scarring and secondary atrophic rhinitis.

The earliest stage of simple swelling is not often seen. Later there is a diffuse or localized submucosal swelling and infiltration. The surface is red, and may be nodular. The lesion is usually unilateral but, if the septum is involved, the swelling is seen on both sides. Tenderness of the nasal bridge is a characteristic sign. As a rule, when first seen, ulceration has already taken place, and a putrid-smelling discharge is escaping from the crusted surface. The crusts should be removed, and bare bone may be felt with a probe. The margins of the ulcers are irregular, overhanging and indurated.

The following are special aids to diagnosis:

1 There is no shrinkage with vasoconstrictors
2 Radiographs show rarefaction of bone, with blurring of the cortical outline
3 Serological tests for syphilis are positive in 90% of cases
4 Biopsy shows the typical syphilitic histological appearances.

This stage has the following complications and sequelae:

1 Secondary infection with pyogenic organisms
2 Sequestration
3 Perforation of the septum, palate or nasal walls
4 Collapse of the nasal bridge, and deformity of the face
5 Scarring and stenosis of the nasal passages

6 Atrophic rhinitis
7 Intracranial complications from involvement of the meninges.

Differential diagnosis

A gumma should be suspected when there is a firm reddened nodular swelling of the bony portion of the septum or nasal wall, with obstruction, nocturnal pain and tenderness of the nasal bridge. Ulceration, fetor and necrosis of bone practically confirm the diagnosis. Serological tests for syphilis are positive. Other blood changes are absent, and the response to treatment is rapid. In all cases of doubt a biopsy should be performed, as the histological appearances in syphilis and in all the conditions given below are characteristic.

Yaws differs from syphilis only in its origin in tropical countries, the onset in childhood by extragenital infection, and the gross skin lesions. Serological tests for syphilis are usually positive and the lesions respond to antisyphilitic treatment.

Lupus vulgaris affects mainly the anterior cartilaginous portion of the septum and anterior ends of the turbinates. There may be associated nodules in the skin. Apple-jelly nodules may be seen, and there is no special odour.

In *tuberculosis* the course is rapid, and the skin is not affected. Typical signs of tuberculosis may be present in the lungs.

Sarcoid resembles tuberculosis, but does not caseate; nodules appear in the skin and other organs. There is anergy to tuberculin, and the Kveim–Siltzbach skin test is usually positive.

In *atrophic rhinitis* the fetor is characteristically offensive and nauseating. The mucosa does not ulcerate deeply, and there is no bone necrosis.

Leprosy occurs only in certain countries, is painless and develops very slowly. Nodules may be present in the skin, and deformity is severe in the late stages. Areas of anaesthesia may be present. *Mycobacillus leprae* may be seen in the discharge.

Scleroma occurs in patients of Central European, Asian, American and African origin. It is slow, painless and does not ulcerate. Stenosis and adhesions are characteristic. Associated lesions are found in the nasopharynx and larynx.

Chronic glanders closely resembles tertiary syphilis, but there is an intermittent pyrexia, and *Burkholderia mallei* may be cultured from the discharge.

Leishmaniasis occurs chiefly in South American countries. It commences as a nodule on the septum, which spreads slowly, destroying cartilage, but not bone. It is followed by fibrosis, and scarring. The histology is characteristic, and the Leishman–Donovan bodies can be identified. Response to tartar emetic is rapid.

Benign neoplasms grow slowly, and are painless. Ulceration and bleeding are rare, except in angioma.

A *malignant neoplasm* is at first unilateral. It grows steadily and ulcerates superficially, and the surface is hard and friable, and bleeds readily on probing. Radiographs show invasion and destruction of bone.

A sequestrum must be distinguished from a foreign body or a rhinolith by probing. The first is always attached deeply at some point, the second and third can always be moved, if only to a slight extent. When bone necrosis is present, only the silent form of osteomyelitis requires to be excluded. In this the swelling is more diffuse; it is associated with sinusitis, there are general signs of infection and a leucocytosis. Radiographs show the typical worm-eaten appearance of the bone.

A septal perforation caused by a gumma is situated posteriorly on the vomer or ethmoid. When due to rhinitis sicca, trauma, lupus vulgaris, leprosy or chrome ulceration it affects the anterior cartilaginous portion.

Treatment

General treatment

General antisyphilitic treatment is given.

Local treatment

The nasal passages must be cleared of crusts and discharge by copious alkaline douches every morning, and repeated if necessary two to three times a day. Dilute mercuric nitrate ointment should be applied freely to the nasal vestibules.

Sequestra should be removed with great care. The free portion may be removed piecemeal but any firmly attached portion should be allowed to separate naturally, as avulsion may cause severe haemorrhage or damage adjacent tissues. Gummas respond rapidly to general antisyphilitic treatment, but atrophic rhinitis and deformity may persist after the disease is cured.

Perforations of the palate and deformities of the face may be repaired by reconstructive surgery.

Hereditary or congenital syphilis

In congenital syphilis, any of the lesions described under the secondary and tertiary forms of syphilis of the nose may occur.

In the infant, 'snuffles' is the most common lesion. This begins about the third week of life, but may appear as late as 3 months after birth. At first it appears as a simple catarrhal rhinitis. In a short time it becomes purulent, with secondary fissuring and excoriation of the nasal vestibule and upper lip. The obstruction may be so severe as to interfere seriously with suckling and nutrition.

Gummatous and destructive lesions occur most commonly at puberty in the 'latent' form of the disease. Mucous membrane, periosteum and bone may all be affected. The resulting ulceration and destruction lead ultimately to atrophy of the mucous membrane, secondary atrophic rhinitis and sinking of the nasal bridge, producing the saddle-nose deformity. Serological tests for syphilis of the patient and parent are positive; biopsy shows the characteristic syphilitic histological picture.

There may be a prenatal and family history of syphilis, miscarriages or stillbirths. Snuffles should be suspected when a severe rhinitis with excoriation of the nares develops about the third week of life, and interferes with suckling. A common cold infection at this age may often produce a severe rhinitis, but there is usually a definite history of exposure to infection; serological tests for syphilis are negative, and cultures may show virulent pyogenic organisms. When obstruction dominates the picture congenital atresia of the choanae or adenoid hypertrophy must be excluded by sounding the nasal passages with a soft catheter.

In the tertiary form, the diagnosis rests on the presence of other stigmata, particularly Hutchinson's incisors and Moon's molars, interstitial keratitis, corneal opacities, sensorineural deafness and the serological reactions.

Treatment

In snuffles the airway must be restored for suckling. The discharge is removed by gentle suction and irrigation and drops of 0.5% ephedrine in normal saline solution should be inserted into the nose, with the head hyperextended, before feeding.

In the tertiary forms simple nasal toilet by syringing with isotonic alkaline douche solution will remove the crusts and discharge, and yellow mercuric oxide ointment may be applied frequently to the nasal vestibules.

In both forms antisyphilitic treatment is essential and rapidly arrests the disease, but the destruction and deformity remain.

Tuberculosis

Tuberculosis of the nose is very rare. It may be nodular or ulcerative. It affects the cartilaginous portion of the nasal septum, and has been reported on the lateral nasal wall. It may be primary but is usually secondary to tuberculosis of the lungs.

The symptoms are discharge, slight pain and partial obstruction. On examination a bright red nodular thickening, with or without ulceration, is seen on the septum. Tuberculosis follows a relatively rapid course, and ulceration leads to perforation of the septum.

Bacteriological examination of the discharge shows tubercle bacilli, and biopsy will confirm the typical appearance of tuberculosis.

Nasal douches may be used to remove the discharge and crusts. Treatment is with antituberculous drugs (rifampicin, ethambutol, isoniazid, pyrazinamide, streptomycin, PAS) in a planned schedule for at least 6 months.

Lupus vulgaris

Lupus vulgaris is an indolent and chronic form of tuberculous infection which affects the skin and mucous membrane.

It is twice as common in women as in men, and is developed most often in early adult life. It is a disease mainly of northern climates and is rare in the tropics. The mucocutaneous junction of the nasal septum is the most common site of inoculation as this is frequently exposed to trauma in patients who have the habit of picking the nose. The nasal lesion is frequently associated with, or a precursor of, nodules on the face.

Sections of tissue show the characteristic appearance of a tuberculous granuloma. In the centre, at first, there is a collection of reticuloendothelial cells which soon necrose and coalesce. Around this necrotic centre there is a ring of living reticuloendothelial cells, and around this ring are lymphocytes, plasma cells and fibroblasts, giant cells scattered throughout the tubercle are found with a peripheral arrangement of nuclei (Figure 8.13).

The early symptoms are those of nasal discharge and obstruction followed by crusting and occasional epistaxis. When the ulceration is established there may be slight fetor and soreness. Ulceration may be followed by fibrosis and contraction, with distortion of the alae nasi. When the turbinates are extensively involved the ciliated epithelium is not renewed and atrophic rhinitis may develop.

The course is very slow, and may last for a life time with periods of regression and healing, alternating with periods of active extension, depending to a great extent on the general health of the patient.

The typical early lesion is a reddish firm nodule at the mucocutaneous junction of the nasal septum. In more advanced cases, there may be extensive involvement of the floor of the nose and the turbinates, spreading backwards from the primary site. The surface shows superficial ulcers and crusts. The septum may perforate, but only in the cartilaginous portion, and there is no sinking of the nasal bridge.

If the disease spreads forwards there may be external scarring and distortion of the nasal vestibule, tip and alae nasi, and nodules may be seen in the skin of the face.

Blanching, bacterial examination and biopsy are of use in diagnosis:

1 To show apple-jelly nodules, the blood is expressed from adjoining tissues by pressure with a glass

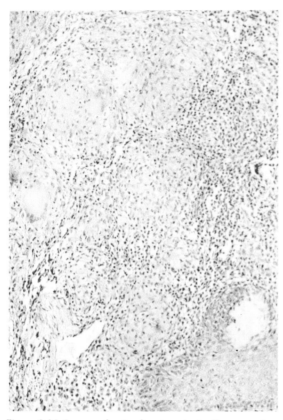

Figure 8.13 Lupus vulgaris, showing giant cells, zones of reticuloendothelial cells, lymphocytes, plasma cells and fibroblasts (× 200)

slide on the skin, or shrinkage with cocaine and adrenalin on the mucous membrane, thus making the pinkish lupus nodules more evident by contrast

2 Bacteriological examination of the discharge may show tubercle bacilli

3 Biopsy will confirm the typical histological picture. For differential diagnosis, see above under tertiary syphilis.

Complications

1 Pulmonary tuberculosis develops in a small proportion of cases

2 Dacryocystitis, corneal ulceration, nasopharyngeal lupus, and lupus of the face may occur

3 Atrophic rhinitis may be a sequel

4 Epithelioma may develop in the infected tissue.

Sudden increase in size and hardness of one area and, in the elderly patient, an increased tendency to bleed should arouse the suspicion that a malignant change has supervened. A biopsy should be taken, and the tissue examined histologically.

Treatment consists of specific antitubercular therapy and calciferol (vitamin D2) 150 000 units daily for 6–9 months. Surgical repair of any residual nasal deformities may be required when the disease has been arrested.

Sarcoidosis (Boeck's sarcoid)

Sarcoidosis is a chronic systemic disease of unknown cause which clinically may involve any organ with a non-caseating granulomatous inflammation closely resembling tuberculosis without caseation. The tubercle consists of a collection of pale-staining epithelioid cells, sometimes surrounded by a thin layer of lymphocytes. Giant cells are present and, in older lesions, contain asteroid intracytoplasmic inclusion bodies which stain with haematoxylin (Schaumann bodies). This histological picture is not, however, specific for sarcoidosis as it may be seen in other granulomas, e.g tuberculosis, leprosy or berylliosis. Before confirming the diagnosis it is therefore important to exclude these other causes.

Nasal sarcoidosis was first described by Boeck (1905), and confirmed by biopsy by Kistner and Robertson (1938).

Aetiology

Two hypotheses have been advanced (Gordon *et al.*, 1976):

1 That sarcoid is a special form of tuberculosis which is the result of an altered bacillus with an atypical host response. Tuberculosis is known to precede, occur with or follow clinical sarcoidosis. However, tubercle bacilli have been reported in only a few cases.

2 That an unidentified organism or agent is responsible, e.g. pine pollen, wood dust, beryllium and silica or tubercle bacilli, *M. leprae*, a protozoon, virus or fungus.

Incidence

Sarcoidosis occurs all over the world but is more prevalent in rural south-eastern USA and Scandinavian countries. Coloured races are more affected than white, and woman more than men. Nasal sarcoidosis occurs in 3–20% of systemic cases. The median age of onset is 25 years, and 50% of cases occur below the age of 30 years.

Clinical picture

Presenting symptoms include nasal discharge which ranges from serosanguineous to mucopurulent, nasal obstruction and epistaxis, facial pain and dryness.

There may be a secondary sinusitis, a result of super-added infection or involvement by the disease. Nasal skin and bone lesions are asymptomatic. There may be a general swelling of the bridge of the nose with discoloration of the overlying skin (Munro Black, 1966).

Examination of the nasal mucosa may reveal tiny, 1 mm, yellow nodules surrounded by hyperaemic boggy granular mucosa. Alternatively the mucosa may be dry, ulcerated and covered with crusts. The anterior septum and inferior turbinates are the most commonly involved areas and adhesions may develop between them, resulting in stenosis of the anterior nares. Septal perforations may arise spontaneously or may occur following septal surgery in the unrecognized case. Nasal skin lesions appear as elevated, yellowish, dry, scaling discrete nodules or plaques. These may coalesce to form large bluish-red granulomas, separated by normal skin, over the tip, alae, columella or dorsum. Violaceous, diffuse bulbous affliction of the nasal tip area in conjunction with other skin and pulmonary lesions was separately described by Besmer in 1889 as *Lupus pernio* (Gordon *et al.*, 1976) and is a manifestation of chronic multi-system sarcoidosis (James, 1959). Weiss (1960) believed that skin and mucosal lesions are completely separate independent lesions.

Nasal lesions may be associated with other lesions in the head and neck which may include tonsil, tongue, salivary glands, lacrimal glands, bronchial mucosa, paranasal sinuses, nasopharynx, or larynx. Heerfordt's syndrome describes a transient bilateral facial palsy associated with fever, parotid enlargement and uveal tract disease.

Diagnosis

The nasal mucous membrane, particularly in the region of the anterior septum and inferior turbinates, can be easily biopsied and will produce valuable diagnostic material. The histological picture is described above. Culture and stains for acid-fast bacilli and fungi should be negative. There is usually an anergy to the tuberculin skin test, but pulmonary tuberculosis develops during the course of the disease in 10% of cases and tuberculin hypersensitivity then develops. The Kveim–Siltzbach skin test (in which a subcutaneous injection of a suspension from a lesion in another case is followed by the development of a sarcoid nodule) is usually positive in all mucosal cases, and in 75% of patients with active sarcoidosis. It is an invaluable aid in the differential diagnosis of granulomas of the nose.

The radiographic changes in cases of involvement of the nasal bones are characteristic and consist of cystic, punched-out lesions with thinning of the cortex of the bone and a reticular pattern in the medulla (Curtis, 1964). Hilar node involvement is shown in radiographs of the chest, and bone cysts are seen in radiographs of the hands and feet.

Serum and urinary calcium levels should be measured to exclude hypercalcaemia. Serum immunoglobulin, particularly IgG, and the erythrocyte sedimentation rate (ESR) may be raised and a mild anaemia, leucocytopenia and eosinophilia may be present. The serum levels of serum angiotensin-I-converting enzyme, which is secreted by the epithelioid cell granuloma, are elevated in about 60% of patients with active sarcoidosis (Studdy *et al.*, 1978).

Differential diagnosis

The differential diagnosis includes:

1 Chronic irritation and foreign body reaction, as in berylliosis
2 Infectious conditions, such as tuberculosis, actinomycosis, rhinosporidiosis, leprosy, syphilis, glanders, histoplasmosis and blastomycosis
3 Other granulomatous conditions such as Wegener's granulomatosis
4 Acquired immune deficiency syndrome (AIDS) may present with a similar granulomatous condition in the nose.

Treatment

There is no specific therapy. Steroids may be used locally or systemically. Local depot steroids (McKelvie, Gresson and Pokhrel, 1968) produce a marked decrease in the size of mucosal lesions, but there is little reduction in the size of lesions in patients with systemic disease. Topical steroid nasal drops are beneficial. Atrophic rhinitis may develop as a result of the disease or secondary to depot steroids. In a series of 53 patients with sarcoidosis of the upper respiratory tract, James *et al.* (1982) found systemic steroids were necessary in 46% of the patients. When steroids alone are insufficient in the management of chronic fibrotic sarcoidosis they can be combined with either chloroquine (adult oral dose of 250 mg on alternate days for about 9 months) or methotrexate (adult oral dose of 5 mg, once weekly for a course of 3 months). The long-term use of chloroquine carries the risk of occasional development of irreversible retinal damage. Cutaneous lesions may be excised and skin grafted (Golding, Jawad and Reid, 1983).

Chronic diphtheritic rhinitis

Chronic diphtheritic rhinitis (fibrinous rhinitis) is an inflammation of the nasal mucous membrane, caused by *Corynebacterium diphtheriae*. Diphtheria is now extremely rare in the UK. More commonly a fibrinous rhinitis may be caused by the pneumococcus, staphylococci or streptococci and is seen very occasionally in debilitated children.

All the changes of a severe chronic inflammation are seen and on the surface there is extensive necrosis and defoliation of the epithelium. The area is covered with a membrane of fibrin and entangled cells. The fibres of fibrin extend deeply into the submucosa and this accounts for the tenacity of its adhesion, and for the bleeding when the membrane is removed. The corynebacteria and pneumococci cause the formation of an adherent membrane, but staphylococci and streptococci produce only a superficial membrane which can be stripped off easily.

The local symptoms are obstruction and discharge which is watery at first and later becomes blood-stained and mucopurulent. The course of the disease is slow, and may go on for 3 months, ending in spontaneous recovery. Paralysis, toxaemia and other general symptoms are absent.

The anterior nares may be excoriated by the acrid discharge. The nasal mucosa is generally congested and swollen, and the inferior turbinates, floor of the nose and sometimes the septum are covered with a greyish adherent membrane. After removing this a raw bleeding surface remains.

Bacteriological examination of the nasal discharge should never be omitted, and if *C. diphtheriae* is present the organism should be tested for virulence.

Treatment consists of systemic antibiotics, usually parenteral penicillin and nasal toilet. Systemic antitoxin is unnecessary but, in the past, local application of antitoxin has been found beneficial. In all cases the patient should be isolated until nose swabs are negative.

Rhinoscleroma

Rhinoscleroma, or scleroma, is a progressive granulomatous disease commencing in the nose and eventually extending into the nasopharynx and oropharynx, the larynx and sometimes the trachea and bronchi (Friedmann, 1966).

Scleroma may occur at any age and in either sex. It is seen mainly in central and south-eastern Europe, North Africa, Pakistan and Indonesia, Central and South America. It may be seen anywhere in the world and people of any race may be affected. There is, in most patients, one common factor – a poor standard of domestic hygiene.

Pathology

Although there is still controversy over the precise pathogenesis of scleroma it is now generally agreed that the causative organism is the Gram-negative Frisch bacillus (*Klebsiella rhinoscleromatis*). That this organism was a secondary invader following an initial filterable virus infection is disputed by the work of Fisher and Dimling (1964) who failed to reveal virus-like particles or inclusion bodies on electron

microscopy. Steffen and Smith (1961) successfully recovered the organism from the lungs of mice previously inoculated with *K. rhinoscleromatis*, and Sinha, Pandhi and Prakash (1969) isolated it from 60% of their cases. A complement fixation test based on the reaction of the patient's serum with suspensions of *K. rhinoscleromatis* was described by Levine (1951) and re-evaluated by Toppozada *et al.* (1983). They found a high titre of antibodies in the serum of patients with rhinoscleroma indicating that humoral immunity was not impaired. Although they recognized that cross-reactions could occur, they concluded that the complement fixation test was valuable in the diagnosis of early unrecognized cases of rhinoscleroma.

Histologically (Figure 8.14) granulomatous tissue infiltrates the submucosa and is characterized by the presence of an accumulation of plasma cells, lymphocytes and eosinophils among which are scattered large foam cells (Mikulicz cells), which have a central nucleus and a vacuolated cytoplasm containing Frisch bacilli (Figure 8.15) and Russell bodies, the latter resembling plasma cells and having an eccentric nucleus and deep eosin-staining cytoplasm.

Friedmann (1963), in an electron microscope study, observed the transformation of plasma cells into Russell bodies. Further ultrastructural work by Toppozada *et al.* (1981) has demonstrated the different stages of distension of the rough endoplasmic reticulum up to the formation of Russell bodies inside the 'reactive' plasma cell, thus supporting the theory of an intracellular formation of Russell bodies. The histochemical studies of Gonzalez-Angulo *et al.* (1965) indicated a high content of mucopolysaccharides around the walls of the *Klebsiella* and inferred that this may be responsible for the protection of the organism against both antibiotic therapy and the patient's own antibodies.

Clinical picture

There are three recognized stages of this chronic and progressive disease:

1 *The atrophic stage.* Changes occur in the mucous membrane of the floor of the nose, septum or turbinates which resemble atrophic rhinitis, with crust formation and foul-smelling discharge (Figure 8.16)
2 *Granulation or nodular stage.* Non-ulcerative nodules develop which at first are bluish-red and rubbery and later become paler and harder
3 *Cicatrizing stage.* Adhesions and stenosis distort the normal anatomy. The coarsening of the external nose has been called a 'tapir' nose. The disease may extend to the maxillary sinus (Mossallam and Attia, 1956; Yasmin and Safwat, 1966), the lacrimal sac (Badraway, 1962), the nasopharynx, hard palate, trachea and main bronchi. Spread to

Mikulicz cell

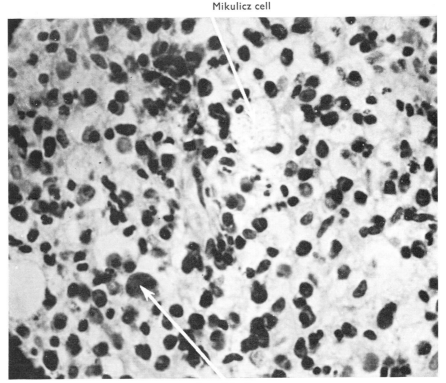

Russell body

Figure 8.14 Scleroma showing infiltration with plasma cells, lymphocytes, eosinophils, Russell bodies and Mikulicz cells (× 800)

lymph nodes has been reported but is extremely uncommon and is thought to be prevented by early fibrous tissue deposition blocking the lymphatics (Badraway and El-Shennawy, 1974). Bone may be extensively involved (Badraway, 1966). Malignant change is uncommon but can occur (Yasmin and Safwat, 1966).

Treatment

Once the diagnosis has been confirmed by biopsy, treatment must be intense and prolonged in order to eradicate the disease completely. Bactericidal antibiotics in large doses are given for a minimum of 4–6 weeks and are continued until two consecutive cultures from biopsy material are proved to be negative (Ssali, 1975). In practice, the most effective antibiotics are streptomycin and tetracyline but Riad (1982) has shown that rifampicin in a daily dose of 450 mg for 6 weeks gives good results in the treatment of both the atrophic and granulomatous stages. Gamea (1988) reported the successful use of local rifampicin. Based on an observation by Rizk (1977) that acriflavine solution *in vitro* killed *K. rhinoscleromatosis*, Shaer *et al.* (1981) treated 50 patients suffering from rhinoscleroma with local applications of differing concentrations of acriflavine solution over an 8-week period. The 2% solution produced a complete cure of the disease in all its stages after 8 weeks, whereas the 5% concentration caused recurrent epistaxis, vestibulitis and an occasional septal perforation, and the 1% solution failed to cure all cases.

Chemotherapy may be combined with surgery to re-establish the airway without causing further atrophic changes. This is most effectively achieved by discrete removal of granulations and dilatation of the airways combined with the insertion of polythene tubes for 6–8 weeks (Ssali, 1975). Various forms of cautery and laser treatment have been recommended. Irradiation to a total dose of 3000–3500 cGy over 3 weeks destroys scleroma organisms (Toppozada and Gaafer, 1986).

In late cases where the disease has been eradicated plastic reconstructive surgery may be required.

Leprosy

Leprosy is a chronic granulomatous disease caused by *Mycobacterium leprae*, an acid-fast bacillus morphologically similar to *M. tuberculosis*. Although *M. leprae* cannot yet be cultured on an artificial medium it can, nevertheless, be inoculated into experimental animals, particularly immunologically deficient mice

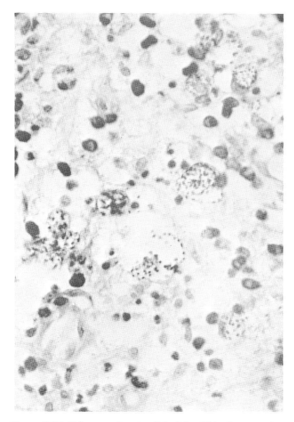

Figure 8.15 Scleroma showing Frisch bacilli in the vacuoles of the Mikulicz cells (× 800)

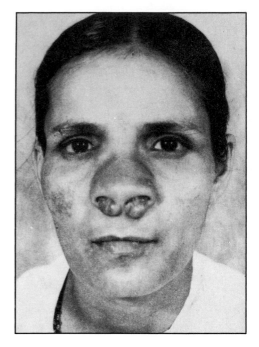

Figure 8.16 A case of rhinoscleroma. (Reproduced by courtesy of Dr Rege, Bombay)

(Rees, 1966), to produce a disease similar to that in man. Worldwide, 12–15 million people suffer from some form of this disease which is particularly prevalent in India, Central Africa, and Central and South America.

Three main types of leprosy are recognized (Barton and Davey, 1976):

1 *Tuberculoid leprosy* in which solitary lesions cause anaesthetic cutaneous patches with involvement of one or more related sensory or motor nerves with possible paralysis of muscles. Cutaneous patches may extend as far as the nasal vestibule but nasal mucosa is not involved bacteriologically or histologically. Isolated cranial nerve palsies (e.g. Vth and VIIth) may occur.

2 *Lepromatous leprosy* in which there is diffuse infiltration of skin, nerves and mucosal surfaces. *M. leprae* favours an environment where the temperature is lower than central (core) temperature. Thus cutaneous infiltration on the face is most apparent on the edges of the pinna, chin, nose and brow. Nasal mucosal involvement occurs early in the disease process and is present in 97% of patients

with lepromatous leprosy (Barton *et al.*, 1973). The nasal discharge in these patients, who frequently have minimal systemic signs, contains millions of potentially infectious bacilli and therefore suggests that this is the principal route of spread of infection. Most commonly there is crust formation, nasal obstruction and blood-stained discharge. Hyposmia may be demonstrated in over 40% of patients with lepromatous leprosy (Barton, 1974).

3 *Borderline leprosy.* The first two types are probably immunologically stable. Patients with borderline leprosy with poor resistance may develop the lepromatous type or less commonly, as the disease is modified by treatment or as immunity is acquired, the tuberculoid type. Skin lesions are more numerous than in tuberculoid leprosy and are frequently seen around the eyes, nose and mouth. In pure borderline leprosy there is no involvement of the mucous membranes of the nose, mouth, pharynx or larynx. A conversion to the lepromatous type is indicated by the appearance of mucosal involvement.

Clinical picture

With lepromatous leprosy the earliest sign is a nodular thickening of the nasal mucosa which appears paler than normal and often has a yellowish tinge. These isolated nodules most commonly first involve the anterior end of the inferior turbinate. The disease progresses to gross inflammation of the nasal mucosa and severe obstruction and is out of proportion to the almost imperceptible clinical changes of lepromatous leprosy elsewhere in the body. Perforation of the cartilaginous portion of the nasal septum is followed by perichondritis and periostitis of the nasal cartilages, inferior turbinates and anterior nasal spine which leads to the typical nasal deformity. Atrophic rhinitis, fibrotic atresia or stenosis of the airway are typical sequelae (Figure 8.17).

McDougall *et al.* (1974) have made an extensive histological study of biopsies of nasal mucosa in patients suffering from leprosy. They found no bacilli or evidence of leprosy infection in the septum and turbinates of borderline cases. However, in lepromatous leprosy bacilli were found in macrophages, fibroblasts, within the cytoplasm of endothelial cells of blood vessels and lymphatics and within the free lumina of secretory gland acini (Figure 8.18).

Diagnosis

Diagnosis of early and intermediate changes in the nose, pathognomonic of lepromatous leprosy, can often be made in the absence of other manifestations of the disease. The presence of atrophic rhinitis and septal perforations is indicative of late disease with other systemic manifestations (Barton, 1976).

Early diagnosis is essential as the nasal component of the infection results in a highly bacilliferous nasal

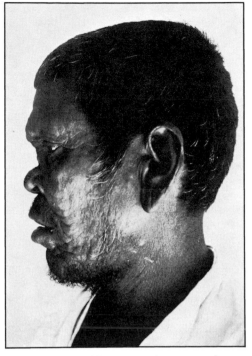

Figure 8.17 Advanced lepromatous leprosy: nasal deformity. (Reproduced by courtesy of Mr R. P. E. Barton, FRCS and the Editor, *Journal of Laryngology and Otology*)

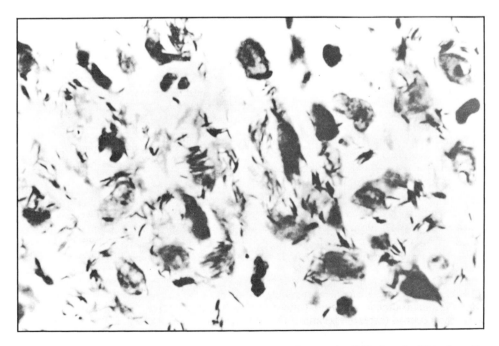

Figure 8.18 From the anterior end of the middle turbinate. Numerous oil immersion fields show bacilli in the mid submucosa with a very high percentage of solid staining forms. The host cell is the macrophage (× 3750). (Reproduced by courtesy of Dr A. C. McDougall and the Editor, *Journal of Pathology*)

discharge which is the principal route of transmission of the disease (Davey and Rees, 1974). Confirmation is by microscopy of the nasal discharge for acid-fast bacilli, microscopy of scrapings of the nasal mucosa (the most positive site being the anterior end of the inferior turbinate) for acid-fast bacilli, and histology of the nasal mucosa. Radiographs of the anterior nasal spine frequently show erosion (Møller–Christensen, Bakke and Melsom, 1952) and in a study of sinus radiographs the most constant finding was mucosal thickening of the maxillary antra on the occipitomental view (Barton, 1979).

It should always be remembered that, with the current patterns of migration, cases of leprosy may be seen in countries where it is no longer endemic (Barton and Davey, 1976).

Treatment

Dapsone remains the standard drug in the treatment of leprosy and will reduce the bacterial count of nasal discharge to zero or near zero within 2 months; however, there are increasing reports of dapsone resistance. The more expensive drugs, rifampicin (Rifadin) and clofazimine (Lamprene), act more rapidly and reduce the count to zero in 10 days; however, their cost precludes their general usage in developing countries. Triple therapy if available reduces the relapse rate and helps to prevent the emergence of drug resistance. The usual regimen is rifampicin 600 mg on the first 2 days of each month, taken before breakfast, clofazimine 100 mg on alternate days 3 times in a week and dapsone 100 mg daily. Local treatment to the nose will help to prevent the external deformity of advanced lepromatous leprosy. Betnovate (one part) in Unguentum (two parts) has been used with good results. In cases of late involvement when the nasal septum has been perforated and atrophic rhinitis is established, careful crust removal is important. The crusts may be softened with a solution of sodium bicarbonate, sodium borate and sodium fluoride 15 g each, dissolved in 500 ml of warm water. After removal of the crusts, the nasal cavities can be painted with a suitable ointment such as Vaseline 1 kg, glycerin 200 g, Vioform 300 g, and crystal violet 5 g (Barton, 1985).

Yaws

Yaws (framboesia) is a disease closely resembling syphilis, if not identical with it, and occurs only in natives of the tropics. It is widespread in Central Africa, Jamaica and the Philippines. The causative organism is *Treponema pertenue*, which is indistinguishable morphologically from *T. pallidum*. Transmission of the disease is by direct contact, which is usually extragenital. There is a high incidence in infancy and childhood.

Clinical picture

Primary, secondary and tertiary stages occur as in syphilis. Characteristically yaws affects principally the skin and only rarely the mucous membranes except at the mucocutaneous junctions. Nasal lesions are very rare and do not differ in appearance from those of syphilis. When very extensive and advanced there may be complete destruction of the nose and palate, involving the whole maxilla, face and pharynx. Clinically this is indistinguishable from true gangosa (Figure 8.19) but in yaws the serological tests for syphilis are positive, and the lesions respond to antisyphilitic treatment.

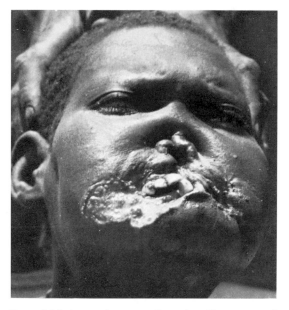

Figure 8.19 A case of gangosa. (Reproduced by courtesy of Professor T. F. Hewer)

Another special form is designated 'goundou'. In this there is a chronic osteitis, forming bilateral rounded swellings of the nasal processes of the maxillae, which may encroach on the orbits and destroy the eyes. In the early months there is pain and serosanguineous nasal discharge.

The lesions in the nose are indistinguishable from syphilis. Some authorities consider that the two diseases are identical, but that their manifestations differ in natives of certain areas of the tropics. Differentiation from syphilis is made on the country of origin, the onset in childhood by extragenital infection, the gross skin lesions, and the fact that it is never congenital and that it does not cause quaternary lesions in the nervous system.

Treatment

The lesions respond rapidly to treatment with a single large dose of long-acting penicillin. Attention must be paid to general nourishment and hygiene. Cosmetic deformities may require surgical correction.

Chronic glanders

Glanders is a specific inflammatory disease due to infection with *Burkholderia mallei* which is parasitic in horses, donkeys and mules. The infection is extremely rare in man. It occurs in both acute and chronic forms in grooms and others who handle horses. The infection is transferred directly from the horse to the human through an abrasion of the skin, or occasionally through the nose or mouth. The incubation period may be a few hours, but is usually 2–6 days in the acute form. In the chronic form it may be as long as a year.

Clinical picture

The disease is usually ushered in with an acute febrile attack, and in some cases a rash develops which resembles smallpox. After a variable length of time, up to 5 years, during which the organisms lie latent, subcutaneous and intramuscular abscesses appear and nodules develop in the skin and in the mucous membrane of the mouth, palate and nose. The nodules ulcerate and later heal, and fresh ones appear and pass through the same stages. The ulceration closely resembles that of tertiary syphilis. In the nose there is also a severe generalized rhinitis, with tenacious mucopus and crusts lying on a reddened and scarred mucous membrane.

Throughout the active stages a variable pyrexia of 1 or 2°C is constant, but periods of complete remission of all signs of the disease are common.

In fatal cases, death is due to toxaemia and pulmonary and intracranial complications. The duration of the disease may be anything from 6 weeks to 15 years. It has been estimated that 6% of cases recover spontaneously.

It is very difficult to distinguish the lesions from those of tertiary syphilis, but in glanders there is usually a characteristic daily intermittent pyrexia and in syphilis the serology is positive. In the latter condition there is prompt response to antisyphilitic treatment, and characteristic papery scars are left after healing.

Any cases diagnosed as tertiary syphilis with a negative serology, and no response to antisyphilitic treatment, should be suspected as possible cases of chronic glanders. Culture and isolation of *Pseudomonas mallei* are often difficult, but intraperitoneal inoculation of the male guinea-pig produces inflammatory changes in the tunica vaginalis of the testis (Straus's reaction). Biopsy may not show any certain points of differentiation.

Treatment

The organism is sensitive to the tetracyclines, streptomycin, chloramphenicol and the sulphonamides.

Pathogenic fungi and yeasts

The classification and pathology of these diseases is complex and the reader is referred to the superb and exhaustive description given by Emmons *et al.* (1977).

Rhinosporidiosis

Rhinosporidiosis is a chronic infestation by the fungus *Rhinosporidium seeberi*, which predominantly affects the mucous membranes of the nose and nasopharynx but occasionally involves the lips, palate, uvula, maxillary antrum, conjunctiva, lacrimal sac, epiglottis, larynx, trachea, bronchus, ear, scalp, skin, penis, vulva and vagina. Osteolytic lesions (Figure 8.20) in the bones of the hands and feet have been reported by Chatterjee *et al.* (1977). Rhinosporidiosis, however, is usually limited to surface epithelium but may on occasions be widespread with visceral involvement. The disease, which is chronic and is characterized by the formation of papillomatous and polypoid

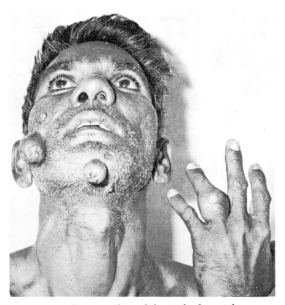

Figure 8.20 Rhinosporidic nodules in the face and nose, and swelling of the finger. (Reproduced by courtesy of Dr. P. K. Chatterjee and the Editor, *Journal of Laryngology and Otology*)

lesions, tends to affect young males and is endemic in many parts of India and Sri Lanka (Satyanarayana, 1966). Very occasionally the disease has been seen in Europeans who have visited India and Sri Lanka, but it is recognized to be rare for the condition to affect people outside these centres although reports of sporadic cases have come from the USA, Brazil, Africa and Europe. The mode of infection is probably by dust from the dung of infected horses and cattle but this has still to be confirmed.

The characteristic lesion is a bleeding polyp. Histologically the polyp has a vascular fibromyxomatous structure. The unique round structures histologically diagnostic for rhinosporidiosis were first described by Seeber (1900) as a protozoon, later by Ashworth (1923) as a sporangium of a fungus he designated *Rhinosporidium seeberi* and recently as lysosomal bodies loaded with indigestible residue somewhat reminiscent of lysosomal storage diseases. 'Sporangia', therefore have been redesignated nodular bodies and 'spores' as spheres of cellular waste (Ahluwalia, 1992). Azadeh, Baghoumian and El-Bakri (1994) have performed immunohistochemical and electron microscope studies which support this view (Figure 8.21). The indigestible residues are cleared via transepithelial elimination or segregated/destroyed by secondary immune/granulomatous responses. Krishnamoorthy *et al.* (1989), however, have succeeded in cultivating the 'spores'. The organism grows better in a pH of 5.8–6.5 at an optimum temperature of 23°C.

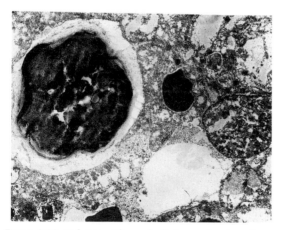

Figure 8.21 End-stage sphere of cellular waste released into tissue showing a dense and fragmented content and a folded periphery possibly caused by destructive inflammatory reactions (× 11 500). (Reproduced by courtesy of Dr Bahram Azadeh, FRCPath. and the Editor, *Journal of Laryngology and Otology*)

Epistaxis is often the only symptom, but in the early stages there is a viscid nasal discharge, with irritation and partial obstruction. With the develop-ment of the characteristic polyps the obstruction gradually increases until it may interfere with swallowing. Constitutional symptoms are rare, and the disease runs a slow course. The polyps may be present for years before the patient seeks advice.

The lesions are friable, in shape and colour resembling a strawberry, with a greyish under-surface studded with sporangia, showing as white dots. When sessile the polyps appear as multiple nodules, or may assume a leaf shape, with rounded or dentate margins. They arise primarily in the vestibule and are usually attached to the septum, but may spread backwards into the nasopharynx, and even hang down into the oropharynx. The nasal mucosa is generally swollen, hyperaemic and covered with copious viscid secretion, containing spores but no pus cells. The lymphatic glands are not affected.

Microscopical examination of the nasal discharge will show spores. Biopsy and histological examination of the polyps reveals the characteristic appearance described above. At first sight carcinoma may be suspected, on account of the friable masses which bleed on contact. The studding of the undersurface with white sporangia should suggest the diagnosis, and this may be confirmed by the special investigations.

The most successful treatment is wide excision with a cutting diathermy and cautery to the base of the lesions, as on occasions excessive bleeding may occur. Medical treatment in the form of local injection of depot corticosteroids into the polypoidal masses and systemic courses of amphotericin (Fungizone) and dapsone (Nair, 1979; Job *et al.*, 1993) may be given in addition.

The phycomycoses

The phycomycoses are a diverse group of mycoses caused by fungi which are traditionally placed in the class Phycomycetes. Although the term is now rejected by the formal taxonomic system it is retained in medical mycology (Emmons *et al.*, 1977). It has since been recommended to revert to the name *mucormycosis* for those mycoses caused by fungi belonging to the order Mucorales and the name *entomophtharamycosis* proposed for those mycoses caused by the fungi which belong to the order Entomophthorales. Certain members of each order can produce nasal disease of which the two major conditions are rhinophycomycosis and rhinocerebral phycomycosis.

Entomophtharamycosis conidiobolae (rhinophycomycosis)

This disease is caused by *Conidiobolus coronatus* and is manifested as prominent nasal polyps and granulomas in the nasal cavity. Most cases have been seen in Central Africa, India, Brazil and the West Indies.

Males are affected more than females. Symptoms consist of nasal obstruction and swelling over the nose and later the cheek and upper lip. Lesions usually begin in the inferior turbinate and spread in the submucosa through the natural ostia to the paranasal sinuses and to the subcutaneous tissues of the face. Histological examination shows a granulomatous reaction with collections of multinucleate giant cells in the centres of which hyphae can be seen. Treatment consists of removal of the tumour masses and systemic amphotericin (Fungizone).

Orbital and central nervous system mucormycosis (rhinocerebral phycomycosis)

Rhinocerebral mucormycosis is an aggressive opportunistic infection due to fungi of the order Mucorales, which include *Rhizopus oryzae*, *Mucor circinelloides*, *Mucor javanicus* and *Absidia corymbitera*. Differentiation between these causative organisms is unnecessary since their behaviour is similar (Shugar, 1987).

Phycomycetes are ordinarily saprophytic organisms existing in soil, manure, fruits and starchy food. They can be cultured from the human nose and gastrointestinal tract. They become pathogenic when the patient's general resistance has been altered by metabolic disorders or chemotherapeutic agents. This is most often associated with diabetic ketosis but can be seen with uraemic acidosis, leukaemia, malnutrition, steroid, antimetabolic or antibiotic therapy, and severe burns. The fungus has a remarkable affinity for arteries and, by dissecting the internal elastic lamina from the media, leads to extensive endothelial damage and thrombosis. Pathologically there is a mixed picture of inflammatory and necrotic changes. Later the veins and lymphatics are involved.

Mucormycosis appears in cerebral, pulmonary ocular, superficial and disseminated forms. Rhinocerebral disease is the commonest clinical form and is further subdivided into rhinomaxillary and rhino-orbitocerebral forms, the latter having a high mortality. The disease usually commences in the nose and extends by direct extension and intravascular propagation to involve the paranasal sinuses, orbit, cribriform plate, meninges and brain. Proptosis, ophthalmoplegia and blindness herald involvement of the central nervous system (Shugar, 1987). Pain in the face and orbit is out of proportion to the physical signs at first but shortly the characteristic rhinological finding of a black necrotic turbinate resembling a mass of dried clotted blood is seen. Unilateral gangrene and perforation of the hard and soft palates may occur from involvement of the palatine arteries. Sinus radiographs show thickening of the lining of the sinuses, no fluid levels and spotty destruction of the bony walls. Magnetic resonance imaging has the advantage of detecting early vascular and intracranial invasion (Yousem *et al.*, 1989).

Early clinical recognition of this potentially fatal disease is essential before irreversible changes occur. The disease is confirmed by biopsy.

Treatment consists of control of the original precipitating condition, heparinization, systemic amphotericin (Fungizone) and local drainage and debridement. Orbital exenteration is mandatory if ophthalmoplegia and loss of vision have occurred (Pillsbury and Newton, 1977) as the orbit is the portal of entry of infection to the central nervous system. Fisher *et al.* (1991) have reported the use of liposomal amphotericin (AmBisome) which is both less toxic and more effective than amphotericin. Bahadur *et al.* (1983) used oral potassium iodide therapy as an alternative treatment. The exact mode of action of the drug is unknown but it is believed to have an antifungal property.

Aspergillosis

Aspergillus is the commonest fungal infection of the nose and sinuses (Stammberger, Jaske and Beaufort, 1984) and seven pathogenic species have been described. Of these *A. fumigatus* accounts for 90%, followed by *A. niger* and *A. flavus*. The latter is the commonest organism isolated from patients in the Sudan (Milosev *et al.*, 1969; Mahgoub, 1977) where the disease is almost endemic and in Saudi Arabia (Kameswaren *et al.*, 1992). *Aspergillus* infection of the nose and sinuses can occur anywhere and at any age. It is a filamentous fungus which occurs as a saprophyte in soil and decaying matter such as fruit and other foods and is probably spread by air-borne transmission. *Aspergillus* reproduces as a sexual conidium and is recognized by septate hyphae and dichotomous branching at an angle of 45° degrees (Figure 8.22) (Milroy *et al.*, 1989).

A number of forms of nasal and paranasal sinus aspergillosis is described: non-invasive (aspergilloma), allergic, invasive and fulminant.

Non-invasive disease results from the formation of an aspergilloma or fungus ball which behaves as a chronic sinusitis and should be suspected in any refractory case. The most characteristic feature is a green-brown sludge which is found filling the sinus cavity, typically the maxillary antrum. Calcium deposits, visible on radiographs, can occur.

Allergic *Aspergillus* sinusitis (AAS), first described by Katzenstein, Sale and Greenberger in 1983, is likened to allergic bronchopulmonary aspergillosis and is thought to be a combination of type I and type III immune responses to *Aspergillus* antigens. It tends to occur in young adults with a history of asthma or polyps. Thick inspissated mucus, found in the sinuses, contains eosinophils and Charcot-Leyden crystals which are recognized as hexagonal strucures in cross-section and bi-pyramidal or rectangular structures in longitudinal section. Fungal hyphae are

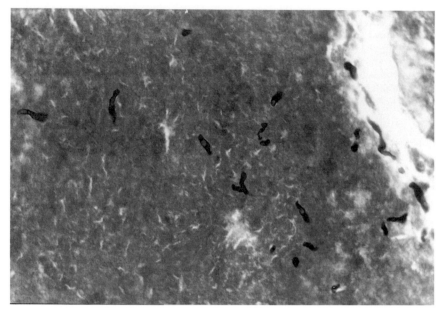

Figure 8.22 Septate *Aspergillus* hyphae branching at 45 degrees (Grocott's silver stain). (Reproduced by courtesy of Dr C. M. Milroy and the Editor, *Journal of Clinical Pathology*)

scanty but may be identified by special stains such as Grocott silver (Figure 8.22).

Both the non-invasive and allergic forms of paranasal aspergillosis are considered saprophytic, extramucosal disease, benign in nature (Hartwick and Batsakis, 1991).

The uncommon invasive form, described by Hora (1965) behaves like a malignant neoplasm and spreads to adjacent structures such as the soft tissues of the cheek and orbit. Proptosis is often a prominent feature. It is slowly progressive and locally destructive. Evidence of bone destruction may be seen radiologically and serology and skin tests for aspergillus antigens may be positive. A progressive fibrotic or sclerosing form can occur.

The fulminant form is a rapid progressive angioinvasive, destructive infection which carries a high mortality and usually affects immunocompromised patients (McGill, Simpson and Healy, 1980). Intracranial extension, either direct or blood-borne is fatal in one-fifth of patients even with treatment. The histological picture shows infiltrating aspergillus hyphae with little inflammatory response which contrasts with the invasive form where there is fibrosis and a granulomatous response to the aspergillus hyphae which are seen in giant cells when fungal stains are used. Fulminant disease can also be seen to arise from slowly progressive invasive lesions.

The four types of paranasal aspergillosis are not confined groups but tend to represent a progressive spectrum of disease as has been described for pulmonary aspergillosis (Gefter *et al.*, 1981). *Aspergillus*

infection may produce marked destruction and erosion of the sinuses without fungal tissue invasion and aspergillomas can destroy sinus bony walls and show evidence of fungal tissue invasion. A range of disease activity may also be found between the invasive form, developing over many months and the typically rapid, angioinvasive fulminant form developing over days. In the immunocompromised patient the disease usually arises *de novo*. Thus the concept of a clinical semi-invasive state may be used to describe how the disease might progress from a longstanding non-invasive form to the semi-invasive and slowly progressing, invasive forms. Rowe–Jones (1993) has suggested the following classification:

1 Non-invasive, either aspergilloma or allergic in type
2 Semi-invasive, being locally destructive without tissue invasion
3 Invasive, representing true fungal tissue invasion either non-fulminant or fulminant in course (Figure 8.23).

In all forms it is important to make the diagnosis from fresh nasal scrapings, mucus and biopsies of sinus mucosa. Non-invasive disease requires surgical debridement and sinus ventilation. Semi-invasive disease should be treated with surgery and adjuvant itraconazole (Sporanox) which penetrates body fluids and tissues well. Allergic *Aspergillus* sinusitis, in addition to surgical debridement, may be treated with systemic corticosteroids. Invasive and fulminant forms require more radical surgery in the form of

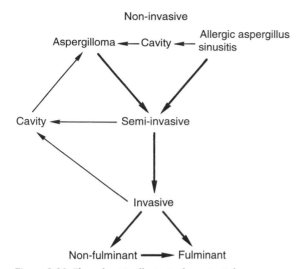

Figure 8.23 Flow chart to illustrate the potential progressive spectrum of disease of paranasal sinus aspergillosis. Aspergilloma may complicate cavities formed by other forms of the disease. (Reproduced by courtesy of Mr J. Rowe-Jones, FRCS and the Editor, *Journal of Laryngology and Otology*)

extenteration of the affected area, which can include craniofacial resection and orbital clearance, combined with intravenous amphotericin (Fungizone) or the less toxic liposomal amphotericin (AmBisome) or with the oral antifungals, ketoconazole (Nizoral) or itraconazole (Sporanox).

Blastomycosis

Blastomycosis is an uncommon fungal infection caused by the organism *Blastomyces dermatidis*, a thermally diamorphic fungus which has been cultured from soil in endemic areas. At room temperature it assumes its mycelial or mold form, which produces spores that can be inhaled into the lungs of the host where the body temperature induces transformation to the thick walled round budding yeast form. The subsequent inflammatory response and lymphohaematogenous spread lead to extrapulmonary manifestations of blastomycosis, typically skin, larynx and less commonly oral and nasal cavities. The disease is practically confined to certain parts of North America, in particular to the Ohio and Mississippi river valleys where it has been endemic. In a series of 102 patients suffering from blastomycosis at the Mayo clinic Redder and Neel (1993) found only 23 with otolaryngological involvement of whom only two had nasal disease. The mucosal lesion, which is near the vestibule or alar rim consists of a papillary hyperplasia with cysts which contain polymorphonuclear leucocytes surrounding the organisms. Dis-

seminated blastomycosis can rarely be fatal. The diagnosis is confirmed by histopathological examination of Gomori-stained or PAS-stained sections and by positive fungal serology for blastomycosis.

Treatment should be matched to the severity or potential morbidity of the disease location. Amphotericin (Fungizone) is the specific drug of choice for severe life-threatening infections, but for less severe disease, the azole oral agents such as ketoconazole (Nizoral) and itraconazole (Sporanox) which are less toxic, should be used.

Cryptococcosis

Cryptococcosis is caused by inhalation or ingestion of *Cryptococcus neoformans*, a yeast-like fungus closely resembling but nevertheless distinct from *Blastomyces dermatidis*. The fungus is found in pigeon or other avian excreta and of the fatal fungal infections in the USA is second only to histoplasmosis (Briggs, Barney and Bahu, 1974). There is, however, a world-wide distribution of the infection, which disseminates after pulmonary infestation to almost any tissue, but particularly to the brain and meninges, to give a chronic meningitis resembling tuberculous meningitis. Isolated lesions may occur in lymph nodes, skin, bone and eye. Nasal involvement is uncommon but external ulceration, nasopharyngitis and pansinusitis have been described. Briggs, Barney and Bahu (1974) described a case of ulceration of the nasal vestibule, biopsy of which revealed focal ulceration of the squamous mucosa and oedematous submucosa containing numerous round-to-oval yeast organisms surrounded by a clear 'halo-like' space caused by the capsule.

Treatment with amphotericin (Fungizone) and flucytosine (Alcobon) can be monitored by a specific slide latex agglutination test. Complete resolution can occur.

Actinomycosis

The genus *Actinomyces* consists of two principal species: *A. bovis*, the cause of actinomycosis or 'lumpy jaw' in cattle; and *A. israelii*, the cause of actinomycosis in man.

The anaerobic fungus, *Actinomyces israelii*, grows in the tissues in the form of colonies composed of branching mycelial threads with clubbed ends – 'ray fungus'. The colonies appear in pus as 'sulphur granules'.

Actinomyces israelii is frequently present as a harmless parasite in the mouths of normal individuals, where it is found around the teeth and in the tonsillar crypts. Trauma is an important predisposing factor in the development of 'cervicofacial' actinomycosis, although the exact conditions necessary to cause an infection are unknown. The infection may originate in a tooth socket and spread to adjacent tissues to produce a large hard, woody mass involving the face, jaw and neck. Softening occurs and multiple sinuses may develop, through which the characteristic pus exudes. The nose is rarely the site of primary infection but nasal actinomycosis has occurred following the implantation of xenologous processed bone for atrophic rhinitis (Thomas, Toohill and Lehman, 1974).

The general symptoms are pyrexia, toxaemia and rarely death. There is extensive tissue destruction and scarring.

Treatment consists of penicillin in large doses for 4–6 weeks and surgical drainage.

Candidiasis (moniliasis)

Candidiasis, commonly known as thrush, is caused by the yeast-like fungus *Candida albicans* which is a common inhabitant of the skin and oral cavity.

The infection occurs very commonly in the mouth and occasionally in the nose in neglected and marasmic infants and old people. It may occur in epidemic form in institutions and may be seen as a complication following courses of broad-spectrum oral antibiotics, long courses of systemic steroids and in immunosuppressed patients. There is a predisposition to candidiasis is in patients suffering from diabetes, tuberculosis and AIDS.

Candidiasis presents as small, discrete, pearly or dirty-white patches in the mucous membrane on a red moist surface. The patches are easily removed without bleeding.

The condition responds to simple cleansing and painting with 1% aqueous solution of gentian violet or the local application of nystatin; alternatively amphotericin (Fungizone) or flucytosine (Alcobon) may be given in severe cases. Any predisposing cause should be sought and corrected.

Histoplasmosis

Histoplasmosis is an infestation due to a yeast-like fungus, *Histoplasma capsulatum*. It is most commonly found in central regions of the USA, but cases have been described throughout the world. Histoplasmosis is a diffuse disease of the reticuloendothelial system and is usually manifest by enlarged spleen, liver and lymph nodes with intestinal ulceration and anaemia. Nasal lesions are rare and may be nodular or infective secondary lymphadenitis develops.

The diagnosis is made by biopsy and the histoplasmin skin test which helps to differentiate pulmonary lesions from tuberculosis.

Treatment is with amphotericin (Fungizone).

Sporotrichosis

This is primarily an infection of the skin, usually of the hand, caused by *Sporothrix schenckii*. It very rarely affects the nasal mucous membrane but could be transposed there either directly from a lesion on the hand or by haematogenous spread. Infection follows a prick with a thorn. After a few days a nodule develops which becomes red and tender finally bursting to discharge viscid yellow mucopus in which organisms may be found. Spread is also by the lymphatics along which secondary nodules develop.

Treatment is with iodides or amphotericin (Fungizone).

Nasopharyngeal leishmaniasis

This condition, sometimes known as American leishmaniasis or espundia, is caused by *Leishmania braziliensis* as distinct from *L. donovani*, the cause of visceral leishmaniasis or *L. tropica*, cutaneous leishmaniasis. It is found chiefly in South and Central America and is transmitted by the sandfly (*Phlebotomus*).

The Leishman–Donovan bodies, which in the mammalian host do not occur in flagellated form, are approximately oval in shape and 2–6 μm in length with an eccentrically placed vesicular nucleus. They may be demonstrated in the discharge from the ulcers and in the reticuloendothelial cells in the granulomatous tissue.

The site of inoculation is usually on the exposed parts where a papule resembling a chancre develops and ulcerates, later healing and leaving a scar. Polypoid growths may form and there may be extensive destructive lesions involving the soft tissues or cartilage of the nasal septum, mouth, pharynx and larynx. Bone is generally not involved. There may be regional lymphadenitis and in untreated cases death follows from exhaustion.

Treatment consists of local cleansing and curettage. Specific treatment is with systemic pentavalent antimony in the form of sodium stibogluconate BP (Pentostam) or in resistant cases with pentamidine isethionate (Pentacarinat). Recently liposomal amphotericin (AmBisome) has been successfully used in visceral leishmaniasis (Davidson and Croft, 1993).

Myiasis

Nasal myiasis, which is not uncommon in hot and humid climates, particularly in India where it is known as Peenash, is a demoralizing condition of infestation of the nasal cavities by maggots, the larvae of a fly (genus *Chrysomyia*).

Myiasis can also affect the ear, mouth or larynx and reaches a peak in the months of September to November. It can affect any age, and both sexes equally. The majority of sufferers live in bad hygienic conditions and have a source of offensive decaying material, e.g. atrophic rhinitis, chronic sinusitis or chronic suppurative otitis media, which provides a suitable environment for the eggs of the fly to hatch into larvae no less than 1.5 cm in length. The eggs may also be deposited in a slight abrasion or crack in the mucous membrane.

The entomological aspects of myiasis are well described by Sood, Kakar and Watlal (1976). The patient complains of a diffuse swelling around the nose and eyes, nasal obstruction, epistaxis or the presence of maggots coming out of the nose. Rhinoscopy reveals a congested oedematous mucosa, necrotic material with embedded maggots, ulcerated mucosa or septal perforations. The disease can spread to the paranasal sinuses and via the nasolacrimal duct to the lacrimal sac. In the later stages the nasal bones may be destroyed and death may result from sepsis, meningitis or suicide.

Treatment is general, with antibiotics and supportive therapy, and local, with olive oil or liquid paraffin or packing with a mixture of chloroform and turpentine (1:4) which stifle the larvae. The nasal cavity is then rinsed with an alkaline douche and the maggots are removed piecemeal. The majority of patients will be maggot free in 4–5 days. To prevent further infestation the predisposing conditions of poor hygiene and a source of chronic infection must be removed. Sharma, Dayal and Argrawal (1989) performed a limited Young's operation (partial closure of both nostrils) in 48% of their series of 252 patients. None of these patients had a recurrence of myiasis compared with 8% of those who refused surgery.

References

ABEL, P. (1895) Die aetiologie der ozaena. *Zeitschrift für Hygiene und Infektionskrankheiten*, **21**, 89–95

AFZELIUS, B. A. (1976) A human syndrome caused by immotile cilia. *Science*, **193**, 317–319

AHLUWALIA, K. B. (1992) New interpretations in rhinosporidiosis – enigmatic disease of the last nine decades. *Journal of Submicroscopic Cytology and Pathology*, **24**, 109–114

ÅKERLUND, A., GRIEFF, L., ANDERSSON, M., BENDE, M., ALKNER, U. and PERSSON, C. G. A. (1993) Mucosal exudation of fibrinogen in coronavirus induced common colds. *Acta Otolaryngologica*, **113**, 642–648

ANDERSEN, I. and PROCTOR, D. F. (1982) The fate and effects of inhaled materials. In: *The Nose, Upper Airway Physiology and the Atmospheric Environment*, edited by D. Proctor and I. Andersen. Amsterdam: Elsevier Biomedical Press. pp. 423–455

ANDERSEN, I., CAMNER, P., JENSEN P.L., PHILIPSON, K. and PROCTOR, D. (1974) Nasal clearance in monozygotic twins. *American Review of Respiratory Disease*, **110**, 301–305

ANDREWES, C. H. (1950) Adventures among viruses III. The puzzle of the common cold. *New England Journal of Medicine*, **242**, 235–240

ANDREWES, C. H. and TYRRELL, D. A. (1965) Rhinoviruses. In: *Viral and Rickettsial Infections of Man*, edited by F. L. Horsfall and I. Tanm. Philadelphia: Lippincott. pp. 546–558

ÅNGGÅRD, A. and MALM, L. (1984) Orally administered decongestant drugs in disorders of the upper respiratory passages: a survey of clinical results. *Clinical Otolaryngology*, **9**, 43–49

ARROWSMITH, H. (1921) Gangosa. *Laryngoscope*, **31**, 843–846

ASHWORTH. J. H. (1923) On *Rhinosporidium seeberi* with special reference to its sporulation and affinities. *Transactions of the Royal Society of Edinburgh*, **53**, 301–342

AXELSSON, A. and BRORSON, J. E. (1973) The correlation between bacteriological findings in the nose and maxillary sinus in acute maxillary sinusitis. *Laryngoscope*, **83**, 2003–2011

AZADEH, B., BAGHOUMIAN, N. and EL-BAKRI, O. (1994) Rhinosporidiosis: immunohistochemical and electron microscopic studies. *Journal of Laryngology and Otology*, **108**, 1048–1054

BACHMANN, R. (1965) Studies on serum alpha A globulin level III. The frequency of A-alpha A-globulinaemia. *Scandinavian Journal of Clinical and Laboratory Investigation*, **17**, 316–320

BADRAWAY, R. (1962) Dacryoscleroma. *Annals of Otology, St Louis*, **71**, 247–254

BADRAWAY, R. (1966) Affection of bone in rhinoscleroma. *Journal of Laryngology and Otology*, **80**, 160–167

BADRAWAY, R. and EL SHENNAWY, M. (1974) Affection of cervical lymph nodes in rhinoscleroma. *Journal of Laryngology and Otology*, **88**, 261–269

BAHADUR, S., GHOSH, P., CHOPRA, P. and RAI, G. (1983) Rhinocerebral phycomycosis. *Journal of Laryngology and Otology*, **97**, 267–270

BARTON, R. P. E. (1974) Olfaction in leprosy. *Journal of Laryngology and Otology*, **88**, 355–361

BARTON, R. P. E. (1976) Clinical manifestation of leprous rhinitis. *Annals of Otology, St Louis*, **85**, 74–82

BARTON, R. P. E. (1979) Radiological changes in the paranasal sinuses in lepromatous leprosy. *Journal of Laryngology and Otology*, **93**, 597–600

BARTON, R. P. E. (1985) Ear, nose and throat involvement in leprosy. In: *Leprosy*, edited by R. C. Hastings. Edinburgh: Churchill Livingstone. pp. 243–252

BARTON, R. P. E. and DAVEY, T. F. (1976) Early leprosy of the nose and throat. *Journal of Laryngology and Otology*, **90**, 953–961

BARTON, R. P. E., DAVEY, T. F., MCDOUGALL, A. C., REES, R. J. W. and WEDDELL, A. G. M. (1973) Clinical and histological studies of the nose in early lepromatous leprosy. Paper 6/47. Tenth International Leprosy Congress, Bergen

BERLINGER, N. T. (1985) Sinusitis in immunodeficient and immunosuppressed patients. *Laryngoscope*, **95**, 29–33

BERNAT, J. (1965) *Ozaena, a Manifestation of Iron Deficiency*. Oxford: Pergamon Press

BÖCKMANN, P., ANDERSSON, L., HOLMER, N-G., JANNERT, M. and LORINC, P. (1982) Ultrasonic versus radiologic investigation of the paranasal sinuses. *Rhinology*, **20**, 111–119

BOECK C. (1905) Fortgetzte untersuchungen uber das multiple benigne sarkoid. *Archiv für Dermatologie und Syphilis*, **73**, 301–332

BRIGGS, D. R., BARNEY, P. L. and BAHU, R. M. (1974) Nasal cryptococcosis. *Archives of Otolaryngology*, **100**, 390–392

CHARLTON, R., MACKAY, I., WILSON, R. and COLE, P. (1985)

Double-blind placebo controlled trial of betamethasone nasal drops for nasal polyposis. *British Medical Journal,* **291,** 788

CHATTERJEE, P. K., KATUA, C. R., CHATTERJEE., S. N. and DASIDAR, N. (1977) Recurrent multiple rhinosporidiosis with osteolytic lesions in hand and foot. *Journal of Laryngology and Otology,* **91,** 729–734

CHATTERJI, P. (1980) Autogenous medullary (cancellous) bone graft in ozeana. *Journal of Laryngology and Otology,* **94,** 737–749

COLE, P. J. (1981) Immunity deficiency states. In: *Scientific Foundations of Respiratory Medicine,* edited J. G. Scadding and G. Cumming. London: William Heinemann. pp. 441–451

COLE, P. J. (1984) A new look at the pathogenesis and management of persistent bronchial sepsis: a 'vicious circle' hypothesis and its logical therapeutic connotations. In: *Strategies for the Management of Chronic Bronchial Sepsis,* edited by R. J. Davies. Oxford: The Medicine Publishing Foundation. pp. 1–20

COLE, P. J. (1985) Investigation of disordered respiratory defences. In: *Clinics in Immunology and Allergy 5: Laboratory Investigation of Immunological Disorders,* edited by R. A. Thompson. Philadephia: W. B. Saunders Company. pp. 549–568

CRUICKSHANK, R. (1942) *Control of the Common Fevers.* London: Lancet Publications

CURTIS, G. T. (1964) Sarcoidosis of nasal bones. *British Journal of Radiology,* **37,** 68–70

DAVEY, T. F. and REES, R. J. W. (1974) The nasal discharge in leprosy: clinical and bacteriological aspects. *Leprosy Review,* **45,** 121–126

DAVIDSON, R. N. and CROFT, S. L. (1993) Recent advances in the treatment of visceral leishmaniasis. *Transactions of the Royal Society of Tropical Medicine and Hygiene,* **87,** 130–131 & 141

DRAF, W. (1983) *Endoscopy of the Paranasal Sinuses.* Berlin: Springer–Verlag. pp. 1–3

DRETTNER, B. (1983) Antral irrigation with an indwelling plastic tube. *Rhinology,* **21,** 369–371

DRUCE, H. M. (1990) Adjuncts to medical treatment for sinusitis. *Otolaryngology, Head and Neck Surgery,* Suppl. **103,** 880–883

ELIASSON, R., MOSSBERG, B., CAMNER, P. and AFZELIUS, B. A. (1977) The immotile cilia syndrome. A congenital ciliary abnormality as an aetiological factor in chronic airway infection and male sterility. *New England Journal of Medicine,* **297,** 1–6

EMMONS, C. W., BINFORD, C. H., UTZ, J. P. and KWOWCHUNG, K. J. (1977) The phycomycoses. In: *Medical Mycology,* 3rd edn, edited by C. W. Emmons. Philadelphia: Lea and Febiger. pp. 254–282

FALCK, B., SVANHOLM, H. and AUST, R. (1990) The effect of xylometazoline on the mucosa of human maxillary sinus. *Rhinology,* **28,** 239–247

FISHER, E. R. and DIMLING, C. S. (1964) Rhinoscleroma. *Archives of Pathology,* **78,** 501–512

FISHER, E. W., TOMA, A., FISHER, P. H. and CHEESEMAN, A. D. (1991) Rhinocerebral mucormycosis: use of liposomal amphotericin B. *Journal of Laryngology and Otology,* **103,** 575–577

FOUAD, H., AFIFI, N., FATT-HI, A., EL-SHEENY, N., ISKANDER, I. and ABOU SAIL, M. N. (1980) Altered cell mediated immunity in atrophic rhinitis. *Journal of Laryngology and Otology,* **94,** 507–514

FREDERICH, J. and BRAUDE, A. (1974) Anaerobic infection of the paranasal sinuses. *New England Journal of Medicine* **290,** 135–137

FRIEDMANN, I. (1963) Electron microscopy of rare diseases of the nose. *Transactions of the American Academy of Ophthalmology and Otolaryngology,* **67,** 261–280

FRIEDMANN, I. (1966) In: *Pathology,* Vol. 1, edited by G. Payling Wright and W. S. Clair Symmers. London: Longmans. pp.295–297

GAMEA, A. M. (1988) Local rifampicin in treatment of rhinoscleroma. *Journal of Laryngology and Otology,* **102,** 319–321

GEFTER, W.B., WEINGRAD, T. R., EPSTEIN, D. M., OCHS, R. H. and MILLER, W. T. (1981) 'Semi-invasive' pulmonary aspergillosis. *Radiology,* **140,** 313–321

GIANCOLI, G. J., MANN, W. J. and MILLER, R. J. (1992) B-mode ultrasonography of the paranasal sinuses compared with CT findings. *Otolaryngology – Head and Neck Surgery,* **107,** 713–720

GODOFSKY, E. W., ZEINREICH, J., ARMSTRONG, M., LESLIE, J. M. and WEIKEL, C.S. (1992) Sinusitis in HIV-infected patients: a clinical and radiographic review. *American Journal of Medicine,* **93,** 163–170

GOLDING, J.H., JAWAD, S. M. A. and REID, A.P. (1983) Cutaneous nasal sarcoidosis – treatment by excision and split skin grafting. *Journal of Laryngology and Otology,* **97,** 1053–1056

GONZALEZ–ANGULO, A., MARQUES–MONTER, H., GREENBERG, S. D and CERBON, J. (1965) Ultrastructure of nasal scleroma. *Annals of Otology, St Louis,* **74,** 1022–1033

GORDON, W. W., COHN, A. M., GREENBERG, S. D. and KOMORN, R. M. (1976) Nasal sarcoidosis. *Archives of Otolaryngology,* **102,** 11–14

GREENSTONE, M., LOGAN–SINCLAIR, R. and COLE, P. J. (1984) An automated method of recording ciliary beat frequency. *IRCS Journal of Medical Science,* **12,** 715–716

GREENSTONE, M., STANLEY, P., COLE, P. and MACKAY, I. (1985) Upper airway manifestations of primary ciliary dyskinesia. *Journal of Laryngology and Otology,* **99,** 985–991

GWALTNEY, J. M. and HAYDEN, F. G. (1982) The nose and infection. In: *The Nose: Upper Airway Physiology and the Atmospheric Environment,* edited by D. F. Proctor and I. Andersen. Amsterdam: Elsevier Biomedical Press. pp. 399–422

HAMORY, B. H., SANDE, M. A., SYDNOR, A. JR, SEALE, D. L. and GWALTNEY, J. H. JR (1979) Etiology and antimicrobial therapy of acute maxillary sinusitis. *Journal of Infectious Diseases,* **139,** 197–202

HARTWICK, R. W. and BATSAKIS, J. G. (1991) Sinus aspergillosis and allergic fungal sinusitis. *Annals of Otology, Rhinology and Laryngology,* **100,** 427–430

HENDRY, W. F., PARSLOW, J. M. and STENDRONSKA, J. (1983) Exploratory scrototomy in 168 azospermic males. *British Journal of Urology,* **55,** 785–791

HENRIKSEN, S. D. and GUNDERSEN, W. B. (1959) The aetiology of ozaena. *Acta Pathologica et Microbiologica Scandinavica,* **47,** 380–386

HOPE-SIMPSON, R. E. (1958a) Symposium on the epidemiology of non-infectious diseases. (a) Common upper respiratory disease. *Royal Society of Health Journal,* **78,** 593–599

HOPE-SIMPSON, R. E. (1958b) Discussion on the common cold. *Proceedings of the Royal Society of Medicine,* **51,** 267–271

HORA, J. F. (1965) Primary aspergillosis of the paranasal sinuses and associated areas. *Laryngoscope,* **75,** 768–773

INGHAM, H.R., SISSON, P. R., THARAGONNET, D., SELKON, J. B.

and CODD, H. A. (1977) Inhibition of phagocytosis in vitro by obligate anaerobes. *Lancet*, ii, 1252–1254

JAMES, D. G. (1959) Dermatological aspects of sarcoidosis. *Quarterly Journal of Medicine*, 28, 109–124

JAMES, D. G., BARTER, S., JASH, D., MACKINNON, D. M. and CARSTAIRS, L. S. (1982) Sarcoidosis of the upper respiratory tract (SURT). *Journal of Laryngology and Otology*, 96, 711–718

JEFFERY, P. K. and REID, L. (1975) New observations of rat airway epithelium: a quantitative and electron microscopic study. *Journal of Anatomy*, 120, 295–320

JENSEN, C. and SYDOW, C. VON (1987) Radiography and ultrasonography in paranasal sinusitis. *Acta Radiologica*, 28, 31–34

JOB, A., VENKATESWARAN, S., MATHAN, M., KRISHNASWAMI, H. and RAMAN, R. (1993) Medical therapy of rhinosporidiosis with dapsone. *Journal of Laryngology and Otology*, 107, 809–812

KAMESWAREN, M., AL-WADEI, A., KHURANA, P. and OKAFOR, B.C. (1992) Rhinocerebral aspergillosis. *Journal of Laryngology and Otology*, 106, 981–985

KARTAGENER, M. (1933) Zur pathogencse der bronkiektasian bei situs viscerum inversus. *Beltrage zur Klinik und Erforshung der Tuberkulose und der Lungen Krankheiten*, 83, 489–501

KATZENSTEIN, A. A., SALE, S. R. and GREENBERGER, P. A. (1983) Allergic aspergillus sinusitis: a newly recognised form of sinusitis. *Journal of Allergy and Clinical Immunology*, 72, 89–93

KERR, W. J. and LAGEN, J. B. (1933–34) Transmissibility of the common cold. *Proceedings of the Society of Experimental Biology, New York*, 31, 713–715

KETLER, A., HAMPARIAN, V. V. and HILLEMAN, M. R. (1962) Characterization and classification of ECHO 28-rhinovirus-coryzavirus agents. *Proceedings of the Society of Experimental Biology and Medicine*, 110, 821–825

KILIAN, M. (1981) Degradation of immunoglobulins A1, A2 and G by suspected principal periodontal pathogens. *Infection and Immunity*, 34, 757–765

KISTNER, F. B. and ROBERTSON, T. D. (1938) Benign granuloma of the nose. *Journal of the American Medical Association*, 111, 2003–2005

KORNFELD, S. and PLAUT, A. G. (1981) Secretory immunity and the bacterial proteases. *Reviews Infectious Diseases*, 3, 521–534

KRISHNAMOORTHY, S., SREEDHARAN, V. P., KOSHY, P., KUMAR, S. and ANILAKUMARI, C. K. (1989) Culture of *Rhinosporidium seeberi*: preliminary report. *Journal of Laryngology and Otology*, 103, 178–181

LEVINE, M. G. (1951) Rhinoscleroma: a complement fixation test. *American Journal of Clinical Pathology*, 21, 546–549

LEVISON, J., MINDORFF, C. M., CHAO, J., TURNER J. A. P., STURGESS, J. M. and STRINGER, D. A. (1983) Pathophysiology of the ciliary motility syndrome. *European Journal of Respiratory Disease*, 64 (suppl. 127), 102–116

LOCKE, A. (1937) Lack of fitness as the predisposing factor in infections of the type encountered in pneumonia and the common cold. *Journal of Infectious Diseases*, 60, 106–110

LOEWENBERG, B. (1894) Le microbe de l'ozene. *Annales de l'Institut Pasteur*, 8, 292–347

LUCAS, A. M. and DOUGLAS, L. C. (1934) Principles underlying ciliary activity in the respiratory tract. *Archives of Otolaryngology*, 20, 518–541

LUND, V. J. and LLOYD G. A. S. (1983) Radiological changes associated with benign nasal polyps. *Journal of Laryngology and Otology*, 97, 503–510

LUND, V. J. and MACKAY, I. S. (1993) Staging in rhinosinusitis. *Rhinology*, 31, 183–184

MCDOUGALL, A. C., REES, R J. W., WEDDELL, A. G. M. and WADJI KANAN, M. (1974) The histopathology of lepromatous leprosy in the nose. *Journal of Pathology*, 115, 215–226

MCGILL, T. J., SIMPSON, G. and HEALY G. B. (1980) Fulminant aspergillosis of the nose and paranasal sinuses: a new clinical entity. *Laryngoscope*, 90, 748–754

MACKAY, I. S. (ed.) (1989) Topical medical management of allergic conditions of the nose. Part 2: Intranasal steroids. In: *Rhinitis. Mechanisms and Management*. London: Royal Society of Medicine Services Limited. pp. 183–204

MACKAY, I. S., STANLEY, P., GREENSTONE, M., HOLMES, P. and COLE, P. (1983) A nose clinic: initial results. *Journal of Laryngology and Otology*, 97, 925–931

MCKELVIE, P., GRESSON, C. and POKHREL, R. P. (1968) Sarcoidosis of the upper air passages. *British Journal of Diseases of the Chest*, 62, 200–205

MCNABB, P. C. and TOMASI, T. B. (1981) Host defence mechanisms at mucosal surfaces. *Annual Review of Microbiology*, 35, 477–496

MAHGOUB, EL S. (1977) Mycoses of the Sudan. *Transactions of the Royal Society of Tropical Medicine and Hygiene*, 74, 162–165

MANN, W., GOBEL, U., PELZ, K. and JONAS, I. (1981) Effect of treatment in maxillary sinusitis. *Journal of Oto-Rhino-Laryngology and Related Specialities*, 43, 274–279

MEIKLE, D., YARINGTON, C. T. and WINTERBAUER, R. H. (1985) Aspergillosis of the maxillary sinus in otherwise healthy patients. *Laryngoscope*, 95, 776–779

MESSERKLINGER, W. (1966) Über die drainage der menschlichen nasennebenhöhlen unter normalen und pathologischen bedingungen 1. Mitteilung. *Monatsschrift für Ohrenheilkunde und Laryngo-Rhinologie*, 100, 56–68

MESSERKLINGER, W. (1967) Über die drainage der menschlichen nasennebenhöhlen unter normalen und pathologischen bedingungen 2. Mitteilung: Die stirnhöhle und ihr ausfuhrungssystem. *Monatsschrift für Ohrenheilkunde und Laryngo-Rhinologie*, 101, 313–326

MESSERKLINGER, W. (1978) *Endoscopy of the Nose*. Baltimore: Urban and Schwartzenberg

MILOSEV, B., MAHBOUG, EL S., AAL, A. and HASSAN, EL A. M. (1969) Primary aspergilloma of the paranasal sinuses in the Sudan: a review of seventeen cases. *British Journal of Surgery*, 56, 132–137

MILROY, C. M., BLANSHARD, J. D., LUCAS, S. and MICHAELS, L. (1989) Aspergillosis of the nose and paranasal sinuses. *Journal of Clinical Pathology*, 42, 123–127

MØLLER–CHRISTENSEN, V., BAKKE, S. N. and MELSOM, R.S. (1952) Changes in the anterior nasal spine and alveolar process of the maxillary bone in leprosy. *International Journal of Leprosy*, 20, 335–337

MOSSALLAM, I. and ATTIA, D. M. (1956) Primary scleroma of the maxillary sinus. *Journal of the Egyptian Medical Association*, 39, 512–515

MUNRO, C. S., STANLEY, P. and COLE, P. J. (1985) Assessment of biological activity of immunoglobulin preparations by using opsonized microorganisms to stimulate neutrophil chemiluminescence. *Clinical and Experimental Immunology*, 61, 183–188

MUNRO BLACK, J. I. (1966) Sarcoidosis of the nose. *Journal of Laryngology and Otology*, 80, 1065–1068

MYERSON, M. C. (1933) Gangosa – occurrence in a white man. *Laryngoscope*, 43, 394–399

MYGIND, N. (1979) *Nasal Allergy*. Oxford: Blackwell Scientific Publications. pp. 257–270

NAIR, K. K. (1979) Clinical trial of diamino-diphenylsulphone (DDS) in nasal and nasopharyngeal rhinosporidiosis. *Laryngoscope*, 89, 291–295

OXELIUS, V. A., LAURELL, A-B., LINQUIST, B, GOLEBIOWSKA, H., AXELSSON, V., BJORKANDER, J. *et al.* (1981) IgG subclasses in selective IgA deficiency: importance of IgG2-IgA deficiency. *New England Journal of Medicine*, 304, 1476–1477

PEDERSEN, H. and MYGIND, N. (1976) Absence of axonemal arms in nasal mucosal cilia in Kartagener's syndrome. *Nature*, 262, 494–495

PEDERSEN, H. and MYGIND, N. (1982) Rhinitis, sinusitis and otitis media in Kartagener's syndrome (primary ciliary dyskinesia). *Clinical Otolaryngology*, 7, 373–380

PEDERSEN, H. and REBBE, H. (1975) Absence of arms in the axoneme of immotile human spermatozoa. *Biology of Reproduction*, 12, 541–544

PETRUSON, B., HANSSON, H. A. and KARLSSON, G. (1984) Structural and functional aspects of cells in the nasal mucociliary system. *Archives of Otolaryngology*, 110, 576–581

PFLEIDERER, A. G., DRAKE-LEE, A. B. and LOWE, D. (1984) Ultrasound of the sinuses: a worthwhile procedure? A comparison of ultrasound and radiography in predicting the findings of proof puncture of a maxillary sinus. *Clinical Otolaryngology*, 9, 335–339

PFLEIDERER, A. G., CROFT, C. B. and LLOYD, G. A. (1986) Antroscopy: its place in clinical practice. A comparison of antroscopic findings with radiographic appearances of the maxillary sinus. *Clinical Otolaryngology*, 11, 455–461

PILLSBURY, H. C. and NEWTON, D. F. (1977) Rhinocerebral mucormycosis. *Archives of Otolaryngology*, 103, 600–604

PROCTOR, D. (1982) The mucociliary system. In: *The Nose. Upper Airway Physiology and the Atmospheric Environment*, edited by D. Proctor and I. Andersen. Amsterdam: Elsevier Biomedical Press. pp. 245–278

PROOPS, D. W. (1983) The unilateral thick walled antrum. A previously unrecognized entity. *Journal of Laryngology and Otology*, 97, 369–373

QIZILBASH, A. A. H. and DAIF, M. (1992) Atrophic rhinitis revisited. *Pakistan Journal of Otolaryngology*, 8, 197–199

QUINLAN, M. F., SALMAN, S. D., SWIFT, D. L., WAGNER, H. N. JR and PROCTOR, D. F. (1969) Measurement of mucociliary function in man. *American Review of Respiratory Disease*, 99, 13–23

REDDER, P. A. and NEEL, B. III (1993) Blastomycosis in otolaryngology: review of a large series. *Laryngoscope*, 103, 53–58

REED, S. E. (1981) The aetiology and epidemiology of common colds, and the possibilities of prevention. *Clinical Otolaryngology*, 6, 379–387

REES, R. J. W. (1966) Enhanced susceptibility of thymectomized and irradiated mice to infection with *M. leprae*. *Nature*, 211, 657–658

RIAD, G. (1982) Comparative study of the effects of rifampicin, tetracycline and combined rifampicin with tetracycline on rhinoscleroma. *Thesis*, Tantra University, Egypt

RIZK, M. (1977) *MD Thesis*, Faculty of Medicine, Mansoura, Egypt

ROSSMAN, C. M., FORREST, J. B., LEE, R. M. K. W. and NEWHOUSE, M. T. (1980) The dyskinetic cilia syndrome. Ciliary motility in the immotile cilia syndrome. *Chest*, 78, 580–582

ROWE-JONES, J. (1993) Editorial. Paranasal aspergillosis – a spectrum of disease. *Journal of Laryngology and Otology*, 107, 773–774

RUTLAND, J. and COLE, P. J. (1980) Non-invasive sampling of nasal cilia for measurement of beat frequency and study of ultrastructure. *Lancet*, ii, 564–565

RUTLAND, J., GRIFFIN, W. M. and COLE, P. J. (1982) Human ciliary beat frequency in epithelium from intra- and extra-thoracic airways. *American Review of Respiratory Disease*, 125, 100–105

SATYANARAYANA, C. (1966) Rhinosporidiosis. In: *Clinical Surgery Ear, Nose and Throat*, edited by M. Ellis. London: Butterworths. p. 143

SCOTT, G. M. (1984) How do viruses overcome mucosal defences? In: *Bacterial and Viral Inhibition and Modulation of Host Defences*, edited by G Falcone, M. Campa, H. Smith and G. M. Scott. London: Academic Press. pp. 25–39

SEEBER, G. R. (1900) *Thesis*. Universidad Nationale, Buenos Aires

SHAER, M., RIZK, M., SHAWAF, I., ALI, M. and HASASH, M. (1981) Local acriflavine: a new therapy for rhinoscleroma. *Journal of Laryngology and Otology*, 95, 701–706

SHARMA, A. N. and SARDANA, D. S. (1966) Stellate ganglion block in atrophic rhinitis. *Journal of Laryngology and Otology*, 80, 184–186

SHARMA, H., DAYAL, D. and AGRAWAL, S. P. (1989) Nasal myiasis: review of 10 years experience. *Journal of Laryngology and Otology*, 103, 489–491

SHUGAR, M. A. (1987) Mycotic infections of the nose and paranasal sinuses. In: *Principles and Practice of Rhinology*, edited by J. L. Goldman. New York: Churchill Livingstone. pp. 717–734

SINHA, A., PANDHI, S. C. and PRAKASH, O. M. (1969) Aetiopathogenesis of scleroma. *Journal of Laryngology and Otology*, 83, 133–139

SINHA, S. M., SARDANA, D. S. and RJVANSHI, V. S. (1977) A nine years' review of 27 cases of atrophic rhinitis and its management. *Journal of Laryngology and Otology*, 91, 591–600

SMALLMAN, L. A., HILL, S. L. and STOCKLEY, R. A. (1984) Reduction of ciliary beat frequencies in vitro by sputum from patients with bronchiectasis: a serine proteinase effect. *Thorax*, 39, 663–667

SMITH W., ANDREWES, C. H. and LAIDLAW, P. P. (1933) A virus obtained from influenza patients. *Lancet*, ii, 66–68

SOOD, V. P., KAKAR, P. K. and WATLAL, B. I. (1976) Myiasis in otolaryngology with entomological aspects. *Journal of Laryngology and Otology*, 90, 393–399

SPENCER, H. (1985) *Pathology of the Lung*, 4th edn. Oxford: Pergamon Press. pp. 517–525

SSALI, C. L. K. (1975) The management of rhinoscleroma. *Journal of Laryngology and Otology*, 89, 91–99

STAMMBERGER, H. (1991) *Functional Endoscopic Sinus Surgery*. Philadelphia: B. C. Decker. pp. 17–47

STAMMBERGER, H., JASKE, R. and BEAUFORT, F. (1984) Aspergillosis of the paranasal sinuses: X-ray diagnosis, histopathology and clinical aspects. *Annals of Otology, Rhinology and Laryngology*, 93, 251–256

STANLEY, P., MACWILLIAM, I., GREENSTONE, M., MACKAY, I. and COLE, P. (1984) Efficacy of a saccharin test for screening to detect abnormal mucociliary clearance. *British Journal for Diseases of the Chest*, 78, 62–65

STANLEY, P. J. and COLE, P. J. (1985) The concentrations of IgA and free secretory piece in the nasal secretions of patients with recurrent respiratory infections. *Clinical and Experimental Immunology*, 59, 197–202

STANLEY, P. J., CORBO, G. and COLE, P. J. (1984) Serum IgG subclasses in chronic and recurrent respiratory infections. *Clinical and Experimental Immunology*, **58**, 703–708

STANLEY, P. J., WILSON, R., GREENSTONE, M., MACKAY, I. S. and COLE, P. J. (1985) Abnormal nasal mucociliary clearance in patients with rhinitis and its relationship to concomitant chest disease. *British Journal for Diseases of the Chest*, **79**, 77–82

STANLEY, P. J., WILSON, R., GREENSTONE., M., MACWILLIAM, L. and COLE, P. J. (1986) Effect of cigarette smoking on nasal mucociliary clearance and ciliary beat frequency. *Thorax*, **41**, 519–523

STEFFEN, T. N. and SMITH, I. M. (1961) Scleroma, *Klebsiella rhinoscleromatis* and its effect on mice. *Annals of Otology, St Louis*, **70**, 935–952

STUDDY, P., BIRD, R., JAMES D. G. and SHERLOCK, S. (1978) Serum angiotensin-converting enzyme (SACE) in sarcoidosis and other granulomatous disorders. *Lancet*, ii, 1331–1334

SYDOW, C. VON, AXELSSON, A. and JENSEN, C. (1982) Acute maxillary sinusitis: a comparison between 27 different treatment modes. *Rhinology*, **20**, 223–229

SYKES, D. A., WILSON, R, GREENSTONE, M., CURRIE, D. C., STEINFORT, C. and COLE P. J. (1987) Deleterious effects of purulent sputum sol on human ciliary function in vitro: at least two factors identified. *Thorax*, **42**, 256–261

TAYLOR, M. and YOUNG, A. (1961) Studies on atrophic rhinitis. *Journal of Laryngology and Otology*, **75**, 574–590

THOMAS G. G., TOOHILL, R. J. and LEHMAN, R. H. (1974) Nasal actinomycosis following heterograft. *Archives of Otolaryngology*, **100**, 377–378

TOPPOZADA, H., RIAD, W., MICHAELS, L., GAAFAR, H. and SID-AHMED, K. (1981) The epithelium and chronic inflammatory cells in scleroma. *Journal of Laryngology and Otology*, **95**, 1049–1057

TOPPOZADA, H., MAZLOUM, H., EL-SAWY, M., MALATIZ, R. and YAKOUT, Y. (1983) The complement fixation test in rhinoscleroma. *Journal of Laryngology and Otology*, **97**, 55–57

TOPPOZADA, H. H. and GAAFER, H. A. (1986) The effect of streptomycin and irradiation on rhinoscleroma (electron microscopic study). *Journal of Laryngology and Otology*, **100**, 809–815

TOS, M. (1982) Goblet cells and glands in the nose and paranasal sinuses. In: *The Nose*, edited by D. Proctor and I. Andersen. Amsterdam: Elsevier Biomedical Press. pp. 99–144

TYRRELL, D. A. J. and BYNDE, M. L. (1961) Some further virus isolations from common colds. *British Medical Journal*, **1**, 393–396

VAN CAUWENBERGE, P. B. (1985) Epidemiology of the common cold. *Rhinology*, **23**, 273–282

WEISS, J. A. (1960) Sarcoidosis in otolaryngology. *Laryngoscope*, **70**, 1351–1390

WILSON, R., ROBERTS, D. and COLE, P. J. (1985) Effect of bacterial products on human ciliary function in vitro. *Thorax*, **40**, 125–131

WILSON, R., SYKES, D. A., CURRIE, D. and COLE, P. J. (1986) Beat frequency of cilia from sites of purulent infection. *Thorax*, **41**, 453–458

WILSON, R., ALTON, E., RUTMAN, A., HIGGINS, P., AL NAKIB, W., GEDDES, D. M. et al. (1987a) Upper respiratory tract viral infection and mucociliary clearance. *European Journal of Respiratory Disease*, **70**, 272–279

WILSON, R., PITT, T., TAYLOR, G., WATSON, D., MACDERMOT, J., SYKES, D. et al. (1987b) Pyocyanin and 1-hydroxy phenazine inhibit the beating of human respiratory cilia in vitro. *Journal of Clinical Investigation*, **79**, 221–229

WILSON, R., SYKES, D. A., CHAN, K. L., COLE P. J. and MACKAY, I. S. (1987c) The effect of head position on the efficacy of topical treatment of chronic mucopurulent rhino-sinusitis. *Thorax*, **42**, 631–632

WILSON, T. G. (1964) Teflon in glycerine paste in rhinology. *Journal of Laryngology and Otology*, **78**, 953–958

YASMIN, A. and SAFWAT, F. (1966) Unusual features of scleroma. *Journal of Laryngology and Otology*, **80**, 524–532

YOUNG, A. (1967) Closure of the nostrils in atrophic rhinitis. *Journal of Laryngology and Otology*, **81**, 515–524

YOUNG, D. (1970) Surgical treatment of male infertility. *Journal of Reproduction and Fertility*, **23**, 541–542

YOUSEM, D. M., GALETTA, S. L., GUSNARD, D. A. and GOLDBERG, H. I. (1989) MR findings in rhinocerebral mucormycosis. *Journal of Computer Assisted Tomography*, **13**, 878–882

ZIMENT, I. (1991) Help for an overtaxed mucociliary system: managing abnormal mucus. *Journal of Respiratory Disease*, **12**, 21–33

ZINREICH, J. (1993) Imaging of inflammatory sinus disease. *Otolaryngologic Clinics of North America*, **26**, 535–547

9

Intrinsic rhinitis

A. S. Jones

Introduction

Terminology

Intrinsic rhinitis is a non-infective, non-allergic condition. Like many diseases whose aetiology is obscure, it has been bedevilled by various names and misconceptions. Some authors use the term perennial rhinitis to describe intrinsic rhinitis. This is unfortunate as perennial rhinitis includes both allergic and non-allergic causes. Even the suffix – itis – is misleading as at least some cases of intrinsic rhinitis have no pathological evidence of inflammation and some authors have thus suggested that intrinsic rhinopathy would be a better term. Other authors have stated that non-infectious, non-allergic perennial rhinitis would be a better name for the condition and of course the old name of vasomotor rhinitis is still perhaps the commonest term. In a disease complex where the aetiology and pathophysiology have not yet been understood there is much to commend a short term and intrinsic rhinitis is not only short, but its meaning is clear.

Background

Intrinsic rhinitis is essentially a medical condition which has been described and treated by, what has until recently, been an almost exclusively surgical discipline. The lack of unequivocal physical signs in this condition has further heightened the veil of mystery that surrounds it. Historically surgical classification has been based on observational data supplemented by the findings of a pathologist. Because gross signs tend not to be present the problem has been exacerbated. Based on present day evidence intrinsic rhinitis consists of at least two separate disease entities and may well represent a symptom complex produced by several pathological conditions.

Two surgically obvious features occur in intrinsic rhinitis. These are inferior turbinate hypertrophy and nasal polyp formation. Inferior turbinate hypertrophy will be discussed in this chapter whereas nasal polyposis is the subject of Chapter 10 in this volume.

Historical background

Various references to rhinology are found in the writings of ancient Egypt and it is of interest that the first physician in history whose name we know was thought to be a rhinologist. His name was Sekhet'enanch and he lived around 3500 BC (Wright, 1902). The earliest writings on medicine are in the Egyptian's papyri and the first complete papyrus is known as the Ebers papyrus dating from about 1550 BC. Nasal catarrh is dealt with by this: it describes rhinorrhoea and bags under the eyes and recommends various methods of treating these symptoms. While the papyri do not specifically describe hypertrophic turbinates these have been discovered in a skull dated 1000 BC and two further skulls of the early centuries of the first millennium BC (Leek, 1986). Nasal polyps were probably described in the Ebers papyrus and their removal is probably also described (Pahor and Kimura 1991).

Hippocrates, born on the Greek island of Kos in 460 BC made further references to rhinology, and his method of removing nasal polyps by means of a sponge tied to a string was in use into the late nineteenth century. Further advances in rhinology were not made until AD 131 when Galen was born. He was educated at Alexandria and later practised in Rome. Galen, like Hippocrates, believed that the nasal secretions originated from the brain, straining through the ethmoid bones into the nasal cavities. He understood the nasal function of air conditioning:

filtering, warming and moistening of inspired air. Little further progress was made in the understanding of rhinitis until Conrad Victor Schneider described the membranes of the nose in *De Catarrhis* in 1660. Schneider believed that nasal secretions arose from the mucous membrane (Weir, 1990). He did not, however, describe the nasal glands, these were described by Gino Santorini in his *Observationes Anatomicae* of 1724. The microscopic appearance of the nasal mucous membrane was noted by Steno in 1662 and he described the nasal vasculature. Nasal polyps have of course attracted considerable interest with St Hilaire in 1698 giving a description of how polyps may develop and various other theories were expounded by several authorities (Weir, 1990). Morgani in the latter half of the eighteenth century described hypertrophy of the inferior turbinates (Weir, 1990).

In 1853 Kohlrausch spoke of cavernous tissue in the inferior turbinate (Weir, 1990) but the erectile tissue of the nasal mucosa was described fully by Zuckerkandl (1882). The connection between rhinitis and asthma was noted by Hack (1882) in a paper entitled *Reflex Neuroses*. This paper attracted considerable attention particularly with regard to mucosal hypertrophy. This being treated with chloroacetic acid or galvanic cautery.

Clinical characterization

Clinical picture

There are six main symptoms of rhinitis. These are congestion, sneezing, nasal itching, rhinorrhoea, hyposmia and postnasal discharge. The latter may be considered as posterior rhinorrhoea. Of these nasal symptoms significant sneezing and nasal itching are highly suggestive of allergic rhinitis and tend not to occur with intrinsic rhinitis. Very marked nasal congestion and significant hyposmia, tend to be symptoms of non-allergic rhinitis. Rhinitis presenting in childhood is almost invariably of allergic aetiology, whereas rhinitis developing for the first time in the adult is more likely to be due to intrinsic rhinitis.

The classification of rhinitis

Seebohm (1978) noted that there was a group of patients with perennial rhinitis who had negative allergy tests and yet had eosinophils in the nasal secretions. Mullarkey, Hill and Webb (1980) evaluated 142 patients with perennial rhinitis. They investigated these patients by a variety of methods including a nasal secretion eosinophil count. This was considered positive when more than 25% of the cells in the nasal smear were eosinophils. They also assessed the allergic status of the patient by history, skin tests and IgE levels. Using this criterion 34% of their patients were classified as definitely allergic and 15% probably allergic suggesting half of the total number of patients with perennial rhinitis were suffering from allergy. Thirty-seven per cent of their patients were suffering from non-eosinophilic intrinsic rhinitis and 15% of patients (with no demonstrable allergies) had significant nasal secretion eosinophilia. Thus perennial rhinitis can be classified according to two parameters. The first is the presence or absence of allergy and the second is the presence or absence of nasal secretion eosinophilia. Allergic rhinitis is always associated with nasal eosinophilia, whereas non-allergic rhinitis may or may not have eosinophilia. Approximately one-third of intrinsic rhinitis patients have nasal secretion eosinophilia.

Clinical characterization of intrinsic rhinitis

Mygind and Weeke (1983) described, in a modification and extension of Seebohm's work (Seebohm, 1978), the various clinical features of eosinophilic and non-eosinophilic intrinsic rhinitis. They noted that the eosinophilic variety of intrinsic rhinitis was characterized by marked nasal congestion, profuse rhinorrhoea, hyposmia, inferior turbinate hypertrophy and mucoid nasal secretion. They also noted, as did Mullarkey, Hill and Webb (1980) that nasal polyposis was a frequent occurrence in the eosinophilic group. Mygind and Weeke (1983) suggested that rhinorrhoea is profuse in both eosinophilic and non-eosinophilic intrinsic rhinitis. However, Borum Mygind and Schultz Larsen (1979), in describing a new treatment for rhinitis, presented a series of patients in whom rhinorrhoea was the predominant symptom. In a discussion of rhinitis Wentges, in 1979, suggested that there were two clinical types of intrinsic rhinitis and he termed these the 'nasal obstruction syndrome' and the 'rhinorrhoea syndrome'. A large number of patients with intrinsic rhinitis fall into one of two categories; those suffering mainly from nasal obstruction and those suffering mainly from rhinorrhoea. Those with nasal obstruction tend to have nasal secretion eosinophilia whereas those with rhinorrhoea do not. The rhinorrhoea group tend to occur in relatively advanced age whereas the nasal obstruction group tend to occur in middle-age. Table 9.1 summarizes the clinical picture of intrinsic rhinitis.

Other clinical differences between eosinophilic and non-eosinophilic intrinsic rhinitis also occur. Marked mucosal thickening frequently occurs in the eosinophilic group and this is often evident on plain radiological examination of the nasal sinuses. These features do not occur in the non-eosinophilic group. Patients with eosinophilic intrinsic rhinitis frequently have asthma and occasionally have aspirin sensitivity neither of which occurs in the non-eosinophilic subgroup. One of the most clinically obvious differences

Table 9.1 Clinical features of eosinophilic and non-eosinophilic intrinsic rhinitis

Symptom	Eosinophilic	Non-eosinophilic
Obstruction	Moderate/severe	Mild
Rhinorrhoea	Mild/moderate	Severe
Sneezing/pruritus	Minimal	Minimal
Hyposmia	Usual	Rare
Sign		
Mucosal swelling	Marked	Mild
Inferior turbinate enlargement	Marked	Mild
Polyps	Frequent	Never
Sinus mucosal thickening	Frequent	Rare

between the two types of rhinitis is the dramatic response of the eosinophilic subgroup to intranasal corticosteroids and the poor response of the non-eosinophilic group to any therapy apart from anticholinergic agents (Borum, Mygind and Schultz Larsen, 1979; Mygind and Weeke, 1983).

This view is not universally shared as at least one group of workers describe profuse watery rhinorrhoea, paroxysms of sneezing and nasal itching in the absence of marked nasal obstruction in patients with nasal eosinophilia and no detectable allergies (Jacobs, Freedman and Boswell, 1981). This series of 52 patients had symptomatology that was far from typical of eosinophilic intrinsic rhinitis and this demonstrates the problem in categorizing and describing intrinsic rhinitis. The difficulty is that the condition is certainly more than one disease and may in fact be several and, until accurate pathophysiological characterization can be completed, the study and treatment of the disease complex will remain unsatisfactory.

Epidemiology and incidence

The epidemiolpogy of perennial rhinitis is difficult to study because of the lack of a consistent definition and the lack of understanding of the pathophysiology. Some studies exist on the incidence of 'allergic rhinitis', although for practical reasons allergy tests are frequently not carried out. A large number of such patients will of course by suffering from seasonal allergic rhinitis as well as a large number of those with intrinsic rhinitis. In several studies of patients in general practice, 'allergic rhinitis' has been defined as 'paroxysmal sneezing and rhinorrhoea with or without conjunctivitis and without signs of infection'.

In 1974, Broder *et al.* studied 10 000 people in a town in Michigan. The incidence rate of 'allergic rhinitis' was 0.5% and the one year prevalence rate 7.5% for males and 8.2% for females. The cumulative prevalence rate was 10% for both sexes.* Edfors-Lubs in 1971 found a cumulative prevalence rate for 'allergic rhinitis' of 14.5% in Sweden. In a national morbidity study in Britain for 1970/72, the one year prevalence rate for 'hay fever' was just over 1% (Office of Population Censuses and Surveys, 1974). In a study of 'hay fever' in general practice, Perki (1972) found a prevalence rate of 2% in British general practice patients. In a Danish population study 2000 adults were investigated using a questionnaire about 'hay fever and hay fever-like disease'. An incidence rate of 1%, a one-year period prevalence rate of 1% and a cumulative prevalence rate of 9% were found (Fry, 1979). From these data it appears that 10% of the population may suffer from 'allergic rhinitis'. It must be accepted that a large number of these patients were, in fact, suffering from intrinsic rhinitis. If the definition of 'allergic-like disease' were extended to include intermittent nasal obstruction as a main symptom, then it is likely that the total number of patients affected would be much increased. In a study carried out in 1989, Jessen and Janzon sent questionnaires to 1469 unselected individuals: 21% suffered from 'non-allergic' nasal complaints and only 5% from 'allergic' complaints. The prevalence of the non-allergic complaints was highest in subjects in their third decade. In 1991, Sibbald and Rink studied a London general practice and found that 13% of the patients had perennial rhinitis of which half were suffering from intrinsic rhinitis.

Another way of attempting to study the incidence of intrinsic rhinitis is to look at those patients suffering from nasal polyposis. Nasal polyposis is almost certainly a part of the disease complex of eosinophilic non-allergic rhinitis, allergy (if present) being incidental (Mullarkey, Hill and Webb, 1980; Jacobs, Freedman and Boswell, 1981). The prevalence of nasal polyposis has been studied in some detail (Settipane and Chafee, 1977). It was found that approximately 30% of patients with the eosinophilic subgroup of intrinsic rhinitis suffered from nasal polyposis and because those with eosinophilic rhinitis form one-third of those patients with intrinsic rhinitis, one can arrive at a figure of 18% for the incidence of intrinsic rhinitis in the population. Although this figure may seem high it should be remembered that symptoms of intrinsic rhinitis, when mild, merge into the normal range of human experience.

In those patients said to be suffering from 'allergic rhinitis' allergy is actually present in 80% of children but in those patients aged over 60 years only 20% demonstrate any evidence of allergy (Mygind, 1978). Those patients defined as having perennial rhinitis

---

* *The incidence rate is the number of new cases per 100 persons. The prevalence rate is the number of active cases during a one year period per 100 persons. The cumulative prevalence rate is the number of persons who have ever had the disease per 100 people.*

who are tested by skin tests to a panel of allergens have allergy demonstrated in only 30–60% of cases (Mygind *et al.*, 1978). In addition, as the patient presenting with perennial rhinitis becomes older so the chance of non-eosinophilic intrinsic rhinitis being the cause increases at the expense of the eosinophilic subgroup.

In summary figures for the prevalence of intrinsic rhinitis vary from 7% to 21%. It is thus a very common disease with considerable social and economic consequences.

Eosinophilia, allergy and hyperreactivity
Nasal secretion eosinophilia

At present, a patient with perennial non-infectious rhinitis is characterized on the basis of allergy assessment and nasal secretion eosinophilia. Because eosinophilia is so central to the present understanding of intrinsic rhinitis this will be dealt with in some detail. The eosinophil was first described by Ehrlich in 1879. It was he who stained and characterized the typical acidophilic granules, but it was nearly 50 years before the first report of eosinophils in nasal secretion smears was published (Eyerman, 1927). Three cell types were noted – neutrophils and epithelial cells being present in addition to eosinophils. From the start it was found that considerable variation occurred in the sampling of nasal secretions and Hansel (1936) suggested specimens should be taken from both nostrils and more recent work has confirmed this (Kaufman *et al.*, 1982). Vaheri (1956) found that nasal biopsies from patients with 'rhinitis' contained eosinophils in the mucosa. The eosinophils were particularly numerous in the middle turbinate and ethmoid regions. Unfortunately he did not carry out nasal secretion sampling at the same time. Phillips *et al.* (1992) have recently shown that there is a close correlation between nasal mucosal eosinophil counts in nasal biopsies and nasal eosinophil counts in nasal secretion smears.

Most of the work on nasal eosinophilia has been carried out on patients with 'allergic rhinitis'. It has been noted that the level of nasal secretion eosinophilia correlates with the severity of the nasal symptoms (Murray, 1971; Holopainen, Malmberg and Tarkiainen, 1977). Recruitment of eosinophils into the nasal mucosa can occur surprisingly quickly; within 1–3 hours in response to nasal allergen challenge, and this may persist for 1–3 days (Mygind, 1978). Studies have demonstrated a reduction in the level of nasal secretion eosinophil numbers following topical nasal steroid treatment and this reduction is associated with a corresponding reduction in nasal symptoms (Holopainen, Malmberg and Tarkiainen, 1977). Eosinophils may be subdivided into those that are active and those that are inactive on the basis of the immunohistochemical staining characteristics of the granules (Lozewicz *et al.*, 1992). In Lozewicz's study the eosinophil count did not fall with topical nasal steroids but the staining characteristics based on the immunohistochemistry of the granules suggested that previously active eosinophils became inactive. This change correlated with a reduction in the nasal symptoms.

The eosinophil contains many enzymes, including aryl sulphatase, histaminase, and phospholipase D. The presence of these enzymes is evidence that the eosinophil may be important in damping down the early phase of the allergic response by inactivating mast cell mediators such as leukotrienes, histamine, and platelet activating factor. On the other hand, eosinophils contain two cytotoxic substances: eosinophil cationic protein and major basic protein. While these agents can cause tissue damage in allergic disease (Nishioka *et al.*, 1993) their original function was probably part of the host defence against parasites; both these agents being highly toxic to helminths.

Nasal secretion eosinophilia appears to be a very common finding. Of 634 students studied by Malmberg (1979), 152 had nasal secretion eosinophilia and, of these, 129 reported a history of 'rhinitis'. Other studies have shown that nasal secretion eosinophilia occurs in 13% of infants (Matheson *et al.*, 1957) and in 20% of young adults (Malmberg, 1979). Not all patients with nasal eosinophilia are symptomatic. Of the infants that were found to have eosinophils in the secretions, most were asymptomatic as were 60% of school children with this finding. Of young adults, on the other hand, only one third were symptom-free. There is some evidence that asymptomatic nasal secretion eosinophilia may indicate a risk of subsequently developing symptomatic rhinitis (Crawford, 1960).

Various factors may affect the expression of eosinophils in the nasal secretions. Obviously in allergic individuals, allergen exposure is important (Mygind, 1978) but infection may also affect the secretion eosinophil count. Such counts may fall in the presence of infection and may be inversely related to the neutrophil count in a secretion smear (Malmberg, 1979).

The sampling of nasal eosinophils is a problem. Eosinophil counts are known to vary between nasal cavities in the same patient (Kaufman *et al.*, 1982) and to vary depending from which part of the nasal cavity the secretion smear is taken. (Phillips *et al.*, 1992). Various methods of sampling nasal secretions have been described. The commonest is to use a cotton swab tightly wound around an applicator. This is passed behind the inferior turbinate and brought forward (Mygind, 1986). This method assumes that the eosinophil distribution is uniform and that the area adjacent to the inferior turbinate is most representative. In an effort to improve sampling Pipkorn, Karlsson and Enerback (1988) described a 'rhinobrush'. This is a plastic coated steel wire with nylon strings (Mellanrumsborste 0.8 mm, Apoteksbolaged, Gothenburg). Other methods include blowing secretions on to wax paper (Miller *et al.*, 1982) or into a polythene bag (Jacobs *et al.*, 1981). Sampling secretions that have not been obtained by a swab or brushing have possible advantages in that the sampling may be more representative and less dependent on variations in eosinophil distribution. The problem, however, is that nasal secretions vary considerably in quantity and viscosity and this makes this technique prone to considerable error and in many patients no sample will be obtained. Phillips *et al.* (1992) found that taking smears from a wide variety of sites within the nose produced results that correlated well with the degree of eosinophilia in nasal biopsy specimens. It thus appears that if nasal secretion samples are taken carefully with a cotton-tipped probe and care is taken to sample a wide area of the nose, a representative set of smears may be obtained.

Another problem is at what level does a nasal secretion eosinophil count become significant? Studies have shown considerable variation. Mygind (1978) considers a positive result if 10% of a diffusely spread smear contains eosinophils or 50% of a single part of a smear contains a large number of eosinophils. Mullarkey, Hill and Webb (1980) consider that eosinophils must make up more than 25% of the total cell count of a nasal secretion smear before nasal secretion eosinophilia is diagnosed. Phillips *et al.* (1992) agreed with the latter view but noted that, of the patients in their study with intrinsic rhinitis two were considered eosinophilic and eight non-eosinophilic using Mullarkey's criteria, whereas six would be classified as eosinophilic and four non-eosinophilic using Mygind's criteria. This is obviously a considerable problem and not easily resolved. As a large number of subjects with nasal eosinophilia are asymptomatic a simple correlation between symptoms and eosinophil count cannot be used to define this latter parameter. Before this problem can be resolved much basic work into the aetiology and pathology of intrinsic rhinitis must be carried out.

It is the author's preference for smears to be taken from several sites within each nasal cavity, transferred to Cytospin fluid and a Cytospin centrifuge is used to produce an even smear on a microscope slide (Pipkorn and Karlsson, 1988). The smear is stained with Mayer's haemalum (taken up by the nuclei) then washed with water and then in 70% ethanol. The smear is then stained with sirius red for 1 hour, washed in water for 10 minutes and dehydrated. The eosinophil count is obtained by counting at least 500 inflammatory cells and expressing the eosinophil count as a percentage (Figure 9.1).

The exclusion of allergy

At present intrinsic rhinitis remains a diagnosis of exclusion. While the broader diagnosis of perennial rhinitis may be made by history and examination, the diagnosis of non-allergic perennial rhinitis

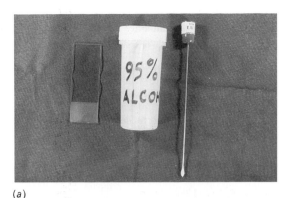

(*a*)

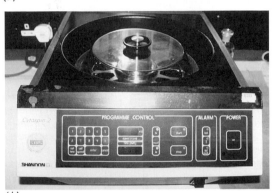

(*b*)

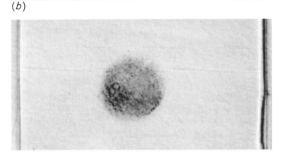

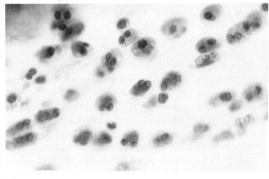

(*d*)

Figure 9.1 Taking a smear for nasal cytology: (*a*) a cotton tipped probe and cytology fluid; (*b*) a Cytospin centrifuge; (*c*) a Cytospin preparation; (*d*) a nasal cytogram

(intrinsic rhinitis) requires that, in addition, a full allergic history and investigations must be negative. For many years skin testing has been the mainstay of allergy diagnosis. A problem with skin testing is that many asymptomatic subjects have positive skin tests and this frequency varies from 6% to 30% (Barbee *et al.*, 1976). Positive skin tests are more likely to occur in young adults and in this group only about half the subjects develop symptoms. Many authorities regard a positive skin test in asymptomatic individuals as evidence of latent allergy or, if local eosinophilia is present, of subclinical allergy. For example, an asymptomatic subject with a positive skin test to grass pollen has a significantly increased risk of subsequently developing hay fever.

Serum IgE concentrations can be measured by immunoassay and while the median values are significantly higher in allergic perennial rhinitis than they are in intrinsic rhinitis or normal subjects, the overlap of values is too big to make it a clinically useful test on its own (Mygind *et al.*, 1978). In the latter paper an elevated serum IgE was taken as greater than 370 units/ml and only 7% of patients with perennial rhinitis had an elevated serum IgE even though 40% of these patients had positive skin tests. In patients with perennial rhinitis and asthma 46% had elevated IgE values. Total serum IgE levels therefore may reflect the size of the 'shock organ' rather than being diagnostic of allergy per se. Workers such as Wittig (Wittig *et al.*, 1980) also demonstrated a wide overlap between serum IgE levels in patients with allergic rhinitis and in normal controls. Measurement of allergen specific IgE by the radio-allergosorbent test (RAST) has been of great value in allergy research (Wide, Bermich and Johansson, 1967). RAST has a very high correlation with skin tests (Mygind, 1978) and has some advantages over skin tests. The test is not invalidated by systemic drugs such as antihistamines and is not affected by any cutaneous hyper-reactivity. In addition, in patients with extensive skin disease, RAST is the only allergy test possible. The disadvantages of RAST are that the results are not immediately available, it is expensive and it is not as sensitive as skin testing.

A history of allergy is important and no test should be interpreted without an adequate history. History on its own may be quite specific as in the case of hay fever or allergy to animal dander. In most cases of perennial rhinitis however, history on its own is of little value (Sibbald and Rink, 1991). Most rhinologists, however, value a full history and various questionnaires have been designed to make it more accurate and standardized (Dirksen, 1982). Nasal allergen challenge preceded and followed by rhinomanometry to assess any change in resistance is the most sensitive method for assessing nasal allergy and is the final arbiter in difficult cases. The technique is, however, extremely time consuming. An additional measurement that can be carried out to assess the nasal response to allergen challenge is to assess any changes in the eosinophil counts in the nasal secretion.

In practice, the combination of a strong history of allergy and positive skin tests perhaps with a high total IgE estimation will diagnose 90% of patients with allergy. It is the author's practice to test for house dust mite, mixed animal dander, fungi and, for completeness, grass and mixed tree pollen. While only one grass pollen need be tested as the pollens cross react the same is not true for tree pollen. A positive result to mixed allergen solutions obviously requires further testing to elucidate the specific allergen responsible for symptoms in that individual.

Allergy and intrinsic rhinitis

The problems in defining intrinsic rhinitis are legion and one of the most serious is the possibility of allergy being present in these patients. In a fascinating study, Sibbald and Rink (1990) found that the month of birth was a risk factor for both allergic and *non-allergic* rhinitis. In 1975, Huggins and Brostoff (1975) described a small group of patients with negative skin tests and negative serum IgE to house dust mite but positive nasal challenges and IgE present in the nasal secretions. It is now generally accepted that nasal polyps occur almost exclusively in patients with eosinophilic intrinsic rhinitis (Caplin, Haynes and Spahn, 1971; Mullarkey, Hill and Webb, 1980; Mygind and Weeke, 1983). The incidence, however, of nasal polyps in allergic rhinitis is approximately 10% and this compares with only 4% in the general population (Settipane and Chafee, 1977). While this may represent sampling error, recent work has suggested that allergy to house dust mite antigen may be more common than expected in patients with nasal polyposis. Mertens, Wellbrock and Feidert (1991) found that 28% of their cases of nasal polyps had an allergy to house dust mite and in the younger patient (below 40 years of age) nearly half of them had such an allergy. The diagnosis in many cases was reached only after nasal challenge testing. In another recent investigation, Moneret-Vautrin, Way off and Hsieh (1988) found that some patients diagnosed as suffering from intrinsic rhinitis with eosinophilia in fact had allergy to house dust mite. They suggested that for the diagnosis of intrinsic rhinitis to be firmly established the degree of nasal secretion eosinophilia following nasal challenge with house dust mite should be studied; an increase indicating allergy. In a later study Moneret-Vautrin *et al.* (1990) were unable to demonstrate allergy to house dust mite in a group of patients with either eosinophilic or non-eosinophilic intrinsic rhinitis. Interestingly they noted an increase in adrenergic hyperreactivity among these patients when they studied the reactivity of the cardiovascular alpha and beta adrenoreceptors. In support of this Deuschl and Johansson (1977) were unable to find any patients whose nasal allergen specific IgE scores exceeded serum levels. Again Swart *et al.* (1991) found no nasal secretion IgE in patients with intrinsic rhinitis.

It thus seems that there is a small group of patients with negative or weakly positive skin tests who have allergy, particularly to house dust mite, on nasal challenge testing. While at face value this may indicate the nasal condition is due to house dust mite allergy, the significance of this finding in response to such a powerful stimulus must be in doubt.

Hyperreactivity

The aetiology of intrinsic rhinitis is obscure but the most frequently cited theory has been that of autonomic imbalance (Malcolmson, 1959). Other theories include allergy to an as yet unidentified allergen and psychosomatic problems. Patients with perennial rhinitis have hyperreactivity demonstrating an increase in nasal resistance to airflow with histamine challenge and an increase in nasal secretion with methacholine challenge (Corrado *et al.*, 1986). Patients with intrinsic rhinitis appear to have two different types of response depending on whether the main symptom is nasal obstruction or rhinorrhoea. A study in 1991 by Gerth-van-Wijk (Gerth-van-Wijk and Dieges, 1991) found that patients with intrinsic rhinitis with rhinorrhoea proved to be hyperresponsive to metacholine challenge compared to normal controls. In contrast, patients with nasal obstruction as the main symptom tended to be hyperresponsive to histamine. In eosinophilic intrinsic rhinitis the cause of the hyperreactivity may be an underlying inflammation within the nasal mucosa (Moneret-Vautrin *et al.*, 1992). Kubo and Kumazawa (1993) experimentally induced nasal hypersensitivity in guinea-pigs and proposed that this was basically due to disturbances of β-receptor function. They proposed four mechanisms for this dysfunction and the ensuing airway hyperreactivity:

1. Down-regulation caused by excess endogenous noradrenaline stimulation
2. Down-regulation and uncoupling of adenylate cyclase produced by the inflammatory mediator induced activation of protein kinase
3. The action of a β-receptor inhibitory factor presumed to be an anti-β-receptor autoantibody
4. Dysfunction of β-receptor kinase which is known to cause short-term desensitization of β-receptors after exposure to β-agonists.

Aetiology

The autonomic nervous system exerts its effects by secreting neurotransmitters at nerve terminals (Bacq, 1975). Until recently it was thought that there were two neurotransmitters: adrenaline secreted by the sympathetic nerve endings and acetylcholine secreted by the parasympathetic nerve endings. Adrenergic receptors may be of two basic types, α and β (Mygind, 1986), the nasal vasculature vasoconstricting following α-receptor stimulation (Aschan and Drettner, 1964). Both α and β-receptors may be further subdivided (into 1 and 2) on the basis of their pharmacological properties and site. β-Receptors are relatively unimportant in the control of nasal airway resistance (Malm, 1974a) but when stimulated may cause vasodilatation (Malm, 1974b). Division of the nasal sympathetic input causes nasal obstruction (Moore, 1954) whereas electrical stimulation causes nasal decongestion (Malm, 1973). It is now known that other neurotransmitters exist, for example vasoactive intestinal polypeptide found in association with parasympathetic nerve endings (Lundberg *et al.*, 1980) and neuropeptide Y with sympathetic nerve endings (Uddman, Sundler and Emson, 1984). Nasal obstruction can occur in patients as a side effect of certain antihypertensive drugs particularly where these agents exert their effect by sympathetic blockade (Gorenberg, 1979). In addition, the long-term use of topical α-adrenoceptor agonists may cause rhinitis medicamentosa; a condition not unlike the nasal congestion found in intrinsic rhinitis (Toohill *et al.*, 1981).

While nasal resistance to airflow is controlled by the sympathetic system, innervation of the nasal glands is subserved by the parasympathetic nerves (Golding-Wood, 1961; Eccles and Wilson, 1973; Wilson and Yates, 1978). Increase in parasympathetic outflow leads to glandular hypersecretion. Vasoactive intestinal polypeptide is liberated during such parasympathetic activity and may be responsible for the associated atropine resistant vasodilatation (Lundberg *et al.*, 1980). Nasal secretion can be reduced to basal levels by the interruption of the nasal parasympathetic supply by vidian neurectomy (Golding-Wood, 1961, 1973).

The evidence thus far presented leads to the generally accepted view of 'vasomotor rhinitis' and this is best expressed in the work of Malcolmson (1959). There is some evidence that *non-eosinophilic* intrinsic rhinitis may in fact be due to such autonomic imbalance. This condition may be relieved by the topical administration of anticholinergic agents such as ipratropium bromide (Borum, Mygind and Schultz Larsen, 1979) as well as by vidian neurectomy (Golding-Wood, 1973). A condition clinically similar to non-eosinophilic intrinsic rhinitis has been reported as a side effect of treatment with β-adrenoreceptor blocking agents (Malm, 1981).

Eosinophilic intrinsic rhinitis is probably a different entity. The fact that inflammatory cells are present suggests the disease process may be taking place at a cellular level in the nasal mucosa. Eosinophilic intrinsic rhinitis responds well to topical inhaled nasal steroids (Mygind and Weeke, 1983) and this again suggests that inflammation plays a part in the disease process. Drake-Lee (1987) demonstrated that nasal mast cells in subjects with nasal polyposis (a disease associated with eosinophilic intrinsic rhinitis) show extensive degranulation both in the polyps and in the mucosa of the inferior turbinate. The structural changes are similar to those seen in patients with allergic rhinitis and has been noted by other workers (Cauna *et al.*, 1972). Eight per cent of subjects with nasal polyposis suffer intolerance to aspirin (Drake-Lee *et al.*, 1984). This proportion rises significantly in patients with nasal polyposis and asthma (Delaney, 1976) and in some studies on patients with intrinsic rhinitis, nasal polyposis and intrinsic asthma 70% have aspirin sensitivity (Samter and Beers, 1968; Spector and Farr, 1983). The prevalence of aspirin intolerance in patients with intrinsic rhinitis alone is, however, probably less than 1% (Chafee and Settipane, 1974). In children aspirin intolerance may be more common (Mygind, Pederson and Nielsen, 1983). It has been demonstrated that inhibition of prostaglandin synthesis by aspirin (Vane, 1971) causes an increase in nasal resistance to airflow in asymptomatic human subjects (Jones *et al.*, 1985). The nasal mucosa is capable of synthesizing and inactivating prostaglandins (Bedwani, Eccles and Jones, 1983a, 1984). In vivo administration of E series prostaglandins decreases nasal resistance to airflow (Anggard, 1969; Bedwani, Eccles and Jones, 1983b; Jackson, 1970; Karim, Adaikan and Kunaratnam, 1978), while prostaglandins D_2 and I_2 cause an increase (Bedwani, Eccles and Jones, 1983b). Subjects with allergic rhinitis have large quantities of E series prostaglandins present in their nasal secretions implying that these agents may be important in nasal inflammation (Okazaki *et al.*, 1977).

Prostaglandins have complex effects, one class of prostaglandins often having opposite effects to another. For instance, the prostaglandin liberated from human mast cells on degranulation, prostaglandin D_2, facilitates mast cell degranulation while prostaglandin E_2 inhibits it (Mygind, 1986). Lipoxygenase products have been isolated from nasal polyps and high levels of leukotrienes B_4 and C_4 have been found. Polyps associated with aspirin intolerance have particularly high levels of arachidonic acid metabolites (Jung *et al.*, 1987). The evidence presented suggests that a defect in eicosanoid metabolism may be one possible abnormality in (eosinophilic) intrinsic rhinitis.

Frequently, inflammatory mediators demonstrate considerable interplay with the autonomic nervous system and prostaglandins are no exception (Wasserman *et al.*, 1977; Ramwell, 1980). Prostaglandin E_2 inhibits adrenergic neurotransmission while prostaglandin $F_{2\alpha}$ facilitates it (Ramwell, 1980). Similarly autonomic outflow can modulate the biological effects of eicosanoids (Wasserman *et al.*, 1977). If intrinsic rhinitis is a defect in eicosanoid metabolism, perhaps being a prostaglandin deficiency disease, then it is possible that pharmacological manipulation of prostaglandin metabolism may prove therapeutically beneficial. Prostaglandin analogues (Brand *et al.*, 1985) could be administered as could non-specific stimulators of prostaglandin synthesis, such as frusemide and low dose paracetamol (Ramwell, 1980).

While the above argument is compelling a recent case report describes a patient whose asthma was improved by aspirin (Imokawa *et al.*, 1992)! In addition recent work has suggested that while prostaglandin D_2 levels are reduced in patients with intrinsic rhinitis, levels of prostaglandin E_2 may be increased (Phillips and Jones, unpublished data) compared with normal subjects.

Autonomic function and asthma have been studied in detail and in this condition it is known that autonomic imbalance plays a part in the airway hyperactivity. The balance is between the moderating effect of the β_2-adrenoreceptor responsiveness on the one hand and the hyperreactivity producing effects of the α-adrenoreceptor and cholinoceptors on the other (Mygind, 1986). In asthma autoantibodies have recently been found to β_2-adrenoreceptors (Wallukat and Wollenberger, 1992). The concept of autonomic imbalance also applies to perennial rhinitis (Corrado *et al.*, 1986) and Kubo and Kamazawa (1993) have shown in guinea-pigs with experimentally induced nasal hypersensitivity that β-receptor function is disturbed.

Stjarne *et al.* (1989) compared the effect of local applied capsaicin, nicotine and methacholine in patients with no symptoms (what the authors term vasomotor rhinitis) and those patients with increased nasal secretion as a main symptom of nasal hyperreactivity. Both capsaicin and nicotine challenge caused a larger secretory response in those patients with rhinorrhoea as their main symptom than in the other two groups. Pre-treatment with muscarinic receptor antagonists abolished the secretory response to capsaicin and nicotine and also blocked the methacholine-induced hypersecretion.

The authors suggested that in patients with rhinorrhoea as the main symptom of their intrinsic rhinitis enhanced secretion may be due to hyperreactive efferent cholinergic mechanisms rather than hypersensitive irritant receptors. In a further study of the rhinorrhoea variant of intrinsic rhinitis Rucci *et al.* (1989) carried out vidian neurectomy in 22 patients and investigated the effect of this operation on histamine levels and metabolism and mast cell numbers in the nasal mucosa. They noted that vidian neurectomy cured the nasal symptoms, decreased the previously high histamine levels and reduced histadine-decarboxylase activity. Interestingly the density and degranulation index of mast cells was significantly lowered. These data suggest that an increase in parasympathetic outflow not only leads to mast cells being less hyperreactive (Mygind, 1986), but also leads to reduced chemotaxis to these cells. The findings of this study also suggest that mast cell activity is important in non-eosinophilic intrinsic rhinitis.

The interplay of cellular recruitment and autonomic imbalance is highly complex. The autonomic nervous system certainly plays an important role in the process of inflammation. α-Receptor agonists and acetylcholine facilitate the release of mediators (including prostaglandin D_2) from mast cells while β_2-adrenoreceptor agonists inhibit the release of mediators (Mygind, 1986). The interplay between the autonomic nervous system and prostaglandins is considerable and has already been discussed. As some of the evidence discussed above suggests, autonomic imbalance may be the only process necessary to cause mast cells to degranulate in response to what would normally be considered trivial stimuli. Recruitment of cells does occur and plays a vital part in the inflammatory response within the nose in intrinsic rhinitis (Cauna *et al.*, 1972; Mygind *et al.*, 1978; Borum,

Mygind and Schultz Larsen, 1979; Mullarkey, Hill and Webb, 1980; Mygind and Weeke, 1983; Drake-Lee, 1987). Furthermore, patients with intrinsic rhinitis have a significantly higher secretory immunoglobulin A to protein ratio than healthy control subjects (Swart *et al.*, 1991).

Patients with intrinsic rhinitis have not only been found to demonstrate nasal hyperreactivity as measured by changes in nasal resistance to airflow, but also generalized autonomic hyperreactivity as assessed by changes in systolic and diastolic blood pressure and pulse rate (unpublished data). The autonomic stress tests used were those employed in the investigation of autonomic dysfunction in patients with diabetes. They included changes in blood pressure and pulse in response to variations in posture, isometric exercise and the cold pressor test. The results suggest that those patients with intrinsic rhinitis not only have nasal hyperreactivity but also have generalized autonomic dysfunction. Provisional work suggests that topical nasal steroids (fluticasone) abolish the nasal hyperreactivity, although this has no effect on the generalized autonomic dysfunction (Figure 9.2) (Cook and Jones, unpublished data).

On the evidence so far it seems that eosinophilic intrinsic rhinitis is associated with both autonomic imbalance and local inflammation with recruitment of inflammatory cells; the main symptom being nasal

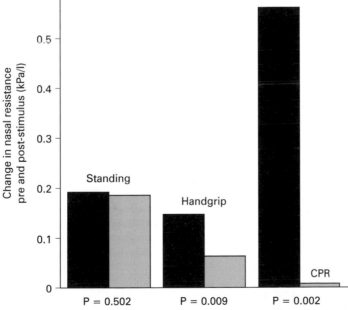

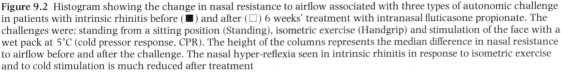

Figure 9.2 Histogram showing the change in nasal resistance to airflow associated with three types of autonomic challenge in patients with intrinsic rhinitis before (■) and after (□) 6 weeks' treatment with intranasal fluticasone propionate. The challenges were: standing from a sitting position (Standing), isometric exercise (Handgrip) and stimulation of the face with a wet pack at 5°C (cold pressor response, CPR). The height of the columns represents the median difference in nasal resistance to airflow before and after the challenge. The nasal hyper-reflexia seen in intrinsic rhinitis in response to isometric exercise and to cold stimulation is much reduced after treatment

obstruction. Non-eosinophilic intrinsic rhinitis, on the other hand, is associated with severe rhinorrhoea as its main symptom and autonomic imbalance as its main pathological feature. Further circumstantial evidence to support this is that corticosteroids have little effect on non-eosinophilic rhinitis (Mygind and Weeke, 1983) while anticholinergic drugs and particularly topical ipratropium control rhinorrhoea in non-eosinophilic intrinsic rhinitis in the majority of subjects (Borum, Mygind and Schultz Larsen, 1979; O'Dwyer *et al.*, 1988).

A further interesting association is that 13% of patients with non-eosinophilic intrinsic rhinitis have asthma as do 14% suffering from the eosinophilic subgroup (Mullarkey, Hill and Webb, 1980). These figures are low compared with the association of allergic rhinitis and asthma occurring in 58% of patients (Mullarkey, Hill and Webb, 1980) and the association of nasal polyps and asthma in 71% (Settipane and Chafee, 1977). In a recent study, Verdiani, Di-Carlo and Buronti (1990) studied bronchial hyperreactivity with carbachol or methacholine challenge in a group of patients with asymptomatic seasonal rhinitis (out of season), a group of patients with symptomatic seasonal rhinitis (during the season) and in patients with perennial rhinitis. Only the perennial rhinitis group exhibited bronchial hyperreactivity. In addition, gas exchange abnormalities have been noted in patients with perennial rhinitis challenged with ultrasonically nebulized distilled water. While this effect was of shorter duration in the rhinitic than in asthmatic subjects, no effect was seen in normal subjects (Dal-Negro, Turco and Allegra, 1992).

Turbinate enlargement

Mucosal swelling and inferior turbinate enlargement

One of the commonest conditions leading to nasal obstruction is the enlarged inferior turbinate. This condition not only affects man but also dogs, cats and horses (Lane, 1982). Enlargement of the inferior turbinates is almost always due to swelling of the submucosa and only rarely due to enlargement of the bone itself. This swelling is caused by the dilatation of the submucosal venous sinusoids (Cauna and Cauna, 1975). In most cases of intrinsic rhinitis the inferior turbinates, although enlarged, are capable of shrinking. The venous sinusoids are under adrenergic control and collapse on sympathetic stimulation (Anggard and Edwall, 1974; Malm, 1977). This shrinking can be facilitated by applying vasoconstrictor drugs containing α-receptor agonists which causes collapse of the venous sinusoids leading to shrinking of the nasal mucosa (Aschan and Drettner, 1964). Sometimes the inferior turbinate is enlarged due to submu-

cosal fibrosis rendering the turbinate incapable of decongestion. In some cases of inferior turbinate hypertrophy the venous sinusoids become atonic (varicose), they then become unresponsive to either endogenous or exogenous adrenergic stimulation (Richardson, 1985). In intrinsic rhinitis the turbinate mucosa may also be oedematous with eosinophils and mast cells present. This tends to be the case in eosinophilic rhinitis rather than the non-eosinophilic subgroup (Cauna *et al.*, 1972; Mygind *et al.*, 1978; Borum, Mygind and Schultz Larsen, 1979; Mullarkey, Hill and Webb, 1980; Mygind and Weeke, 1983; Drake-Lee, 1987; Phillips and Jones, unpublished data).

The diagnosis of intrinsic rhinitis

As in other diseases the diagnosis is based on history, examination and investigations. In a case of intrinsic rhinitis the differential diagnosis is between non-allergic and allergic perennial rhinitis. The distinction is made as discussed above on the basis of history and allergy testing. A summary of the investigations that may be performed in a patient with intrinsic rhinitis are shown in Table 9.2. The patient should have a nasal secretion smear taken and examined for eosinophils. Some objective assessment of nasal patency should be made as should some objective assessment of nasal secretion. Subjective assessments should be made either using a five point scale or a visual analogue scale and diary cards may be useful for the patient to complete.

If sinusitis is suspected then plain radiographs may be obtained but will only demonstrate gross pathology (Stammberger and Wolf, 1988). For more subtle changes and in patients with facial pain, CT scanning will be necessary (Zinreich *et al.*, 1977; Stammberger and Wolf, 1988).

Examination of the nose with Hopkin's rod telescopes should be carried out with particular reference to the ostiomeatal complex (Stammberger and Wolf, 1988).

Objective measures of nasal patency and secretion together with subjective measures are useful in assessing and monitoring response to therapy.

While it is tempting to discharge a patient with intrinsic rhinitis as soon as the diagnosis has been made, perhaps with a prescription of a favourite remedy, these patients are liable to suffer from the disease for some considerable length of time, if not life, and the condition although not serious, causes much misery. In addition poor or casual treatment of such patients leads to repeated 'new patient' consultations which becomes extremely expensive. Better to investigate fully and treat properly such a patient early on in the disease process, than to treat a patient with indifference who then becomes dissatisfied and a repeated attender.

Table 9.2 Investigation and clinical characterization of intrinsic rhinitis

			Factors in favour of intrinsic rhinitis or comments
Diagnosing intrinsic rhinitis	History (see text)		No seasonal or diurnal variation No family history No allergies as a child Adult onset No itching or sneezing No associated asthma or conjunctivitis
	Examination (see text)		No structural abnormality No signs of infection Inflamed mucosa Swollen mucosa Inferior turbinate hypertrophy Nasal polyps
	Radiology (see text and Chapter 3)	Plain X-ray, CT	No gross evidence of sinus disease Mucosal thickening common
	Bacteriology (see Chapter 8)		No bacterial rhinitis
	Allergy testing (see Chapter 6)	IgE (total) Skin prick test RAST Challenging testing	Below 350 iu/l Negative or very weakly positive compared with histamine reference Negative or very weakly positive Negative – particularly to house dust mite allergen
Baseline characterization and monitoring treatment	Secretion eosinophilia (see text)		Eosinophilic if > 25% inflammatory cells
	Diary card		Obstruction, secretion, sneezing Postnasal discharge Hyposmia
	Nasal patency (see Chapter 4)	Rhinomanometry Acoustic rhinometry Peak flow	Normally above 0.5 kpal/s
	Nasal secretion	Weigh paper handkerchiefs	

Treatment

Most patients' symptoms are controlled by medical means and only the minority require surgical treatment. Medical treatments are summarized in Table 9.3 and surgical treatments in Table 9.4.

Like most aspects of intrinsic rhinitis the treatment is controversial. Topical α-adrenoreceptor agonists are effective nasal decongestants (Aschan and Drettner, 1964) but should not be used for any length of time because of the risk of rhinitis medicamentosa (Capel and Swanston, 1986). Systemic sympathomimetics have been shown to be effective in the short term (Broms and Malm, 1982) but tachyphylaxis develops after a variable length of time. Systemic sympathomimetics also have serious potential side effects, although it must be admitted they are rare. These include hypertension and urinary retention in adults, and behavioural disturbances and night terrors in children (Anggard and Malm, 1984). Tricyclic antidepressants have been tried because they have anticholinergic and sympathomimetic properties (Laurence and Bennett, 1980) but long-term results have proved disappointing. Some of the older H_1 antagonists such as chlorpheniramine have anticholinergic and sympathomimetic properties which may make them useful for treating intrinsic rhinitis. Hyoscine either orally or as a cutaneous patch occasionally proves useful in patients with severe rhinorrhoea. Some authorities feel that cromoglycate may be useful in intrinsic rhinitis (Wentges, 1979) and it is possible that newer mast cell stabilizing agents such

Table 9.3 Medical treatment of intrinsic rhinitis

	Type of drug	Drug and administration
Eosinophilic	Steroids	Topical, e.g. fluticasone, beclomethasone, budesonide, flunisolide
		Systemic (for short course)
	α-Receptor agonists	Systemic, e.g. pseudoephedrine
		Topical, e.g. xylometazoline (short courses only)
	Mast cell stabilizers	Topical, cromoglycate solution
		Ketotifen orally
Non-eosinophilic	Anticholinergic	Topical, e.g. ipratropium
		Hyoscine (orally or patch)
	Anticholinergic/ sympathomimetic	Imipramine orally
		Chlorpheniramine orally

NB: The table is a guide only and, for example, some patients with non-eosinophilic intrinsic rhinitis will respond to topical steroids or to mast cell stabilizing agents.

Table 9.4 Surgical treatment of intrinsic rhinitis

Symptom	Type of procedure	Procedure
Nasal obstruction	Turbinate reduction	Submucosal diathermy
		Cryosurgery
		Laser cautery
	Turbinate resection	Partial excision
		Submucosal turbinectomy
		Radical turbinectomy
Rhinorrhoea	Vidian neurectomy	Excision of vidian nerve
		Diathermy/division to vidian nerve

as ketotifen may prove more beneficial in this respect (Talaat *et al.*, 1991). The mainstay of treatment, however, is by topical nasal steroids or ipratropium.

Eosinophilic intrinsic rhinitis responds dramatically to topical intranasal steroids (Mullarkey, Hill and Webb, 1980; Mygind and Weeke, 1983). New agents in use include beclomethasone, budesonide, flunisolide and fluticasone. All these agents are potent steroids and are destroyed by first pass metabolism, thereby giving no measurable systemic side effects (Brown, Storey and George, 1972; Pipkorn *et al.*, 1980; MacKenzie, 1991; Bryson and Faulds, 1992). Fluticasone may be absorbed less than the other topical steroids (MacKenzie, 1991). Topical nasal steroids are also useful in reducing the recurrence rate

after nasal polypectomy (Drettner, Ebbsen and Nilsson, 1982) and may induce small polyps to regress (Mygind *et al.*, 1975). Inhaled steroids have been said to be associated with posterior subcapsular cataracts and this may be dose related (Stead and Cooke, 1989), but more recent work has suggested that this risk is in fact minimal and that topical steroids are extremely safe (Toogood *et al.*, 1993). A topical anticholinergic agent, ipratropium, is the most useful treatment in patients with rhinorrhoea as their main complaint and has, therefore, revolutionized the treatment of non-eosinophilic intrinsic rhinitis (Borum, Mygind and Schultz Larsen, 1979; O'Dwyer *et al.*, 1988; Druce *et al.*, 1992; Meltzer *et al.*, 1992).

The general rule in the treatment of intrinsic rhinitis is that a thorough trial of medical treatment, particularly steroids, or ipratropium should be continued for a protracted length of time before surgery is considered (Jones and Lancer, 1987b). Patients with obstruction due to refractory hypertrophic inferior turbinates should be considered for some form of turbinate reduction.

Various surgical treatments for enlarged inferior turbinates that have been tried over the centuries including linear thermal cautery and silver nitrate cautery. Laser cautery is the most recent addition to this list (McCombe, Cook and Jones, 1992). Most rhinologists, however, would consider treatment in the first instance by submucosal diathermy or cryotherapy, both are probably equally effective (Wengraf, Gleeson and Siodlak, 1986). Submucosal diathermy leads to a dramatic fall in nasal resistance to airflow at 2 months postoperatively and this is accompanied by a fall in the subjective sensation of nasal obstruction.

It has been shown, however, that in patients who do not have concurrent medical treatment the inferior turbinates re-hypertrophy within 15 months (Jones and Lancer, 1987a). This finding merly reinforces the assertion that swelling of the inferior turbinates is primarily a medical condition and medical treatment should be continued even after surgical reduction.

Many rhinologists only advocate submucosal diathermy in those cases where the inferior turbinate shrinks with an α-receptor agonist. While this is indeed a good predictor of a satisfactory outcome of diathermy (Jones *et al.*, 1989) it is not diagnostic and many cases not exhibiting decongestion nevertheless gain a good result from diathermy. It is reasonable practice to carry out submucosal diathermy as an initial procedure in all patients with inferior turbinate hypertrophy unresponsive to medical treatment.

If inferior turbinate hypertrophy recurs following submucosal diathermy a radical trimming of the inferior turbinates should be considered (Figure 9.3). There seems little doubt that this procedure used to be accompanied by an unacceptable incidence of atrophic rhinitis but there is good evidence that this is no longer the case (Martinez *et al.*, 1983). Radical trimming of the inferior turbinates typically halves nasal resistance to airflow (Wight, Jones and Beckingham, 1990). Nasal symptom scores for obstruction also fall dramatically. Unlike submucosal diathermy, radical trimming of the inferior turbinates is associated with recurrence of the symptoms of reduced nasal patency in only 20% of patients within 2 years (Wight, Jones and Beckingham, 1990). Additionally nasal crusting may be a problem in up to 20% of patients. This symptom can be irritating and reinforces the idea that radical trimming should not be undertaken as a primary procedure.

Hypertrophic inferior turbinates cause most obstruction at the pyriform aperture (Haight and Cole, 1983; Jones *et al.*, 1988). With this in mind it is obviously important to pay particular attention to the anterior end of the inferior turbinate whichever method of reduction is being used. Anterior trimming is almost equally effective at reducing nasal resistance to airflow as the radical operation (Wight, Jones and Clegg, 1988), but is not associated with a subjective improvement (Wight, Jones and Clegg, 1988). Even in patients who have had a useful relief of symptoms the turbinate soon re-hypertrophies.

Radical trimming of the interior turbinates is a safe procedure with minimal side effects (Wight, Jones and Beckingham, 1990). The procedure is, however, attended by a risk of reactionary haemorrhage which may be severe and occurs in a significant number of patients. The complication of atrophic rhinitis following this procedure appears to have been overrated or in any event does not seem to be a problem nowadays even in tropical countries (Ophir, Shapira and Marshak, 1985; Odetoyinbo, 1987; Wight, Jones and Beckingham, 1990).

It should be emphasized that neither submucosal diathermy nor radical trimming of the inferior turbinates significantly reduces any other nasal symptom apart from obstruction.

Middle turbinate enlargement

Nasal obstruction due to middle turbinate hypertrophy is relatively uncommon (Richardson, 1948). The

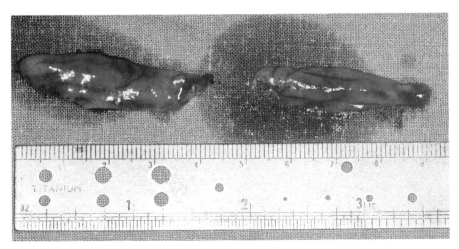

Figure 9.3 Enlarged inferior turbinates removed by radical turbinectomy

turbinate can be trimmed or treated with diathermy but the safest technique is probably to reduce it with punch forceps (Fry, 1973).

Concha bullosa may be similarly reduced or trimmed with turbinectomy scissors. There is little information on the objective affects of middle turbinate reduction but some patients seem to benefit from the procedure. Functional endoscopic nasal surgery is now frequently employed to carry out surgery in this region.

Vidian neurectomy

In contrast to the success of the surgical treatment of nasal obstruction, that for rhinorrhoea is disappointing. Vidian neurectomy (Golding-Wood, 1973) should be reserved for those patients with severe rhinorrhoea who do not respond to ipratropium and other medical treatments. The operation is complex to perform, is not without complications and has a high relapse rate. Experimental evidence suggests that after division of the autonomic nerves reinnervation occurs within a year (Grote, 1974). The operation described by Golding-Wood is complex and involves a transantral approach to the pterygopalatine fossa. Simpler methods have been suggested (Minnis and Morrison, 1971) and good results are claimed, although it seems unlikely that recurrence of symptoms will not eventually occur. Polyps unresponsive to steroids should, of course, be removed and this is discussed in Chapter 10 of this volume.

If all else fails Zeiger and Schatz (1982) suggest that vigorous exercise should be prescribed for the patient in the hope that it improves his general vasomotor tone!

Summary

Intrinsic rhinitis is a common disease. If the otolaryngologist devotes the same care and attention to its diagnosis and treatment that he does with other diseases, such as otosclerosis, treatment should be rewarding. A thorough history and examination must be taken and every effort made to come to a positive diagnosis of intrinsic rhinitis. Allergy must, of course, be excluded and the various precipitating factors should be identified. Local eosinophilia should be assessed and baseline nasal investigations including some measure of objective nasal patency should be made. Apart from general advice and treatment of any coexistent conditions, a patient with eosinophilic intrinsic rhinitis should be treated in the first instance with a topical intranasal steroid, whereas those with non-eosinophilic rhinitis should be treated with ipratropium. Various other drugs should be considered as discussed in the text before recourse to surgery is made.

References

ANGGARD, A. (1969) The effect of prostaglandins on nasal airway resistance in man. *Annals of Otology, Rhinology and Laryngology*, **78**, 657–662

ANGGARD, A. and EDWALL, L. (1974) The effects of sympathetic nerve stimulation on the tracer disappearance rate and local blood content in the nasal mucosa of the cat. *Acta Otolaryngologica*, **77**, 131–139

ANGGARD, A. and MALM, L. (1984) Orally administered decongestant drugs in disorders of the upper respiratory passages: a survey of clinical results. *Clinical Otolaryngology*, **9**, 43–49

ASCHAN, G. and DRETTNER, B. (1964) An objective investigation of the decongestive effect of xylometazoline. *Eye, Ear, Nose, Throat Monthly*, **43**, 66–74

BACQ, Z. (1975) *Chemical Transmission of Nerve Impulses.* Oxford: Pergamon Press

BARBEE, R. A., LEBOWITZ, M. D., THOMPSON, H. C. and BURROWS, B. (1976) Immediate skin-test activity in a general population. *Annals of Internal Medicine*, **84**, 129–133

BEDWANI, J. R., ECCLES, R. and JONES, A. S. (1983a) The isolation of prostaglandin E from pig nasal mucosa. *Clinical Otolaryngology*, **8**, 159–163

BEDWANI, J. R., ECCLES, R. and JONES, A. S. (1983b) The effect of prostaglandins E_2, I_2 and D_2 on pig nasal vasculature. *Clinical Otolaryngology*, **8**, 337–341

BEDWANI, J. R., ECCLES, R. and JONES, A. S. (1984) A study on the synthesis and inactivation of prostaglandin E by pig nasal mucosa. *Acta Otolaryngologica*, **98**, 308–314

BORUM, P., MYGIND, N. and SCHULTZ LARSEN, F. (1979) Intranasal ipratropium: a new treatment for perennial rhinitis. *Clinical Otolaryngology*, **4**, 407–411

BRAND, D. L., ROUFAIL, W. M., THOMSON, A. B. R. and TAPPER, E. J. (1985) Misoprostol, a synthetic PGE_1 analog, in the treatment of duodenal ulcers. *Digestive Disorders Science*, **30**, 147S

BRODER, I., HIGGINS, M. W., MATHEWS, K. P., and KELLER, J. B. (1974) Epidemiology of asthma and allergic rhinitis in a total community, Tecumseh, Michigan. *Journal of Allergy and Clinical Immunology*, **54**, 100–110

BROMS, P. and MALM, L. (1982) Oral vasoconstrictors in perennial non-allergic rhinitis. *Allergy*, **37**, 67–74

BROWN, H. M., STOREY, G. and GEORGE, W. H. S. (1972) Beclomethasone dipropionate: a new steroid aerosol for the treatment of allergic asthma. *British Medical Journal*, **1**, 585–590

BRYSON, H. M. and FAULDS, D. (1992) Intranasal fluticasone proprionate. A review of its pharmacodynamic and pharmacokinetic properties and therapeutic potential in allergic rhinitis. *Drugs*, **43**, 760–775

CAPEL, L. H. and SWANSTON, A. R. (1986) Beware congesting nasal decongestants. *British Medical Journal*, **293**, 1258–1259

CAPLIN, L., HAYNES, J. T. and SPAHN, J. (1971) Are nasal polyps an allergic phenomenon? *Annals of Allergy*, **29**, 631–634

CAUNA, N. and CAUNA, D. (1975) The fine structure and innervation of the cushion veins of the human nasal respiratory mucosa. *Anatomy Research*, **181**, 1–16

CAUNA, N., HINDERER, K. H., MANZETTI, G. W. and SWANSON E. W. (1972) Fine structure of nasal polyps. *Annals of Otology, Rhinology and Laryngology*, **81**, 41–58

CHAFEE, F. H. and SETTIPANE, G. A. (1974) Aspirin intolerance

I. Frequency in an allergic population. *Journal of Allergy, and Clinical Immunology*, **53**, 193–199

CORRADO, O. J., GOULD, C. A. L., KASSAB, J. Y. and DAVIES, R. J. (1986) Nasal response of rhinitic and non-rhinitic subjects to histamine and methacholine: a comparative study. *Thorax*, **41**, 863–868

CRAWFORD, L. V. (1960) A study of the nasal cytology in infants with eczemoid dermatitis. *Annals of Allergy*, **18**, 502–509

DAL-NEGRO, R. W., TURCO, P. A. and ALLEGRA, L. (1992) Blood gas changes in nonasthmatic rhinitis during and after nonspecific airway challenge. *American Review of Respiratory Disorders*, **145**, 337–339

DELANEY, J. C. (1976) Aspirin idiosyncracy in patients admitted for nasal polypectomy. *Clinical Otolaryngology*, **1**, 27–30

DEUSCHL, H. and JOHANSSON, S. G. O. (1977) Specific IgE antibodies in nasal secretion from patients with allergic rhinitis and with negative or weakly positive RAST on the serum. *Clinical Allergy*, **7**, 195

DIRKSEN, A. (1982) Clinical vs paraclinical data in allergy. *Danish Medical Bulletin*, **29** (suppl. 2), 5–72

DRAKE-LEE, A. B. (1987) Nasal mast cells: a preliminary report on their ultrastructure. *Journal of Laryngology and Otology*, Suppl. 13, 1–17

DRAKE-LEE, A. B., LOWE, D., SWANSTON, A. and GRACE, A. (1984) Clinical profile and recurrence of nasal polyps. *Journal of Laryngology and Otology*, **98**, 783–793

DRETTNER, B., EBBSEN, A. and NILSSON, M. (1982) Prophylactic treatment with flunisolide after polypectomy. *Rhinology*, **20**, 149–158

DRUCE, H. M., SPECTOR, S. L., FIREMAN, P., KAISER, H., MELTZER E. O., BOGGS, P. *et al.* (1992) Double-blind study of intranasal ipratropium bromide in non-allergic perennial rhinitis. *Annals of Allergy*, **69**, 53–60

ECCLES, R. and WILSON, H. (1973) The parasympathetic secretory nerves of the nose of the cat. *Journal of Physiology*, **230**, 213–223

EDFORS-LUBS, M. L. (1971) Allergy in 7000 twin pairs. *Acta Allergologica*, **26**, 249–285

EHRLICH, P. (1879) Uber die spezifischen Granulationen des Blutes. *Archives für Anatomie und Physiologie Leipzig*, **3**, 531

EYERMAN, C. H. (1927) Nasal manifestation of allergy. *Annals of Otology, Rhinology and Laryngology*, **36**, 808–815

FRY, H. J. (1973) Judicious turbinectomy for nasal obstruction. *Australia and New Zealand Journal of Surgery*, **42**, 291–294

FRY, J. (1979) Hay fever. In: *Common Diseases*, 2nd edn. Lancaster: MTP Press

GERTH-VAN-WIJK, R. and DIEGES, P. H. (1991) Nasal hyperresponsiveness to histamine, methacholine and phentolamine in patients with perennial non-allergic rhinitis and in patients with infectious rhinitis. *Clinical Otolaryngology*, **16**, 133–137

GOLDING-WOOD, P. H. (1961) Observations on petrosal and Vidian neurectomy in chronic vasomotor rhinitis. *Journal of Laryngology and Otology*, **75**, 232–247

GOLDING-WOOD, P. H. (1973) Vidian neurectomy: its results and complications. *Laryngoscope*, **83**, 1673–1683

GORENBERG, D. (1979) Rhinitis medicamentosa. *Western Journal of Medicine*, **131**, 313–314

GROTE, J. J. (1974) The autonomic innervation of the nasal mucosa. *Thesis*, Nijmegen, The Netherlands

HACK, W. (1882) Reflex neuroses. *Berliner Klinische Wochenschrift*, **19**, 379

HAIGHT, J. S. J. and COLE, P. (1983) The site and function of the nasal valve. *Laryngoscope*, **93**, 49–55

HANSEL F. K. (ed.) (1936) *Allergy of the Nose and Paranasal Sinuses*. St Louis: C. V. Mosby Co. p. 379

HOLOPAINEN, E., MALMBERG, H. *and* TARKIAINEN, E. (1977) Experiences of treating allergic rhinitis results with intranasal beclomethasone dipropionate. *Acta Allergologica*, **32**, 263–277

HUGGINS, K. G. and BROSTOFF, J. (1975) Local production of specific IgE antibodies in allergic rhinitis patients with negative skin tests. *Lancet*, ii 148–150

IMOKAWA, S., SATO, A., TANIGUCHI, M., TOYOSHIMA, M., NAKAZAWA, K., HAYAKAWA, H. *et al.* (1992) A case of asthma relieved by aspirin the first case in Japan and investigation of its mechanism. *Arerugi*, **41**, 1597–1604

JACKSON, R. T. (1970) Prostaglandin E, as a nasal constrictor in normal human volunteers. *Current Therapeutic Research*, **12**, 711–717

JACOBS, R. L., FREEDMAN, P. M. and BOSWELL, R. N. (1981) Nonallergic rhinitis with eosinophilia (NARES syndrome). *Journal of Allergy and Clinical Immunology*, **61**, 253–262

JESSEN, M. and JANZON, L. (1989) Prevalence of non-allergic nasal complaints in an urban and a rural population in Sweden. *Allergy*, **44**, 582–587

JONES, A. S. and LANCER, J. M. (1987a) Does submucosal diathermy to the inferior turbinates reduce nasal resistance to airflow in the long term? *Journal of Laryngology and Otology*, **101**, 448–451

JONES, A. S. and LANCER, J. M. (1987b) Vasomotor rhinitis. *British Medical Journal*, **294**, 1505–1506

JONES, A. S., LANCER, J. M., MOIR, A. A. and STEVENS, J. C. (1985) Effect of aspirin on nasal resistance to airflow. *British Medical Journal*, **290**, 1171–1173

JONES, A. S., WIGHT, R. G., STEVENS, J. C. and BECKINGHAM, E. (1988) The nasal valve: a physiological and clinical study. *Journal of Laryngology and Otology*, **102**, 1089–1094

JONES, A. S., WIGHT, R. G., KABIL, Y. and BECKINGHAM E. (1989) Predicting the outcome of submucosal diathermy to the inferior turbinates. *Clinical Otolaryngology*, **14**, 41–44

JUNG, T. T. K., JUHN, S. K., HWANG, D. and STEWART, R. (1987) Prostaglandins, leukotrienes and other arachidonic acid metabolites in nasal polyps and nasal mucosa. *Laryngoscope*, **97**, 184–189

KARIM, S. M. M., ADAIKAN, P. G. and KUNARATNAM, N. (1978) Effect of topical prostaglandins on nasal patency in man. *Prostaglandins*, **15**, 457–462

KAUFMAN, H. S., ROSEN, I., SHAPOSHNIKOV, N. and WAI, M. (1982) Nasal eosinophilia. *Annals of Allergy*, **49**, 270–271

KUBO, N. and KUMAZAWA, T. (1993) Functional disturbances of the autonomic nerves in nasal hyperreactivity: an up-to-date review. *Acta Otolaryngologica*, Suppl. **500**, 97–108

LANE, J. E. (ed.) (1982) Canine and feline nasal disorders. In: *ENT and Oral Surgery of the Dog and Cat*. Bristol: Bristol PSG. pp. 41–79

LAURENCE, D. R. and BENNETT, P. N. (1980) Drugs and mental disorder. In: *Clinical Pharmacology*. Edinburgh: Churchill Livingstone. pp. 506–546

LEEK, F. F. (1986) Cheops courtiers: their skeletal remains. In: *Science in Egyptology*, edited by A. R. David. Manchester: Manchester University Press. p. 183

LOZEWICZ, S., WANG, J., DUDDLE, J., THOMAS, K., CHALSTREY, S., REILLY, G. *et al.* (1992) Topical glucocorticoids inhibit activation by allergen in the upper respiratory tract. *Journal of Allergy and Clinical Immunology*, **89**, 951–957

LUNDBERG, J.M., ANGGARD, A., FAHRENKRUG, J., HOKFELT, T. and MUTT, V. (1980) Vasoactive intestinal polypeptide in cholinergic neurones of exocrine glands: functional significance of coexisting transmitters for vasodilation and secretion. *Proceedings of the National Academy of Science USA*, **77**, 1651–1655

MCCOMBE, A.W., COOK, J.A. and JONES, A.S. (1992) A comparison of laser cautery and sub-mucosal diathermy for rhinitis. *Clinical Otolaryngology*, **17**, 297–299

MACKENZIE, C.A. (1991) Growth in asthmatic children – clinical experience with inhaled fluticasone propionate. *European Respiratory Journal*, Suppl. 4, 171s–637s

MALCOLMSON, K.G. (1959) The vasomotor activities of the nasal mucous membrane. *Journal of Laryngology and Otology*, **73**, 73–98

MALM, L. (1973) Stimulation of sympathetic nerve fibres to the nose in cats. *Acta Otolaryngologica*, **75**, 519–526

MALM, L. (1974a) Responses of resistance and capacitance vessels in feline nasal mucosa to vasoactive agents. *Acta Otolaryngologica*, **78**, 90–97

MALM, L. (1974b) Beta adrenergic receptors in the vessels of the cat nasal mucosa. *Acta Otolaryngologica*, **78**, 242–246

MALM, L. (1977) Sympathetic influence on the nasal mucosa. *Acta Otolaryngologica*, **83**, 20–21

MALM, L. (1981) Propanolol as a cause of watery nasal secretion. *Lancet*, i, 1006

MALMBERG, H. (1979) Symptoms of chronic and allergic rhinitis and occurrence of nasal secretion granulocytes in university students, school children and infants. *Allergy*, **34**, 389–394

MARTINEZ, S.A., NISSEN, A.J., STOCK, C.R. and TESMER, T. (1983) Nasal turbinate resection for relief of nasal obstruction. *Laryngoscope*, **93**, 871–875

MATHESON, A., ROSENBLUM, A., GLAZER, R. and DECANAY, E. (1957) Local tissue and blood eosinophils in newborn infants. *Journal of Pediatrics*, **51**, 502–509

MELTZER, E.O., ORGEL, H.A., BRONSKY, E.A., FINDLAY, S.R., GEORGITIS, J.W., GROSSMAN, J. *et al.* (1992) Ipratropium bromide aqueous nasal spray for patients with perennial allergic rhinitis: a study of its effect on their symptoms, quality of life and nasal cytology. *Journal of Allergy and Clinical Immunology*, **90**, 242–249

MERTENS, J., WELLBROCK, M. and FEIDERT, F. (1991) Correlation between nasal polyposis and perennial allergy exemplified by house dust mite and house dust allergy. *HNO*, **39**, 307–310

MILLER, R.E., PARADISE, J.L., FRIDAY, G., FIREMAN, P. and VOITH D. (1982) The nasal smear for eosinophils. *American Journal of Diseases in Childhood*, **136**, 1009–1011

MINNIS, N. L. and MORRISON, A. W. (1971) Trans-septal approach for Vidian neurectomy. *Journal of Laryngology and Otology*, **85**, 255–260

MONERET-VAUTRIN, D. A., WAYOFF, M. and HSIEH, V. (1988) Non-allergic eosinophilic rhinitis. From clinical diagnosis to pathogenic study. *Annals Otolaryngologie Chirurgie Cervicofaciale*, **105**, 553–557

MONERET-VAUTRIN, D. A., HSIEH, V., WAYOFF, M., GUYOT, J.L., MOUTON, C. and MARIA, Y. (1990) Nonallergic rhinitis with eosinophilia syndrome a precursor of the triad: nasal polyposis, intrinsic asthma and intolerance to aspirin. *Annals of Allergy*, **64**, 513–518

MONERET-VAUTRIN, D. A., JANKOWSKI, R., BENE, M. C., KANNY, G., HSIEH, V., FAURE, G. *et al.* (1992) NARES a model of

inflammation caused by activated eosinophils? *Rhinology*, **30**, 161–168

MOORE, D. C. (1954) *Stellate Ganglion Block*. Springfield, Illinois: Charles C Thomas

MULLARKEY, M. F., HILL, J. S. and WEBB, D. R. (1980) Allergic and non-allergic rhinitis: their characterisation with attention to the meaning of nasal eosinophilia. *Journal of Allergy and Clinical Immunology*, **65**, 122–126

MURRAY, A. B. (1971) Nasal secretion eosinophilia in children with allergic rhinitis. *Annals of Allergy*, **28**, 142–148

MYGIND, N. (ed.) (1978) *Nasal Allergy*. Oxford: Blackwell Scientific Publications. p. 231

MYGIND, N. (ed.) (1986) Examination of the nose. In: *Essential Allergy*. Oxford: Blackwell Scientific Publications. pp. 305–306

MYGIND, N. and WEEKE, B. (1983) Allergic and non-allergic rhinitis. In: *Allergy Principles and Practice*, 2nd edn, edited by E. Middleton Jr, C. E. Reed and E. F. Ellis. St Louis: C. V. Mosby Co. pp. 1101–1117

MYGIND, N., PEDERSEN, M. and NIELSEN, M. H. (1983) Primary and secondary ciliary dyskinesia. *Acta Otolaryngologica*, **95**, 688–694

MYGIND, N., BRAHE PEDERSEN, C., PRYTZ, S. and SORENSEN, H. (1975) Treatment of nasal polyps with intranasal beclomethasone dipropionate aerosol. *Clinical Allergy*, **5**, 159–164

MYGIND, N., DIRKSEN, A., JOHNSEN, N. J. and WEEKE, B. (1978) Perennial rhinitis: analysis of skin testing, serum IgE, and blood and smear eosinophilia in 201 patients. *Clinical Otolaryngology*, **3**, 189–196

NISHIOKA, K., SAITO, C., NAGANO, T., OKHNO, M., MASUDA, Y. and KURIYAMA, T. (1993) Eosinophil cationic protein in the nasal secretions of patients with mite allergic rhinitis. *Laryngoscopy*, **103**, 189–192

ODETOYINBO, O. (1987) Complications following total inferior turbinectomy: facts or myths? *Clinical Otolaryngology*, **12**, 361–363

O'DWYER, T. P., LEE, R. J., KAYE, J. and FENNELL, G. (1988) Ipratropium bromide in the treatment of the 'rhinorrhoea syndrome'. *Journal of Laryngology and Otology*, **102**, 799–801

OFFICE OF POPULATION CENSUSES AND SURVEYS (1974) Morbidity statistics from general practice. Second national study 1970–71. *Studies on Medical and Population Subjects*. no. 26. London: HMSO

OKAZAKI, T., REISMAN, R. E. and ARBESMAN, C. E. (1977) Prostaglandin E in the secretions of allergic rhinitis. *Prostaglandins*, **13**, 681–690

OPHIR, D., SHAPIRA, A. and MARSHAK, G. (1985) Total inferior turbinectomy for nasal airway obstruction. *Archives of Otolaryngology*, **111**, 93–95

PAHOR, A. L. and KIMURA, A. (1991) History of removal of nasal polyps. *A Folha Medica (Brazil)*, **102**, 183–186

PERKI, J. M. (1972) Allergy in general practice. *Practitioner*, **208**, 776–783

PHILLIPS, D. E., JONES, A. S., HOFFMAN, J. and GILLIES, J. (1992) Distribution of eosinophils in the nose in patients with perennial rhinitis. *Clinical Otolaryngology*, **17**, 478–481

PIPKORN, U. and KARLSSON, G. (1988) Methods for obtaining specimens from the nasal mucosa for morphological and biochemical analysis. *European Respiratory Journal*, **1**, 856–862

PIPKORN, U., RUNDCRANTZ, H., LINDQVIST, S. and LINDQVIST, N. (1980) Budesonide – a new nasal steroid. *Rhinology*, **18**, 171–175

PIPKORN, U., KARLSSON, G. and ENERBACK, L. (1988) A brush method to harvest cells from the nasal mucosa for microscopic and biochemical analysis. *Journal of Immunological Methods*, **112**, 37–42

RAMWELL, P. (ed.) (1980) General introduction to clinical implications of prostaglandin synthetase inhibition. In: *Prostaglandins and Related Lipids*. New York: Alan R. Liss Inc. vol 1, pp. xi–xviii

RICHARDSON, J. (1948) Turbinate treatment in vasomotor rhinitis. *Laryngoscope*, **58**, 834–847

RUCCI, L., MASINI, E., ARBI-RICCARDI, R., GIANNELLA, E., FIORETTI, C., MANNAIONI, P. F. *et al.* (1989) Vidian nerve resection, histamine turnover and mucosal mast cell function in patients with chronic hypertrophic non-allergic rhinitis. *Agents-Actions*, **28**, 224–230

SAMTER, M. and BEERS, R. F. JR. (1968) Intolerance to aspirin. *Annals of Internal Medicine*, **68**, 975–983

SEEBOHM, P. M. (1978) Allergic and nonallergic rhinitis. In *Allergy: Principles and Practice*, edited by E. Middleton Jr, C. E. Reed and E. F. Ellis. St Louis: C. V. Mosby Co. p. 868

SETTIPANE, G. A. and CHAFEE, F. H. (1977) Nasal polyps in asthma and rhinitis: a review of 6037 patients. *Journal of Allergy and Clinical Immunology*, **59**, 17–21

SIBBALD, B. and RINK, E. (1990) Birth month variation in atopic and non-atopic rhinitis. *Clinical and Experimental Allergy*, **20**, 285–288

SIBBALD, B. and RINK, E. (1991) Epidemiology of seasonal and perennial rhinitis: clinical presentation and medical history. *Thorax*, **46**, 895–901

SPECTOR, S. L. and FARR, F. S. (1983) Aspirin idiosyncracy asthma and urticaria. In: *Allergy: Principles and Practice*, 2nd edn, edited by E. Middleton JR, C. E. Reed and E. F. Ellis. St Louis: C. V. Mosby Co. pp. 1249–1273

STAMMBERGER, H. and WOLF, G. (1988) Headaches and sinus disease: the endoscopic approach. *Annals of Otology, Rhinology and Laryngology*, **97** (Suppl. 134), 3–23

STEAD, R. J. and COOKE, N. J. (1989) Adverse effects of inhaled corticosteroids. *British Medical Journal*, **298**, 403–404

STJARNE, P., LUNDBLAD, L., LUNDBERG, J. M. and ANGGARD, A. (1989) Capsaicin and nicotine-sensitive afferent neurones and basal secretion in healthy human volunteers and in patients with vasomotor rhinitis. *British Journal of Pharmacology*, **96**, 693–701

SWART, S. J., VAN DER BAAN, S., STEENBERGEN, J. J., NAUTA, J. J., VAN KAMP, G. J., BIEWENGA, J. (1991) Immunoglobulin concentrations in nasal secretions differ between patients with an IgE-mediated rhinopathy and a non-IgE-mediated rhinopathy. *Journal of Allergy and Clinical Immunology*, **88**, 612–619

TALAAT, M. A., INAAM, P. K., MOHAMMED, M. H. and IBRAHIM, T. E. (1991) The histological and histochemical effects of ketotifen in allergic rhinitis. *Journal of Asthma*, **28**, 117–128

TOOGOOD, J. H., MARKOV, A. E., BASKERVILLE, J. and DYSON, C. (1993) Association of ocular cataracts with inhaled and oral steroid therapy during long-term treatment of asthma. *Journal of Allergy and Clinical Immunology*, **91**, 571–579

TOOHILL, R. J., LEHAM, R. H., GROSSMAN, T. W. and BELSON, T. P. (1981) Rhinitis medicamentosa. *Laryngoscope*, **91**, 1614–1621

UDDMAN, R., SUNDLER, F. and EMSON, P. (1984) Occurrence and distribution of neuropeptide-Y-immuno-reactive nerves in the respiratory tract and middle ear. *Cell and Tissue Research*, **237**, 321–327

VAHERI, E. (1956) Nasal allergy with special reference to eosinophilia and histopathology. *Acta Allergologica*, **10**, 203–211

VANE, J. R. (1971) Inhibition of prostaglandin synthesis as mechanism of action for aspirin-like drugs. *Nature*, **231**, 232–235

VERDIANI, P., DI-CARLO, S. and BARONTI, A. (1990) Different prevalence and degree of nonspecific bronchial hyperreactivity between seasonal and perennial rhinitis. *Journal of Allergy and Clinical Immunology*, **86**, 576–582

WALLUKAT, G. and WOLLENBERGER, A. (1991) Autoantibodies to beta 2-adrenergic receptors with antiadrenergic activity from patients with allergic asthma. *Journal of Allergy and Clinical Immunology*, **88**, 581–587

WASSERMAN, M. A., DUCHARME, D. W., GRIFFIN, R. L., DEGRAAF, G. L. and ROBINSON, F. G. (1977) Bronchopulmonary and cardiovascular effects of prostaglandin D_2 in the dog. *Prostaglandins*, **13**, 255–269

WEIR, N. (1990) *Otolaryngology: an Illustrated History*. London: Butterworth Ltd.

WENGRAF, C. L., GLEESON, M. J. and SIODLAK, M. Z. (1986) The stuffy nose: a comparative study of two common methods of treatment. *Clinical Otolaryngology* **11**, 61–68

WENTGES, R. TH. R. (1979) Allergic and vasomotor rhinitis. In: *Clinical Otolaryngology*, edited by A. G. D. Maran and P. M. Stell. Oxford: Blackwell Scientific Publications. pp. 226–238

WIDE, L., BENNICH, H. and JOHANSSON, S. G. O. (1967) Diagnosis of allergy by an in-vitro test for allergen antibodies. *Lancet*, ii, 1105–1107

WIGHT, R. G., JONES, A. S. and CLEGG, R. T. (1988) A comparison of anterior and radical trimming of the inferior nasal turbinates and the effects on nasal resistance to airflow. *Clinical Otolaryngology*, **13**, 223–226

WIGHT, R. G., JONES A. S. and BECKINGHAM, E. (1990) Trimming of the inferior turbinates a prospective long-term study. *Clinical Otolaryngology*, **15**, 347–350

WILSON, H. and YATES, M. S. (1978) Sympathetic nerves and nasal secretion in the cat. *Acta Otolaryngologica*, **85**, 426–430

WITTIG, H. J., BELLOIT, J., FILLIPPI, I. D. and ROYAL, G. (1980) Age-related serum immunoglobulin levels in healthy subjects and in patients with allergic disease. *Journal of Allergy and Clinical Immunology*, **66**, 305–313

WRIGHT, J. (1902) The nose and throat. In: *Medical History*. Philadelphia: Lee & Febiger

ZEIGER, R. S. and SCHATZ, M. (1982) Chronic rhinitis: a practical approach to diagnosis and treatment. *Immunology and Allergy Practice*, **4**, 26–36

ZINREICH, S. J., KENNEDY, D. W., ROSENBAUM, A. E., GAYLER, B. W., KUMAR, A. J. and STAMMBERGER, H. (1987) Paranasal sinuses: CT imaging requirements for endoscopic surgery. *Radiology*, **163**, 761–765

ZUCKERKANDL, E. (1882). *Normale und pathologische der nasen höhle*. Wien: W. Braumüller

10

Nasal polyps

A. B. Drake–Lee

Benign, mucous or simple nasal polyps are an easily recognizable clinical entity. They result from the prolapsed lining of the ethmoid sinuses and block the nose to a variable degree depending on their size. On examination polyps appear as pale bags which arise most commonly from the middle meatus and are relatively insensitive when probed: this helps to differentiate polyps from mucosa of the middle turbinate which may be polypoid. The pale colour is due to the poor blood supply but, in the presence of repeated trauma and inflammation, they may become reddened. They are commonly bilateral and, when unilateral, require histological examination to exclude the transitional cell papilloma (Ringert's tumour, inverted papilloma) or malignancy.

Antrochoanal polyps are similar in colour to ethmoid ones, but are a different disease affecting the maxillary sinus, where the lining prolapses through the middle meatus backwards into the postnasal space. Simple polyps may arise at any time after the age of 2 years, and if seen before this age, a meningocoele or encephalocoele should be excluded and the floor of the anterior cranial fossa examined radiographically. It is unusual for simple nasal polyps to arise before the age of 10 years and if found may be the presenting complaint of cystic fibrosis (Schwachman *et al.*, 1962). Any child with nasal polyps should have cystic fibrosis excluded by sweat tests. It is much more common for polyps to arise in established cases (Schwachman *et al.*, 1962; Drake–Lee and Pitcher Wilmott, 1982).

Although polyps are a disease of the ethmoid sinuses, the mucosal changes frequently extend further in the nose and into the other paranasal sinuses. The maxillary sinuses are affected more commonly than the frontal and sphenoid sinuses. The extent of these changes may be seen radiographically. The mucosal changes may not be limited to the nose since patients may have coexisting asthma.

There are three factors which may be involved in the pathogenesis of nasal polyps; the mucosal reactions at the cellular level, the relatively poorly developed blood supply of the ethmoid sinuses and finally the complex anatomy of the ethmoid labyrinth.

Treatment is a combination of surgery to the polyps and medical therapy with systemic or topical corticosteroids. Whatever therapeutic regimen is used, nasal polyps are a chronic condition prone to recurrence and in some cases, with embarrassing frequency.

Historical background

The condition was first recognized in India and by 1000 BC curettes had been devised to remove them (Vancil, 1969). Ancient Egyptian skulls show the grosser features of nasal polyps. Hippocrates (BC 460–370) recognized them as well and devised a method using a piece of string which was passed through the nose into the nasopharynx. A piece of sponge was attached to the postnasal end and the sponge was then pulled through the nose removing the polyps before it. The word polyp comes from the Greek, although it was subsequently latinized and means many-footed (poly-pous). Snares and forceps similar to those used today were developed in the middle ages.

All polypoidal conditions were initially grouped together until histological classification helped to differentiate them from the neoplastic conditions (Berdal, 1954). Billroth, who described their histological characteristics in the middle of the nineteenth centry, still considered them neoplastic (Berdal, 1954). Zuckerkandl understood that they were an inflammatory condition. He also demonstrated that the histological changes in the sinuses were the same as those in polyps (Berdal, 1954).

The first advance in treatment was the introduction of cocaine local anaesthesia. In addition to the anaesthetic properties, it is also a vasoconstrictor. It is still widely used today and may be used in combination with a general anaesthetic. More extensive surgery is better performed under general anaesthesia. Better illumination has aided surgery. With a more controlled technique of anaesthesia, removal with the aid of a microscope and by endoscopy may be favoured.

Aetiology

There have been a number of different theories put forward for the pathogenesis of nasal polyps. Although a single aetiology would be attractive this may not be the case but it appears that patients may be divided clinically into several groups. There are five main theories of pathogenesis: the Bernouilli phenomenon, polysaccharide changes, vasomotor imbalance, infection, and allergy. All may contribute to polyp formation, but none is obviously the commonest aetiology.

Bernouilli phenomenon

The Bernouilli phenomenon results in a pressure drop next to a constriction. This sucks the mucosa of the ethmoids into the nose. If this were the only factor, then the mucosa nearest the nasal valve would be polypoidal in the normal nose.

Polysaccharide changes

An alteration in the polysaccharides of ground substances has been postulated by Jackson and Arihood, 1971, but analysis of polyps have shown them to be oedematous (Taylor, 1963) with little alteration in the collagen. The collagen appears normal on analysis, although it tends to be recently formed and therefore less mature.

Vasomotor imbalance

Vasomotor imbalance is implied because the majority of cases are not atopic and no obvious allergen can be found. Patients frequently have a prodromal period of rhinitis prior to occurrence of polyps. Polyps themselves often have a very poor nerve supply since they may be palpated freely and insensitively. Blood vessels are encountered in polyps but they are infrequent and are usually capillaries. Larger ones have little smooth muscle within them. Vasomotor problems may cause polyps, but this is conjecture alone.

Infection

In the nineteenth century, there were two main types of maxillary sinusitis – purulent and hyperplas-

tic. It became increasingly clear that some authors interchanged the terms failing to understand the difference between the two conditions.

Purulent sinusitis results from infection usually by bacteria following a viral upper respiratory infection. The inflammatory changes may extend into the ethmoids and cause the mucosa to become polypoidal. It is encountered today usually as unilateral sinus disease. Hyperplastic sinusitis is associated with mucus hypersecretion in which organisms may be found and cultured. Infection may exacerbate the condition as in chronic bronchitis, but it does not cause it. Inappropriate surgery on the maxillary sinus leaves an intranasal antrostomy through which the new mucosa undergoes the same changes and subsequently prolapses through the artificial ostium. Polyps now appear from both the middle and inferior meatus.

The cause of inflammatory reactions is uncertain. Unfortunately because there are mucosal changes in the maxillary sinus in the majority and these are labelled sinusitis, it is frequently inferred that the sinuses are 'infected'. Indeed mucus is washed out and when cultured a significant proportion grow an organism. The commonest organism is the non-capsulated *Haemophilus influenzae* (Majumdar and Bull, 1982). This study was confirmed by Dawes *et al.* (1989) who also showed that pus cells and bacteria were only found in 16 out of 100 antral irrigations. Pus cells were found in 25 and bacteria were cultured in 31: both were found together in 16 wash outs.

Non-capsulated *Haemophilus influenzae* is a common commensal organism in the nose and oropharynx and is frequently cultured from the sputum of chronic bronchitis. There it exacerbates the condition and it may do so in cases with nasal polyps. Unfortunately, it is difficult to implicate any further relationship because antibiotics have little effect on the course or recurrence of the disease and merely modify the infectivity of the mucus. The actions of corticosteroids allow no place for infection as a primary cause. Corticosteroids improve the condition in over one-half of cases and, where they do not improve, they certainly do not exacerbate it as expected if infection plays an important role. It may be possible that patients are allergic to bacteria but no evidence has been found nor any mechanism shown (Table 10.1).

Allergy

Allergy has been implicated because of three factors: the histological picture where 90% or more of nasal polyps have an eosinophilia, the association with asthma and, finally, the nasal findings which may mimic allergic symptoms and signs.

The term allergy is used in a variety of ways. It was originally used by von Pirquet in 1906 to describe the altered host reactivity to an antigen which,

Table 10.1 Comparison of bacterial cultures from the nose and paranasal sinuses (%)

| | Normal nose | | Maxillary sinuses | | Tissue |
	Anterior	Posterior	Acute	Polyposis	Nasal polyps
Staphylococcus aureus	30	10	4	–	12
Streptococci (all)	–	15	30	10	25
Gram-negative bacteria	1	10	10	–	10
Haemophilus influenzae	–	40	20	10	–
Anaerobes	–	–	6	–	5

These figures are presented as percentages for comparison. Figures are derived as follows: the normal nose, Gwaltney and Hayden (1982); acute maxillary sinusitis, aggregated figures, chronic sinus disease in patients with nasal polyps, Dawes *et al.* (1989); polyp homogenates, Dunnette *et al.* (1986).

in today's terms, is any immune response. It is now used more commonly to mean hypersensitivity. The immune reactions involved cause tissue damage and are mainly mediated by the immunoglobulin IgE which is attached to the mast cell. Two molecules of allergen specific IgE need to be adjacent and the reaction with the allergen causes the cell membrane to alter and calcium ions to enter the mast cell.

Degranulation is a rapid event and is complete within 30 minutes. Arachidonic acid from the cell surface membrane is metabolized by two pathways to produce prostaglandins and leukotrienes. Further mediators come from the cytoplasm. The early phase produces blockage, running and sneezing in the nose. Following this cells are attracted into the site of the reaction and lymphocytes and eosinophils amplify the response releasing further mediators. This phase produces mainly nasal obstruction and mucous hypersecretion.

It is now clear that mast cells may be triggered by other reactions including those involving IgG, complement activation, some drugs, chemicals and non-specific factors. The resulting degranulation produces similar symptoms whatever the trigger. The mast cell releases preformed elements, histamine, heparin and other vasoactive and chemotactic factors and generates the metabolies of arachidonic acid, the prostaglandins and leukotrienes, the latter including slow reacting substance of anaphylaxis (SRS-A).

Clinically it is easy to consider symptoms such as attacks of anterior rhinorrhoea, sneezing and blockage as allergic when no obvious cause is found and the patients have one or more positive skin tests (Table 10.2).

Conditions associated with polyps
Asthma and nasal polyps

The association of nasal polyps and asthma has long been accepted and has been reviewed (Maloney and Collins, 1977). Of patients with polyps 20–40% have coexisting asthma and it appears that a similar propor-

Table 10.2 The incidence (%) of allergic and respiratory diseases in nasal polyps

	Polyp patients	Normal population
Hayfever	10	10
Childhood asthma	5	5
Eczema	11	3
Penicillin allergy	7	< 15
Positive skin tests	25	20–25
Non-allergic diseases		
Late onset asthma	> 25	3
Aspirin intolerance	8	0.1

The figures of the controls are gathered from a number of different studies and referenced in Drake-Lee *et al.* (1984).

tion of adults with asthma have nasal polyps. Unfortunately earlier work suggested that polypectomy caused asthma, but studies were anecdotal.

Late onset asthma rather than childhood asthma is associated with nasal polyps. The incidence of childhood asthma is about 5% of the population and it was 3.5% in a study of cases with nasal polyps (Drake-Lee *et al.*, 1984). Asthma usually developed around the onset of nasal polyps with over one-half developing either polyps or asthma within 5 years of each other. Surgery has little effect on asthma, if anything patients notice a subjective improvement in their asthma (Maloney, 1977). It has been suggested that patients with asthma may be a distinct subgroup within the disease because proportionately a greater number of patients with asthma and polyps are women whereas polyps usually occur more frequently in men.

Aspirin hypersensitivity

Patients with aspirin hypersensitivity, asthma and nasal polyps are a well-recognized subgroup (Samter and Beers, 1968) which occurs in up to 8% of patients with nasal polyps. The mechanism for both aspirin hypersensitivity and asthma is unclear, but it is not an allergic reaction and there is some suggestion that there is an alteration in prostaglandin synthesis (Sczeklik, Gryglewski and Czerniawski–Mysik, 1975).

Cystic fibrosis

Cystic fibrosis is a multisystemic disease affecting the exocrine glands. It is an autosomal recessive disease occurring in one in 2000 live births. The abnormality lies in the seventh chromosome in three-quarters of the cases. The exocrine glands are unable to produce dilute sweat and values of above 60 mmol of sodium on two consecutive tests are diagnostic.

Transepithelial electrolyte transport controls the quantity and composition of the respiratory tract fluid and so is important in mucociliary clearance. Cystic fibrosis epithelia have defective electrolytic transport especially of the chloride ion. This results in the airway secretions being thick and dehydrated.

The disease produces gastrointestinal and respiratory symptoms. The gastrointestinal symptoms may present at birth with failure of the neonate to pass meconium ileus or subsequent failure to thrive. Conversely some children have little in the way of gastrointestinal symptoms and present with recurrent respiratory tract infections, which may result in severe lung damage produced by persistent colonization by staphylococci and pseudomonas.

Although the pathological changes in the sinuses were first described in detail by Bodian in 1952, the first description of polyps was made by Lurie in 1959. Bilateral nasal polyps are unusual in children and if they are discovered after 2 years and before 10 years of age then they suggest the diagnosis of cystic fibrosis. It is much more common for polyps to develop in children who are known to have the disease rather than polyposis to be the first manifestation of the disease. Schwachman and his colleagues made the first extensive study of relationship between cystic fibrosis and nasal polyps in 1962. A similar study was reported 10 years later by Neely and others who found polyps in 15 of 93 patients (Neely *et al.*, 1972). The true incidence is uncertain and reports have varied from 3 to 48%. The larger studies suggest that nasal symptoms are troublesome in one-third of cases and polypectomy is required in about 10%. A study that compared polyp patients with a control group found that there was no greater incidence of allergic diseases and positive skin tests in the polyp patients (Drake–Lee and Pitcher Willmott, 1982).

Occasionally, the nasal symptoms may occur first as was confirmed by two cases in a study, but usually the other manifestations occur first (Drake-Lee and Pitcher Willmott, 1982). Males predominate, as is found in adults, with a ratio of five to one which appears to be real, even though cystic fibrosis is slightly more common in males.

Although Schwachman and his colleagues noted that 8% of children with cystic fibrosis had polyps, they felt that the incidence would increase as the survival improved (Schwachman *et al.*, 1962). Improved survival has occurred in patients who present with meconium ileus, the commonest presenting symptom, and those with gastrointestinal problems during the first year of life. Polyp patients have significantly less gastrointestinal trouble which is why the incidence of polyps does not appear to have increased (Drake–Lee and Pitcher Willmott, 1982). Lung function deteriorates with age in all cases, but with modern conservative therapy, children live to adulthood when heart and lung transplantation may be required. The incidence and severity of polyposis decreases with advancing age (Drake–Lee and Morgan, 1989).

Bodian who noted that the sinuses were filled with secretions in the cases studied at postmortem, did not infer that the patients had sinusitis (Bodian, 1952). Schwachman *et al.* (1962) found that the sinus radiographs were always opaque but felt that this was not diagnostic since some degree of mucosal thickening was present in one-third of normal children. Since many of the patients require long-term antibiotics it is not surprising that the sinuses are often sterile. Bacteria were cultured in only five out of 11 patients who had antral irrigations (Drake–Lee and Morgan, 1989). The presence of relatively sterile sinuses does not support the hypothesis that the sinuses act as a reservoir for descending infection. This is further supported by the differences between the organisms cultured from the sputum and the sinus irrigations, in only one case was it the same and the organism cultured was *Pseudomonas*.

Other respiratory diseases

While the deficit in cystic fibrosis is in the function of the exocrine glands, other abnormalities in the respiratory mucosa may result in polyp formation. Primary ciliary dyskynesia (immotile cilial syndrome, Kartagener's syndrome) can eventually result in polyps because of stasis of mucus, as can hyperviscous mucus seen in Young's syndrome (bronchiectasis, sinusitis and azoospermia). These two are very rare causes of polyps in adults and often follow a long period of respiratory illness in childhood which should alert the clinician.

Age

Nasal polyps are a disease of adults although children with cystic fibrosis and occasionally teenagers develop them. The incidence every 10 years is equal between the ages of 30 and 60 years and then the chance of developing polyps decreases. Patients who are atopic and asthmatic do not develop polyps any earlier.

Incidence

The true incidence is difficult to assess but it may be inferred from the incidence of asthma since the incidence of nasal polyps in late onset asthmatics is the same as the incidence of late onset asthma in patients with nasal polyps. The incidence of asthma is about 5% with over one-half of the patients developing asthma during childhood. It would be expected that between one in 1000 and 20 in 1000 of the adult population would have nasal polyps once or more in their life. This would fit with the general prevalence of nasal disease in the UK where about 10% of the population suffers from seasonal allergic rhinitis (hay fever), about 5% suffers from perennial allergic or vasomotor rhinitis and of these only a proportion would develop nasal polyps.

Sex

There is a strong male predominance in patients who have polyps; figures range between 2:1 to 4:1 depending on the study. The male predominance is present also in children with cystic fibrosis (even though more males have cystic fibrosis). The sex incidence of patients with asthma and nasal polyps is equal which suggests a different clinical subgroup.

Racial groups

Nasal polyps have been reported in all major racial groups though the comparative incidence has not been documented.

Animals

The only other animal to have nasal polyps is the chimpanzee and polyps occur infrequently with only two cases being reported in the last 50 years. Although cattle may develop polypoid lesions of the nasal septum and cats can present with eustachian tube polyps they are different lesions so it appears that this disease is virtually confined to humans.

Genetic predisposition

As mentioned before, cystic fibrosis is an autosomal recessive disease which is associated with a gene defect on the seventh chromosome but it is not known which phenotype is associated with nasal polyps. Cystic fibrosis gene probes have been used in

seven patients with nasal polyps but without cystic fibrosis (Burger *et al.*, 1991). G551D mutation was found to be higher than expected in this small study so this work suggests that nasal polyps are associated with a higher incidence of this gene mutation.

Maloney and Oliver (1980) looked at the HL-A classification of 29 patients with nasal polyps and found that there was a higher incidence of A1/B8 in patients with nasal polyps, asthma and aspirin hypersensitivity.

Several members of a family may be affected with nasal polyps but there is little evidence for a genetic basis for this. Some evidence to support a genetic predisposition comes from the development of polyps in identical twins (Drake-Lee, 1992).

Macroscopical features

Polypoidal lesions may arise from the nasal mucosa particularly the middle and inferior turbinate and also from any respiratory mucosa in the nose. The classical and commonest situation for their development is the ethmoid sinuses, they arise from beneath the middle turbinate anteriorly and above the middle turbinate posteriorly. Polyps may occur in the other sinuses particularly the maxillary antrum and, following surgery, they may prolapse through an antrostomy. The colour of nasal polyps varies but it is usually a translucent white swelling that blocks the nose to a variable degree, and polyps may become red with repeated trauma and nasal infection, and in the most florid cases prolapse through the anterior nose. The degree of development varies from side to side and without therapy the size may also vary considerably; up to one-quarter will regress spontaneously without treatment. Polyps are usually multiple (Figure 10.1).

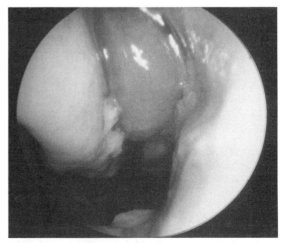

Figure 10.1 A nasal polyp seen lying between the nasal septum and the inferior turbinate

Histology

Tissue removed from the maxillary sinuses, nasal polyps and the bronchi (from patients dying from status asthmaticus) are similar. Nasal polyps usually have a respiratory epithelium with ciliated columnar and goblet cells. If there has been repeated trauma, squamous metaplasia occurs. The gross oedema will give rise to artefact when polyps are processed for scanning electron microscopy since this process involves the dehydration of material. As the polyp shrinks the surface epithelium is lost to a variable extent and this has been described as 'cobblestones'. There is apparent thickening of the basement membrane which will vary from area to area and polyp to polyp.

The submucosal tissue is grossly oedematous and contains few blood vessels which are mainly capillaries and the occasional nerve fibre. The cellular infiltrate is mainly plasma cells, small lymphocytes, macrophages and the most striking feature is an eosinophilia. The eosinophilia may be very variable not only from patient to patient but also between polyps in the same patient. Eosinophils are found in 90% of polyps, the majority of the remaining cells in the other polyps are neutrophils. Occasionally some of the stroma cells may show marked atypia (Friedman and Osbourne, 1982). Their part in the pathogenesis of polyps remains unclear. Sensitized eosinophils are believed to be important in the initiation of mucosal oedema in patients with aspirin hypersensitivity (Sasaki and Nakahara, 1989).

Further work

Mast cells

Mast cells are a heterogeneous collection of cells and have been divided in animals into two main groups: mucosal and connective tissue types; in addition, circulating basophils may also enter the tissue. Ultrastructural analysis showed that mast cells were degranulated (Cauna *et al.*, 1972) and this has been confirmed, but further comment on the granule morphology and cell structure suggests that the features may not be consistent with those described in the allergic nose (Drake–Lee, Barker and Thurley, 1984). The mast cells are also degranulated on the inferior turbinate of over one-half of patients. It suggests that mast cell reactions within the nose as a whole may be important in the development of polyps in these cases. Mast cell reactions occurring within the polyps would lead to construction of oedema once the condition has started (Figures 10.2 and 10.3).

Nasal polyp oedema

Histological examination has demonstrated that polyps are mainly oedamatous (Taylor, 1963) and the extracellular oedema is easy to extract and has been analysed in different studies (Berdal, 1954; Donovan *et al.*, 1970; Drake–Lee and McLaughlan, 1982). After they are removed, polyps may be coarsely minced and centrifuged and the resulting oedema is

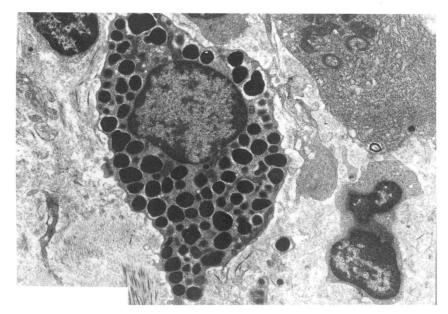

Figure 10.2 The normal ultrastructure of a mast cell with its electron dense granules

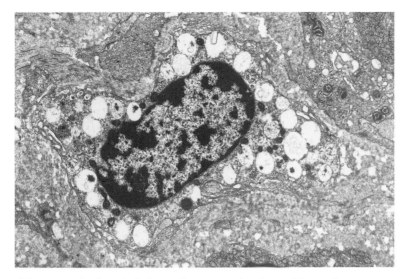

Figure 10.3 A mast cell from a nasal polyp which shows ultrastructural evidence of degranulation

collected and analysed. Matched serum may be taken at the same time. Berdal (1954) injected polyp fluid subcutaneously and repeated skin tests. Those patients who had a positive skin test tended to have greater reactions when tested again at the site of injection. Donovan *et al.* (1970) showed that the level of IgE was raised in polyp fluid irrespective of the results of skin tests.

Immunoglobulins

Nasal polyp tissue continues to behave like normal respiratory mucosa in some respects and it is able to produce immunoglobulins from the plasma cells present. All immunoglobulins are found in polyp oedema with both IgA and IgE levels tending to be higher in polyp fluids than in sera. The levels of IgG, IgA and IgM are variable and elevated levels probably represent a recent upper respiratory tract infection. IgA is a dimeric immunoglobulin which has a junctional chain and secretory piece which makes it stable in mucus. It is the surface immunoglobulin of the respiratory and gastrointestinal tract. The levels are higher in polyp fluid and so it could be argued that this causes polyps in a similar manner to that advocated for IgE.

Allergen-specific IgE

IgE was discovered as the main immunoglobulin in immediate hypersensitivity (Ishizaka and Ishizaka, 1967), and soon afterwards the radioallergosorbent test (RAST) was developed to detect allergen specific IgE in serum (Wide, Bennich and Johansson, 1967). Mixed grass pollens and house dust mite are the commonest allergens to cause allergic rhinitis. Only 25% of patients with nasal polyps have positive skin tests to these allergens (Drake-Lee *et al.*, 1984). Since these are the two most commonly positive skin tests in patients with nasal polyps it would seem logical to expect these to be the commonly raised levels of allergen-specific IgE. RAST levels in polyp fluid and sera are raised only infrequently (John and Merret, 1979). This would suggest that allergic reactions may occur but are infrequently encountered in patients with nasal polyps.

Local nasal allergy

It is possible that even though the patients are no more allergic as a group, a local allergy occurs in the nasal cavity that is not manifest systemically. If this were to be the case then a local allergic reaction should occur in the nose.

Levels of IgE in polyp oedema have been shown to be higher than the corresponding values in serum in several studies (Donovan *et al.*, 1970; Drake-Lee and McLaughlan, 1982). Although some authors feel that this may be related to the presence of an allergic response, others feel that the production is purely a function of local plasma cells, because elevated levels of IgE may be found in nasal secretions in non-atopic subjects (Mygind, Weeke and Ullman, 1975). Polyps are capable of local production and this has been shown by comparing the levels of IgE with those of either albumin or α_2 macroglobulin which are produced elsewhere. Serum values for these compounds are usually below those in polyp oedema.

Free histamine in polyp fluid

When mast cells degranulate a variety of products is produced of which histamine is easiest to measure and has been measured in polyp oedema (Drake-Lee and McLaughlan, 1982). Levels which are between 100 and 1000 times the serum level are encountered. This would suggest that when mast cells degranulate local homeostatic mechanisms may be overcome. This occurs most easily in the ethmoid sinuses, partly because of the anatomy, which allows the mucosa to prolapse into the nose, and partly because the blood supply is less well developed here and so is less able to remove vasoactive compounds. This is a dynamic state so that polyps will vary in size.

The presence and release of other vasoactive compounds and mediators

Arachidonic acid metabolites are not easy to quantify since they are relatively unstable and may be generated by trauma. The results from the four main studies which looked at these compounds are difficult to interpret (Nigam *et al.*, 1986; Salari *et al.*, 1986; Jung *et al.*, 1987; Smith, Gerrard and White, 1987), since there is little work on normal levels in nasal tissues and two of the studies induced the generation of metabolites by challenge. It appears that the levels of thromboxanes are elevated and that challenge will produce 5, 12 and 15 hydroxyeicosatetraenoic acid (HETE), the most elevated being 15-HETE. There is some suggestion that levels are higher in patients with aspirin sensitivity, but whether this is due to a more severe inflammation is not clear. Leukotrienes C4 and D4 may be demonstrated in polyp oedema fluid (see above). Prostaglandins E2, F2α and 6 keto are also present in the oedema.

Allergen challenge to polyp tissue

Bacterial challenge has been discussed already. The first report of pollen allergen challenge to nasal polyp tissue was by Kaliner, Wasserman and Frank Austin in 1973. They used a heterogeneous collection of tissue, including that taken from children with cystic fibrosis, and either challenged allergic tissue or passively sensitized non-allergic tissue with pollen extract and demonstrated that it was possible to release histamine. Challenge to non-sensitized tissue with mixed grass pollen and house dust mite extracts has shown that it is possible to release tissue histamine. Polyp tissue is less reactive than peripheral blood and then only releases histamine rarely on direct

challenge suggesting that allergic reactions are not common.

Culture

Nasal polyp homogenates have been cultured for organisms and 24 out of the 40 grew aerobic bacteria, Gram-negative cultures were obtained in six cases whereas 14 were completely sterile (Dunnette *et al.*, 1986). Streptococci were cultured most frequently and were more common in asthmatics and patients on inhaled steroids. If the polyps showed a polymorph infiltration then bacteria were more likely to be cultured. Cultures were completely negative for mycobacteria, mycoplasmas and viruses.

The presence of bacterial specific IgE in nasal polyp oedema fluid has been investigated by Calenoff *et al.* (1983). They stated that 59 of the 61 patients had bacterial-specific IgE in the polyp oedema and the most commonly raised immunoglobulin was to *Proteus*. They defined a positive result on the basis of a count of 150% above background noise. It would appear from their studies that the activity was lost on incubation of sera at 56°C. They gave no information on the anti-IgE used and some of the commercial anti-IgEs have had purity and specificity problems. The results appear to be inconclusive.

Nasal polyp tissue has been challenged with bacteria to release histamine (Baenkler, Schaubschlager and Behnsen, 1983) and a wide and variable release of histamine occurred with anti-IgE. The study concluded that although there was some response to challenge with streptococcal and staphylococcal extracts bacterial allergy was only a possibility.

Vascular development

There has been little work done on the vascular flow through the nose and sinuses and that which has, has used relatively insensitive techniques.

Direct inspection of the nasal cavity will show the well-developed blood supply which can be compared directly by endoscopy with the sinus mucosa both in the ethmoid complex and the maxillary antrum. The sinus mucosa is a pale almost transparent lining and the feeding vessels can be seen through the yellowish mucosa.

This picture is confirmed by histological examination. Sections through the nasal cavity show how well adapted the mucosa is to fulfill its physiological function of warming and humidifying the inspired air. The blood supply has both capacitance and resistance vessels together with venous sinusoids, whereas the vascularity of the sinuses is much less well developed. This means that there is less reserve in the blood supply in the sinuses to transport away compounds released by cellular reactions: homeostasis is reached less easily. Venous congestion is a feature of intranasal disease whereas persistent oedema is found in sinus conditions.

Nasal symptoms

Almost without exception all patients suffer from nasal blockage. This is constant although it will vary with the size and position of polyps. The mildest form of complaint is congestion. Patients will often complain they feel as though they have a cold at times and this may be socially embarrassing. Usually there is some nasal breathing. It may be that following surgery with the improvement of nasal function with adequate warming and humidification of the air that those patients with asthma notice an improvement in their chest symptoms.

Running and sneezing

About one-half of the patients suffer from attacks of either running and/or sneezing and this may be helped with surgery when large areas of oedematous mucosa are improved. Patients who suffer with these symptoms will often say that they have hay fever. This is because the symptoms are the same but they are perennial and even if intermittent have no obvious triggers.

Sense of smell

Partial loss of the sense of smell and alterations in taste are common complaints. These do not tend to recover following treatment except in some cases treated by corticosteroids, particularly when taken orally, when there may be a general improvement in respiratory function.

Pain

Although not frequent, pain does occur in patients with polyps and is usually over the bridge of the nose, the forehead and cheeks. It is worse when the nose is congested or when the postnasal drip changes in colour and the sinuses are infected secondarily.

Postnasal drip

Most patients will complain of some postnasal drip. It is usually white but may become green or yellow particularly with maxillary pains or following exacerbation of nasal symptoms. Alteration of the mucus and its hypersecretion is a consequence of inflammation irrespective of cause, since nasal polyps are an inflammatory condition then mucus hypersecretion occurs. A severe eosinophilia may change the colour of the mucus from white to yellow or a yellow/green colour and was called allergic pus in the 1930s. The postnasal drip may improve following surgery or if the mucus changes to green may become normal following antibiotic therapy.

Epistaxis

It is infrequent and follows extensive clearing of the nose, if it does occur as a major symptom then it may indicate a more sinister underlying pathology.

Signs

Patients have a distinctive hyponasal voice and when the blockage is severe, polyps may be seen externally. Mouth breathing and occasionally flaring of the alar cartilages occur with complete obstruction. This later sign is usually produced by the polyps themselves. If polyps develop before the nasal facial bones fuse, hypertelorism will develop in more florid cases: it is seen in children with cystic fibrosis. The intranasal signs have been discussed previously.

Investigations

There are no specific haematological, biochemical or immunological investigations that are required apart from those involved in the general work up of cases prior to surgery. Skin tests have been widely used to investigate nasal cases but the incidence of positive skin tests is no greater than expected in the general population (Pepys and Duveen, 1951; Settipane and Chafee, 1977; Drake–Lee *et al.*, 1984). Those with positive skin tests do not present any earlier nor have more severe recurrence. Cases with hayfever and dust mite allergy should have these treated in their own right.

If patients had anterior mucoid rhinorrhoea or have developed polyps at an early age then they should be investigated for cystic fibrosis, ciliary dysfunction or immune deficiency.

Radiology

Plain radiographs of the paranasal sinuses demonstrated by the conventional three views will show the extent of the disease in the nose and paranasal sinuses to some extent. A CT scan will give more information, particularly the anatomical detail. Other features seen include, loss of radiotranslucency in the nose, hypertrophy of the turbinates and deviation of the bony septum and intranasal masses. The ethmoid complex is usually opaque to a variable extent on the side of the polyps and these changes may occur on the other side where there are no visible polyps. The maxillary sinus will have changes in most cases with mucosal thickening of a variable degree until the antrum becomes opaque. Fluid levels are encountered and may be due to retained secretion alone or purulent material, since blockage of the maxillary ostium by polyps will prevent the migration of mucus from the sinus.

Expansion of the ethmoids will be encountered in those patients with polyps which developed before the bones fused. Bony erosion, although highly suggestive of malignancy, may be found in patients who have polyps and is ususally due to previous surgery. Previous surgery is often implicated when mucocoeles develop. They are most commonly frontal or ethmoid; primary sphenoid mucocoeles are rare (Lund and Lloyd, 1983).

Anatomical variations

Considerable attention has been paid in the past few years to the variation of the middle meatus of the nose and its impact on the presentation of nasal disease. The collective term for the area is the ostio-meatal complex. Some surgeons consider that the variations here are the most important factor in the development of nasal polyps and that the correction of these variations is the main stay of therapy.

Variations include agger nasi cells, concha bullosa, paradoxical middle turbinate, over-pneumatized ethmoid bulla and bent uncinate process. The frequency of these variations would seem similar in patients with and without nasal polyps (Lloyd, 1990). A similar anatomical approach is advocated by those who believe that the junction of the nose and the ethmoid sinus is the area that polyps start. Surgical treatment is aimed at correcting the anatomical variations and opening out the ethmoid cells into a large unit, an ethmoidectomy, often aided by the endoscope. Correct radiographic imaging with CT is essential before surgery but a limited series of cuts of four or five coronal sections at 5-mm intervals and two axial cuts through the orbits may be all that is necessary (White, Cowan and Robertson, 1991). Any CT scan increases the dose of radiation to the orbit but is limited by decreasing the number of sections.

Treatment

Most surgeons today treat polyps surgically but many polyps are sensitive to corticosteroids and where polyps are not obstructing the nose completely a trial of corticosteroids preoperatively is worthwhile.

Treatment is a combination of medical and surgical modalities following the assessment of the patient.

Unfortunately much of what is written on the treatment of polyps is anecdotal and has not been subject to useful trials and scrutiny. Very limited disease associated with an anatomical abnormality of the middle meatus may not respond to medical treatment. It is the author's view that unless any operation has been shown to be more effective than another then it is best to perform the simplest operation with the best illumination available and with least risk of harm to the patient.

Medical treatment can be conveniently divided into two areas, first inducing remission and second preventing recurrence (Table 10.3).

Table 10.3 Summary of medical treatment

Preoperative therapy
Intranasal corticosteroids
   Trial of therapy for one month since one-half of patients respond
   Betamethasone nose drops, two drops each side twice a day
or
   Aqueous beclomethasone, flunisolide, budesonide, fluticasone two puffs each side twice a day

Postoperative therapy
Intranasal corticosteroids
   Indicated in patients with severe recurrence or symptoms
   Intranasal corticosteroids, e.g. beclomethasone first, if patients do not respond then,
   Betamethasone nose drops, two drops each side twice a day for one month, if patients do not respond then,
Oral corticosteroids
   Prednisolone, between 5 and 30 mg daily for 10 days with topical treatment which should be continued

Diets
May help those with aspirin hypersensitivity

Allergy control
If patients have allergic rhinitis therapy may be required

Preoperative medical treatment

About one-half of cases respond to corticosteroids. Polyps regress when corticosteroids are given orally which are as effective as surgery (Lildholdt *et al.*, 1988). Because of the risk of side effects, corticosteroids are usually given intranasally.

It is worth trying intranasal corticosteroids on all patients since they will prevent surgery in up to one-half of patients. Betamethasone drops 0.1% where available, two each side twice a day with retention should be tried for a month. An aqueous spray such as beclomethasone, flunisolide, budesonide or fluticasone may be used as an alternative therapy and should also be given for a month when the response can be reassessed (Charlton *et al.*, 1985; Dingsor *et al.*, 1985). Beclomethasone diproprionate, 400 μg daily, two puffs each side twice a day is a typical treatment.

Medical treatment must be given in a way which will ensure contact for a reasonable length of time. Nose drops may be given in either the head down and forward position or lying prone with the head dependent and the patient should stay in the position for at least a minute, preferably longer. Systemic absorption occurs with betamethasone. Cushing's syndrome has been described following betamethasone abuse (Stevens, 1988), so this should be given carefully if used on a continuous basis.

Sprays are easier to use and probably have a better compliance. Betamethasone has yet to be produced as a spray. Although it is felt that the position of a nasal spray is important, so long as the spray ends on the ciliary epithelium, ciliary action will transport the spray posteriorly and cover the nasal lining. Although it will not be transported into the ethmoids, it will cover the polyps.

If the polyps do not respond after a month then they may be removed surgically. As more patients are given medical treatment before they reach the specialist, the proportion of 'steroid resistant' polyps will rise.

Surgical treatment

Anatomical considerations

The anatomy of the nose and ethmoids has been considered elsewhere but there are several points which should be highlighted. The middle turbinate is the key to nasal surgery. If surgery is performed medially then the cribriform plate may be breached and the anterior cranial fossa entered. If surgery is lateral then the ethmoid complex may be entered. Extensive intranasal operations on the ethmoids renders the middle turbinate unstable; if it is lost or removed it makes subsequent orientation difficult. Since many operations are performed subsequently by junior surgeons the risk of complications is greater. Stenosis of the middle meatus can occur following endoscopic surgery.

The eye is the lateral relation of the ethmoids and the lamina papyracea is very thin, it is easy to enter the orbit if ethmoid surgery is vigorous. The simplest complication is herniation of orbital fat but more extensive surgery may injure the medial rectus anteriorly and the optic nerve posteriorly.

Preoperative preparation

The keys to good and safe surgery are good illumination and minimal bleeding. The nose should be prepared adequately before surgery to cause vasoconstriction and shrinkage of the mucosa. Drier fields are obtained under local anaesthesia alone. Various methods are used to prepare the nose and each will give a good field if used well. The author's technique is outlined below. If nasal surgery is performed under local anaesthesia, patients should be admitted and sedated with an adequate parenteral premedication. Surgery should be performed in theatre where all facilities are available.

Cocaine 10% spray is given on the ward 15 minutes before local anaesthesia. This allows a much more thorough local anaesthetic to be given. Cocaine paste 25% is used on cotton wool loaded wires and the mucosa is painted thoroughly. Anterior nerve block is obtained with one wire between the nasal bones and septum. Posteriorly, a wire is inserted as far back as possible under the middle turbinate to block the sphenopalatine nerve. If the inferior meatus is to be entered, a further probe is inserted here as well. If this technique is used as well for cases operated on under a general anaesthetic, then bleeding is reduced and the need to pack the nose afterwards is removed.

Silver is used for the wires since it is malleable and bends if the patients were to have a vasovagal attack. These are prevented by premedication and performing the local with the patient lying flat. Adequate time should be left for the local anaesthetic to work. When general anaesthesia is used in addition, an endotracheal tube or laryngeal mask is required.

Surgical procedures

Simple polypectomy

There are different views on the type of surgery required for nasal polyps. Many patients will have infrequent recurrence and to advocate an extensive operation initially before the problem of recurrence is evident is illogical. The majority of patients who have occasional recurrences every few years may be treated very effectively by simple polypectomy.

Polyps may be removed by either an avulsion or cutting snare or forceps such as Tilley Hinkells. Care must be taken when using forceps not to go either too medially or too laterally. All polypoidal mucosa should be removed from the ethmoids, the lower border of the middle turbinate and the inferior turbinate and the forceps should be pushed first before they are pulled anteriorly. The ipsilateral eye should be left exposed at all times and inspected before any material is pulled from the nose (Figure 10.4).

Intranasal ethmoidectomy

Modern diagnostic techniques including endoscopic examination of the nose and computerized evaluation of the nose and paranasal sinuses have shown the site of disease more accurately. The endoscope can be used to undertake a more thorough endonasal ethmoidectomy. It can also be used to monitor the postoperative course. Polypoidal mucosa can be

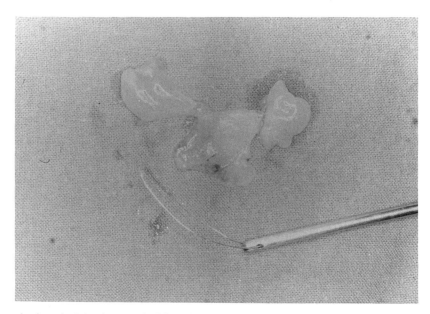

Figure 10.4 A nasal polyp which has been avulsed from the ethmoid sinuses. More of the polyp is in the sinuses than prolapsing into the nasal cavity

shrunk by preoperative oral corticosteroids and some surgeons advocate very large doses of over 30 mg of prednisolone a day in reducing doses over 10 days prior to surgery.

Although intranasal ethmoidectomy is advocated by some authors for all polyp patients, it is neither a complete nor safe operation. It is impossible to remove all the anterior and posterior ethmoidal air cells without making the middle turbinate unstable unless an endoscope is used. If the middle turbinate is lost, so is the main intranasal landmark.

External ethmoidectomy

External ethmoidectomy is performed through an incision medial to the inner canthus of the eye (Howarths) or through an incision in the natural skin crease below the infraorbital margin (Pattersons). All the ethmoid cells may be removed once the orbit has been displaced laterally with the lacrimal apparatus. The anterior ethmoidal vessels are divided. The anterior ethmoidal vessels provide a landmark for the level of the cribriform plate. All the ethmoidal cells should be removed and the sphenoid sinus may be entered if desired. Care should be taken to open the ostium of the frontal sinus widely to prevent future mucocoeles which are a late complication of surgery. There have been no trials to see if external ethmoidectomy prevents recurrence, although it has some advocates (Hughes, 1973). It may delay recurrence for a number of years until the area has been filled with oedematous mucosa.

The mucosal changes may extend into the maxillary sinus and some surgeons advise the Jansen–Horgan procedure. This is the combination of a Caldwell–Luc operation with a posterior ethmoidectomy through the antrum combined with an intranasal anterior and middle ethmoidectomy. It is rarely performed today.

A Caldwell–Luc procedure may be undertaken alone for maxillary mucosal disease but polypoidal mucosa prolapses through the antrostomy in the inferior meatus when frequent recurrence is a problem. This is exceptionally difficult to treat.

Complications of surgery

The main immediate complication is haemorrhage. This occurs at the time of surgery and is usually minimized if the operation is performed with suitable preparation. It is often not necessary to pack the nose when a good local preparation is used and the patient feels the immediate benefit of the improved airway. Packing will control the haemorrhage in virtually every case particularly when simple polypectomy alone is performed. Slight ooze and serosanguineous discharge occur from the raw areas for the next few postoperative days.

Crusting occurs as the blood and mucus dries but this will separate by 2 weeks after surgery leaving the area healed. Surgeons who advocate endosopic sinus surgery may follow up patients at frequent intervals to remove debris and crusts and any small polyps that recur.

The main complications occur from damage to the cribriform plate and the orbit. The anterior cranial fossa may be entered and this may result in CSF leakage only or, more importantly, meningitis and abscess formation. Complete anosmia is rare since the olfactory bulb will remain undamaged. The orbit may be entered through the lamina papyracea or through the posterior ethmoid air cells. Damage to the orbital periostium may cause herniation of periorbital fat, medial rectus palsy, damage to the anterior of posterior ethmoidal arteries and division of the optic nerve.

Endoscopic surgery has been associated with an increase in complications and litigation (Levine, 1990). Before any surgeon uses the endoscope for intranasal surgery, they should be familiar with the anatomy, have practised on cadavers and attended a course. Although a useful tool, its efficacy at preventing recurrence has yet to be evaluated.

Recurrence of nasal polyps is not a complication of surgery since it is a feature of the disease. Even though surgery is meticulous it is most frustrating to see polyps at the first postoperative visit.

Postoperative medical care

There is no single approach to care. Some surgeons advocate a 10-day course of decongestants and steam inhalations for all patients who have undergone nasal surgery. The role of long-term medical treatment with corticosteroid sprays has yet to be fully evaluated but evidence suggests recurrence may be controlled (Mygind *et al.*, 1975; Deuschl and Drettner, 1977). There are two main reasons to give corticosteroid sprays: to control the symptoms of rhinitis and to prevent recurrence.

Patients who have rhinitis and polyps do not as a group seem more prone to recurrence. Any trial that groups control of these symptoms together with recurrence is open to question. There is only one true test of control and that is the regimen which gives rise to fewer operations. There would seem to be no case for giving all patients who present for the first time with nasal polyps long-term steroids until the results of large clinical trials are available. In those patients with established disease, a 1-year trial of medical treatment would seem to be appropriate. It is sometimes necessary to combine corticosteroid nose drops with an aqueous-based corticosteroid spray.

Antihistamines have virtually no place in the management of recurrence. The sedation caused by some products is unacceptable and although non-sedating antihistamines are available, enzyme induction occurs in the liver after 6 weeks and so the effect of the antihistamine is reduced. A short course may be prescribed if the rhinitis is difficult to control.

Diets

There has been much enthusiasm recently in 'allergy' to foods, which means food sensitivity and may be treated by exclusion diets. Tartrazine dyes are linked to aspirin pharmacologically and since a group of patients have aspirin hypersensitivity it would seem logical to exclude tartrazine dyes from their diet. No controlled trials have been performed but patients say frequently that they feel better and have fewer nasal symptoms. The treatment does not harm the patient, has no side effects and may help some of those who want to try to do something themselves to prevent recurrence.

Recurrence

Recurrence of nasal polyps is one of the problems facing every otolaryngologist in management of cases. The rate of recurrence is variable and a 2-year study showed that just over 40% presented for the first time and 5% had had five or more previous polypectomies (Drake-Lee *et al.*, 1984). It is difficult to study factors which are associated with recurrence well but several factors are important. As expected if a patient develops polyps when younger and if there is a long history of nasal complaints then recurrence tends to be more severe. Patients with severe nasal disease often have more extensive surgery but this has not been shown to improve the recurrence rate in this study. Perhaps the single most easily detectable aetiological factor is the association with asthma. Patients with asthma suffer more severe recurrence in general and if they have aspirin hypersensitivity then this is even more so. Since women have a higher incidence of asthma, then they may be more prone to recurrence.

It is noteworthy that hay fever, childhood asthma, penicillin allergy and multiple positive skin tests, all manifestations of allergic diatheses, are in no way associated with severe recurrence.

The treatment of nasal polyps in patients with cystic fibrosis

The best method of treatment is debated. Crockett *et al.* (1987) advocated extensive sinus surgery where as Donaldson and Gillespie (1988) recommended the use of intranasal corticosteroids and noted that spontaneous resolution of polyps occurred even without using corticosteroids. Donaldson and Gillespie believed that intranasal steroids are the first line of treatment in controlling polyps. Both these studies suggest that significant control may gained in up to 60% of cases. The exact method depends both on the age and compliance of the child and family. If there has been improvement corticosteroid nose drops such as betamethasone with or without neomycin may be tried for a period of up to 2 months. This may be followed by long-term corticosteroid sprays (beclomethasone, budesonide, flunisolide, fluticasone).

Others have stated that simple polypectomy is associated with a high rate of recurrence (Stern *et al.*, 1982), or that the extent of intranasal surgery is inversely proportional to recurrence. Extensive surgery is associated with blood loss which may require transfusion as in three of the 40 cases treated by Crockett and his associates. Functional endoscopic sinus surgery (FESS) under local anaesthesia may have a place in the older child. The local anaesthesia prevents the possible complications of performing general anaesthesia on patients with compromised pulmonary function. Functional endoscopic sinus surgery allows removal of the diseased mucosa with minimal disruption of the normal anatomy. In a recent study of 18 cases who required surgery, only two had 10 or more recurrences and 13 had had one or two polypectomies only. The average time between recurrences requiring surgery was 18 months and the age of first operation varied between 2 and 15 years with a mean of 7.5 (Drake–Lee and Morgan, 1989).

Since many patients may develop severe lung damage, the shortest anaesthetic possible should be used which means that simple polypectomy would appear to be the method of choice, if intranasal steroids are unsatisfactory in the first instance.

Antrochoanal polyps

These polyps arise in the maxillary antrum and prolapse through the ostium of the sinus in the middle meatus. They hang either in the nose or if larger into the posterior choana. The choanal part of the polyp may be seen in the oropharynx where it pushes the soft palate forward.

Antrochoanal polyps (Killians polyps) are rare and probably occur in all racial groups. Like benign nasal polyps they are more common in men than women. The onset is usually before 40 years although they may be found at all ages. The polyps tend to be dumb-bell in shape with a constriction where they pass through the ostium (or accessory ostium) of the sinus. They occur usually either from the left or right maxillary sinus alone, but may be bilateral rarely. Attempts have been made to define from where in the maxillary antrum they arise. The floor and lateral wall are common, although their site of origin frequently cannot be determined. The polyp is similar in colour to the simple types being pale white or translucent in appearance.

Histology shows a respirating epithelium over a normal basement membrane. The interstitium is grossly oedematous and the cellular infiltrate is similar to ordinary polyps except that there is no eosinophilia. There have been no ultrastructural studies of these polyps.

The commonest symptom is unilateral nasal blockage, although when very large they may cause bilateral blockage. The blockage may be greater on expiration than on inspiration due to the ball-valve effect. Other nasal symptoms are uncommon except for anterior nasal discharge which is usually mucoid. The polyp may not be visible on anterior rhinoscopy but is usually seen posteriorly, occasionally without the aid of the mirror. Rigid endoscopy will show the polyp.

Radiographs of the sinuses may show mucosal thickening or a completely opaque antrum. The sinuses are almost never normal on the affected side. The lateral view may show the polyp in the postnasal space.

Aetiology

Antrochoanal polyps are an entity of unknown aetiology. They are not associated with allergy, lower respiratory tract disease or sinusitis. Proetz suggested that they may be due to a faulty development of the maxillary sinus ostium since it is always large. The ostium may be large because of expansion by the polyp but this is unlikely since there is no expansion of the posterior choana by large polyps nor is there any erosion or displacement of the middle turbinate medially.

Treatment

There is no medical treatment either preoperatively or postoperatively.

Preoperatively nasal preparation with a vasoconstrictor is essential. It is necessary to remove both parts of the polyp. There has been debate on the best method of removal of polyps. The approach is dictated by the age of the patient. Simple intranasal polypectomy alone will almost always result in recurrence. Many of the patients are young and dentition is incomplete so that a Caldwell–Luc procedure is not indicated. An antral wash out may produce straw-coloured fluid and should be performed since it may help in the dissection of the antral mucosa if simple polypectomy is performed. It is often impossible to remove the polyp through the nose so that it has to be delivered through the oropharynx. Larger polyps may be difficult to remove because they develop adhesions in the nose which have to be broken by blunt dissection.

A Caldwell–Luc antrostomy is the treatment of choice in adults since recurrence will be reduced. In children, once dentition is complete then simple polypectomy is replaced by the more radical procedure. All the lining of the sinus is removed together with the polyp. It is debatable whether an antrostomy into the inferior meatus is required.

References

BAENKLER, H., SCHAUBSCHLAGER, W. and BEHNSEN, H. (1983) Antigen induced histamine release from the mucosa in nasal polyposis. *Clinical Otolaryngology*, **8**, 227–230

BERDAL, P. (1954) Serological examination of nasal polyp fluid. *Acta Otolaryngologica*, **115**

BODIAN, M. (1952) *Pathology in Fibrocystic Disease of the Pancreas*. London: Heinemann Medical Books. ch. 5 pp. 67–146

BURGER, J., MACEK, M., STUHRMANN, M., REIS, A., KRAWCZAK, M. and SCHMIDTKE, J. (1991) Genetic influences in the formation of nasal polyps (letter). *Lancet*, i, 974

CALENOFF, E., GUILFORD, T., GREEN, J. and ENGELHARD, C. (1983) Bacterial specific IgE in patients with nasal polyps. *Archives of Otolaryngology*, **109**, 372–375

CAUNA, N., HINDOVER, K. H., MANZETHI, G. W. and SWANSON, E. W. (1972) Fine structure of nasal polyps. *Annals of Otolaryngology*, **81**, 41–58

CHARLTON, R., MACKAY, I., WILSON, R. and COLE, P. (1985) Double blind placebo controlled trial of beclamethesone nose drops for nasal polyposis. *British Medical Journal*, **2**, 788–798

CROCKETT, D., MCGILL, T., HEALY, G., FRIEDMAN, E. and SALKELD, L. (1987) Nasal and paranasal sinus surgery in children with cystic fibrosis. *Annals of Otorhinolaryngology*, **96**, 367–372

DAWES, P., BATES, G., WATSON, D., LEWIS, D., LOWE, D. and DRAKE-LEE, A. (1989) The role of bacterial infection of the maxillary sinus in nasal polyps. *Clinical Otolaryngology*, **14**, 447–450

DEUSCHL, L. H. and DRETTNER, B. (1977) Nasal polyps treated by beclamethasone nasal aerosol. *Rhinology*, **15**, 17–23

DINGSOR, G., KRAMER, J., OLSHOLT, R. and SONDERSTOM, J. (1985) Flunisolide nasal spray 0.025% in the prophylactic treatment of nasal polyposis after polypectomy. A randomized, double blind, parallel, placebo controlled study. *Rhinology*, **23**, 49–58

DONALDSON, J. and GILLESPIE, C. (1988) Observations on the efficacy of intranasal beclomethasone diproprionate in cystic fibrosis patients. *Journal of Otolaryngology*, **17**, 43–45

DONOVAN, R., JOHANSSON, S. G. O., BERNICH, H. and SOOTHILL, J. P. (1970) Immunoglobulins in nasal polyp fluid. *International Archives of Allergy and Applied Immunology*, **37**, 154–166

DRAKE-LEE, A. (1992) Nasal polyps in identical twins. *Journal of Laryngology and Otology*, **106**, 1084–1085

DRAKE-LEE, A. B. and MCLAUGHLAN, P. (1982) Clinical symptoms, free histamine and IgE in patients with nasal polyps. *International Archives of Allergy and Applied Immunology*, **69**, 268–271

DRAKE-LEE, A. B. and MORGAN, D. (1989) Nasal polyps and sinusitis in children with cystic fibrosis. *Journal of Laryngology and Otolaryngology*, **103**, 753–755

DRAKE-LEE, A. B. and PITCHER WILLMOTT, R. (1982) The clinical and laboratory correlates of nasal polyps in cystic fibrosis. *International Journal of Paediatric Otolaryngology*, **4**, 209–214

DRAKE-LEE, A. B., BARKER, T. H. W. and THURLEY, K. (1984) Nasal polyps II. Fine structure of mast cells. *Journal of Laryngology and Otology*, **98**, 285–292

DRAKE-LEE, A. B., LOWE, D., SWANSTON, A. and GRACE, A. (1984) Clinical profile and recurrence of nasal polyps. *Journal of Laryngology and Otology*, **98**, 783–793

DUNNETTE, S., HALL, M., WASHINGTON, J., KERN, E., MCDONALD, T., FACER, G. et al. (1986) *Journal of Allergy and Clinical Immunology*, **78**, 102–108

FRIEDMAN, I. and OSBOURNE, D. A. (1982) Miscellaneous granulomas and nasal polyposis. In: *Pathology of Granulomas and Neoplasms of the Nose and Paranasal Sinuses*. ch. 2. Edinburg: Churchill Livingstone. pp. 28–35

GWALTNEY, J. and HAYDEN, F. (1982) The nose and infection. In: *The Nose. Upper Airway Physiology and the Atmosphere and Environment*, edited by D. Proctor and I. Anderson, Amsterdam: Elsevier. ch. 16, pp. 399–422

HUGHES, R. G. (1973) The role of radical surgery in the treatment of recurrent nasal polyposis. *Journal of Laryngology and Otology*, **87**, 117–122

ISHIZAKA, K. and ISHIZAKA, T. (1967) Identification of γE antibodies as a carrier of reaginic activity. *Journal of Immunology*, **99**, 1187–1198

JACKSON, R. J. and ARIHOOD, S. A. (1971) The acid mucopolysaccharides and collagen content of human nasal polyps, and perinasal nasal mucosa. *Annals of Otolaryngology*, **80**, 586–592

JOHN, A. C. and MERRETT, T. G. (1979) The radioallergosorbent test (RAST) in nasal polyposis. *Journal of Laryngology and Otology*, **93**, 889–898

JUNG, T., JUHN, S., HWANG, D. and STEWART, R. (1987) Prostaglandins, leukotrienes and other arachidonic acid metabolites in nasal polyps and nasal mucosa. *Laryngoscope*, **97**, 184–189

KALINER, M., WASSERMAN, S. and FRANK AUSTIN, K. (1973) Immunologic release of chemical mediators from human nasal polyps. *New England Journal of Medicine*, **289**, 277–281

LEVINE, H. (1990) Functional endoscopic sinus surgery: evaluation, surgery and follow up of 250 patients. *Laryngoscope*, **100**, 79–84

LILDHOLDT, T., FORGSTRUP, J., KORTHOLM, B. and ULSOE, C. (1988) Surgical versus medical management of nasal polyps *Acta Otolaryngologica*, **105**, 140–143

LLOYD, G. A. S. (1990) CT of the paranasal sinuses: study of a control series in relation to endoscopic sinus surgery. *Journal of Laryngology and Otology*, **104**, 477–481

LUND, V. J. and LLOYD, G. A. S. (1983) Radiological changes associated with benign nasal polyps. *Journal of Laryngology and Otology*, **97**, 503–510

LURIE, H. (1959) Cystic fibrosis of the pancreas and the nasal mucosa. *Annals of Otology, Rhinology and Laryngology*, **68**, 478

MAJUMDAR, B. and BULL, P. D. (1982) The incidence of maxillary sinusitis in nasal polyposis. *Journal of Laryngology and Otology*, **96**, 937–941

MALONEY, J. R. (1977) Nasal polyps, nasal polypectomy, asthma and aspirin sensitivity. *Journal of Laryngology and Otology*, **91**, 837–846

MALONEY, J. R. and COLLINS, J. (1977) Nasal polyps and bronchial asthma. *British Journal of Diseases of the Chest*, **71**, 1–6

MALONEY, J. and OLIVER, R. (1980) HLA antigens, nasal polyps and asthma. *Clinical Otolaryngology*, **5**, 183–189

MYGIND, N., PEDERSEN, C. B., PRYTZ, S. and SORESEN, H. (1975) Treatment of nasal polyps with intranasal beclomethasone diproprionate aerosol. *Clinical Allergy*, **5**, 159–164

MYGIND, N., WEEKE, B. and ULLMAN, S. (1975) Quantitative determination of immunoglobulins in nasal secretion. *International Archives of Allergy and Applied Immunology*, **49**, 99–102

NEELY, J., HARRISON, G., JERGER, J., GREENBERGER, S. and PRESBERG, H. (1972) The otolaryngologic aspects of cystic fibrosis. *Transactions of the American Academy of Ophthalmology and Otorhinolaryngology*, **76**, 313–324

NIGAM, S., KUNKEL, G., HEROLD, D., BAUMER, F. and JUSUF, L. (1986) Nasal polyps and their content of arachidonic acid metabolites. *New England and Regional Allergy Proceedings* **7**, 109–112

PEPYS, J. and DUVEEN, G. E. (1951) Negative skin tests in allergic rhinitis and nasal polyps. *International Archives of Allergy*, **2**, 147–160

SALARI, H., BORGEAT, P., STEFFENRUD, S., RICHARD, J., BEDARD, P., HEBERT, J. *et al.* (1986) Immunological and non-immunological release of leukotrienes and histamine from human nasal polyps. *Clinical and Experimental Immunology*, **63**, 711–717

SAMTER, M. and BEERS, R. F. (1968) Intolerance to aspirin. Clinical studies and consideration of its pathogenesis. *Annals of Internal Medicine*, **68**, 975

SASAKI, Y. and NAKAHARA, H. (1989) Granule core loss in eosinophils from a patient with aspirin induced asthma: an electron microscope study. *Annals of Allergy*, **63**, 306–308

SCHWACHMAN, H., KULCZYCHI, I. L., MUELLER, H. L. and FLAKE, C. G. (1962) Nasal polyposis in patients with cystic fibrosis. *Paediatrics*, **30**, 389–410

SCZEKLIK, A., GRYGLEWSKI, R. J. and CZERNIAWSKA-MYSIK, G. (1975) Relationship of inhibition of prostaglandin biosynthesis by analgesics to asthma attacks in aspirin-sensitive patients. *British Medical Journal*, **1**, 67–69

SETTIPANE, G. A. and CHAFFEE, F. G. (1977) Nasal polyps in asthma and rhinitis. *Journal of Allergy and Clinical Immunology*, **58**, 17–21

SMITH, D., GERRARD, J. and WHITE, J. (1987) Comparison of arachidonic acid metabolites in nasal polyps and eosinophils. *International Archives of Allergy and Applied Immunology*, **82**, 83–88

STERN, R. C., BOAT, T. F., WOOD, R. E., MATTHEWS, L. W. and DOERSHUK, C. F. (1982) Treatment and prognosis of nasal polyps in cystic fibrosis. *American Journal of Diseases of Children*, **136**, 1067–1070

STEVENS, D. (1988) Cushings's syndrome due to the abuse of betamethasone nasal drops. *Journal of Laryngology and Otology*, **102**, 219–221

TAYLOR, M. (1963) Histochemical studies on nasal polyps. *Journal of Laryngology and Otology*, **77**, 326–341

VANCIL, M. E. (1969) A historical survey of treatment for nasal polyposis. *Laryngoscope*, **79**, 435–445

WHITE, P., COWAN, I. and ROBERTSON, M. (1991) Limited CT scanning techniques of the paranasal sinuses. *Journal of Laryngology and Otology*, **105**, 20–23

WIDE, L., BENNICH, H. and JOHANSSON, S. (1967) Diagnosis of allergy by and in-vitro test for allergen antibodies. *Lancet*, ii, 1105–1107

11

The nasal septum

David Brain

Injuries to the septum

The anterior part of the nasal septum projects in front of the plane of the pyriform aperture and is frequently damaged when the nose is injured. This may result in a haematoma formation and/or septal deviations.

Septal haematoma

When the septum is subjected to a sharp buckling stress, submucosal blood vessels are frequently torn and, if the mucosa remains intact, this will result in the formation of a haematoma. If the injury is severe enough to fracture the septal cartilage, the blood will often pass through to the other side and produce a bilateral haematoma. The blood mainly accumulates in the subperichondrial layer and this will usually interfere with the vitality of the cartilage which becomes compromised, as it depends on the perichondrium for its nutrition. The cartilage can probably remain viable for 3 days, but after this the chondrocytes die, and absorption of the cartilage follows. Cartilage absorption can occur with alarming rapidity and Fry (1969) has suggested that the process is hastened by enzyme action, probably in the form of one of the tissue collagenases. Small haematomas will not cause this necrosis of cartilage, but may slowly absorb leading to permanent thickening of the septum with gross fibrosis.

Symptoms and signs

The dominant symptom is nasal obstruction, and initially there may be some discomfort. Examination is best made without a speculum, and will reveal a smooth rounded bilateral septal swelling which often extends to the lateral nasal walls causing complete obstruction (Figure 11.1).

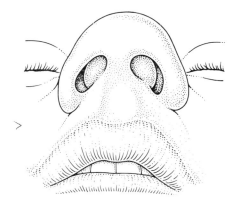

Figure 11.1 Septal haematoma

Treatment

Fry (1969) has shown that early surgical drainage of the haematoma reduces the risk of cartilage necrosis, and is therefore always indicated. A long hemitransfixation incision is made (see Figure 11.27) and usually the haematoma will have elevated the perichondrium from the cartilage. Blood is aspirated, together with any necrotic material. The state of the cartilage is carefully assessed and, if a defect is present, it is advisable to support the defect with homograft cartilage (Masing, 1965). This should be cut to a size slightly greater than the perforation and, after insertion, a small drain is inserted into the bottom of the cavity, and the mucosa is replaced and maintained in this position by nasal packing.

Cartilage grafts can be used even if abscess formation has occurred, as Masing (1965), Hellmich (1970) and Vase and Johannessen (1981) have all shown that these grafts take well, and effectively prevent the saddling deformities which otherwise invariably occur.

Complications

External deformity of the nose

The cartilaginous dorsum of the nose is supported by the septal cartilage and, if this support is lost, dorsal saddling in the supratip area will result (see Figures 11.9 and 11.10). If this type of injury occurs during childhood, it may also affect the development of the whole of the mid-third of the face with resulting maxillary hypoplasia.

Septal abscess

A haematoma may easily become infected and this can lead to abscess formation. This complication is commonly associated with an increase in the severity of the pain, together with the usual manifestations of toxaemia, such as pyrexia and a raised pulse rate. The advent of secondary infection makes extensive cartilage necrosis virtually inevitable, and is an even more pressing indication for surgical drainage.

Certainly 75% of septal abscesses are traumatic in origin (Ambrus *et al.*, 1981). Septal abscess formation may however complicate ethmoidal (Beck, 1945) and sphenoidal (Collins, 1985) sinus infections and a septal abscess has been reported in a patient with AIDS (Henry, Sullivan and Crossley, 1988). Spread of the infection from the septum can then occur to the orbit, meninges, cavernous sinuses and brain. In a recent paper (Chukuezi, 1992), three fatalities are reported due to brain abscesses which have complicated septal abscesses. These all occurred in a continent where AIDS is very common and this may possibly be an additional causative factor.

Septal deviation

Septal deviations are extremely common, but are not usually severe enough to affect nasal function. The incidence of these deformities is much higher in the leptorrhine type of nose found in the Caucasian races.

Aetiology

Many septal deviations are due to direct trauma and this is frequently associated with damage to other parts of the nose such as fractures of the nasal bone.

In many patients with septal deviations there is no obvious history of trauma. Gray (1972) explains these cases by means of the birth moulding theory (Figures 11.2 and 11.3). Abnormal intrauterine posture may result in compression forces acting on the nose and upper jaws (the widest part of the face). Displacement of the septum can result and the nose can be exposed to further torsion forces during parturition. Moulding pressures vary with the type of delivery and are minimal in cases of elective Caesarian section, moderate with normal vertex presentation and severe with a persistent occipitoposterior presentation. A careful study of the obstetric data should provide confirmatory evidence for this theory. However, in a recent extensive study carried out in Birmingham (Kent *et al.*, 1988), it was found that the type of delivery, the presentation, the parity, the birthweight, and gestation period did not have any significance with regard to the frequency of these lesions. This is in agreement with the findings of Jazbi (1974), Pease (1969) and Hartikainen-Sorri *et al.* (1983). Moulding pressures should produce asymmetry of the palate in some neonates with septal deviations. A recent study by Kent *et al.* (1991) failed to confirm this fact.

Quite marked septal deviations have been recorded in neonates who have been delivered by elective Caesarian section, where there has been no possibility of birth trauma, both by Kent *et al.* (1988) and Harkavy and Scanlon (1978).

There is no doubt that many septal deviations we see at birth arise during the prenatal period. Ruano-Gil, Montserrat-Viladin and Vilanova-Treas (1980) found that 4% of a series of fetuses had septal deviations and that this was present at a time before either compression or birth trauma could be implicated as possible causative factors.

In 1875, Sir Francis Galton advocated the study of identical twins as a means of differentiating between deformities caused by genetic and environmental factors. Such a study was recently carried out by Grymer and Melsen (1989) who were able to examine 41 pairs of identical twins. They found that 21% of these individuals had an anterior septal deviation and that some sort of deformity was present in the posterior part of the septum in 74%. The distribution of the deviations within the twins suggested that anterior lesions were due to an external cause (trauma) whereas the posterior lesions were due to genetic factors.

The incidence of these neonatal septal deviations is about 4% (Kent *et al.*, 1988). Although these lesions may be due to both trauma and genetic factors, recent research tends to suggest that the role of trauma is less important than was once believed.

Pathological anatomy

Deformity of the nasal septum can be classified into the following types.

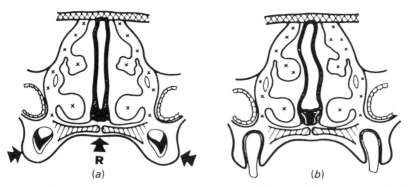

Figure 11.2 Combined septal deformity. Diagrammatic representation of effect of equal pressures on septal growth, producing deviation deformity and splaying out of vomer-cartilage junction. Note irregular hypertrophy of lateral nasal wall. (From *Modern Trends in Diseases of Ear, Nose and Throat*, 1972. London: Butterworths. Reproduced by permission of Mr Lindsay Gray)

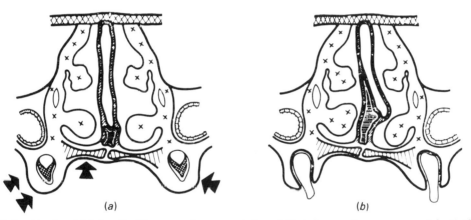

Figure 11.3 Combined septal deformity. Diagrammatic representation of effect of unequal pressure on septal growth producing spur deformity. Note elevation of palate, with tilting of vomer to opposite side, unequal growth of the vomer, irregular hypertrophy of the lateral nasal wall and changed alignment of teeth. (From *Modern Trends in Diseases of Ear, Nose and Throat*, 1972. London: Butterworths. Reproduced by permission of Mr Lindsay Gray)

Spurs

These are sharp angulations which may occur at the junction of the vomer below, with the septal cartilage and/or ethmoid bone above. This type of deformity is usually the result of vertical compression forces. Fractures through the septal cartilage may also produce sharp angulations. These fractures heal by fibrous union and the fibrosis extends to the adjacent mucoperichondrium. This increases the difficulty of the flap elevation in this area (Figure 11.4).

Deviations

These lesions are characterized by a more generalized bulge. 'C'- or 'S'-shaped deviations occur which can be either in the vertical or horizontal plane, and they usually involve both the cartilage and the bone.

Dislocations

Here the lower border of the septal cartilage is usually displaced from its medial position and projects into one of the nostrils (Figure 11.5).

Septal deviations are also frequently associated with anatomical abnormalities in adjacent areas.

The lateral nasal wall

A compensatory hypertrophy of the turbinates and ethmoidal bulla usually occurs on the side of the septal concavity.

Maxilla

The compression forces which are responsible for the septal deviations are often asymmetrical and may

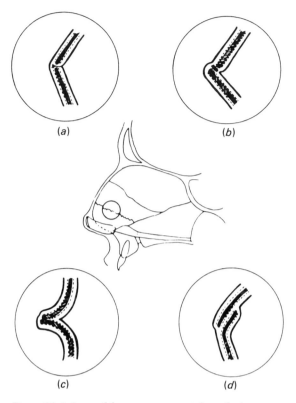

Figure 11.4 Some of the commoner septal cartilaginous fractures. (*a*) Edge-to-edge angulation; (*b*) angulation with overlap; (*c*) bowing of both edges at the fracture line; (*d*) duplication. If a fracture-dislocation occurs during the growth period, the displaced edge continues to grow and usually increases the deformity. (From Bernstein, 1973b. Reproduced by permission of W. B. Saunders & Co.)

also involve the maxilla, producing flattening of the cheek, elevation of the floor of the affected nasal cavity, distortion of the palate and associated orthodontic abnormalities. The maxillary sinus is usually slightly smaller on the affected side.

The external nasal pyramid

Anterior septal deviations are often associated with deviations in the external nasal pyramid. Deviations may affect any of the three vertical components of the nose and there are three common types which are listed in order of severity.

Cartilaginous deviations

In these cases, the upper bony septum and the bony pyramid are central, but there is a deviation of the cartilaginous septum and vault (Figure 11.6).

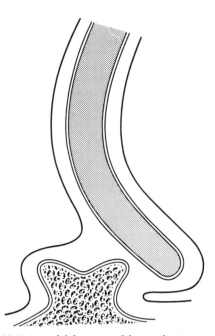

Figure 11.5 A caudal deviation of the cartilaginous septum

The C deviation

In this lesion, there is displacement of the upper bony septum and the pyramid to one side and the whole of the cartilaginous septum and vault to the opposite side.

The S deviation

Here the deviation of the middle third (the upper cartilaginous vault and associated septum) is opposite to that of the upper and lower third.

With deviations of the nose, the dominant factor is the position of the septum. Beekhuis (1973) has succinctly summarized this principle with the dictum, 'as the septum goes, so goes the nose'. The first step, therefore, in treating the twisted nose is to straighten the septum, and if this objective is not achieved, there is no hope of successfully straightening the external pyramid (see Figure 11.6).

There is therefore a sound pathological basis to the concept of straightening a twisted nose by means of a one-stage septorhinoplasty procedure.

The effects of septal deviations

Only the more severe deviations affect nasal function and therefore require treatment.

Nasal obstruction

This is always found on the side of the deviation and is also often present on the opposite side as a result of the hypertrophic changes in the turbinates.

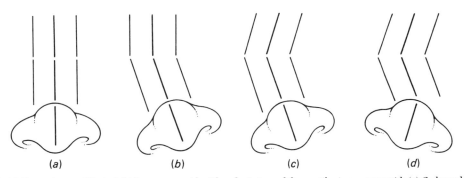

Figure 11.6 (*a*) Normal nose; (*b*) straight bony pyramid with a deviation of the cartilaginous pyramid; (*c*) C-shaped deviations of both bony and cartilaginous pyramids; (*d*) S-shaped deviations of both bony and cartilaginous pyramids

Nasal obstruction can cause snoring and its relief will sometimes cure this troublesome condition. In a recent study (Ellis *et al.*, 1992) it was found that, in a group of snorers with nasal obstruction, 31% no longer snored after the nasal obstruction had been successfully surgically treated, and that the most common cause of this obstruction was a deviated nasal septum.

Mucosal changes

The inspiratory air currents are often abnormally displaced and frequently become concentrated on small areas of nasal mucosa, producing an excessive drying effect. Crusting will then occur, and the separation of the crusts often produces ulceration and bleeding. The protective mucous layer may then be lost and resistance to infection reduced. The mucosa around a septal deviation may become oedematous as a result of Bernouilli's principle, which states that when there is a flow of gas through a constriction lateral pressure drops which will, in turn, predispose to mucosal oedema in the affected area, thus further increasing the obstruction.

Neurological changes

It is possible that the pressure exerted by septal deviations on adjacent sensory nerves can produce pain. This concept was first elaborated by Sluder (1927) and the resultant condition has been called 'the anterior ethmoidal nerve syndrome' (Shalom, 1963). In addition to their direct neurological effects, reflex changes perhaps may result from septal deformities which affect the nasopulmonary and nasal reflexes.

In 1943, McAuliffe, Goodell and Wolff studied the sensitivity of the nasal cavities and the paranasal sinuses using mainly faradic stimulation and found that the lateral wall of the nasal cavity was much more sensitive than the septum. The clinical studies of Masing (1977) and Schonsted-Madsen *et al.* (1986) show that the very severely impacted nasal septum can exert pressure on the more sensitive structures of the lateral nasal wall and cause referred trigeminal pain and chronic headache.

Symptoms

The symptoms caused by septal deviations are entirely the result of their effects on nasal function. The dominant symptom is nasal obstruction but this is rarely severe enough to cause anosmia. Douek (1974), in a review of many patients suffering from anosmia, never found this symptom to be the consequence of an uncomplicated septal deviation.

Signs

Septal deviations are usually quite obvious on anterior rhinoscopy. It is important first to inspect the nasal vestibule without using a speculum because the blade of this instrument can easily straighten the septum and thus hide a caudal deviation. Local anaesthesia with cocaine may facilitate the inspection of some of the more posterior deviations and here the use of a nasal endoscope can be invaluable. Sometimes the patient complains of unilateral nasal obstruction and anterior rhinoscopy will reveal that the septal deviation is to the opposite side. This phenomenon has been called 'paradoxical nasal obstruction' (Arbour and Kern, 1975). These patients have a long-standing, fixed, unilateral nasal obstruction to which they may have become accustomed, and of which they are no longer aware. The mucosal swelling associated with the nasal cycle, results in an additional intermittent nasal obstruction on the wider side of the nose, and this becomes the dominant symptom to be appreciated by the patients.

Septal deviations in the region of the nasal valve area cause the greatest obstruction, because this is at the narrowest part of the nasal cavity. The Cottle test (Figure 11.7) will confirm the fact that the obstruction is in the valve area. In this useful and simple test, the patient pulls the cheek outwards and opens up the internal nares and thus reduces the blockage.

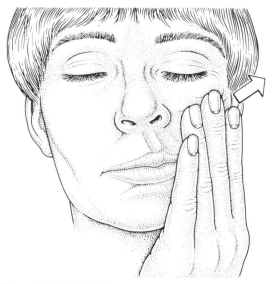

Figure 11.7 Cottle's test

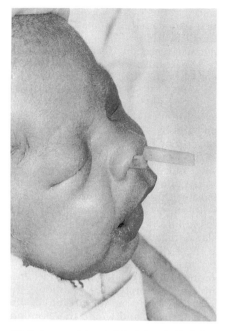

Figure 11.8 A neonatal septal deviation to the left, demonstrated by the use of Gray's struts

In a recent excellent experimental study by Cole *et al.* (1988) on the effect of simulated deviations on nasal airflow resistance, it was found that 'small septal deviations in the anterior part of the nose can cause significant obstruction, whereas large deviations can be present in the cavum without affecting airflow resistance. Furthermore, the mucosal components of resistance, which are contributed by erectile tissue of the anterior part of the septum and the turbinates, are of particular importance in the anterior part of the nose, where, in health, half the total airflow resistance is located'.

The septum cannot be considered in isolation and it is therefore necessary to perform a careful inspection of the lateral nasal wall to determine the size of the turbinates. Examination must also include the external nasal pyramid, the palate and the teeth, as these structures are often also involved to some degree with septal deformities. Whenever sinus complications are suspected, CT scanning of the paranasal sinuses are indicated.

Septal deviation in the newborn is sometimes associated with asymmetry of the nostrils, an oblique columella and tip which points in the direction which is opposite to the deviation. The nostril on the affected side may look distinctly flattened. These characteristic features are rarely present, and most cases are diagnosed by anterior rhinoscopy and the use of Gray's struts (Figure 11.8). These struts are 4 mm wide and 2 mm thick and, after lubrication, are inserted into the nostrils, and then gently pushed backwards along the floor of the nose, hugging the septum. Normally the struts can be introduced for a distance of 4 or 5 cm, but in cases of deviation, a frank obstruction is encountered, usually 1.5–2 cm back from the nostril. This is the most reliable test and is well tolerated during infancy. Less frequently, the compression test may be positive. In this test the nasal tip is pushed backwards and if there is a septal dislocation, it will collapse against the philtrum of the upper lip.

Indications for submucous operations on the nasal septum

Septal deviations

Cottle has classified septal lesions into three types.

Simple deviations

Here there is a mild deflection of the septum which does not cause obstruction. The majority of Caucasians have this type of septum, and it certainly does not require any surgical treatment.

Obstruction

This is a more severe deviation of the nasal septum which may touch the lateral wall of the nose, but on vasoconstriction the turbinates shrink away from the septum.

Impaction

This is a very marked angulation of the septum with a spur which lies in contact with the lateral nasal wall, even after the application of a vasoconstrictor. Surgical treatment is reserved for some of the obstructing lesions and most of those associated with impaction, the essential indication being a skeletal septal obstruction.

In many patients with septal deviations there is also some generalized mucosal pathology in the form of a perennial rhinitis, and this will not be corrected by septal surgery. Thomas (1978) has shown that the most common cause of poor results following a submucous resection operation is the presence of a coexisting perennial rhinitis. A test that would differentiate between the obstruction caused by a skeletal septal deviation and that as a result of mucosal pathology, would therefore be very helpful in assessing the suitability of patients for septal surgery (Cottle, 1968). Claims that this can be achieved by performing measurements of nasal resistance before and after vasoconstriction with drugs or following physical exercise have been made by Broms (1982) and by Jessen and Malm (1984). Unfortunately, McCaffrey and Kern (1979) did not find these tests of much help for this purpose.

Closure of septal perforations

Most techniques which have been described for the closure of septal perforations involve the submucous elevation of the flaps for this purpose.

Source of grafting material

Submucous resection of nasal cartilage and, less commonly, vomerine bone, is sometimes required to obtain graft material for such operations as rhinoplasty and tympanoplasty.

To obtain surgical access

Submucous resection of the septum has been advocated as giving the necessary access for the following surgical operations to be performed:

1 Hypophysectomy (Hirsch, 1952)
2 Vidian neurectomy (Minnis and Morrison, 1971).

The development of septal surgery

The study of the history of septal surgery is both interesting and instructive. It clarifies the basic problems encountered in treating septal deviations, and demonstrates the limitations of the various techniques which have been evolved to solve them. During the nineteenth century, surgeons started tackling these problems by a variety of techniques which have now been completely abandoned. Acute spurs and angulations were removed either by shaving down the convexities (Langenbeck, 1843; Dieffenbach, 1845; Chassaignac, 1851), or by performing a complete removal of the deviation by punch forceps (Rubrecht, 1868). The usual result of these operations was to exchange a septal deviation for a perforation. These techniques are only of historical interest, and there is little doubt that the first major breakthrough in surgical therapy occurred around the turn of the century with the development of the submucous resection operation.

As so often happens, the idea of effecting a submucosal removal of the deviation occurred to several surgeons working independently at the same time. Probably the earliest was Ingalls in 1881, but the names of Killian and Freer are usually associated with the refinement and popularization of the actual procedure (Ingalls, 1882). It was Killian (1904) who described the technique which is most commonly practised today, with a retention of both dorsal and caudal struts of cartilage to prevent any subsequent change in the external shape of the nose. Freer (1902) adopted a much more radical approach as, in his view, the septal cartilage did not contribute to the support of the nasal pyramid and could be completely removed if necessitated by the extent of the pathology. He admitted that 'saddling' of the dorsum did sometimes occur in the supratip region, but said that this was always due to rough surgery, which had damaged or partly removed the upper lateral cartilages.

The submucous resection operation was undoubtedly a great advance and was widely adopted throughout the world. With subsequent experience, however, it was evident that there were certain associated problems. For surgical purposes, the septum can be divided by a vertical line drawn from the frontal nasal spine to the maxillary nasal spine (see Figure 11.16). Deviations posterior to this line can be treated by the submucous resection technique. The problems occur when using this technique in the anterior part of the septum. All too frequently, the operation was followed by a supratip depression and columellar retraction (Figures 11.9 and 11.10). To minimize these complications, most surgeons adopted the conservative Killian technique, but retention of dorsal and caudal struts does not ensure complete immunity; in addition, the deviations may be found in the region of the dorsal and caudal struts, and would therefore not be corrected by this operation. These complications occur much more frequently than is generally realized because they often take many months to develop. Immediate saddling is rare; usually it occurs as a result of scar contraction in the septum (Figure 11.11). Some surgeons have attempted to solve the problem of scar contraction by replacing all or part of the excised cartilage, while others have avoided producing a large defect in the

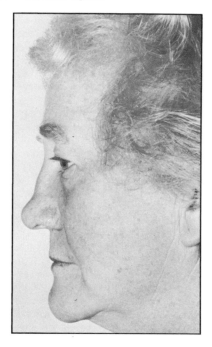

Figure 11.9 Gross supratip saddling and retraction of the columella following a submucous resection

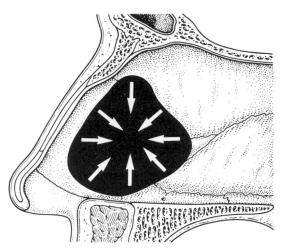

Figure 11.11 The contracting scar which develops after a submucous resection

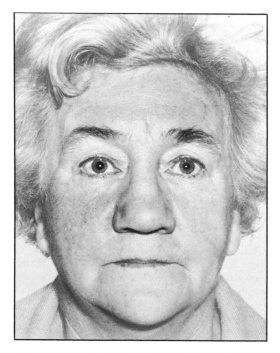

Figure 11.10 Widening and bulbosity of the nasal tip following submucous resection

cartilaginous septum by mobilizing and repositioning the septum in the central position, so that the bulk of the cartilage is retained and is still attached to its mucoperichondrium as part of a compound flap.

The first significant improvement was made by Metzenbaum (1929) in Chicago, using the latter concept. The operation was applicable only to caudal dislocations of the septum without fragmentation of the cartilage and gross fibrosis (Figure 11.12). He likened the principle to that of a swinging door, but late failures were fairly common. A swinging door has a hinge on one side and free edges on the other three borders. In the Metzenbaum operation, the hinge was effectively produced by the incision at the level of the deviation. There was an existing free border inferiorly and one was produced posteriorly by separation of the cartilage from the vomer. There was not, however, a free border anteriorly where the septum was often tethered to displaced upper lateral cartilages (Figure 11.13) and the traction from this source, and also sometimes from the mucoperichondrium which was liberated only on one side above the incision, produced increased tension on the unfreed side during healing, which was prone to cause a recurrence of the deflections.

To overcome these problems, Peer, in 1937, completely excised the deviated caudal segment of the cartilage. If possible, he reinserted it as a free graft, but if the tissue was either unsuitable or inadequate, he obtained a similar sized graft resecting cartilage from the central or more posterior part of the quadrilateral cartilage (Figure 11.14). This operation developed the concept of cartilage excision followed by cartilage replacement. The original Peer operation was extended to include removal of the entire cartilaginous septum. This concept reached its logical

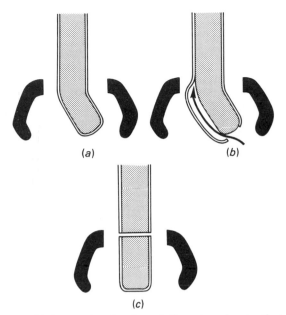

Figure 11.12 Metzenbaum's operation. (*a*) A coronal section through the septum showing the type of caudal deviation for which the Metzenbaum operation was designed; (*b*) the unilateral elevation of the mucoperichondrium to just above the level of the deviation; (*c*) division of the cartilage at the level of the deviation and its repositioning in the midline

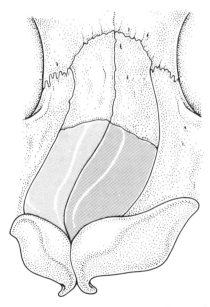

Figure 11.13 A deviated nasal septum with secondary deviations in the upper lateral cartilages

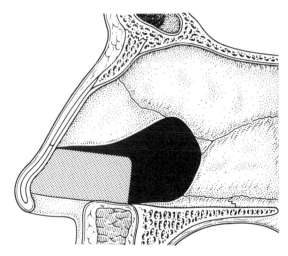

Figure 11.14 Peer's operation. Removal of a caudal septal deviation and the replacement of cartilage as a free graft. The resected area is shown in black and the graft as the dotted area

conclusion in the Galloway operation (1946). Galloway removed the entire nasal cartilage, and replaced the anterior septum with a single free autograft cut from the excised cartilage. He also described a useful detail of operative technique, in the manner in which

he facilitated the placing of the graft with traction sutures (Figure 11.15).

Afterwards, the graft was held in place with mattress sutures, and the traction sutures were removed.

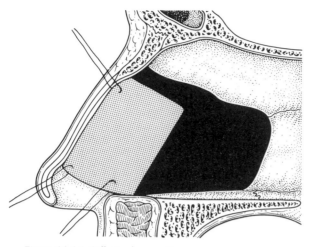

Figure 11.15 Galloway's operation

Subsequent experience with this operation showed that it was by no means always successful because:

1 Unequal scar contraction between the two septal flaps sometimes led to a recurrence of the deviation
2 Absorption of the autograft sometimes occurred leading to saddling of the supratip region
3 The lower end of the graft sometimes immobilized the membranous septum and gave it a rather peculiar and unnatural appearance.

In 1948, Fomon *et al.* and later Rees (1986) endeavoured to solve the first and third of these problems by the use of small autografts. The whole principle of septal removal, followed by septal replacement, has some inherent drawbacks and consequently the alternative solution of mobilization and repositioning of septal cartilage has been revived and further developed. This septoplasty concept, in particular, has been popularized by Cottle *et al.* (1958).

More recently, the permanent change in the shape of cartilage by morselization has been advocated by Rubin (1983). The deviated cartilage is crushed by a morselizer after the mucosal flaps have been elevated on both sides, and it is claimed that the new flattened shape of the cartilage is retained on a permanent basis.

The principles of septal surgery

From the experience over the last 90 years, it is evident that, from a surgical point of view, the septum can be divided into anterior and posterior segments by a vertical line drawn between the nasal processes of the frontal and maxillary bones (Figure 11.16). Deviations in the posterior segment can be easily and

effectively treated by the classic Killian submucosal resection operation, whereas those in the anterior segments should be treated by a more conservative septoplasty technique.

Anaesthesia for septal operations

Septal surgery can be satisfactorily performed under either local or general anaesthesia. General anaesthesia is preferred in the UK. A general anaesthetic is also invariably required for children and nervous adults. The nose should be sprayed with a decongestant about 10–15 minutes before the induction of a general anaesthetic. This will greatly diminish the amount of bleeding at operation. The postural nerve block technique described by Curtiss (1952) is easily the best of the local anaesthetic methods. It was

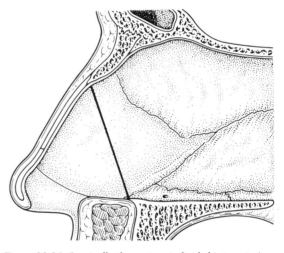

Figure 11.16 Surgically the septum is divided into anterior and posterior segments by a vertical line passing between the nasal processes of the frontal and maxillary bones

evolved from the earlier technique of Moffett (1941), but is much simpler and quicker, and is quite as effective. The patient is placed in the Proetz position with the chin and external auditory meatus in the same vertical plane. Then 2 ml of 4% cocaine solution are introduced into each nostril using a special angulated needle. The cocaine gravitates into the superior and middle meatus where it blocks both the ethmoidal and sphenopalatine nerves. The patient is kept in this position for 10 minutes. A small quantity of 2% lignocaine is finally injected into the columella. This method gives far better results than the older technique of using cocaine and adrenaline packs as it is often difficult to push these packs beyond the septal deviations.

Septoplasty

Septoplasty is an operation which should be performed under direct vision. To achieve this it is necessary to obtain adequate illumination. A satisfactory headlight is therefore essential and can also be supplemented by using an expanding nasal speculum fitted with a light carrier. Bleeding can obscure the operative field, and it is therefore very important to obtain maximum vasoconstriction of the mucosa before making the first incision. Traditionally, adrenaline has usually been used for this purpose, often in combination with 2% lignocaine. However, there is a risk of producing cardiac dysrhythmias when adrenaline is injected into a patient receiving halothane anaesthesia (Millar, Gilbert and Brindle, 1958). This prompted Katz, Matteo and Papper (1962) to recommend substituting vasopressin for adrenaline in these circumstances. Vasopressin has been shown to be an inferior vasoconstrictor to adrenaline (McClymont and Crowther, 1988).

This operation should not be a single standardized procedure, but should be tailored to the needs of the individual patient. For example, if the deviation is confined to the caudal border of the septum anteriorly, there is no need to touch the posterior part of the septum. There are however, certain general principles and these include:

1 Incision.
2 Exposure: the cartilaginous and bony septum is exposed by the complete elevation of a mucosal flap on one side only. Contact between the cartilaginous septum and the mucoperichondrial flap on the other side is maintained as much as possible because, in addition to ensuring the viability of cartilage, it also greatly reduces the risks of complications such as haematoma and abscess formation, perforation and overriding of the different segments of the cartilages.
3 Mobilization and straightening: the septal cartilage is then freed from all its attachments apart from the mucosal flap on the convex side. Many deviations are maintained by extrinsic factors such as the caudal dislocation of the cartilage from the vomerine groove (see Figure 11.5). Mobilization alone will often correct this type of problem. When deviations are due to intrinsic causes, for example healed fractures, it is necessary to combine mobilization with some direct surgery on the cartilage such as a strip excision of the fracture line. Bony deviations are treated either by fracture and repositioning or by submucous resection of the deviation.
4 Fixation: the septum is then maintained in its straightened position during the healing phase by sutures and/or splints.

Incision

The incision is best made at the lower border of the septal cartilage as was originally advocated by Freer (1902). A unilateral (hemitransfixation) incision (see Figure 11.27) is adequate for a septoplasty and, for the right-handed surgeon, this is usually most conveniently made on the left side. The advantages of this incision have been tabulated by Bernstein (1973a) in the following fashion:

1 The incision is placed in a relatively avascular plane.
2 The mucosal edges here are both thick and tough, thus reducing the risk of tears. If tears do occur, a satisfactory repair is normally quite easily performed.
3 It provides easy access to the whole of the septum, including the caudal septal border, and the region of the anterior nasal spine with its associated premaxillary crest.
4 If the septoplasty is to be combined with a rhinoplasty, it is easy to extend the incision through to the opposite side and thus produce a full transfixation incision. It is important to make the incision as high as possible because a low incision through the membranous septum may be followed by a retraction of the columella (Figures 11.17 and 11.18). The first step is therefore to displace the columella downwards and to the opposite side by means of traction, exerted with dissecting forceps or a Cottle columella clamp. The lower border of the septal cartilage will then be plainly visible and the incision made down to the perichondrium, which is incised and the subperichondrial flap elevation then commenced.

Exposure

It is usually best to expose the cartilaginous and bony septum by elevating the mucosal flap on the concave side. The difficulties of the flap elevation are partly a result of the anatomy of the various tissue layers and can often be greatly increased by fibrosis and scarring in these layers following previous trauma. The surgical anatomy of this region is of extreme importance and must be clearly understood if mucosal tears are to be avoided. It is easy to elevate the mucosal flaps across both the ethmoid-vomerine suture and the ethmoid-septal cartilage suture, because very few periosteal or perichondrial fibres pass into either of these suture lines (Figure 11.19). The difficulties of flap elevation occur mainly at the junction of the septal cartilage above, with the anterior nasal spine, premaxillary crest and vomer below. This is because the perichondrium encloses the cartilage in a complete envelope which does not fuse with the periosteum. The periosteum forms another inferior envelope over the adjacent bony septum and may result in a pseudo-joint capsule which can

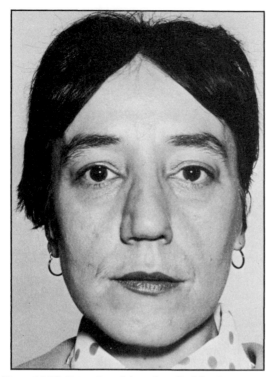

Figure 11.17 Retraction of the columella following a submucous resection (front view)

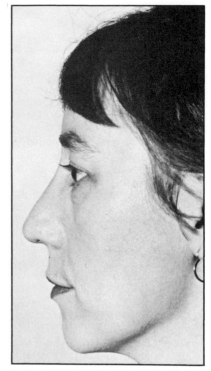

Figure 11.18 Retraction of the columella following a submucous resection (side view)

permit a side-to-side movement of the septal cartilage (see Figure 11.19). The subperichondrial plane over the septal cartilage is therefore not continuous with the subperiosteal plane below and the difficulty in uniting these two planes can easily lead to tears. For this reason, most iatrogenic perforations occur along the chondrovomerine suture particularly anteriorly because the bony groove is widest here, and the problems are greatest.

As a general principle of flap elevation, it is usually best to leave the most difficult areas to last, since they can then be approached from several directions and under direct vision. A suitable technique for dealing with these problems has been evolved by Cottle *et al.* (1958) who started the elevation over the septal cartilage and worked upwards and backwards always keeping above the chondrovomerine junction. This step in the operation was called the production of the 'anterior tunnel'. Once this had been accomplished, attention was then directed to the posterior end of the incision, and the periosteum over the anterior nasal spine was incised and then elevated backwards on both sides over the premaxillary crest, then the vomer, again keeping below the chondrovomerine suture. These were the so-called 'inferior tunnels' (Figure 11.20). Finally, the most difficult elevation was per-

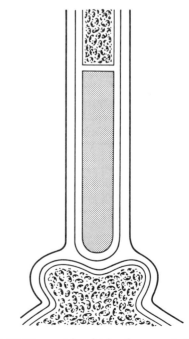

Figure 11.19 Mucoperichondrial and mucoperiosteal layers in the septum

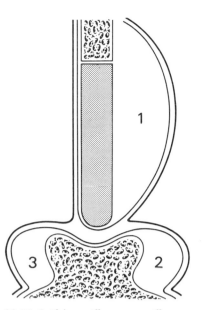

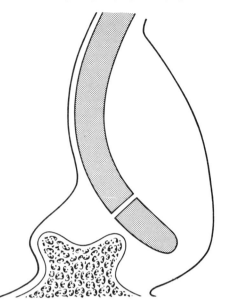

Figure 11.20 Cottle's maxillary-premaxillary approach to extensive nasal surgery. (1) The left anterior tunnel; (2) the left inferior tunnel; (3) the right inferior tunnel

Figure 11.21 Removal of a strip of cartilage from the lower border of the septum thus enabling the dislocation to be reduced

formed which involved uniting the anterior and inferior tunnels under direct vision using a sharp dissector or knife. This is the so-called 'maxilla-premaxilla' approach of Cottle.

It is unusual for all the steps in this particular technique to be required, but in the really difficult demanding case, and particularly when performing revision surgery, it is the method of choice.

Mobilization and straightening

The first step is to separate the lower border of the septal cartilage from its osseous base. In many cases, this lower border has been dislocated from its osseous groove and there is also a considerable amount of fibrosis which can greatly distort the anatomy. A sharp dissector knife is always required. The lower border of the septal cartilage is encased in a perichondrial envelope, and it is usually possible to continue the subperichondrial elevation downwards over the concave side of the septum, then around its lower border and upwards for a few millimetres on the convex side of the septum. When the cartilage has been freed, an attempt is made to reposition it back into the midline where it should rest in its osseous groove. Usually this is impossible because of the excess height of the septal cartilage and it is then necessary to remove a strip of cartilage about 3–4 mm wide from its lower border (Figure 11.21). This excised cartilage is part of the quadrilateral plate and may be up to 4 cm long. It can make an ideal

autograft, should one be required at a later stage in the operation. It should therefore be kept in sterile saline during the rest of the operation in case the need arises. It is usually also necessary to straighten and lower the vomerine crest in order to make a suitable bed to accommodate the septal cartilage. When the anterior spine is deviated it can be fractured and repositioned in the midline. If the bony septum is deviated, it is sometimes possible in the less severe cases to reposition it in the midline with a heavy elevator after preliminary fracture. However, this technique is inadequate for the angulated spurs which are often encountered at the junction between the ethmoid plate and vomer. Here a vertical incision is made through the septal cartilage, just behind the line joining the nasal process of the frontal and maxillary bone. The mucosal flap is then elevated off the cartilage and bone on the opposite side, and the deviated cartilage and bone may be removed back to the face of the sphenoid. When making this vertical incision through the cartilage, it is important not to make it too anteriorly, as otherwise the nasal dorsum will only be supported by a narrow strip of cartilage, and this can fracture superiorly and lead to a saddling deformity (Figure 11.22).

If the external nasal pyramid is twisted, it is important to separate the skin and subcutaneous tissue off the underlying upper lateral cartilages. This will allow the skin to be draped easily over the straightened cartilaginous dorsum without the risk of cutaneous traction on the upper lateral cartilages producing a recurrence of the deviation.

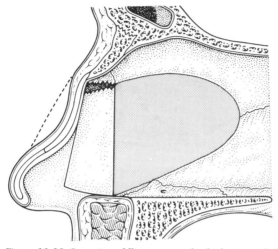

Figure 11.22 Supratip saddling as a result of a fracture of the dorsal septal strut

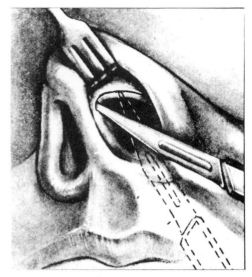

Figure 11.23 Intercartilaginous incision at the level of the internal nares. (From Selzer, 1949, and reproduced by kind permission of J. B. Lippincott & Co)

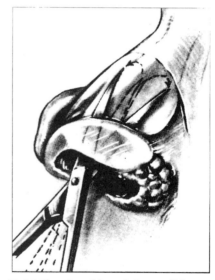

Figure 11.24 Elevation of the soft tissues off the upper lateral cartilages. (From Selzer, 1949, and reproduced by kind permission of J. B. Lippincott & Co)

This uncovering of the cartilaginous dorsum is easily performed through the classic intercartilaginous incision (Figure 11.23). Usually a 15 blade Bard Parker knife is used to make the incision at the level of the internal nares. Anteriorly, each intercartilaginous incision is united with a transfixation incision. A series of opening and closing movements with a pair of Knapp scissors will enable the elevation of the subcutaneous tissues off the cartilaginous dorsum to be easily effected (Figure 11.24).

The plane of dissection should be directly above the perichondrium as most of the blood vessels are found in the more superficial layers. The upper lateral cartilages are firmly united to the cartilaginous septum. There are often secondary changes in the upper lateral cartilages associated with a twisted nose. When this occurs it is necessary to separate the upper lateral cartilages from the septum and this is best done submucosally. By now the septal cartilage has been fully mobilized and, in the absence of intrinsic deviations, should be easily repositioned in the midline. A careful examination should be made at this stage and the mobility of the septum checked by moving it from side to side with a septal elevator. If there is any reduced mobility, its exact site should be noted and further trimming at this point may be necessary.

Other possible factors include a large turbinate, which will require treatment, the details of which are given in Chapter 9.

At times, the mucosa on the narrow side of the nose is too short to allow the septum to return to the midline. This problem can be solved by cutting through the mucosa at the junction of the nasal floor and the septum. There will be a residual dehiscence on the floor of the nose after the septum has been repositioned into the midline, but this will re-epithelialize quite rapidly, afterwards. Any residual obstruction is usually the result of intrinsic deviations in the septal cartilage. Old fractures in the cartilage often heal by fibrous union and this may result in severe angulations, which are best treated by the removal of a narrow strip of cartilage along the line of the deviation. This will break the spring of the cartilage which can then usually be repositioned into the midline (Figure 11.25).

Sometimes the septal lesion is so severe, either because of previous disease (for example, a septal

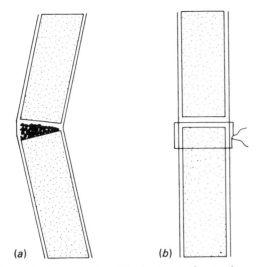

Figure 11.25 (*a*) Excision of the fracture in the septal cartilage; (*b*) use of a Wright suture to prevent overlap

haematoma), or where extremely radical surgery is necessary to correct the deviation, that too little supporting cartilage remains anteriorly to maintain the normal shape of the nasal pyramid and the columella. In such a nose, the anterior residual septal cartilage can be supported with a free bone graft, taken preferably from the thinner part of the perpendicular plate of the ethmoid or, if this is impossible, from the rather thicker vomer. A suitable piece of bone can be obtained with a pair of heavy angled Fomon scissors and chisel. It can then be cut to the shape of the dorsocaudal septum, and two holes drilled in it to accommodate the fixation sutures. The bone graft is placed alongside the residual septal cartilage and sutured in position. Bernstein (1973b)

has shown that bone is much more satisfactory when used in this supporting role than cartilage, which frequently becomes absorbed (Figure 11.26).

Fixation

At the end of the operation, the septum should be lying freely in the midline and if this objective has not been achieved, neither suturing nor splinting will prevent subsequent failure. If it has been necessary to make multiple incisions in the cartilage, overriding of the segments can be a problem and this is best corrected by a Wright (1967) suture (see Figure 11.25). Here, a through-and-through mattress suture is used, with one arm passing between the segments of the cartilage, and the other through all three layers of the septum. A figure-of-eight suture, immobilizing the lower border of the septum to the anterior nasal spine, is then inserted. Finally, the septocolumellar incision is closed with a few sutures.

In the past it has been traditional to insert splints and/or packs into the nose after septal operations. Splints were first described by Salinger and Cohen in 1955 and now a wide range is available commercially. Recently, the advisability of using these splints and/or packing has been challenged. There is uniform agreement that postoperative pain is increased by their use (Campbell, Watson and Shenoi, 1987; Cook *et al.*, 1992; Schoenberg, Robinson and Ryan, 1992). In a controlled study by Cook *et al.*, in 1992, splints were shown to offer no additional help in stabilizing the septum postoperatively and, finally, there is the very slight but definite risk of developing the toxic shock syndrome. This syndrome was first reported by Todd *et al.*, in 1978, and is a multisystem disease characterized by fever, rash, hypotension, mucosal hyperaemia, vomiting, diarrhoea and

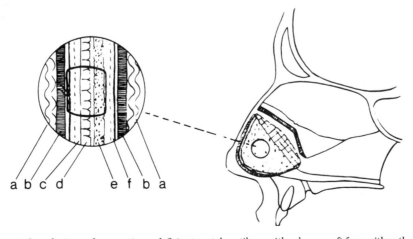

Figure 11.26 Bernstein's technique of supporting a deficient septal cartilage with a bone graft from either the ethmoid or the vomer. (*a*) Nasal packing; (*b*) Silastic splint; (*c*) mucoperichondrium attached to (*d*) cross-hatched cartilage; (*e*) bone graft; (*f*) freed perichondrium. (Reproduced by kind permission of W. B. Saunders & Co)

laboratory evidence of multisystem organ dysfunction. It is caused by enterotoxin-producing *Staphylococcus aureus* infections and there have been numerous reports in the literature of this very serious, and sometimes fatal, condition complicating operations where intranasal splints and/or packs have been used (Thomas, 1982; Barbour, 1984; Wagner and Toback, 1986).

There is no doubt, however, that intranasal splints are very effective in the prevention of nasal adhesions. Adhesion formation is common after turbinate surgery and when combined procedures on the septum and turbinates are necessary, it is the practice of the author routinely to use Silastic nasal splints, but not when septal surgery alone is performed, because here the risk of adhesion formation should be minimal.

The use of fibrin glue in septal surgery has been advocated by Hayward and Mackay (1987). In addition to their adhesive properties, they are also haemostatic agents and can be used to stick the septal flaps together and thus reduce the risk of haematoma formation. A commercial preparation is available (Tisseel by Immuno Ltd) which incorporates the use of bovine thrombin. Allergic reactions can occur to the bovine thrombin and there is also the theoretical risk of transmitting such viral infections as hepatitis and HIV. For this reason, the use of an autologous fibrin glue (Siedentop, Harris and Sanchez, 1985) is undoubtedly safer but is less convenient as it entails obtaining 100 ml of whole blood from the patient about a week before the operation. In a personal series of 30 operations (Brain, D. J., 1991, unpublished data), the author did not find the advantages of this preparation justified the extra effort, cost and inconvenience involved.

The classic submucous resection operation

The Killian incision (Figure 11.27) is most commonly used for this operation. This is an oblique incision about 5 mm above the caudal border of the septal cartilage. Elevation of the mucosal flap through this incision is usually easier than with the hemitransfixation incision, although this can also be used for this particular operation. The exposure stage is similar to that for septoplasty. Afterwards, an incision is made through the septal cartilage about 1 cm above and parallel to its lower border. The incision should be made through the cartilage, but not through the opposite perichondrium. The mucoperichondrium can then be elevated off the far side of the cartilage through this incision. A pair of angled scissors is introduced and used to cut through the septal cartilage in a direction which is parallel to and at least 1 cm posterior to the nasal dorsum. It is then possible to remove the obstructing cartilage and bone leaving these dorsal and caudal struts of cartilage to maintain

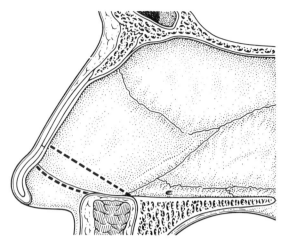

Figure 11.27 Incisions for septal surgery. Upper incision described by Killian and the lower incision by Freer. Freer incision sometimes also called the hemitransfixation incision

the support of the nasal dorsum and columella. The cartilage is removed with Luc's forceps or a Ballenger's swivel knife. Any deviated bone in the region of the vertical plate of the ethmoid is then removed. The next step is to elevate the flaps off the maxillary crest and vomer. The periosteum covering this is not in the same plane of cleavage as the cartilaginous dissection. A separate breakthough has to be made with a knife or dissector on to the bone to elevate the periosteum. The crest is finally removed with a hammer and gouge or with Jansen-Middleton bone forceps.

If the flap is torn, this does not matter unless there is another tear on the other side exactly opposite, when a septal perforation will inevitably result unless a satisfactory repair is effected. The site of the tear is first reinforced by the introduction of a small autograft of septal cartilage or bone between the flaps and the lacerations are then sutured (Figure 11.28). Some surgeons routinely replace septal cartilage and bone after performing the classic Killian technique. The almost universal use of central heating in North America tends to produce atrophic changes in the nasal mucosa and Briant (1977, personal communication) considers there is a very definite risk that this is increased after the loss of support of the septal cartilage and bone, and that septal perforations for this reason can sometimes follow a perfectly performed Killian-type operation. Therefore, he advocates that the excised cartilage and bone be straightened in a Cottle's crusher and then re-inserted between the flaps.

Postoperative care

Packs, if used, are removed after 24 hours and splints after 7 days. Antibiotics are not usually required.

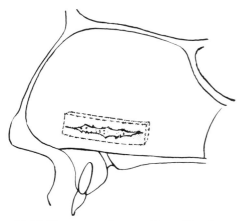

Figure 11.28 The support of mucosal tear with a free cartilage or bone graft prior to suture of the tear. (From Bernstein, 1973b. Reproduced by kind permission of W. B. Saunders & Co)

Septal surgery in the growing nose

Since the turn of the century, it has been widely believed that the nasal septum plays an important role in the development of the facial skeleton and, in particular, the nose. For this reason most surgeons have avoided performing surgical operations on the growing septum for fear of producing some retardation of growth.

Some of the earliest work was undertaken by Hayton (1948), who made a careful study of 31 patients aged between 6 and 14 years who had been treated in Logan Turner's clinic in Edinburgh by the classic Killian operation. In 10 of the patients, there was some broadening of the nose, which was associated with supratip depression.

Septal surgery performed during childhood carries with it the additional problem that it may interfere with the subsequent growth of the nose. Because of this risk, it was the usual practice to postpone all septal surgery until after the age of 16 years but, more recently, this view has been challenged by Cottle (1951), Jennes (1964), Huizing (1979) and others. Attempts have been made to elucidate this matter by animal experimentation (Ismail, 1964; Hartenstrom, 1970), and by observing the effects of injuries and operations performed during childhood.

Verwoerd, Urbanus and Nijdam (1979), Rhys-Evans and Brain (1981) and Sarnat and Wexler (1961, 1967) have all shown that removal of cartilage in experimental animals interferes with the subsequent development both of the nose and of the maxilla. Brain and Rock (1983) performed a cephalometric study of 29 adult patients awaiting surgical treatment for injuries which had occurred during childhood, and demonstrated significant differences in nasal and orthodontic development compared with a control population.

A septal abscess occurring during childhood invariably leads to a saddle deformity, and Hayton (1948) showed that this also frequently follows the Killian submucous resection operation. In addition to the saddling of the dorsum, damage to the caudal septum can interfere with the development of the nasal tip (Figure 11.29). There is, therefore, universal agreement that no operation which involves radical removal of cartilage should be performed on the septum during childhood. Any surgery performed at this age should be of a very conservative nature, and should be confined to the repositioning of the septum. It may be necessary to incise the cartilage in order to achieve this. Verwoerd, Urbanus and Nijdam (1979) considered it advisable to avoid actually performing the operation during either of the two nasal growth spurts. The results of these conservative operations are far from good. The experimental work on rabbits by Rhys-Evans and Brain (1981) showed that a recurrence of the deviation often occurs and, in clinical practice, it is found that frequently up to 50% of these patients need revision procedures when they reach the age of 16 years.

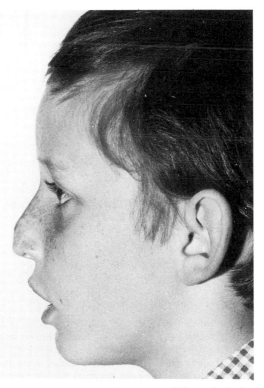

Figure 11.29 Photograph of a 12-year-old boy who had surgery to the caudal septum performed when he was nine, and who subsequently developed shortening of the columella with greatly reduced projection of the nasal tip

Reduction of septal dislocation in the newborn

This should be undertaken as early as possible as it becomes increasingly difficult with the passage of time (Metzenbaum, 1936). The present author considers it to be usually impossible after about the age of 3 months (Figure 11.30), although Gray (1972) has had successes up to the age of 9 months. No anaesthetic is necessary, and both the instrumentation and technique have been developed by Gray, who inserts a special pair of neonatal nasal septal forceps into the nose (Figure 11.31). The middle of the palate is then firmly pressed downwards for about 15–20 seconds to pull the septum straight. The septum is then manipulated into the midline (Figure 11.32).

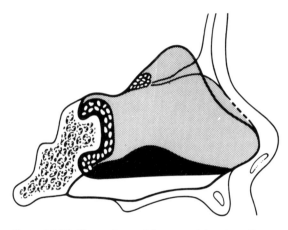

Figure 11.30 The anatomy of the neonatal septum. Bony septum shown in black with the light shaded area representing the cartilaginous septum

The septum in rhinoplasty

It is necessary to consider the septum in rhinoplastic surgery because it is of great importance:

1 In the deviated nose
2 In reduction rhinoplasty
3 As a support to the nasal dorsum
4 As a source of graft material for augmentation
5 There may be an unrelated septal problem requiring surgical treatment.

The septum is the central supporting strut of the nasal pyramid and it participates in every external nasal deviation. A look at a cross-section of the deviated nose (see Figure 11.6) shows that it is impossible to straighten the external pyramid by any combination of osteomies without straightening the nasal septum, and it is for this reason that the most important skill required to correct a deviated nose is a capacity to deal with difficult septal problems, and

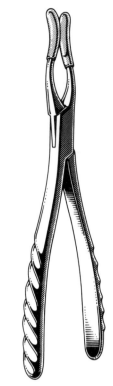

Figure 11.31 Gray's modification of Walsham's forceps

this is why the author believes that this type of case is best treated by an otolaryngologist trained in rhinoplastic techniques.

The septum is also of importance in a reduction rhinoplasty. After the removal of a nasal hump, the nose, on cross-section, resembles a truncated cone (Figure 11.33). It is then necessary to narrow the external pyramid, the result of which is that a modest septal deviation, which preoperatively was of no functional importance, will now produce obstruction and unfortunately, it is by no means uncommon for a patient with a previously normal functioning nose to develop iatrogenic obstruction after a cosmetic rhinoplasty.

Ulceration and perforation of the septum

These are usually different stages in the same pathological process and, apart from the traumatic cases, septal perforations are usually preceded by ulceration. Successful treatment of a septal ulcer will therefore prevent the development of perforation, and this is particularly important in the case of children, as the development of perforated septum in the growing nose will often retard grow both of the nose and of the mid-third of the face.

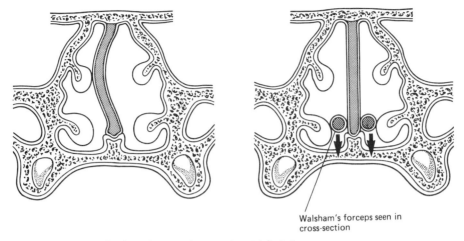

Walsham's forceps seen in cross-section

Figure 11.32 Gray's technique for the reduction of neonatal septal deviation

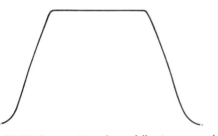

Figure 11.33 Cross-section of nose following removal of nasal hump

Causes of septal perforation

1 Trauma
   a surgical
   b repeated cautery
   c digital trauma ('nose picking')
2 Malignant disease
   a malignant tumours
   b malignant granuloma
3 Chronic inflammation
   a Wegener's
   b syphilis
   c tuberculosis
   d candida
   e lupus erythematosus
   f rheumatoid arthritis
4 Poisons
   a industrial
   b cocaine addicts
   c topical corticosteroids
   d topical decongestants
5 Idiopathic

Apart from syphilis which normally attacks the bony septum, most perforations are found anteriorly, in the septal cartilage. Unfortunately, most are iatrogenic in origin and usually occur as a complica-

tion of septal surgery, particularly when the Killian submucous resection technique is used. Although the septoplasty procedure does not give complete immunity against this complication, perforations are a rarity following this operation. A recent survey of the world literature (Schonsted-Madsen, Stoksted and Outzen, 1989) gives the average incidence of perforation following the Killian submucous resection operation as 6.91% compared with 0.86% in the case of septoplasty. Perforations result from mucoperichondrial tears, particularly when they are bilateral and overlapping. Gross post-traumatic fibrosis increases the risk, and the site of the perforation is usually along the line of the chondrovomerine suture where the anatomy of perichondrial and periosteal layers also increases the difficulty of flap elevation. When mishaps of this kind occur during a submucous resection operation, every effort should be made to prevent this complication by inserting a bony or cartilaginous autograft between the torn flaps and also by closing the tears with catgut sutures (see Figure 11.28).

Repeated cautery of the septum can lead to perforations. The risk is much greater when both sides of the septum are cauterized at one sitting, and it is therefore wise to have an interval of 3–4 weeks between the two treatments. In the author's experience, patients who suffer from Osler's disease are lucky to escape this complication.

Septal perforations are sometimes occupational in origin and the commonest such cause is penetration of the nasal mucosa by one of the hexavalent forms of chromium. In addition to its role in plating processes, this metal is used in certain tanning, dyeing and photographic processes. Workers engaged in the manufacture of dichromates are particularly at risk. Other causes include exposure to anhydrous sodium carbonate (soda ash), arsenic and its compounds, organic compounds of mercury, particularly mercury fulminate, alkaline dusts such as soap powders, hydrofluoric acid and fluorides, capsacin, the pungent active principle of capsicum (chillies), vanadium, dimethyl sulphate, cocaine and other drugs taken as snuff, copper salts (rarely), and lime (rarely).

Chromium has an irritant effect on the respiratory mucous membrane which can result in ulceration and perforation of the nasal septum, pulmonary fibrosis and emphysema. Nasal disease in chrome workers was first reported by Newman in 1890. The incidence of perforation depends on the intensity and duration of the exposure. It has been greatly reduced by the use of exhaust ventilation and seromists. Survey of the literature by Sanz, in 1989, regarding the incidence of septal perforations in chrome workers, shows marked variations from 14.9% to 63%. Water soluble chromates are carcinogenic and the incidence of both lung and nasal cancer in chromate workers is raised. As a result of these hazards, chromate workers should be screened for septal ulceration at regular monthly intervals.

Cocaine abuse is a rapidly increasing cause of septal perforation. The National Institute on Drug Abuse (NIDA) estimated that by 1985, over 22 million Americans had tried cocaine and 5 million were using the drug regularly (Schade, 1988). The toxic effect of cocaine on the nose was first reported by Owens, a US Navy Surgeon, in 1912. Most addicts start by administering the drug intranasally using a technique known as 'snorting'. A 'quill' usually in the form of a plastic straw is used to insert the irritant powder as high into the nasal cavity as possible and against the septum. The cocaine causes intense vasoconstriction as well as topical anaesthesia and the trauma of the 'quill' leads to ulceration followed by chondritis and ultimately septal necrosis. The problem is further compounded by the fact that illicit cocaine varies in purity from 10 to 70% and is always mixed with a wide range of adulterants which contribute both to mucosal irritation and systemic toxicity. In exceptional and severe cases, the tissue necrosis can extend to the turbinates, ethmoid sinuses and hard palates (Kuriloff and Kimmelman, 1989). Rhinological examination of a large series of drug addicts revealed an incidence of 4.8% of septal perforations (Messinger, 1962). The frequency of perforations among female addicts are five times that of the males. This is probably due to the fact that most males much more rapidly graduate to the intravenous administration of the drug. Perforations have developed within 3 weeks of the commencement of the addiction.

Chronic inflammatory diseases, such as syphilis and tuberculosis, have been known as rare causes of septal perforations for many years. More recently a high incidence of spontaneous perforations has been reported in association with classic systemic lupus erythematosus (Willkens *et al.*, 1976) and with rheumatoid arthritis (Mathews *et al.*, 1983).

There have been several case reports in the literature of septal perforations occurring following the prolonged use of topical steroids (Miller, 1975; Jones, Spector and English, 1979; Soderberg-Warner, 1984). Decongestants are another rare iatrogenic cause, although this would appear only to occur when a virtual addiction becomes established with a resulting grossly excessive dosage (Vilensky, 1982).

Symptoms and signs

Apart from the traumatic causes, septal perforations are usually preceded by ulceration. There are often four well-marked stages, starting with redness and congestion of the mucosa producing irritation and rhinorrhoea. Shortly afterwards the mucosa becomes blanched and anaemic; later it undergoes necrosis as revealed by the development of tough adherent crusts over the affected area. Finally, the crusting extends into the substance of the cartilage and a perforation results. Septal perforations are quite often asymptomatic, but the development of large crusts may cause obstruction and the separation of these crusts may lead to bleeding. Patients not infrequently complain of abnormal dryness in the nose, and sometimes of a dull discomfort over the bony dorsum. The passage of respiratory air often produces a whistling noise. Crusting problems are usually much worse when there is any interference with the normal respiratory air currents, as may occur with such obstructive lesions as septal deviations behind the perforations. Phonation can be affected as a result of the impaired resonance associated with the disturbed anatomy of the nasal cavities and voice changes were found by Younger and Blokmanis (1985) in 2% of patients with symptomatic septal perforations.

Brain (1980) has shown, in a series of 69 septal perforations, that 62.4% were completely free from any symptoms. The two main factors found to affect the function of the nose and produce symptoms, were the size and position of the perforation. Septal perforations become symptomatic when the mucociliary clearance mechanism no longer functions adequately. The mucus stagnates, dries and forms crusts inside the perforation which, when extruded, traumatize the mucosa and cause bleeding. Crusts, clotted blood and mucosal oedema obstruct the nasal airflow, which becomes increasingly turbulent, and this in turn leads to further excessive drying with more loss of ciliary function and a vicious circle is established. The mucous membrane lining the nose is relatively inactive anteriorly. The extent of this inactive zone varies greatly according to individual anatomical characteristics but it often occupies up to the anterior third of the nasal cavity. The drainage from this inactive zone depends entirely on the traction exerted by the cilia further back. Clearance from the anterior inactive zone is 15 times slower than from the active region. The anterior zone is therefore much more vulnerable to any pathological reduction in mucociliary activity and this is why anterior perforations are much more likely to be symptomatic (Table 11.1). Apart from position, any large loss of mucosa will reduce mucociliary function, and this is why the large perforations are more often symptomatic (Table 11.2). The problems of a large perforation are therefore somewhat similar to those of atrophic rhinitis. Removal of yet more nasal mucosa is likely therefore to increase the problems of these patients and yet the surgical enlargement of these perforations was advocated in a standard textbook by Jackson and Coates in 1922.

Table 11.1 Symptoms in relation to position of perforation

Area 1	
present in 1 out of 1	(100%)
Area 2	
present in 4 out of 8	(50%)
Area 3	
present in 5 out of 42	(11.9%)
Area 4 and area 5	
all perforations present in these areas also extended anteriorly to involve other areas	

Cottle's topographical classification used to record location of perforation

Table 11.2 Symptoms in relation to size of perforation

1	Small	
	troublesome in 2 out of 20	(10%)
2	Medium	
	troublesome in 11 out of 33	(33.3%)
3	Large	
	troublesome in 13 out of 16	(81.25%)

The state of the residual nasal mucosa is also of importance. Some cases of perforation are due to malignant disease or to a midline granuloma and may have been heavily irradiated, and this does often lead to a severe atrophic rhinitis which greatly increases the crusting problem.

Diagnosis

The history is of importance in the diagnosis of traumatic and occupational cases. When the edge of the lesion looks raised or hypertrophic, a biopsy should be performed to exclude malignancy. A biopsy is also essential in suspected cases of Wegener's granuloma. Serological tests for syphilis should always be performed if the lesion is involving the bony septum, and the erythrocyte sedimentation rate is invariably raised in cases of Wegener's granuloma; this can be a useful confirmatory diagnostic test for this condition, together with the biopsy. When it is suspected,

but not admitted by the patient, that the illicit use of cocaine is the cause of the perforation, then a urine drug screen test should be performed (EMIT).

More recently, the use of CT scanning and/or MRI in selected cases has been advocated, both to assess the extent of bone erosion and to measure the size of the perforation (Frank, Kern and Kispert, 1988).

Treatment

The first objective in the management of septal ulcers and perforations is to cure the causative disease process. Conditions such as malignant tumours, malignant granuloma, and chronic infections are discussed in other chapters. In the occupational cases, it will be necessary to obtain the cooperation of the industrial medical officer to prevent further exposure to the toxic agent. Most recent cases have occurred when the exhaust ventilation system in the chrome plant has become defective. When the perforation is due to cocaine it is of paramount importance that the addiction should be cured before any surgical treatment is even considered.

The second objective is to encourage natural healing of the lesion and, if this does not occur, to consider performing a surgical repair. The patient must be told to treat his nose with great care, and to avoid traumatizing actions such as vigorous blowing and nose picking. The patient should also apply some Cicatrin cream on the tip of the little finger to the lesion, twice daily. This treatment will heal most ulcers, although the original area will often permanently remain white, dry and scarred.

Perforations never heal spontaneously, but fortunately most do not cause symptoms, and therefore do not require any treatment. Crusting and bleeding are the main problems associated with the more troublesome minority. Less severe cases can be satisfactorily controlled by the use of a nasal douche (Collunarium alkalinus), but should this prove to be inadequate, the closure of the perforation, either by filling it with an obturator, or by means of a surgical operation, will have to be considered. Obturators (Figure 11.34) are a simple, safe, and reliable method of closing almost any septal perforation. Cooperation with a specialist in dental prosthetics is essential. The obturators are constructed from Silastic and are made from an impression of the perforation.

The author has closed over 200 perforations using this technique, the full details of which have already been published (Davenport, Brain and Hunt, 1984). It is easy to close perforations of up to 3 cm in diameter and it has proved to be always possible, but technically more difficult to close larger perforations. The largest was in fact 5 × 3.5 cm. The long-term results of this treatment have now been carefully studied in the first 102 cases and for this purpose the perforations were classified according to size (Table 11.3).

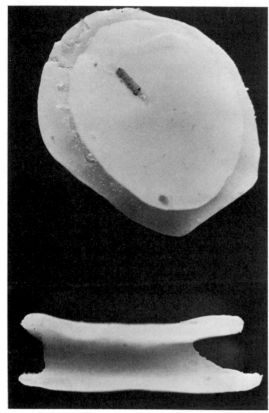

Figure 11.34 A Silastic obturator for the closure of a septal perforation. There is a millimetre scale on the left side

Table 11.3 Size of perforations

Small	Up to 1 cm in diameter
Medium	1–2 cm in diameter
Large	Over 2 cm in diameter

The criteria used to assess the results are shown in Table 11.4).

Table 11.4 Symptoms

1	None
2	Minimal symptoms controlled by douching
3	Troublesome symptoms not controlled by douching

Very few small perforations cause symptoms and therefore require treatment as shown by the number of cases treated (Table 11.5).

Table 11.5 Cases treated

Small	2
Medium	63
Large	37

Whistling was the main indication for closure in the two small perforations treated and here the results were excellent. The same unfortunately cannot be said for medium sized and large perforations and it is evident that therapeutic success bears an inverse relationship with the size of the perforation (Table 11.6).

Table 11.6 Results of obturator closure

	Medium-sized perforations (%)	*Large perforations (%)*
Good	44.4	32.4
Fair	38.1	16.2
Poor	17.5	51.4

Retention of these obturators is on the whole good but in nine cases there were problems. Usually the obturator became loose and had to be replaced. An obturator will reliably close almost any perforation, and eliminate the crusting which occurs around its edges. What it does not do is to replace the normal functioning septal mucosa. In the smaller and medium-sized perforations, the compensatory capacity of the residual mucosa is sufficient to overcome this deficiency, whereas this is not the case with 50% of the larger perforations. This is a very unfortunate finding, because the difficulties in effectively closing a septal perforation surgically are directly proportional to the size of the perforation.

Another problem with surgery is the fact that, not infrequently, an unsuccessful operation actually enlarges the perforation and can make the patient considerably worse. It has been the author's policy to close all troublesome septal perforations with obturators, and only to consider surgical closure as a secondary treatment when the obturator fails to reduce dramatically the symptoms. Acrylic obturators are also used to close septal perforations (McKinstry and Johnson, 1989). In our experience the rigidity of this material makes it less satisfactory than Silastic both from the point of view of its insertion and retention.

If the services of a specialist in dental prosthetics are not available it may be possible to close the perforation with prefabricated Silastic buttons, which have been popularized by Kern, Facer and McDonald (1977). The retention of this type of device is, however, far less satisfactory.

The operative closure of septal perforations is a rather unsatisfactory chapter in the subject of nasal surgery. It is extremely difficult to close surgically any perforation larger than 2 cm in diameter. Masing

(1965) has shown that the partial anterior closure of larger perforations does frequently greatly reduce the symptoms.

These operations are technically difficult to perform, and it is therefore important to effect an adequate exposure of the perforation and this is not generally possible with the usual endonasal approach. When the upper limit of the perforation is 2 cm or less from the nasal floor, it is usually possible to obtain a reasonably good exposure by making an incision through the alar facial crease (Figure 11.35). Higher perforations are best reached through the external rhinoplasty approach (Figure 11.36), which has been popularized by Goodman and Strelzow (1978). Undoubtedly the widest exposure can be obtained by the midfacial degloving technique (Romo *et al.*, 1988) which is described elsewhere. This is, however, a very radical procedure and as the author has been satisfied with the external rhinoplasty approach he has never resorted to it.

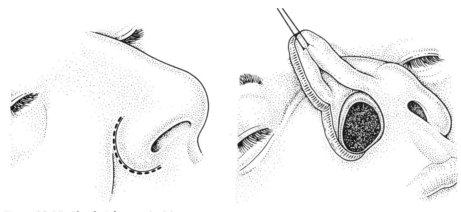

Figure 11.35 Alar-facial crease incision

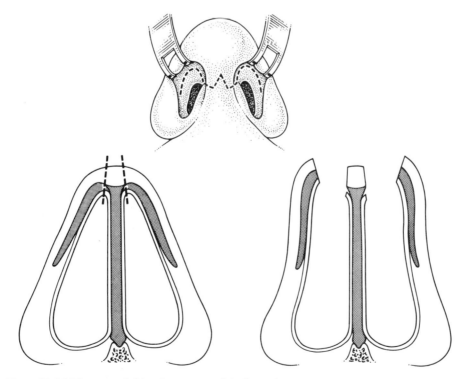

Figure 11.36 The external rhinoplasty approach to the septum

Perforations can be closed by grafts or by flaps, and in the case of large perforartions, a combinartion of grafts and flaps is necessary. Good results have been obtained by Fairbanks and Fairbanks (1973), using temporalis facial grafts. An alternative graft is the three-layer composite graft from the pinna, using the technique popularized by Walter (1969). Free grafts taken from the turbinates have been employed to close small septal perforations (Ismail, 1964; Seiffert, 1967), but unfortunately the amount of tissue available is extremely limited, and it is impossible to close a defect which is 1 cm or more in diameter with this technique. These small perforations rarely need treatment and should this be necessary, they usually do well with obturators.

The mucosal flaps can be cut from the septum, the inner surface of the upper lip, or the lateral nasal wall. Septal mucosal flaps are rarely satisfactory as the mucosa around the perforation is usually thin and atrophic. Cartilage has often been extensively removed and the normal tissue planes have often been completely obliterated with fibrous tissue. The amount of the mucosa available for closure is inversely pro-

portional to the diameter of the perforation (Figure 11.37). It is possible, however, to elevate widely the mucosa from the nasal floor and lower lateral wall in addition to the septum. A broad bipedicled flap, 2.5 cm in width, is created which is based on the branches of the sphenopalatine and superior labial arteries. This can then be rotated medially and superiorly to close the septal defect (Figure 11.38).

The operative technique found most satisfactory by the author is basically that described by Fairbanks and Fairbanks (1973) which is really similar to an underlay myringoplasty. Bipedicle advancement flaps are used together with a fascial graft. Fairbanks and Fairbanks use temporalis fascia but the author has preferred to use fascia lata which is available in greater quantity and can be conveniently harvested by an assistant. The beauty of this method is that complete closure of the flaps on both sides is not essential as the mucosa can regenerate over the fascial graft. It is important not to suture the edges of the perforation under tension, and closure is facilitated by the use of short straight needles, and by the use of tissue glues which reduce the number of

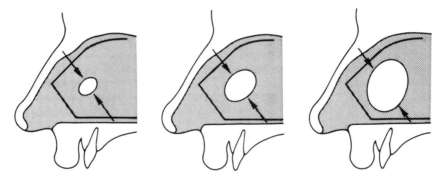

Figure 11.37 The amount of septal mucosa available for the closure of a perforation is inversely proportional to the size of the defect

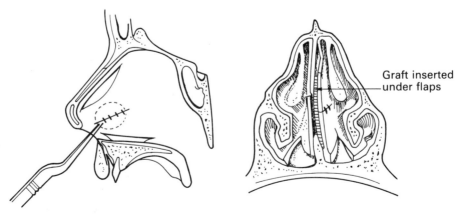

Graft inserted under flaps

Figure 11.38 Completed closure with fascia graft inserted under left septal flaps. Left, left lateral view; right, cross-section. (Based on Fairbanks and Fairbanks, 1973)

sutures required, help to fix the fascial graft in place and also have a haemostatic effect.

As an alternative method, a buccal flap from the inner margin of the upper lip can be brought through a stab incision in the floor of the nose and used to close septal perforations (Figures 11.39 and 11.40) (Tipton, 1970). The maximum width of the flap is, however, only 2 cm and this limits the size of perforation which can be treated by this technique which was popularized by Tardy (1973).

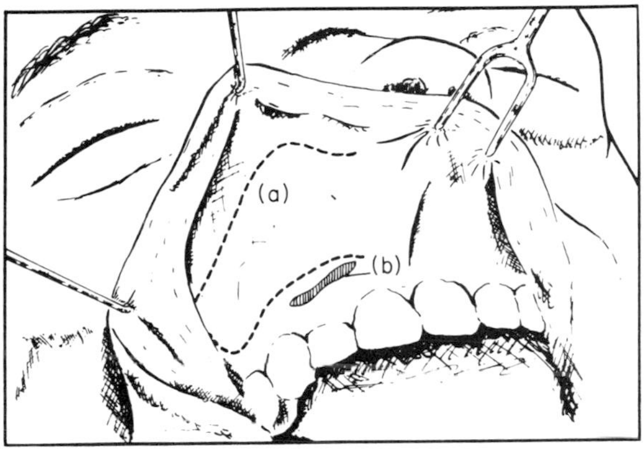

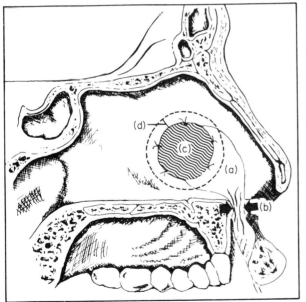

Figure 11.39 Closure of a septal perforation by a labial flap. (*a*) Design of labial flap; (*b*) small incision in floor of nose. (From Tipton, 1970. Reproduced by kind permission of *Plastic and Reconstructive Surgery*)

Figure 11.40 Labial flap in place closing off the septal perforation (*c*) with its distal edges tucked in under the edges of the septal mucosa around the defect (*d*). (From Tipton, 1970. Reproduced by kind permission of *Plastic and Reconstructive Surgery*)

After the operation, crusting inside the nose can prejudice the result by traumatizing the suture line. For this reason Fairbanks advises preventing the formation of crusts by occluding the nostrils for 1 month postoperatively.

References

AMBRUS, P. S., EAVEY, R. D., BAKER, A. S., WILSON, W. R. and KELLY, J. H. (1981) Management of nasal septal abscess. *Laryngoscope*, **91**, 575–582

ARBOUR, P. AND KERN, E. B. (1975) Paradoxical nasal obstruction. *Canadian Journal of Otolaryngology*, **4**, 333–338

BARBOUR, S. D. (1984) Toxic shock syndrome associated with nasal packing: analogy to tampon associated illness. *Pediatrics*, **73**, 163–165

BECK, A. L. (1945) Abscess of the nasal septum complicating acute ethmoiditis. *Archives of Otolaryngology*, **42**, 275–279

BEEKHUIS, G. J. (1973) Nasal septoplasty. *Otolaryngologic Clinics of North America*, **6**, 693

BERNSTEIN, L. (1973a) Early submucous resection of nasal septal cartilage. *Archives of Otolaryngology*, **97**, 273

BERNSTEIN, L. (1973b) Submucous operations on the nasal septum. *Otolaryngologic Clinics of North America*, **6**, 675

BRAIN, D. J. (1980) Septo-rhinoplasty: the closure of septal perforations. *Journal of Laryngology and Otology*, **94**, 495–505

BRAIN, D. J. and ROCK, W. P. (1983) The influence of nasal trauma during childhood on growth of the facial skeleton. *Journal of Laryngology and Otology*, **97**, 917–923

BROMS, P. (1982) Rhinomanometry, procedures and criteria for distinction between skeletal stenosis and mucosal swelling. *Acta Otolaryngologica*, **94**, 361–370

CAMPBELL, J. B., WATSON, M. G. and SHENOI, P. M. (1987) The role of intranasal splints in the prevention of postoperative nasal adhesions. *Journal of Laryngology and Otology*, **101**, 1140–1143

CHASSAIGNAC, C. (1851) *Gazette des Hopitaux, Paris*, 419

CHUKUEZI, A. B. (1992) Nasal septal haematoma in Nigeria. *Journal of Laryngology and Otology*, **106**, 396–398

COLE, P., CHABAN, R., NAITO, K. and OPRYSK, D. (1988) The obstructive nasal septum. *Archives of Otolaryngology*, **114**, 410–412

COLLINS, M. P. (1985) Abscess of the nasal septum complicating isolated acute sphenoiditis. *Journal of Laryngology and Otology*, **99**, 715–719

COOK, J. A., MURRANT, N. J., EVANS, K. L. and LAVELLE, R. (1992) Intranasal splints and their effects on intranasal adhesions and septal stability. *Clinical Otolaryngology*, **17**, 24–27

COTTLE, M. H. (1951) Nasal surgery in children. *Eye, Ear, Nose and Throat Monthly*, **30**, 32–38

COTTLE, M. H. (1968) Rhino-sphygmo-manometry and aid in physical diagnosis. *International Rhinology*, **6**, 7

COTTLE, M. H., FISCHER, G. G., GAYNOR, I. E. and LORING, R. M. (1958) The maxilla-pre-maxilla, approach to extensive nasal septum surgery. *Archives of Otorlaryngology*, **68**, 301

CURTISS, E. S. (1952) Postural nerve block for intranasal operations. *Lancet*, i, 989

DAVENPORT, J. C., BRAIN, D. J. and HUNT, A. J. (1984) Laboratory techniques for the construction of intranasal prosthesis. *Journal of Prosthetic Dentistry*, **51**, 477–585

DIEFFENBACH, J. (1845) *Die Operative Chirugie*. Leipzig: F. A. Brockhans. p. 366

DOUEK, E. (1974) *The Sense of Smell and its Abnormalities.* London, Churchill Livingstone

ELLIS, P. D. M., HARRIES, M. L. L., FFOWCS WILLIAMS, J. E. and SHNEERSON, J. M. (1992) The relief of snoring by nasal surgery. *Clinical Otolaryngology*, **17**, 525–527

FAIRBANKS, D. N. F. and FAIRBANKS, G. R. (1973) Surgical management of large nasal septum perforations. *British Journal of Plastic Surgery*, **24**, 382–387

FOMON, S., GILBERT, J. G., SILVER, A. G. and SYRACUSE, V. R. (1948) Plastic repair of the obstructing nasal septum. *Archives of Otolaryngology*, **47**, 7

FRANK, D. A., KERN, E. B. and KISPERT, D. B. (1988) Measurement of large or irregular-shaped septal perforations by computed tomography. *Radiologic Technology*, **59**, 409–412

FREER, O. (1902) The correction of deflections of the nasal septum with a minimum of traumation. *Journal of the American Medical Assocation*, **38**, 636

FRY, J. H. (1969) The pathology and treatment of haematoma of the nasal septum. *British Journal of Plastic Surgery*, **22**, 331

GALLOWAY, T. (1946) Cited by Bolotow, N., Fomon, S., Pullen, M. and Syracuse, V. R. Plastic repair of the deflected nasal septum. *Archives of Otolaryngology*, **44**, 141

GALTON, F. (1875) The history of twins as a criteria of the relative power of nature and nurture. *Frazer's Magazine*, 12th November

GOODMAN, W. S. and STRELZOW, V. V. (1978) Nasoseptal perforation: closure by external septorhinoplasty. *Journal of Otolaryngology*, **7**, 43–48

GRAY, L. P. (1972) Early treatment of septal deformity and associated abnormalities. In: *Modern Trends in Diseases of the Ear, Nose and Throat*, edited by M. Ellis, London: Butterworths, pp. 219–236

GRYMER, L. E. and MELSEN, B. (1989) The morphology of the nasal septum in identical twins. *Laryngoscope*, **99**, 642–646

HARKAVY, K. L. and SCANLON, J. W. (1978) Dislocation of the nasal triangular cartilage after Caesarian section for breech presentation without labour. *Journal of Pediatrics*, **92**, 162–165

HARTENSTROM, D. F. (1970) Facial Growth Effects of Nasal Septal Cartilage Resection in Beagle Pups. *Thesis.* University of Iowa, Iowa City

HARTIKAINEN-SORRI, A. L., SORRI, M., VAINIO-MATTILA, J. and OJALA, K. (1983) Aetiology and detection of congenital nasal septal deformities. *International Journal of Paediatric Otorhinolaryngology*, **1**, 83–88

HAYTON, C. H. (1948) Quoted by St Clair Thomson and V. E. Negus *Diseases of the Nose and Throat* London: Cassell. p. 193

HAYWARD, P. J. and MACKAY, I. S. (1987) Fibrin glue in nasal septal surgery. *Journal of Laryngology and Otology*, **101**, 133–138

HELLMICH, S. (1970) Die Verträglichkeit konservieter homioplastischer knorpelimplantate in der Nase. *Zeitschrift für Laryngologie-Rhinologie-Otologie and ihre Grenzgebeite*. **49**, 742–749

HENRY, K., SULLIVAN, C. and CROSSLEY, K. (1988) Nasal septal abscess due to *Staphylococcus aureus* in a patient with Aids. *Reviews of Infectious Diseases*, **10**, 428–429

HIRSCH, O. (1952) Symptoms and treatment of pituitary tumours. *Archives of Otolaryngology*, **55**, 268

HUIZING, E. H. (1979) Septum surgery in children: indications, surgical techniques and long term results. *Rhinology*, **17**, 91–100

INGALLS, E. F. (1882) Deflection of the septum narium. *Archives of Laryngology*, **3**, 291–298

ISMAIL, H. K. (1964) Closure of septal perforations. A new technique. *Journal of Laryngology and Otology*, **78**, 620

JACKSON, C. L. and COATES, G. M. (1922) *Diseases of the Throat, Nose and Ear*, Philadelphia: W. B. Saunders

JAZBI, B. (1974) Nasal septum deformity in the newborn: diagnosis and treatment. *Clinical Paediatrics*, **13**, 953–956

JENNES, M. K. (1964) Corrective nasal surgery in children. *Archives of Otolaryngology*, **79**, 145–151

JESSEN, M. and MALM, L. (1984) The importance of nasal airway resistance and nasal symptoms in the selection of patients for septoplasty. *Rhinology*, **22**, 157–164

JONES, L. M., SPECTOR, S. L. and ENGLISH, G. M. (1979) Treatment of perennial rhinitis with flunisolide corticosteroid spray. *Annals of Allergy*, **34**, 107

KATZ, R. L., MATTEO, R. S. and PAPPER, E. M. (1962) The injection of epinephrine during general anaesthesia with halogenated hydrocarbons and cyclopropane in man. *Anesthiology*, **23**, 597–600

KENT, S. E., REID, A. P., NAIRN, E. R. and BRAIN, D. J. (1988) Neonatal septal deviations. *Journal of the Royal Society of Medicine*, **81**, 1258–1262

KENT, S. E., ROCK, W. P., NAHL, S. S. and BRAIN, D. J. (1991) The relationship of nasal septum deformity and palatal symmetry in neonates. *Journal of Laryngology and Otology*, **105**, 424–427

KERN, E. B., FACER, G. M. and MCDONALD, T. J. (1977) Closure of nasal septum perforations with a sialastic button. *Otorhinolaryngology Digest*, **39**, 9–17

KILLIAN, G. (1904) Die submucöse Fensterresektion der Nasen-scheidewand. *Archivs für Laryngologie und Rhinologie*, **16**, 362

KURILOFF, D. B. and KIMMELMAN, C. P. (1989) Osteocartilaginous necrosis of the sinonasal tract following cocaine abuse. *Laryngoscope*, **9**, 918–924

LANGENBECK, B. (1843) *Handbuch der Anatomie*. Göttingen;

MCAULIFFE, G. W., GOODELL, H. and WOLFF, H. G. (1943) Experimental studies on headache: pain from the nasal and paranasal structures. *Research Publication of the Association for Research into Nervous and Mental Disease*, **23**, 185–206

MCCAFFREY, T. and KERN, E. (1979) Clinical evaluation of nasal obstruction. *Archives of Otolaryngology*, **105**, 542–545

MCCLYMONT, L. G. and CROWTHER, J. A. (1988) Local anaesthetic with vasoconstrictor combinations in septal surgery. *Journal of Laryngology and Otology*, **102**, 793–795

MACHLE, W. M. and GREGORIOUS, F. (1948) Cancer of the respiratory system in the United States chromate producing industry. *Public Health Report*, **63**, 1114–1127

MCKINSTRY, R. E. and JOHNSON, J. T. (1989) Acrylic nasal septal obturators for nasal septal perforations. *Laryngoscope*, **99**, 560–563

MASING, H. (1965) Zur plastische-operativen Versorgung von Septumhamotomen und abscessen. *HNO*, **13**, 235–240

MASING, H. (1977) Functional aspects into septal plasty. *Rhinology*, **15**, 167–172

MATHEWS, J. L., WARD, J. R., SAMUELSON, C. O. and KNIBBE, W. P. (1983) Spontaneous nasal septal perforation in patients with rheumatoid arthritis. *Clinical Rheumatology*, **2**, 13–18

MESSINGER, E. (1962) Narcotic septal perforations due to drug addiction. *Journal of the American Medical Association*, **179**, 964–965

METZENBAUM, M. (1929) Replacement of the lower end of the dislocated cartilage versus submucous resection of the dislocated end of the septal cartilage. *Archives of Otolaryngology*, 9, 282

METZENBAUM, M. (1936) Dislocation of the lower end of the septal cartilage. *Archives of Otolaryngology*, 24, 78

MILLAR, R. A., GILBERT, R. G. B. and BRINDLE, G. F. (1958) Ventricular tachycardias during halothane anaesthesia. *Anaesthesia*, 13, 164–172

MILLER, F. F. (1975) Occurrence of nasal septal perforation with use of intranasal dexamethasone aerosol. *Annals of Allergy*, 34, 107–109

MINNIS, N. L. and MORRISON, A. W. (1971) Trans-septal approach for vidian neurectomy. *Journal of Laryngology and Otology*, 85, 255

MOFFETT, A. J. (1941) Postural installation – a method of inducing local anaesthesia in the nose. *Journal of Laryngology and Otology*, 56, 429

NEWMAN, D. (1890) A case of adenocarcinoma of the left inferior turbinate body and perforation of the nasal septum in the person of a worker in chrome pigments. *Glasgow Medical Journal*, 33, 469–470

OWENS, W. D. (1912) Signs and symptoms presented by those addicted to cocaine: observations in a series of 23 cases. *Journal of the American Medical Association*, 58, 329–330

PEASE, W. S. (1969) Neonatal nasal septal deformities. *Journal of Laryngology and Otology*, 83, 271–274

PEER, L. (1937) An operation to repair lateral displacement of the lower border of the septal cartilage. *Archives of Otolaryngology*, 25, 475

REES, T. D. (1986) Surgical correction of the severely deviated nose by extra mucosal excision of the osteocartilaginous septum and replacement as a free graft. *Plastic and Reconstructive Surgery*, 78, 320–330

RHYS EVANS, P. H. and BRAIN, D. J. (1981) The influence of nasal osteotomies and septum surgery on the growth of the rabbit snout. *Journal of Laryngology and Otology*, 95, 1109–1119

ROMO, T., FOSTER, C. A., KOROVIN, G. W. and SACHS, M. E. (1988) Repair of nasal septal perforation utilizing the midfacial degloving technique. *Archives of Otolaryngology and Head and Neck Surgery*, 114, 739–742

RUANO-GIL, D., MONTSERRAT-VILADIN, J. M. and VILANOVA-TREAS J. (1980) Deformities of the nasal septum in human foetuses. *Rhinology*, 18, 105–109

RUBIN, F. F. (1983) Controlled tip sculpturing with the morselizer. *Archives of Otolaryngology*, 109, 160–163

RUBRECHT, W. (1868) *Weiner medizinische Wochenschrift*, 18, 1157

SALINGER, S. and COHEN, D. M. (1955) Surgery of the difficult septum. *Archives of Otolaryngology*, 61, 419–421

SANZ, P. (1989) Nasal septum perforation in chromate-producing industry in Spain. *Journal of Occupational Medicine*, 12, 1013

SARNAT, B. G. and WEXLER, M. R. (1961) Growth of the face and jaws after resection of the septal cartilage in the rabbit. *American Journal of Anatomy*, 118, 755

SARNAT, B. G. and WEXLER, M. R. (1967) Rabbit snout growth after resection of the central linear segments of nasal cartilage. *Acta-Oto-laryngologica*, 63, 467–478

SCHADE, C. P. (1988) *Smoking More Now and Enjoying it Less: the Epidemiology of Cocaine Abuse in the United States in the late 1980s*. Rockville, Md: National Institute on Drug Abuse

SCHOENBERG, A., ROBINSON, P. and RYAN, R. (1992) The morbidity from nasal splints in 105 patients. *Clinical Otolaryngology*, 17, 528–530

SCHONSTED-MADSEN, U., STOKSTED, P., CHRISTENSEN, P. H. and KOCH-HENRIKSEN, N. (1986) Chronic headache related to nasal obstruction. *Journal of Laryngology and Otology*, 100, 165–170

SCHONSTED-MADSEN, U., STOKSTED, P. E. and OUTZEN, K. E. (1989) Septorhinoplastic procedures versus submucous resection of the septum, using septum perforation as an indicator. *Rhinology*, 27, 63–66

SEIFFERT, A. (1967) Quoted in *Plastic Surgery of Head and Neck*. edited by H. J. Denecke and R. Meyer. New York: Springer-Verlag. p. 139

SELZER, (1949) *Plastic Surgery of the Nose*.

SHALOM, A. S. (1963) The anterior ethmoid nerve syndrome. *Journal of Laryngology and Otology*, 77, 315

SIEDENTOP, K. H., HARRIS, D. M. and SANCHEZ, B. (1985) Autologous fibrin tissue adhesive. *Laryngoscope*, 95, 1074–1079

SLUDER, G. (1927) *Nasal Neurology, Headaches and Eye Disorders*. London: Kimpton

SODERBERG-WARNER, M. L. (1984) Nasal septal perforation associated with topical corticosteroid therapy. *Journal of Pediatrics*, 105, 840–841

TARDY, M. E. (1973) Septal perforations. *Otolaryngologic Clinics of North America*, 6, 711

THOMAS, J. N. (1978) SMR – a two-year follow-up survey. *Journal of Laryngology and Otology*, 92, 661–666

THOMAS, S. (1982) Toxic shock syndrome following submucous resection and septorhinoplasty. *Journal of the American Medical Association*, 247, 2403–2404

TIPTON, J. B. (1970) Closure of large septal perforation with a labial-buccal flap. *Plastic and Reconstructive Surgery*, 46, 514

TODD, J., FISHAUT, M., KAPRAL, F. and WELCH, T. (1978) Toxic shock syndrome associated with phase group I staphylococcus. *Lancet*, i, 1116–1118

VASE, P. and JOHANNESSEN, J. (1981) Homograft cartilage in the treatment of an abscess in the nasal septum. *Journal of Laryngology and Otology*, 95, 357–359

VERWOERD, C. D. A., URBANUS, N. A. M. and NIJDAM, D. C. (1979) The effects of nasal surgery on the growth of the nose and maxilla. *Rhinology*, 17, 53–63

VILENSKY, W. (1982) Illicit and licit drugs causing perforation of the nasal septum. *Journal of Forensic Science*, 27, 958–962

WAGNER, R. and TOBACK, J. M. (1986) Toxic shock syndrome following septoplasty using plastic septal splints. *Laryngoscope*, 96, 609–610

WALTER, C. (1969) Composite grafts in nasal surgery. *Archives of Otolaryngology*, 90, 622–630

WILLKENS, R. F., ROTH, G. J., NOVAK, A. and WALIKE, J. (1976) Perforation of the nasal septum in rheumatic disease. *Arthritis and Rheumatology*, 19, 119–121

WRIGHT, W. K. (1967) Study on hump removal in rhinoplasty. *Laryngoscope*, 77, 508

YOUNGER, R. and BLOKMANIS, M. B. (1985) Nasal septal perforations. *Journal of Otolaryngology*, 14, 125–131

12

Surgical management of sinusitis

I. S. Mackay and V. J. Lund

There can be few other areas of otorhinolaryngology which in the last decade have witnessed such a fundamental change in emphasis than the surgical management of rhinosinusitis. The underlying pathophysiological concepts are not new but there has been a resurgence of interest largely initiated by the new technology of rigid endoscopy and CT scanning which has improved visualization and surgical access. One of the most important things to emerge from this change in emphasis is the use of endoscopes for diagnosis and interest in the aetiology of sinus pathology. This has focused attention to that area of the middle meatus, the 'ostiomeatal complex' into which maxillary, frontal and anterior ethmoid sinuses open and where malfunction of drainage, for whatever reason, will have the maximum impact upon these dependent sinuses (Figure. 12.1). It is on this area that therapeutic attention has recently focused and whether this is effected medically or surgically, by endoscope, microscope, illuminated speculum or headlight, is less important than the underlying philosophy. Thus the concept of 'irreversibly damaged' mucosa has come to be seriously questioned.

Despite the unprecedented rise in popularity of endoscopic sinus surgery around the world, not every patient is suitable for this and although our approach may have become more conservative, with a general move away from the more radical procedures, it is still necessary to employ these in certain circumstances.

Embryological considerations (Schaeffer, 1920; Wolf, Anderhuber and Kuhn, 1993)

The maxillary sinus is first recognizable as a shallow groove expanding laterally from the ethmoidal infundibulum in the fourth intrauterine month (Figures 12.2 and 12.3). Extension laterally to reach the lateral cartilaginous plate is followed by absorption and expansion so that, at birth, there is a small sinus cavity with its lower border about 4 mm above the nasal floor. Expansion and pneumatization continue until 8–9 years of age when the floors of the sinus and nasal cavity are roughly equal and the sinus is $2 \times 2 \times 3$ cm in dimension. Growth continues at

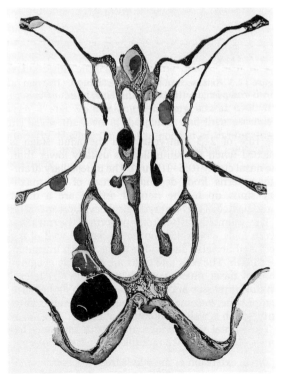

Figure 12.1 Coronal section through adult midfacial block (H and E)

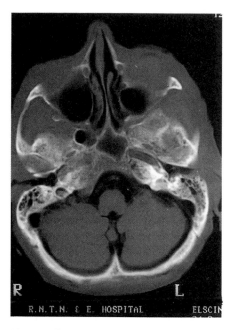

Figure 12.5 Axial CT scan showing nasolacrimal duct

The anterior superior alveolar nerve derives from the infraorbital nerve and contributes to the superior dental plexus. It is related to the anterior attachment of the inferior turbinate where a nasal branch is given to the mucosa of the lateral wall as high as the maxillary ostium. Damage to this nerve during anterior enlargement of an inferior meatal antrosotomy results in changes in dental sensation. Paraesthesia can also result from direct damage to the infraorbital nerve during a Caldwell–Luc approach. The infraorbital canal represents a constant thinning of the bone in the orbital floor and may be dehiscent. The nerve may also be damaged as it leaves the infraorbital foramen to supply the soft tissue of the anterior cheek (Figure 12.6).

The configuration of the middle meatus is complex and subject to considerable variation (Figure 12.7). The middle turbinate provides the key to understanding the surgical anatomy Anteriorly it attaches by a vertical strut to the skull base and posteriorly to the maxilla and lamina papyracea by a horizontal attachment. Joining the two is an oblique lamella of bone, the ground lamella, which divides the drainage of the ethmoid complex into anterior and posterior.

The uncinate process is a thin crescent of ethmoid bone which attaches to the anterior edge of the maxillary hiatus but in life variable areas of the hiatus anterior and posterior to this attachment are filled with mucosa and membrane and are termed respectively the anterior and posterior fontanelles. It is in these natural areas of weakness that accessory ostia are found. The relationship of maxillary ostium to frontonasal recess will depend upon the superior

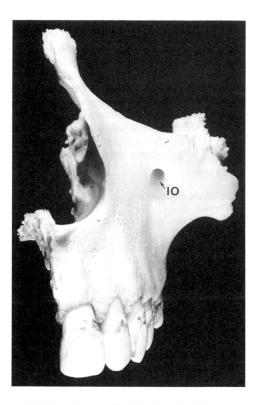

Figure 12.6 Anterior maxilla. IO: infraorbital foramen

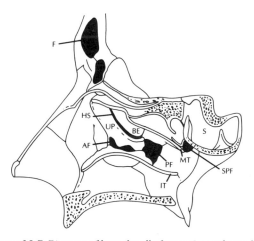

Figure 12.7 Diagram of lateral wall of nose. S = sphenoid sinus; F = frontal sinus; MT = middle turbinate attachment; IT = inferior turbinate attachment; AF = anterior fontanelle; PF = posterior fontanelle; BE = bulla ethmoidalis; UP = uncinate process; HS = hiatus semilunaris; SPF = sphenopalatine foramen

attachment of the uncinate process. If the uncinate joins the lamina papyracea, a separate cul-de-sac results, the terminal recess. Adjacent to the uncinate and just anterior to the anterior attachment of the middle turbinate, the agger nasi area is found, which may be pneumatized. Just anterior to the attachment of the uncinate process to the maxilla is the nasolacrimal duct, generally lying in thick bone, but occasionally encroached upon by the agger nasi cells.

The ethmoidal bulla is a fairly constant feature, containing anterior ethmoidal cells, though it can be poorly pneumatized or completely unpneumatized in 8% (Stammberger, 1991). The hiatus semilunaris is a two-dimensional space between the posterior edge of the uncinate process and the anterior face of the bulla. Through it the ethmoidal infundibulum is entered, the funnel-shaped space leading to the maxillary ostium. Posteriorly the bulla may fuse with the ground lamella of the middle turbinate or there may be a cleft, the lateral sinus.

The frontal recess is preferred to the term 'frontonasal duct' as it is usually an hour-glass shaped constriction and not a true duct. It is found in the most anterosuperior part of the middle meatus, often lying medial to the ostium of a suprabullar cell. However, accessory channels are found in 12% of the Caucasian population.

The ethmoid bone is a complex bone composed of clefts and cells. It is completed superiorly by the frontal bone which is generally thicker bone, resistant to disease and trauma. However, an area of weakness exists where the frontal bone joins the ethmoid, particularly medially, which is further endangered by the passage of the anterior ethmoidal artery. It is at this point that the anterior cranial fossa may be readily entered. The vessel may also be damaged as it traverses the roof and lateral wall, from which it may retract, producing, in the worst instance, a rapidly developing orbital haematoma. The posterior ethmoidal vessel by contrast is usually more protected, running within bone.

The level of the ethmoidal roof varies in 12% of the population between right and left, with the right side being more usually the lower (8%) (Dessi *et al.*, 1994). This may in part explain the tendency for the right side to be the site of iatrogenic CSF leaks.

The posterior ethmoid cells are generally larger, pyramidal and fewer in number. They drain via the superior meatus. A supreme turbinate is discernible in two-thirds of subjects (Schaeffer, 1920). The sphenoethmoidal recess lies medial to the superior turbinate and is the location of the ostium of the sphenoid sinus. The most posterior ethmoidal cell can extend lateral to the sphenoid, a variant described by Onodi (1910). The optic nerve is particularly vulnerable in such cells and even under normal circumstances bone overlying the nerve has been estimated to be clinically dehiscent in 6% of the normal Caucasian population (Kennedy, 1990). Ethmoidal cells may also pneumatize the floor of the orbit, forming Haller cells, which can encroach on the ethmoidal infundibulum (Haller, 1769 in Stammberger, 1991).

This pneumatization can occur from the anterior system (70%) or posterior (30%).

The sphenoid sinus is also intimately related to the optic nerve and the internal carotid artery may be prominent on the posterior wall. The bone overlying it can be extremely thin or dehiscent in 25% of the population.

Diagnosis

While a careful clinical history remains the cornerstone of diagnosis, and all patients will undergo a general otorhinolaryngological examination, the emphasis has moved towards endoscopy supported by appropriate imaging to confirm the diagnosis, define the extent of pathology and demonstrate relevant anatomy.

Endoscopy

Historical aspects

Endoscopy was first performed by Hirschmann in 1903 using a modified Nitze cystoscope which he used in the nasal cavity and in the maxillary sinus via a tooth socket. This cystoscope had a diameter of 5 mm and an electric bulb deflected 90° by a distal prism with 180° rotation. Reichert (1902), Sargon (1908) and Imhofer (1910) all used similar instruments and even attempted removal of foreign bodies. Speilberg in 1922 was the first to introduce an endoscope into the maxillary sinus via the inferior meatus, but it was Maltz who, in 1925, commissioned Wolf to make a dedicated endoscope and who introduced the term 'sinoscopy'. These endoscopes using a series of small lenses continued in use until Hopkins, Professor of Optics at Reading, invented a far superior system in the 1950s, based on solid glass rods, which is now universally utilized.

The technique is described in Chapter 1 but a few specific points should be made:

1 A careful endoscopic examination will reveal disease not visualized by conventional anterior or posterior rhinoscopy, but it is not always possible to enter the middle meatus, either from anteriorly or medially

2 Even when the middle meatus is readily examined, only the 'tip of the iceberg' is visible and the mucosa may appear normal even in the presence of sinus disease

3 Particulaly with the wide-angled lenses, there is a flattening effect on the mucosal surface.

However, the diagnostic role of endoscopy cannot be too strongly emphasized and it should be available for routine clinical use.

Radiology

The role of plain sinus X-rays has been the subject of

considerable discussion as false positives and false negatives can occur, particularly in infants and children (McAlister, Lusk and Muntz, 1989). Neither is it possible adequately to visualize the ostiomeatal area, identify anatomical variants or judge important surgical features such as prominent or dehiscent optic or carotid canals.

Zinreich *et al.* (1987) have popularized a protocol for computer assisted tomography (CT) using sections taken in the coronal plane with 'wide window' settings to show optimally fine bone detail (2000–4000 HU). For coronal sections, the patient must hyperextend the head but the coronal plane approximates closest to the surgical field and best demonstrates the ostiomeatal complex, and base of skull. However, when pathology is present in the posterior ethmoids and sphenoid, axial views are required adequately to show the optic nerve and carotid artery. Slices of 4 mm thickness are taken. Exact settings will vary from one machine to another, but Zinreich *et al.* (1987) have recommended the following settings using a Siemens Somatron DR 3 scanner: kVp = 125, mAs = 450, scan time 5 s with window widths at + 2000, centred at − 200 (Figure 12.8). With these settings, and centring of the film, metallic dental fillings do not produce too serious an artefact. Reconstructed coronals can be obtained from the axials but are reserved for those patients unable to extend the neck.

While plain radiographs are inferior to CT, it is inappropriate to scan all patients with rhinological complaints. The use of a plain lateral sinus X-ray taken at 145 kV will predict the presence of ethmoidal opacification with a 90% correlation with subsequent CT scanning (Lloyd, Lund and Scadding, 1991) though both right and left sides are superimposed and cannot, therefore, be distinguished.

Surgical approaches

Historical aspects

The first clear indication of the existence of the paranasal sinuses was provided by Berenger del Carpi, anatomist and surgeon at Bologna in the early sixteenth century (Wright, 1914). Fallopius (1600) referred to the maxillary sinus and suggested that the sinuses were absent in children until they reached maturity. Apart from the quotation, 'In a person having a painful spot in the head, with intense headaches, pus or fluid running from the nose removes the disease' (Hippocrates, 5 BC) which may be inferred as describing a sinus infection, the maxillary sinus and associated suppuration were not adequately described until 1651 when they were reported by Nathaniel Highmore and for some time the sinus was referred to by his eponym.

The treatment of maxillary sinusitis by opening and irrigating the sinus via a variety of routes has a long and varied history. Highmore himself advocated decompression by thrusting a silver bodkin through an empty tooth socket. Many of the earliest writers such as Cowper (1707) and Meibomius (1718) recom-

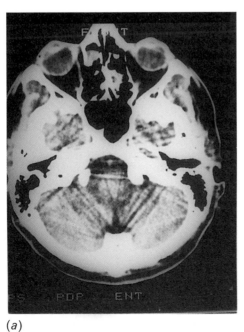

(*a*)

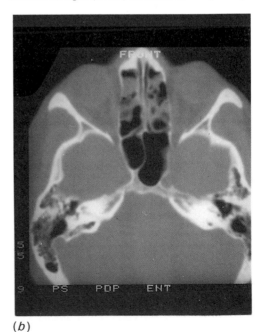

(*b*)

Figure 12.8 (*a*) Axial CT scan of patient performed using narrow window widths. (*b*) Axial CT scan of same patient performed using wide window widths showing greater detail within ethmoids

mended irrigation through the alveolar tooth margin after molar tooth extraction, while Lamorier (1743) and Desault (1798) preferred the canine fossa approach. John Hunter (1835) was one of the first proponents of the intranasal approach and Zuckerkandl (1893) initially advocated perforation of the middle meatus, but later abandoned the technique because of the potential for orbital damage. It is of interest that sporadic interest continued in middle meatal antrostomy, predating the introduction of endoscopic visualization (Lavelle and Spencer Harrison, 1971).

The first description of the inferior meatal antrostomy was probably by Gooch in 1770 (Cordes, 1905) but routine puncture of the inferior meatus was not common until advocated by Krause (1887), Mickulicz (1887) and Lichtwitz (1890), using needle, trocar and stylette, respectively. Thus began the first attempts at diagnosis by proof puncture followed by irrigation. In 1890 Lichtwitz invented the cannula which accompanied the perforating needle.

Mickulicz understood the anatomical and physiological pitfalls of the inferior meatal antrostomy, including its propensity to closure. Shortly after its introduction, it was largely superseded by the more radical canine fossa approach described by Caldwell (1893), Spicer (1894) and Luc (1897). This differed from that already described by Lamorier and Desault in that a nasal counter-opening was included. The Caldwell–Luc approach was the primary operation during the first part of the twentieth century but there began an increasing trend towards lavage, followed by inferior meatal antrostomy with Caldwell–Luc reserved for any failures. This situation pertained up to the early 1980s in the UK when endoscopic surgery first made its appearance.

From the outset, operations on the frontoethmoid complex fell into two groups (Macbeth, 1954): those designed to enhance drainage while preserving facial contour; and those aimed at eradicating diseased mucosa disregarding cosmesis. As with the maxillary sinus, initial surgical treatment of the infection concentrated on opening and draining the frontal sinus by trephination (Wells, 1870; Ogston, 1884). A more extreme procedure was described by Riedel in 1898 in which inferior and anterior walls were removed leading to severe cosmetic deformity.

To overcome some of these problems, Killian (1903) proposed removal of the anterior and inferior walls but with preservation of the supraorbital rims. Later he extended dissection to include the frontal process of the maxilla to facilitate drainage through the anterior ethmoidal cells and this procedure remained popular during the beginning of the twentieth century. It was, however, criticized by Howarth (1921), among others, for leaving a 'dead-space', for closure of the frontonasal recess. Howarth proposed an alternative operation which was synchronously described by Lynch (1921) in the USA in which all diseased frontal sinus mucosa was removed, and the

sinus drained via an ethmoidectomy. This operation gained considerable popularity and dominated the first half of the twentieth century though interest centred on methods to maintain patency of the frontonasal recess, ranging from mucoperiosteal flaps (Sewall, 1935; Ogura, Watson and Jurcina, 1960; Baron, Dedo and Henry, 1973), split skin around a rubber tube (Smith, 1934; Howarth, 1936; Negus, 1947), tantalum (Goodale, 1945), and silastic. However, a high recurrence rate of problems led Boyden (1952) to conclude that closure of the frontonasal recess was the main reason for failure and resulted in an increasing popularity for the osteoplastic flap, with (Goodale and Montgomery, 1958) and without obliteration (Macbeth, 1954). This operation has remained popular in the USA, whereas the Lynch–Howarth external frontoethmoidectomy was favoured in the UK.

Mosher (1913) is credited with the first description of an intranasal ethmoidectomy but by 1929 he concluded that while theoretically easy, this operation had in practice, proven to be one of the easiest operations with which to kill the patient!

Endoscopic surgery has traditionally been divided into two schools, though in practice the distinction is less definite. The primary objective of the 'Messerklinger' approach, championed by Stammberger (1985a, b; 1991), is the removal of pathology in the ostiomeatal complex, sufficient to achieve ventilation and drainage, thereby addressing the underlying pathophysiology by a conservative technique; hence the term 'functional' (Kennedy, 1985; Kennedy *et al.*, 1985). A more radical extirpation of disease has been proposed by Draf (1983) and Wigand (1981, 1990), particularly related to polyposis, in which an absence of surgical landmarks and profuse pathology determines a 'back to front' approach. The title 'FESS' (functional endoscopic sinus surgery) is therefore only appropriate when performing limited surgery with preservation of existing structures and should not be used for the many surgical indications for which the endoscope may now be utilized, e.g. orbital decompression, dacrocystorhinostomy, etc.

A recent questionnaire survey showed the rapid increase in surgeons performing endoscopic surgery in the UK with an exponential increase in numbers between 1986 and 1992 but notwithstanding this, by 1993 only 38% of those otolaryngologists who returned the questionnaire claimed to be performing this surgery (Cumberworth and Mackay, 1994) and this has not substantially changed since that time.

Surgical procedures (Table 12.2)
Antral lavage
Indications

Antral lavage has been used both in the diagnosis and treatment of sinusitis. Its previous diagnostic role

Table 12.2 Operations on the paranasal sinuses for chronic rhinosinusitis

Maxillary sinus

Conservative

> Antral washout
> Intranasal antrostomy
> > middle meatal (endoscopic)
> > inferior meatal

Radical

> Caldwell–Luc

Frontoethmosphenoid

Conservative

> Trephination of the frontal sinus or sphenoid washout
> Intranasal ethmoidectomy
> Endoscopic uncinectomy, ethmoidectomy, clearance of the frontal recess, opening of the sphenoid ostium (functional endoscopic sinus surgery)
> Transantral ethmoidectomy (Jansen Horgan)

Radical

> External frontoethmosphenoidectomy (Lynch–Howarth, Patterson)
> Osteoplastic flap (with or without obliteration)

to clarify plain sinus X-ray by proof puncture is somewhat obsolete. Therapeutically it may still be used in the treatment of acute and subacute maxillary sinusitis and pansinusitis which has failed to respond to conservative medication.

Antral puncture is usually performed through the inferior meatus and in the past was often performed several times before proceeding to formal inferior meatal fenestration. One alternative to repeated puncture is the insertion of an indwelling catheter through which daily irrigation can be performed until the quantity and quality of secretion improves (Goode, 1970). The frequency with which antral washout is performed will vary between surgeons, with many now rarely employing the technique and preferring a definitive endoscopic middle meatal approach to enlarge the natural ostium.

Perforation of the anterior wall through the canine fossa is another route by which lavage may be performed though this has generally been used for sinoscopy.

Contraindications

The proximity of the orbital floor and the teeth in the small maxillary sinus of a child under the age of 3 years makes antral puncture hazardous and is, therefore, rarely performed. Similarly in the hypoplastic maxilla with thick bony walls, puncture may be technically difficult. Antral puncture and lavage in acute febrile maxillary sinusitis untreated by antibiotics is theoretically associated with osteomyelitis and

septicaemia. In the presence of trauma which may have disrupted the orbital floor, antral washout is contraindicated and if drainage of a haematoma is deemed necessary, a formal antrostomy is safer.

Anaesthesia

Antral washout can be performed under local or general anaesthesia.

Local anaesthesia

The nasal cavities are first sprayed with 10% cocaine and 1:1000 adrenalin solution and left for 3–4 minutes. This leads to shrinkage of the mucosa and facilitates insertion of cotton wool into the inferior meatus and drainage from the middle meatus through the natural ostium. Pledgets of cotton wool soaked in 10% cocaine and 1:1000 adrenalin solution can be placed along the inferior meatus and left for a further 4 minutes. Alternatively 25% cocaine paste on silver wire wool carriers or Tumarkin wires can be placed, ideally at the genu of the inferior turbinate and close to the sphenopalatine ganglion at the posterior end of the middle meatus.

Cocaine can cause adverse side effects and there has been some recent discussion concerning the safety of its use in combination with adrenalin. Gastric absorption is more rapid than that from the nasal mucosa so excessive cocaine trickling down the nasopharynx should be avoided. The maximal dose of cocaine for an adult is usually between 100 and 200 mg or up to 3 mg/kg. Malleable silver wires should be used in the nose, so that if the patient collapses this does not result in damage from the wires being pushed through the cribriform plate.

General anaesthesia

This is rarely required for antral washouts alone unless dealing with children or anxious adults. A cuffed oral endotracheal tube is employed and haemostasis and access facilitated by additional local anaesthetic vasoconstricting agents such as 25% cocaine paste, which can be spread in the surgical field with a cotton wool bud, under ECG monitoring. Alternatively Moffatt's solution (1941) can be instilled by the anaesthetist. This is composed of 2 ml of 2% sodium bicarbonate, 2 ml of 10% cocaine and 1 ml of 1:1000 adrenaline, half in each nostril.

Surgical technique

With the patient seated comfortably, the wool carriers or pledgets are removed and the inferior meatus visualized using a Thudicum speculum or a rigid endoscope. A Tilley-Lichtwitz trocar and cannula are used for the puncture and it is advisable to check that the instruments match, engaging smoothly and with a sharp trocar end protruding 3 mm from the cannula. This is passed under the attachment of the inferior turbinate up to the genu where it will naturally come to rest. The instruments are held with the body of the trocar in the palm of the hand and the index finger running along the shaft so movement is controlled. Holding the patient's head steady, the trocar is directed towards the tragus of the ipsilateral ear.

Moderate pressure accompanied by a gentle boring action is usually sufficient to perforate the inferior meatal wall at its thinnest point. The trocar is advanced until it abuts the opposite antral wall and then is withdrawn several millimetres (Figure 12.9). The trocar is then removed. The patient now leans forwards, holding a bowl beneath the chin to collect the washings and is instructed to breathe through the mouth and to mention any discomfort as the lavage proceeds. The washout is performed using a Higginson syringe and sterile normal saline or water at 37°C. As fluid is flushed into the sinus, the majority returns via the anterior nares, but any running posteriorly readily runs out of the mouth into the bowl. Washings can be sent for bacteriological and cytological examination though it may be preferable to aspirate with an empty syringe before attachment of the Higginson apparatus to obtain an undiluted specimen.

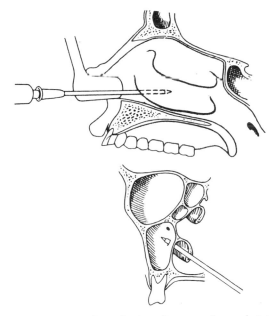

Figure 12.9 Line of introduction of trocar and cannula into maxillary sinus

If the procedure is performed under general anaesthesia, the patient is placed in the tonsil position, with a Boyle-Davis gag in place or in reverse Trendelenberg position with 15° of head flexion and a throat pack. In either case lavage is achieved with an ordinary hypodermic syringe containing 5–10 ml of fluid which are introduced and then aspirated to avoid unnecessary overflow into the nasopharynx. If the natural ostium is occluded, drainage may be facilitated by the introduction of a second cannula alongside the first. Excessive pressure should never be used. Care should also be taken not to introduce air during the procedure as fatal air embolus has been described (McNab Jones, 1976).

If a purulent washout is obtained, lavage is continued until it is clear. If the washout is initially clear, instillation should continue as mucoid material may require some loosening. Following adequate lavage, the cannula is removed and the patient warned that fluid may continue to drain from the nose over the next few hours.

Complications

Mild haemorrhage may occur from the puncture site which can be stopped with a temporary nasal pack during which time the patient must remain in hospital.

Incorrect positioning of the cannula should not occur if the technique described is followed. However, the anterior wall can be breached leading to pain and swelling of the cheek. This is rapidly noticed in the conscious patient but, under general anaesthesia, requires observation and palpation. Similarly, perforation of the orbital floor leads to immediate pain. Under general anaesthesia, bulging of the orbital contents may be observed, and for this reason the eyes must always be left untaped and the upper lids gently elevated by an assistant. In the presence of a dehiscent infraorbital canal, even a correctly placed cannula can produce this complication. Excessive zeal on introduction of the cannula can lead to penetration of the lateral or posterolateral wall, but this is rare. In all these circumstances the procedure should be abandoned and antibiotics given.

Inferior meatal antrostomy

Indications

This operation has traditionally been used in the treatment of acute, recurrent and chronic maxillary sinusitis which has failed to respond to conservative management. In 1986 it was the commonest operation performed by British otolaryngologists for chronic sinusitis but recent figures suggest that it is being superseded by middle meatal surgery (Cumberworth and Mackay, 1994). It relies upon gravitational drainage and aeration to effect improvement in sinus mucosa. It may therefore be of specific benefit in cases of primary mucociliary abnormality such as cystic fibrosis and primary ciliary dyskinesia.

Anaesthesia

Although the operation can be performed under local anaesthesia, general anaesthesia with a cuffed oral endotracheal tube (or laryngeal mask) and pharyngeal pack is preferable. The use of topical anaesthetic agents such as Moffatt's solution are useful in preparing the nasal mucosa prior to surgery.

Surgical technique

The patient is prepared and towelled with 15° of head flexion, in a reverse Trendelenberg position. A headlight, illuminated Killian speculum, microscope or rigid endoscope can be used for illumination. The inferior turbinate is elevated with a Hill elevator. This instrument is then used to perforate the inferior meatus at the highest point under the genu of the turbinate where the bone is thinnest. Enlargement is then performed in all directions using a variety of instruments, e.g. posteriorly with Grunwald nasal turbinate forceps, anteriorly with Seymour Jones antrum forceps and superiorly and inferiorly with a Hayek antrum punch forceps, either up- or down-cutting (Lund, 1986). The Ostrom forceps which are frequently used to cut anteriorly, were designed to perform middle meatal antrostomies and it is therefore, not surprising that they frequently break when incorrectly used on the hard bone of the inferior meatus (Ostrom, 1913).

Anatomical constraints limit the size of the antrostomy but, ideally, at least 2 cm × 1 cm windows are fashioned if long-term patency is desired (Figure 12.10). Care should be taken to lower the inferior edge as much as possible to minimize the inevitable sump which results between the floor of the nasal cavity and that of the maxillary sinus. Some authors have described covering the inferior edge with a mucosal flap (Reynolds and Brandow, 1975; Buiter, 1988). While discrete polyps can be removed via the antrostomy, blindly curetting with a Mackie curette is not recommended. A rigid endoscope may, however, be inserted to inspect directly the antrum and pathology removed under direct vision.

The inferior turbinate should be repositioned at the end of the procedure and a pack may be placed in the nasal cavity overnight. Suction cleaning and douching may be used postoperatively.

Complications

If the antrostomy is extended too far posteriorly, the inferior meatal branch of the lateral sphenopalatine artery is encountered, resulting in significant haemorrhage.

Anterior extension may damage branches of the anterior superior alveolar nerve plexus leading to altered dental sensation, the incidence of which has been underestimated in the past. Damage to the nasolacrimal duct orifice is fortunately rare due to its position and the thickness of the surrounding bone.

After initial fashioning, all inferior meatal antrostomies undergo some circumferential closure due to healing, on average 0.4 cm. However, complete closure may be anticipated if the antrostomy is made 1 cm or less in diameter (Lund, 1988).

Caldwell–Luc procedure

Indications

The operation was designed to remove 'irreversibly' damaged mucosa of the maxillary sinus and to facilitate gravitational drainage and aeration via an inferior meatal antrostomy. It has predominantly been used for persistent chronic sinusitis when medication, lavage and inferior meatal antrostomy has failed. However, it is not normal ciliated respiratory epithelium which replaces diseased mucosa and the cavity becomes partially obliterated by fibrous tissue which may be associated with the formation of retention cysts. The numbers of this procedure performed in the UK have gradually fallen and although the following list gives the range of potential indications, in reality it is principally utilized as a route of access.

1 Chronic maxillary sinusitis
2 Removal of foreign bodies, such as a dental root or amalgam
3 Closure of an oroantral fistula
4 Dental cysts involving the antrum
5 Access to the pterygomaxillary fissure and pterygopalatine fossa
6 Removal of recurrent antrochoanal polyps
7 Elevation and stabilization of orbital floor fractures or removal of the orbital floor in decompression

It is not recommended as a route for biopsy of antral malignancy as it potentially opens a hitherto unaffected area to contamination.

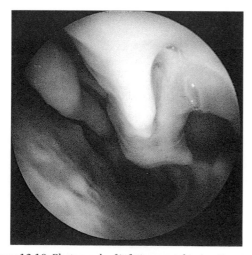

Figure 12.10 Photograph of inferior meatal antrostomy showing abnormal mucociliary pathways

Contraindications

It is rarely performed in children as damage to the secondary dentition can result.

Anaesthesia

While the operation may be performed under local anaesthesia (using a maxillary nerve block) it is commonly carried out under general anaesthesia with a cuffed endotracheal tube (or laryngeal mask) and pharyngeal pack. The use of topical local anaesthesia within the inferior meatus and injection of $1:200\,000$ adrenalin into the gingivolabial sulcus and soft tissues of the canine fossa is recommended.

Technique

The headlight or illuminated speculum is used with the patient positioned in a reverse Trendelenberg position with 15° of head flexion. An incision is made down to the bone in the gum margin, 3 mm above and parallel to the gingivolabial fold from the posterior edge of the lateral incisor to the first or second molar tooth (3–4 cm). It is advisable that the incision does not directly overlie the opening in the anterior face of the maxilla to lessen the risk of a fistula.

The mucoperiosteal flap is then dissected superiorly with a periosteal elevator to expose the anterior wall of the sinus, taking care to avoid damage to the infraorbital nerve arising from its foramen just below the orbital rim, either directly or indirectly from retraction. The anterior wall is opened in the canine fossa where the bone is relatively thin (see Figure 12.6) with a 5 mm Jenkins gouge or more precisely with a drill. The opening can be enlarged with Hayek or Kerrison punch forceps to produce a hole sufficiently large to allow removal of the sinus mucosa (approximately 1–1.5 cm diameter). Inferior extension may lead to damage to the teeth and their nerve supply and laterally bleeding may be encountered from the anterolateral branches of the sphenopalatine artery. Bleeding from the bony edge can be controlled by crushing the bone with punch forceps or by diathermy, but usually settles once the mucosa is removed.

As originally described, the entire lining of the sinus is dissected and removed and the success of the operation in chronic sinusitis was thought to depend upon complete extirpation of the mucosa which can be difficult to achieve in the inferolateral angle and roof.

A large inferior meatal antrostomy (2 × 1 cm) is fashioned as previously described. Packing of the nasal cavity and occasionally of the antrum via the antrostomy is sometimes required though in the latter circumstance care must be taken on its removal to ensure that no strands are caught on the bony edges of the antrostomy. Suturing of the buccal incision is recommended with absorbable suture material to de-crease the risk of fistula formation but should be sufficiently loose to allow drainage of blood.

The patient should be advised against overenthusiastic blowing of the nose for at least a week and should replace upper dentures within 24 hours to avoid obliteration of the labioalveolar sulcus.

Complications

Pain and soft tissue swelling are minimized by attention to surgical technique. Haemorrhage can occur from both the anterior bony wall or inferior meatal antrostomy but is rarely a problem.

Paraesthesia due to damage of the infraorbital nerve may be temporary or permanent but should not occur with careful dissection and retraction. In the long term, patients may complain of significant neuralgia in the distribution of the infraorbital nerve. Damage to the teeth and their innervation can lead to alteration in dental sensation and occasionally devitalization and discoloration of the tooth.

Oroantral fistula occasionally occur particularly if care is not taken with siting of the incision. The fistula may be temporary or permanent, requiring subsequent surgical intervention.

The mucosa which regrows in the maxillary sinus is abnormal both histologically and functionally (Benninger, Sebek and Levine, 1989; Kennedy and Shaalan, 1989). In addition, retention cysts, sufficiently large to fill and expand the sinus have been described, particularly in the Japanese literature (Hasegawa *et al.*, 1979).

Intranasal ethmoidectomy

Indications

The principal indication for this procedure has been chronic sinusitis associated with nasal polyposis. As originally described and performed with headlight illumination, it provides an inadequate approach for complete exenteration of the ethmoid complex.

Contraindications

The procedure has largely been superseded by an endoscopic approach to this area as without adequate visualization it is particularly hazardous.

Surgical technique

The operation is generally performed under general anaesthesia with topical vasoconstrictors to improve haemostasis and in a reverse Trendelenberg position with 15° of head flexion.

Essentially the ethmoidal labyrinth is cleared between the vertical attachment of the middle turbinate medially and the lamina papyracea laterally using small Tilley Henckel forceps. Care is taken not to open these towards the lamina. The ethmoids may be cleared superiorly until the hard white bone of the fovea ethmoidalis is seen. The posterior system may be entered by traversing the ground lamella of the middle turbinate and the turbinate is preserved as a surgical landmark for this or future procedures. The sphenoid may also be entered, though taking care to do so as inferiorly and medially as possible from the posterior ethmoid system. All material removed should be examined for the presence of orbital fat (by seeing if it floats in water).

Complications

Injury to the lamina papyracea may lead to haemorrhage which can produce a periorbital haematoma (Harrison, 1981), erroneously considered by some as the hallmark of a successful operation. Posterior tracking of the haematoma leads to proptosis and risks visual loss, necessitating removal of packing and orbital decompression via an external approach (Leopold, Kellman and Gould, 1980).

Direct injury to the orbital periosteum can lead to prolapse of fat into the surgical field, followed by direct damage to the medial rectus muscle and optic nerve. Dural injury via the medial ethmoidal roof can result in a cerebrospinal fluid leak which can be repaired in a number of ways. Thus both blindness and meningitis are possible sequelae of this surgery and careful monitoring of the patient must be instituted postoperatively.

Transantral ethmoidectomy – Jansen Horgan procedure (Jansen, 1902; Horgan, 1926)

Indications

This operation, which combines a Caldwell–Luc approach with access to the ethmoids was originally described for the chronic antroethmoiditis. It has also been used as a route for orbital decompression.

Contraindications

The inadequate approach afforded to the ethmoids has significantly limited its use.

Surgical technique

After performing a routine Caldwell–Luc approach, the posterior ethmoid cells are opened through the antrum by pushing a closed Tilley Henckel forceps upwards, medially and posteriorly at the upper and inner angle of the antrum, in the direction of the opposite parietal eminence. Those cells which can be safely reached are cleared though the angle of approach will inevitably limit access. It may be combined with an intranasal ethmoidectomy to clear the anterior cells more effectively.

Complications

These are as for intranasal ethmoidectomy and Caldwell–Luc procedures.

External frontoethmoidectomy

Indications

This approach was designed to offer access, illumination and perception of depth which overcame many of the disadvantages of the less 'open' operations. It converts the ethmoidal labyrinth into a single cavity which can include the frontal and sphenoid sinuses and has been used in the following circumstances:

1 Chronic sinusitis unresponsive to conservative medication
2 Complications of acute ethmoiditis such as orbital cellulitis, in which it is a useful approach for decompression and drainage
3 Recurrent polyposis, especially when previous nasal surgery has destroyed useful landmarks
4 Frontoethmoidal mucocoeles
5 Access to the ethmoidal arteries for ligation in epistaxis, transethmoidal hypophysectomy, dacrocystorhinostomy, repair of cerebrospinal fluid leaks and decompression of the orbit for malignant exophthalmos
6 It has no place alone in the definitive oncological treatment of sinus malignancy.

Lynch-Howarth procedure (Lynch, 1921; Howarth, 1921)

The operation is best performed under general anaesthesia via an oral tube, with pharyngeal pack and the application of topical vasoconstrictors. The patient lies in the reverse Trendelenberg position, with 15° of head flexion. A temporary tarsorrhaphy should be performed initially to protect the eye.

The incision is made slightly curved medial and concave towards the medial canthus of the eye, straight down to bone. The incision may be extended under the eyebrow to facilitate access to the frontal sinus (Figure 12.11). Bleeding from the angular vessels is often encountered. The periosteum is elevated with care to reveal the nasal process of the maxilla, frontal bone and medial wall of orbit. The lacrimal sac is elevated and displaced laterally.

Dissection continues posteriorly to reveal the anterior ethmoidal vessels which are ligated, coagulated with bipolar diathermy or neurosurgical clips. The posterior ethmoidal vessels approximate to the posterior limit of the ethmoidal cells and are also ligated. Dissection is aided by the use of 1-cm ribbon gauze soaked in topical adrenalin (1:1000) and retraction is best performed with a malleable copper spatula.

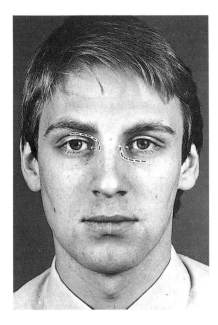

Figure 12.11 Position of Lynch–Howarth incision (superiorly) and Patterson's incision (inferiorly)

The thin medial wall of the orbit is perforated with ease, entering the ethmoidal system which may be progressively exenterated under direct vision, bearing in mind the level of the cribriform plate. It is important that the clearance continues up to and including the sphenoid, allowing removal of all diseased mucosa if this is felt to be appropriate. Similarly the frontal recess can be cleared and the frontal sinus entered. The amount of frontal sinus floor removed will depend on the access required and the extent of disease in the sinus. It is advisable to retain as much bony support of the recess as possible to prevent subsequent prolapse of the orbital contents into this area. Patency of the frontal recess is the key to successful treatment and many methods have been used to achieve this. Stenting in the form of silastic tubes or sheets have traditionally been used and left in place for up to 3–5 months. However, on removal there is a tendency for circumferential scarring to occur and the lining of the surgical channel is rarely functioning respiratory epithelium. Other methods such as split skin grafts and mucoperiosteal flaps are equally unsuccessful. However, a better compromise is to combine an endoscopic and external approach in selected cases, when it may be possible to avoid any form of stenting if there is sufficient bony support for the recess (Lund, 1990).

The periosteum, subcutaneous tissues and skin are sutured carefully with catgut and silk. A single non-resorbable suture (e.g. Prolene) is used to secure the periosteum in the region of the trochlea (see below). The eye should be washed with saline at the end of the procedure to remove blood and chloramphenicol ointment instilled to prevent conjunctivitis. A pressure dressing may be applied for 24 hours. The skin sutures are removed after 4–5 days.

Complications

Problems may result from the incision itself, including oedema and infection, paraesthesia of the skin, damage to the medial palpebral ligament and webbing of the wound. This cosmetic deformity has been made much of in the American literature but careful placement of the incision renders this a minor problem (Rubin, Lund and Salmon, 1986).

Haemorrhage can occur pre- or postoperatively associated with retraction of the ethmoidal vessels before adequate haemostasis is achieved but it is usually self-limiting. If the incision is continued too far laterally the supraorbital nerves may be damaged resulting in a variable area of paraesthesia of the medial forehead.

Dural exposure, either surgically or by the pathology itself, is not uncommon, but any evidence of a cerebrospinal fluid leak, should be treated with appropriate antibiotic cover and primary closure of the defect with a free mucosal flap, e.g. from the middle turbinate, dermal fat, split skin or fascia lata held in position with tissue glue or closure with a septal mucosal flap. These may be held in place with Gelfoam and/or a Whiteheads varnish pack.

Significant damage to the periorbita should be repaired immediately to avoid prolapse of fat into the surgical field. Periorbital swelling is minimized with a pressure dressing and any resultant epiphora and diplopia are usually transient. Temporary diplopia may also result if the globe is decompressed surgically after accommodating to long-term displacement for example with a frontoethmoidal mucocoele. However, a prospective study on 22 patients confirmed that a significant number of patients experience long-term diplopia after a Lynch–Howarth approach due always to superior oblique underaction (Lund and Rolfe, 1989). This results from disturbance of the trochlea and this area of the periosteum should be formally reattached at the end of the operation with a non-resorbable suture to restore the mechanical integrity of the pulley.

Serious visual loss is unusual but can obviously result if the globe is injured. It is a theoretical complication of sudden decompression after long-standing displacement, and may be treated with prophylactic steroids.

Failure to maintain the patency of the frontal recess may be associated with subsequent mucocoele formation (Schenck, 1975) and/or recurrence of the original disease process. This led to the operation being supplanted by the osteoplastic flap in the USA.

Transorbital ethmoidectomy

Patterson's operation (1939)

The indications for this operation are similar to those for the Lynch–Howarth procedure, but in addition, it allows access to the orbital floor which is of use in orbital trauma or decompression.

Patterson also described a similar incision to the Lynch–Howarth but his name has been associated with an incision, 2 cm in length, made in a natural crease line below the inferior orbital margin (see Figure 12.11). The orbicularis muscle is split and the periosteum incised and elevated to the orbital margin. Meticulous care is required to avoid tearing the periosteum and the inferior oblique muscle is detached (except in 9% of the population where the muscle is intraperiosteal (Harrison, 1981)). Care is also taken to preserve the lacrimal sac and duct. The orbital floor is removed laterally as far as the infraorbital nerve, and may in selected cases be removed lateral to the nerve, though only 1 or 2 mm of extra decompression can be obtained. The bone is removed posteriorly from behind the nasolacrimal duct as far as the hard bone of the sphenoid surrounding the optic apex. Bone can be removed superiorly as high as the ethmoidal vessels. Thus the ethmoids can be removed under direct vision both transnasally and externally but for even better visualization a rigid endoscope can be used for the most posterior part of the dissection and for clearance of the frontonasal recess which is difficult to approach by this technique. In decompression procedures the periosteum must be incised in a horizontal and vertical fashion to release the fat into the space created.

Complications are similar to those for the Lynch–Howarth procedure with recurrence of disease and transient epiphora associated with oedema of the orbicularis fibres and/or stretching of the nasolacrimal duct being the commonest. Paraesthesia can also result from damage to the infraorbital nerve. Diplopia may occur from detachment of the inferior oblique muscle and particularly after the periosteal incisions during orbital decompression.

Frontal sinus washout

Indications

This procedure is performed when acute suppurative frontal sinusitis has failed to respond to antibiotics (oral and parenteral), decongestants and topical vasoconstrictors. By draining pus under pressure, it aims to avoid mucosal necrosis and bone resorption, oste(omyel)itis and intracranial complications. It should only be undertaken after adequate antibiotic therapy has been given but should not be delayed if the situation is deteriorating or fails to resolve rapidly. Essentially the operation provides an immediate resolution to an acute problem but may not overcome an underlying cause such as obstruction of sinus outflow so a more formal procedure is often required secondarily. As a consequence some surgeons prefer to do the latter from the outset.

Contraindications

Radiological examination to establish the existence and extent of the frontal sinus should precede any surgery in this region.

Surgical technique

The operation is usually carried out under general anaesthesia, in the reverse Trendelenberg position, with 15° of head flexion, an oral tube and pharyngeal pack. A temporary tarsorrhaphy protects the eye. A small incision is made 1 cm below the medial end of the eyebrow, straight down to bone. The sinus is usually entered with ease, using a drill with rose-head burr or small gouge and hammer and the purulent contents released. The entry hole may be enlarged further with Citelli or Hayek punch forceps to allow adequate visualization of the sinus cavity and a drainage tube can be inserted and sutured in place. Some authors have recommended regular lavage through this tube over the following 48–72 hours or until the return is clear and fluid begins to drain into the nose, suggesting restored function of the frontal recess. Failure of normal drainage to be re-established may necessitate further surgical intervention such as an external and/or endoscopic frontoethmoidectomy.

In the presence of a pansinusitis, which is usually the case, antral lavage may also be indicated and, postoperatively, intravenous antibiotics should be continued.

Complications

Careful placing of the incision avoids damage to the trochlea, supraorbital and supratrochlear nerves. Care should be taken with anteriorly placed dura behind the frontal sinus which may have been exposed by the infection or natural dehiscences in the bone.

Osteoplastic flap procedure

Indications

This procedure was primarily designed for chronic suppurative frontal sinusitis which had failed all other means of treatment. It has been used to access large osteomas, for the repair of trauma in this region and in the treatment of frontoethmoidal mucocoeles.

Contraindications

If the ethmoids are extensively involved, it can be difficult to gain access to this region via the osteoplastic flap alone.

Preoperative preparation and surgical technique

X-rays of the frontal region are taken to determine the extent of the sinuses and the pathological changes. From the X-ray, a template of the sinus can be made using silastic sheeting which can be sterilized. Prophylactic broad-spectrum antibiotics are recommended which can be modified if necessary depending on subsequent bacteriological findings.

The operation is performed under general anaesthesia, in the reverse Trendelenberg position, with 15° of head flexion. The head should be positioned so that the plane of the forehead is horizontal. The skin should be shaved in a 2.5 cm strip within the hairline and prepared with aqueous preparation solution such as Hibitane. If the obliteration is to be performed, the abdomen must also be prepared. Temporary tarsorraphies are performed and infiltration with lignocaine and adrenalin is helpful.

A coronal incision is made, through the skin, subcutaneous tissue and frontalis muscle, behind the hairline, but taking care not to incise the periosteum. The flap is elevated inferiorly in the plane between the frontalis muscle and the periosteum down to the supraorbital rims and glabella. Neurosurgical clips are useful for haemostasis and the incision is extended inferiorly to a point just anterior to the root of the helix to provide wide exposure (Figure 12.12).

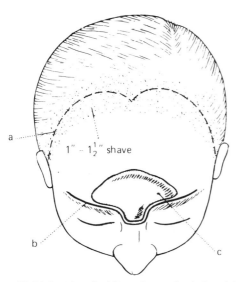

Figure 12.12 Incisions for bilateral osteoplastic flap. (*a*) Coronal incision, (*b*) eyebrow incision (*c*) X-ray template

The sterilized template is then placed over the frontal sinuses, aligning the supraorbital rims exactly and the lateral and superior margins of the sinus are marked with methylene blue. The periosteum may then be incised along this line down to bone. The periosteum is elevated for 2–3 mm either side of the incision to facilitate closure.

Using a fissure burr or oscillating saw, a cut is made round the outline, cutting just inside the line to ensure the incision is within the sinus and bevelling it obliquely to prevent the bone falling into the cavity on replacement. The entire margin is cut around, including the supraorbital rims, leaving only the soft tissue attachment at the glabella. It is often necessary to cut through the intersinus septum with a chisel to free the anterior wall which can then be prised down and forwards, so that the flap is hinged along the floor of the frontal sinus just posterior to the supraorbital rim (Figures 12.13 and 12.14).

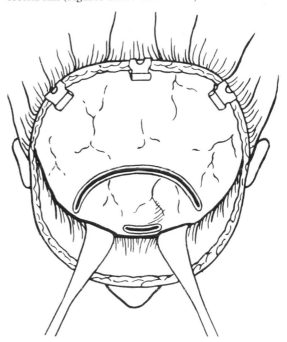

Figure 12.13 The coronal flap has been reflected inferiorly: incisions through the periosteum and bone are shown

All diseased mucosa can be removed completely and the bone burred to remove all traces of mucous membrane. The last vestiges are inverted down into the frontal sinus ostium. If an attempt is being made to obliterate the sinus, fat from the left lower quadrant of the anterior abdominal wall is removed as atraumatically as possible. (The right side is not used to avoid confusion with an appendicectomy scar.) The abdominal wound is closed in layers after achieving haemostasis. The fat is placed in the sinus cavity which should be filled completely.

The bony flap is replaced, and the periosteal layer repaired meticulously to avoid cosmetic deformity. The skin is sutured in two layers and a pressure dressing applied for 24 hours. An alternative incision can be made just above or below the eyebrows and connected across the glabella (spectacle incision). This is suitable when the sinus is small or in men with male-pattern baldness. The eyebrows should never be shaved.

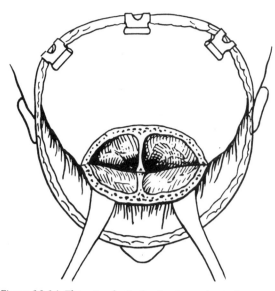

Figure 12.14 The osteoplastic flap has been elevated exposing the contents of the frontal sinuses

The preceding description applies to operations for bilateral disease, but it is possible to open one sinus alone by cutting parallel and lateral to the intersinus septum, the position of which can be determined from the radiology (Figures 12.15 and 12.16).

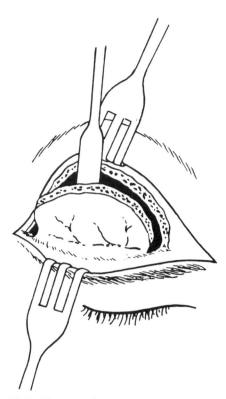

Figure 12.16 Elevation of unilateral osteoplastic flap to expose right frontal sinus

Complications

Cosmetic problems associated with the incision and repair are not uncommon and haematoma collection under the flap may occur. Frontal bossing, depression of the bone flap and nasal skin necrosis have been reported (Sessions *et al.*, 1972; Ward and Bauknight, 1973; Schenck, 1975; Hardy and Montgomery, 1976) and may require subsequent cranioplasty and bone grafting. In middle-aged men with receding hair lines even the best coronal scar may become obvious with time so a spectacle incision may be preferred.

Osteomyelitis can develop in the bone flap and both primary and donor sites can become infected. The dura may be torn if the template is incorrectly drawn or copied leading to a cerebrospinal fluid leak and, as with all operations for sinusitis, the possibility of recurrence of disease has been reported to be as high as 25% (Schenck, 1975).

Endoscopic sinus surgery

Indications

The following list of conditions are amenable to an endoscopic approach:

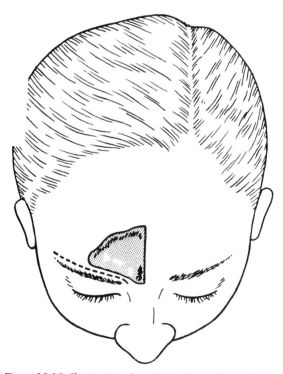

Figure 12.15 Skin incision for unilateral osteoplastic flap

- Chronic sinusitis
- Acute recurrent sinusitis
- Nasal polyposis
- Frontoethmoidal mucocoeles
- Allergic fungal sinusitis and mycetoma
- Repair of CSF leaks
- Orbital and optic nerve decompression
- Repair of blow-out fractures
- Dacrocystorhinostomy
- Choanal atresia
- Hypophysectomy
- Septal and turbinate surgery
- Management of epistaxis
- Drainage of periorbital abscess
- Management of circumscribed benign tumours.

Only the treatment of *chronic* and *acute recurrent sinusitis* could be regarded as exercising a 'functional' approach, i.e. attempting to reverse pathophysiological processes by conservative surgery in defined areas dictated by disease. It should only be offered after an adequate trial of medical treatment and wherever possible treatment of any underlying factors. If such predisposing conditions exist, they will require long-term management and this is also true of conditions such as nasal polyposis. The rest of the list represent conditions which may be successfully approached in many cases with an endoscope.

Nasal polyposis in particular represents a considerable spectrum of disease, from a small area of localized oedema where mucosal surfaces touch (Figure 12.17) to diffuse change throughout the nose and sinuses (Figure 12.18), in their most aggressive form associated with asthma, aspirin idiosyncrasy or cystic fibrosis. It may be possible to perform conservative surgery within the middle meatus but it was for the more extensive disease which had already undergone repeated surgery, with loss of surgical landmarks

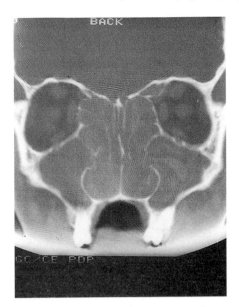

Figure 12.18 Coronal CT scan showing gross polyposis

that Wigand advocated defining the skull base in the sphenoid and working from posterior to anterior (1981, 1990).

Frontoethmoidal mucocoeles can be eminently suitable for an endoscopic approach (Figure 12.19) (Kennedy *et al.*, 1989) but are not always accessible by this approach for technical reasons. Endoscopic marsupialization offers the advantage of avoiding a scar and are associated with less diplopia as the

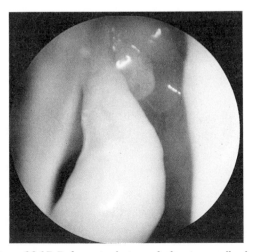

Figure 12.17 Endoscopic photograph showing small polyp in the middle meatus

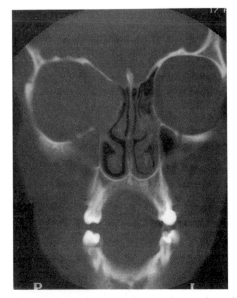

Figure 12.19 Coronal CT scan showing frontoethmoidal mucocoele accessible to an endoscopic approach

trochlea is not disturbed and bone remodelling may mean complete orbital repositioning is less immediate. However, by the same token, the orbital displacement due to bony expansion may take some months to resolve completely. It is particularly suitable in the young and avoids unphysiological stenting of the frontal recess but the patient should be available for follow up. It can also be combined with an external approach when necessary.

When gross polyposis is found associated with quantities of thick green-brown sludge, the possibility of an allergic reaction to fungus should be considered. This will require specific histological stains as it is rare for the microbiologist to culture the offending organism. *Allergic fungal sinusitis* is thus becoming increasingly recognized, having been first described by Katzenstein, Sale and Greenberger (1983), similar in aetiology to allergic aspergillus bronchopulmonary asthma. The treatment is by ventilation and drainage, by a variety of techniques (Waxman *et al.*, 1987; Jonathen, Lund and Milroy, 1989) of which an endoscopic approach has been most successfully applied (Stammberger, 1984, 1985c). It is important, however, to distinguish between this condition where the fungal hyphae are exclusively extramucosal within the secretions and invasive fungal sinusitis which is potentially a fatal disease requiring radical drainage and systemic antifungals.

The endoscope may facilitate access to the skull base for defining the origin and *repair of cerebrospinal fluid leaks* (Figure 12.20) (Papay *et al.*, 1989; Mattox and Kennedy, 1990; Stankiewicz, 1991) and to the orbit for *decompression* or repair of the medial and lateral walls (Yamaguchi *et al.*, 1991) and direct

decompression of the optic canal in selected cases of trauma. Similarly it is an extremely elegant approach for *dacrocystorhinostomy* (Figure 12.21) both in primary and secondary cases and is of particular value in children and young adults, avoiding a facial scar.

Access to *choanal atresia* and the *pituitary gland* via the sphenoid can also be achieved in many cases endoscopically, with bleeding and individual anatomy being the main limiting factors.

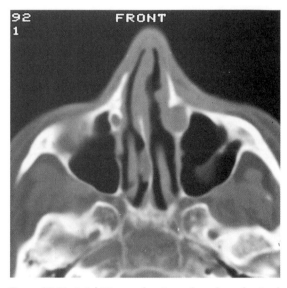

Figure 12.21 Axial CT scan showing enlarged nasolacrimal duct

There has been a tendency to move away from indiscriminate *septal correction*, which has been supported by subsequent surgical results, towards only removing those parts of the septum which limit access to the middle meatus (Figure 12.22). Thus it is per-

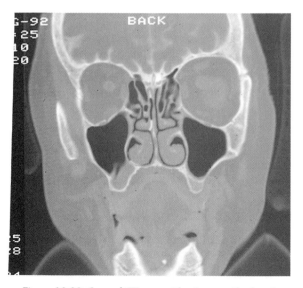

Figure 12.20 Coronal CT scan with nitressamide showing CSF leak from anterior base of skull

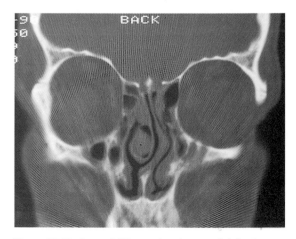

Figure 12.22 Coronal CT scan showing septal deflection impinging on middle meatus

fectly possible to remove a localized spur, usually at the junction of vomer and perpendicular plate of ethmoid under endoscopic control, by cutting directly down onto the deflection.

The endoscope can be combined with other instrumentation such as the *laser* (KTP, Holmium YAG or argon)(Levine, 1989; Shapshay, Rebeinz and Bohigian, 1991) with some success in treating mild to moderate *epistaxis* in hereditary haemorrhagic telangiectasia and reduction of the inferior turbinate. The latter can be done either as for linear cautery or preferably by a cross-hatching technique which produces maximum contraction while preserving islands of normal mucosa. In recurrent epistaxis, the bleeding area may be determined (though this may be difficult in the acute situation) and the lateral sphenopalatine artery can be reached directly as it enters the lateral wall of the nose and liga clipped or diathermied under endoscopic control.

Considerable caution must be exercised in recommending an endoscopic approach for cases of complicated sinusitis. If an *orbital abscess* is extraperiosteal and accessible, an experienced endoscopic sinus surgeon may choose this route for drainage and the treatment of associated sinus infection but wherever vision is potentially at risk, a conventional external approach plus antral drainage is recommended. The acutely infected nose and sinus offers the worst surgical field and the opportunity to save vision should not be compromised by any delay.

Concern has also been strongly expressed regarding recommendations to manage *sinonasal neoplasia* endoscopically. It should be categorically stated that the first removal of a sinonasal tumour is the best opportunity to cure. Therefore, only if there is definite evidence both endoscopically and on imaging of a limited lesion should an endoscopic removal be used for lesions such as inverted papilloma. This situation is rarely encountered at presentation and there are presently insufficient long-term studies to support this approach; suffice to say that a recurrence rate of 50% existed with external frontoethmoidectomy and Caldwell–Luc approaches in contradistinction to 13% or less with a lateral rhinotomy or midfacial degloving approach (Harrison and Lund, 1993). Thus only an experienced endoscopic surgeon should consider it.

These comments apply even more so to malignant disease, with one exception; in addition to allowing careful follow up, occasionally localized recurrence may occur within the surgical cavity which for various reasons cannot be given further radical treatment. Under these circumstances cryosurgery or laser treatment can be given under endoscopic control.

Contraindications

As stated above, Stammberger (1991) considered that, in the presence of an orbital extension of acute sinusitis if there is the slightest suggestion of an intracranial complication such as meningitis, subperiosteal or epidural abscess or cavernous sinus thrombosis or with any visual loss, the Messerklinger technique is contraindicated. He also concluded that this approach is contraindicated as the route to the maxillary antrum when a mycotic mass completely fills the sinus which cannot be removed even through an enlarged ostium or in certain cases of revision surgery when the antrum has become 'compartmentalized'.

Pathology in the frontal sinus is notoriously difficult to treat. If the frontal recess cannot be accurately identified for whatever reason (osteitic change, gross inflammatory change, scarring, previous surgery or trauma), the nasal route should be abandoned. A 'combined approach' using a burr-hole in the anterior wall of the frontal sinus may be useful in some cases with angled endoscopes introduced and controlled from above. Pathology localized in the lateral frontal sinus may not be technically accessible and widely based osteomas cannot be approached endoscopically.

As previously indicated the endoscope is not indicated when dealing with malignant tumours other than for diagnosis or endoscopic control at follow up.

Anaesthesia

Endoscopic surgery can be performed under local or general anaesthesia. Stammberger (1991) and Kennedy (1985) have declared a preference for local anaesthesia, believing that it is safer and associated with less bleeding while Anand and Panje (1992) state that 'efficiency, reduced pain, controlled ventilation, especially for asthmatics and avoidance of aspiration are our primary reasons for the choice of general anaesthesia'. It is difficult to refute the suggestion that local anaesthesia is safer, though generally complications are more likely to occur in those patients with more advanced pathology such as nasal polyposis and it is this group which is more likely to be selected for general anaesthesia.

The authors' preference is for general anaesthesia except in those cases with minimal pathology, when the patient has particularly requested a local anaesthetic or occasionally when their general state of health is so poor that general anaesthesia is contraindicated.

Local anaesthesia is carried out in a similar manner to that for antral lavage except that further injections are made with 2% lignocaine (with 1:80 000) into the uncinate process, greater palatine foramen and middle turbinate (up to 4 ml).

With general anaesthesia, Moffatt's solution is instilled in the anaesthetic room (2 ml of 2% sodium bicarbonate, 2 ml of 10% cocaine and 1 ml of 1:1000 adrenalin), half in each nostril. The patient's head is left hyperextended for 10 minutes before he is transferred to the main operating room where he is placed on the operating table in the supine position. If the surgeon prefers to sit, the table is kept low and horizontal. If the surgeon wishes to stand, the left elbow can be supported on a Loewy support placed towards the head of the table and the patient put in a head-up position which aids haemostasis. Further vasoconstriction can be achieved with ribbon gauze soaked in 1:1000 adrenalin packed around the middle meatus and surgical cavity.

The CT scan should always be available in theatre.

In either case, the patients are usually kept in hospital over night and discharged the following day (usually less than 24 hours admission). Packing is avoided if possible though sometimes a small temporary Telfa or Merocel pack is placed in the surgical cavity.

Surgical technique

A zero degree 4 mm Hopkins rod telescope should be used for most of the surgery, as it is easy to become disorientated with angled endoscopes though the latter are necessary for inspecting recesses and performing middle meatal antrostomy or operating in the frontonasal recess.

An infundibulotomy is then performed by incising the anterior attachment of the uncinate process with a sickle knife. A Freer elevator can be used to lift the uncinate process and it is then grasped with forceps, the upper and lower attachments cut with fine scissors and the process detached with a twisting motion. Care is taken with the site of incision. If this is made too far anteriorly, the bone is hard overlying the nasolacrimal duct. Any residual rim can be removed secondarily with back-biting forceps, again with care to avoid damage to the nasolacrimal duct.

The ethmoidal bulla is opened with a fine straight Blakesley-Wilde forceps and removed piecemeal. The lamina papyracea is extremely thin, through which the yellow orbital fat can often be discerned. Slight pressure on the globe will demonstrate whether the lamina is dehiscent. Behind the bulla, one enters a variable space, the lateral sinus, while superiorly the skull base should be visible and the anterior ethmoidal artery may be identified.

In many cases, this may be all that is required and the decision as to whether to continue to open the maxillary antrum, explore the frontal recess, the posterior ethmoids and sphenoid will depend upon the extent of disease as evidenced by the CT scan and operative findings. The posterior ethmoids are entered by piercing the ground lamella, the lateral attachment of the middle turbinate, 3–4 mm above the horizontal attachment of the turbinate. The posterior cells are generally larger and pyramidal in shape. The optic nerve can be prominent in the lateral wall and the overlying bone extremely thin. The sphenoid can be opened from the posterior ethmoid, by entering it as

inferiorly and medially as possible from the last cell. However, mucociliary clearance occurs into the sphenoethmoidal recess, and it is more logical to enlarge the natural ostium of the sinus. The ostium in the bone of the sphenoid is usually 3–4 mm in diameter and can usually be found by blunt probing approximately 1cm up on the anterior face of the sphenoid, adjacent to the septum. Great care must be exercised in the sphenoid sinus which is variable in size and shape and intimately related to the carotid artery and optic nerve. It is also worth checking the superior meatus and clearing any local pathology so that there is free access into the posterior ethmoidal system.

Middle meatal antrostomy is not necessary if the natural maxillary ostium is patent when uncovered by removal of the uncinate process. If an accessory ostium is present, it should be joined to the natural ostium to avoid abnormal circulation of mucus. As a principle, it is better to enlarge the ostium inferiorly and anteriorly into the respective fontanelles rather than posteriorly to prevent disruption of mucus clearance over the posterior ostial edge. If the ostium is not readily visible after uncinectomy, palpation of the lateral wall with a blunt probe, 'J' curette or curved sucker will usually identify the position, or a few bubbles of mucus may be seen. Once identified, the ostium can be enlarged with fine forward-biting Grunwald forceps ('chompers'), anteriorly and inferiorly with Stammberger Ostrom type back-biting and down-biting punches, again taking care to avoid the nasolacrimal duct and/or lateral sphenopalatine artery. If the ostium cannot be found, the posterior fontanelle can be perforated just above the attachment of the inferior turbinate.

It is advisable to limit removal of mucosa in the frontal recess to avoid scarring and to rely upon medication instilled postoperatively to effect improvement. To avoid bleeding running into the operative field, it is best to reserve surgery in this area to the end of the operation. The uncinate process may attach laterally onto the lamina papyracea. Under these circumstances, the infundibulum leads into the blind-ending terminal recess. When the uncinate process attaches superiorly or rarely medially to the middle turbinate, it is possible directly to visualize the frontal recess with a 30° scope in most cases (preferably with the light cable entering at 90°). A number of angled instruments and curettes have been devised for surgery in this area, which is certainly the most challenging surgically. The frontal recess is usually an hour-glass restriction rather than a 'duct' and is often found situated medial to an opening of a suprabullar ethmoidal cell which extends over the orbital roof. Care should always be taken operating in this area to avoid damage to the anterior ethmoidal artery and entry into the anterior cranial fossa where the artery traverses the medial superior ethmoidal cavity.

Postoperative management

A significant component in the success of endoscopic surgery is meticulous postoperative cleaning of the surgical cavity. This represents an important commitment on the part of the surgeon. It is the authors' practice to give all patients prophylactic broad spectrum antibiotics for 2 weeks postoperatively, combined with alkaline nasal douche and an intranasal steroid preparation. All patients with diffuse polyposis receive a course of oral steroids in reducing dosage (prednisolone 30 mg/20 mg/10 mg each for one week or dexamethasone 12 mg × 3 days, 8 mg × 3 days, 4 mg × 3 days) if there are no contraindications. In severe cases, a similar course is given preoperatively and all patients remain on intranasal steroids prior to surgery,

The patients are usually seen 7–10 days after the surgery and then as often as necessary, usually on a 1–2 weekly basis until the cavities are well-healed. For the purposes of audit, the patients are seen at least at 3, 6, 12, and 24 months postoperatively. On each visit the cavity is cleaned under endoscopic control following application of topical local anaesthetic at which any adhesions are divided, debris removed, further polypoid mucosa removed and additional medication prescribed.

Complications

Such is the excellent visualization provided by an endoscopic approach that a false sense of security may lead the unwary into problems. In the hands of the experienced, reported complications are surprisingly few and similar to those reported by other approaches (Table 12.3). In a series of over 4000 cases, Stammberger and Wolf (1988) reported only two cases of cerebrospinal fluid (CSF) rhinorrhoea, no intracranial complications and no ophthalmic problems. Wigand (1990) reporting on 220 patients undergoing complete ethmoidectomy mainly for polyposis, reported a CSF leak in two (0.9%) and one case of an orbital haematoma (0.5%).

Stankiewicz (1989) suggested that the complication rate decreases with increasing experience, reporting a rate of 29% in the first 90 cases which he performed compared with only 2.2% in the subsequent 90. Most of the cases were minor, such as adhesions but there were two cases of CSF rhinorrhoea and one case of temporary blindness. 'Conventional' surgery is not immune from these problems and Maniglia (1989) reported seven cases of blindness, four cases of CSF rhinorrhoea and two deaths following intranasal ethmoidectomy while a 2.8% complication rate was reported for this operation by Freedman and Kern (1979).

In a group of 650 consecutive patients operated on by the authors, one patient developed a CSF leak on the third postoperative day, after he sneezed. This was managed endoscopically with a free mucoperichondrial graft from the opposite side of the septum. One further case required an external ethmoidectomy at the time of the surgery due to an orbital haematoma resulting from bleeding from the anterior ethmoidal artery which retracted into the orbit. Both cases underwent satisfactory and uneventful postoperative recovery. There have been no cases of diplopia, blindness, meningitis or death.

In a survey of British otolaryngologists (Cumberworth and Mackay, 1994), a questionnaire sent to 653 members of the British Association of Otolaryngologists, received a 57% response of whom 38% were reportedly routinely undertaking functional endoscopic sinus surgery. The estimated complication rate was 0.24%, predominantly CSF leaks, followed by problems related to bleeding. All occurred in patients with diffuse polyposis.

A Working Party of the Royal College of Surgeons

Table 12.3 Complications following sinus surgery

Authors	Operation	No. patients	CSF leak	Intracranial infection	Orbital complications	Haemorrhage	Death
Stankiewicz (1987)	FESS	90	1	—	1	2	—
Stankiewicz (1989)	FESS	90	1	—	—	—	—
Stammberger and Wolf (1988)	FESS	4000 +	2	—	—	—	—
Schaefer *et al.* (1989)	FESS	100	—	—	—	—	—
Levine (1990)	FESS	250	—	—	3	—	—
Levine *et al.* (1990)	FESS	100	1	—	—	—	—
Wigand and Hoseman (1991)	FESS	1000 +	10	2	—	1	1
Danielsen (1992)	FESS	100	—	—	—	—	—
Lazar, Younis and Long (1993)	FESS	773	2	1	—	—	—
Freedman and Kern (1979)	INE	1000	1	1	—	12	—
Watson and Griffiths (1988)	INE	105	—	—	1	—	—
Lund (1990)	EE	320	—	—	—	—	—

FESS = functional endoscopic sinus surgery; INE = intranasal ethmoidectomy; EE = external ethmoidectomy.

of Edinburgh (Maran *et al.*, 1993) was set up to consider ways of reducing complications associated with endoscopic sinus surgery. Among the various conclusions it included the following suggestions:

1 The operator should have experience of at least a 100 diagnostic endoscopic procedure before attempting surgery.
2 The surgeon should attend and participate in a course or workshop that allows hands-on experience.
3 Where possible a proctor system should be encouraged with an experienced surgeon attending initial operations.
4 Follow-up and assessment clinics should wherever possible be separate from the general clinics and should be used for training and audit purposes.
5 CT scan facilities should be available.

Concerns have been raised regarding the long-term effects of such surgery, as to whether surgery in the frontal recess may lead to frontoethmoidal mucocoele formation in the future and in particular the effects of endoscopic surgery in children on facial growth. There have not been any hard data to support the propositions so far and indeed the latter is unlikely given that major sinus procedures such as external ethmoidectomy, lateral rhinotomy and craniofacial resection appear to have no detrimental effect in the long term. The patency of the middle meatal antrostomy appears more reliable that that of the inferior meatus despite its smaller size (Figure 12.23) (Kennedy *et al.*, 1987). This is probably related to its action as a natural physiological fistula made predominantly in membrane rather than bone and generally not enlarged circumferentially (Lund, 1993).

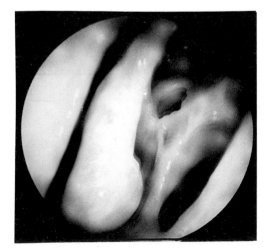

Figure 12.23 Endoscopic photograph of middle meatal antrostomy

Results

Excellent results have been reported by many authors (Stammberger and Posawetz, 1990; Wigand, 1990; Lund, Holmstrom and Scadding, 1991; Stammberger, 1991) following endoscopic sinus surgery, Wigand (1990) reported the subjective assessment of symptoms following endoscopic ethmoidectomy primarily for polyposis in 220 answers returned from 310 questionnaires. Eighty-five per cent rated the procedure successful overall and facial pain and headache were assessed as better by 93.4%. Stammberger (1991) reported similar results on a more heterogeneous group of 500 patients with follow up of between 8 months and 10 years, with 85% having very good improvement.

In a study of 650 of the authors' patients with follow up in excess of 6 months, who fell into two broad categories of chronic rhinosinusitis (51%) or nasal polyposis (48%), individuals were assessed overall as cured, improved, unchanged or worsened by surgery and by individual symptom (ranked into first, second or third) (Lund and Mackay, 1994). Discharge and nasal blockage were the commonest symptoms, with blockage being the most frequent first symptom (Figure 12.24). Eighty-seven per cent regarded themselves as cured or improved, 11% were unchanged and 2% worse. Similar results pertained to both polyposis and chronic rhinosinusitis and were achieved irrespective of many of the systemic conditions such as asthma and immune deficiency which might have had an adverse effect (Table 12.4). However, those polyp patients with cystic fibrosis, especially those who had undergone heart-lung transplants, rated the operation a success in only 54%. All individual symptoms improved significantly, of which nasal blockage (92% cure or improvement) and facial pain (86% cure or improvement) did particularly well and this applied whether the symptom was first, second or third in importance to the patient.

Evaluation of success is however, beset with difficulties as patients may feel well despite a surgical cavity which on endoscopic examination reveals obvious disease (Kennedy, 1992) and neither endoscopic nor

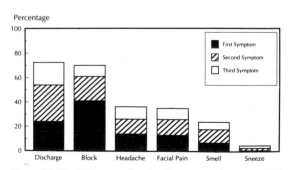

Figure 12.24 Histogram showing frequency of preoperative symptoms in patients undergoing endoscopic sinus surgery.

Table 12.4 Systemic diagnosis in patients undergoing endoscopic sinus surgery

	Number	*Percentage*		
		Improved	*Same*	*Worse*
Asthma	81	94	6	0
(Asthma/ASA	19)			
Cystic fibrosis	28	54	46	0
(CF/HLT	10)			
Immune deficiency (primary and secondary)	14	79	14	7
Bronchiectasis	13	85	15	0
Myeloma	1			
Wegener's granuloma	1			
Sarcoid	2			

21% of series with contributory systemic diagnosis
ASA: asthma and aspirin sensitivity
CF/HLT: cystic fibrosis/heart-lung transplantation

CT findings correlate with symptoms. In an attempt to overcome some of these problems, an objective assessment was conducted on 200 patients with chronic rhinosinusitis, with between 1 and 4 years' follow up. Symptoms were assessed by visual analogue scoring (VAS), nasomucociliary function by ciliary beat frequency (CBF), olfaction by quantitative olfactometry (UPSIT: University of Pennsylvania Smell Identification Test) and olfactory threshold assessment (Olfacto-Labs; pm-carbinol), nasal airway by nasal forced inspiratory peak flow, anterior rhinomanometry, and in selected cases acoustic rhinometry which provides topographical information on the nasal cavity. All tests were performed preoperatively and postoperatively when the surgical cavities were healed as much as possible, usually at around 3 months. There was a significant improvement in all symptom VAS, in CBF and both olfactory tests. As expected, neither nasal inspiratory peak flow nor airway resistance altered. The acoustic rhinometry allowed some quantification of the surgical cavities created.

The dramatic improvement in the subjective sensation of nasal obstruction, despite nasal airflow remaining unchanged may be explained by the removal of inflammatory tissue within the middle meatus and indicates why many of these patients had already undergone unsuccessful septal and turbinate surgery to improve this symptom.

These results must be put into perspective and compared with other surgical procedures designed to treat the same condition. Although several studies comparing endoscopic surgery with inferior meatal antrostomy and a Caldwell–Luc procedure have been performed (Arnes, Anke and Mair, 1985; Stammberger *et al* 1987), they suffer from the disadvantage that they do not compare like with like, either surgically or in patient population. If an historical comparison is made between two prospective groups of chronic rhinosinusitics (65 undergoing inferior meatal antrostomy (Lund, 1988) and 650 undergoing functional endoscopic sinus surgery (Lund and Mackay, 1994) similar overall rates of subjective improvement are obtained (84% versus 87% respectively). However, when the percentage of symptoms which are the same or worse following the surgery are compared, the functional endoscopic sinus surgery patients do significantly better in all cases (Table 12.5). Once the cavity has healed well (Figure 12.25) it generally remains healthy.

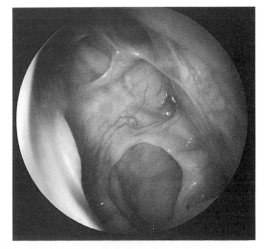

Figure 12.25 Well healed ethmoidal cavity following endoscopic sinus surgery

Table 12.5 Symptoms the same or worse (%)

	Endoscopic sinus surgery (n = 650)	Inferior meatal antrostomy (n = 65)
Discharge	22	62
Block	8	20
Headache	17	42
Facial pain	14	38

Staging of rhinosinusitis

Some of the problems encountered in result assessment may be overcome by accurate staging of the extent of sinusitis. This has been addressed by several authors (Gaskins, 1992; Kennedy, 1992) but suffers from a complexity which has precluded its entering routine clinical practice. A simplified approach has been devised (Lund and Mackay, 1993) which produces a numerical score for four aspects of the condition.

1 The preoperative CT findings are assessed using a scoring system for each of the sinus systems (maxilla, anterior ethmoids, posterior ethmoids, frontal and sphenoid) of 0–2, where 0 = no abnormality, 1 = partial opacification and 2 = total opacification and 0 or 2 for the ostiomeatal complex. A maximum score of 24 is thus possible and each side can be considered separately. Anatomical variants can also be scored on a 0 or 1 basis but are not included in the CT score.
2 The symptoms are evaluated on a visual analogue score (VAS) of 0–10 (where 0 = none and 10 = the most severe) for:
  a Nasal congestion
  b Headache
  c Facial pain
  d Sense of smell
  e Nasal discharge
  f Overall symptomatic assessment.
The VAS is performed pretherapy and at regular intervals post-treatment.
3 A surgical score is derived for each manoeuvre of an endoscopic operation (0 = not performed, 1 = undertaken), producing a maximum score of 14.
  a Uncinectomy
  b Reduction of middle turbinate
  c Middle meatal antrostomy
  d Anterior ethmoidectomy
  e Posterior ethmoidectomy
  f Sphenoidotomy
  g Frontal recess surgery
4 Endoscopic appearances are quantified on a 0–2 point basis for the presence of polyps, discharge, oedema, scarring or adhesions and crusting and this is also performed pre- and post-therapy.

The development of any staging system is an evolutionary process and the simplicity of the above may be criticized for over-diagnosing disease extent when secretion rather than mucosal change produces sinus opacification. Indeed it ultimately may be that those with limited disease, as evidenced by a 'black halo' appearance on CT scanning (Mackay, 1994) do well (Figure 12.26) and patients with complete opacification (or 'white-out') do badly. However, unless attempts are made to quantify sinusitis, contention will continue to surround the results of any treatment modality.

Endoscopic dacryocystorhinostomy

(McDonogh and Meiring, 1989; El-Khoury and Rouvier, 1992)

The nasolacrimal duct and sac are readily accessible from the nasal cavity, running just anterior to the anterior end of the middle turbinate and attachment of the uncinate process. The mucosa can be incised in an 'I' over this region and the mucosal flaps elevated. Bone is removed using an angled drill. The exact site of the sac can be located with a single light

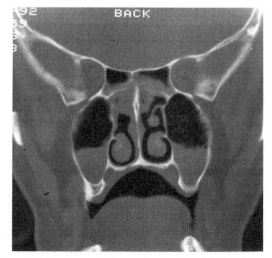

Figure 12.26 Coronal CT scan showing 'black halo' of air around central opacification

fibre inserted via either the upper or lower medial canthal punctum. Once an adequate area of the nasolacrimal system is exposed, it can be incised either with a Beaver myringotome, angled sickle knife or argon laser. The mucosal edges of the duct and nasal lining can be approximated with liga clips and a temporary stent may be inserted.

An endoscopic technique is particularly suitable for secondary procedures or primary operations in children and young adults though so far the published long-term results are not as quite as good as those for conventional external approaches.

Endoscopic orbital decompression
(Kennedy *et al.*, 1990)

The main indication is for malignant exophthalmos in thyroid eye disease. The medial and inferior orbital wall can be removed successfully by an endoscopic approach. It is necessary to make an extremely large middle meatal antrostomy in order to reach as far laterally as the infraorbital nerve but has the advantage of avoiding an external scar, detachment of the inferior oblique muscle and less potential damage to the nasolacrimal duct. It also provides safe access to the thick sphenoid bone around the orbital apex which can be removed in cases of severe optic nerve compression and visual deterioration. Periosteal incisions can be readily effected with an angled sickle knife or myringotome.

The optic nerve may also be decompressed in cases of trauma associated with visual loss. A special drill with irrigation to prevent overheating of the tissues is required accurately to remove the hard sphenoidal bone. Incision of the perineurium is somewhat contentitious as it may lead to a CSF leak or actually damage the nerve but has been advocated by some. However, optic nerve decompression is generally only effective when some residual vision is present.

Endoscopic repair of cerebrospinal fluid leaks

Defects in the skull base, either congenital or acquired, are often amenable to an intranasal endoscopic approach which, if successful, avoids the inconveniences of an external ethmoidectomy or anterior craniotomy. The exact site may be better defined by a nitressamide CT scan or the use of intrathecal fluorescien (Mattox and Kennedy, 1990). The latter must be used under the following strict precautions:

1 Five per cent sodium fluorescin for intravenous use may be used but must be checked for the presence of bacterial pyrogens which sterilization does not eradicate and which are responsible for the pyrexia which can sometimes follow its use.

2 A small test dose of the fluorescien (0.2ml) is administered intravenously in the anaesthetic room immediately prior to intrathecal use with full resuscitation equipment available, in particular to deal with a grand mal episode.

3 A low lumbar puncture is performed, at L3/4 or L4/5, never in the thoracic or cervical region.

4 Ten millilitres of CSF are withdrawn and mixed with 0.2–0.75 ml of fluorescien which is then reintroduced. The patient may then be returned to the ward for 2 hours prior to the repair and kept horizontal.

5 Some authors have also recommended the use of systemic antihistamines preoperatively and with the premedication.

A blue filter can be used in the endoscope system which may enhance the yellow fluorescence in difficult cases. It may be necessary to open the ethmoid system to visual the skull base or enlarge the sphenoidal ostium. The dehiscent area is then repaired with a free mucosal flap taken from the middle turbinate or septum, though dermal fat and fascia have also been employed. The graft may be positioned with tissue glue, synthetic glues and/or a variety of packings. Prophylactic antibiotics should be administered.

Sinusitis in children

The management of children with recurrent or chronic sinus infections has always been a source of debate. Radical surgery is generally avoided because of concerns regarding the long-term effects on dentition. In most cases when medical treatment failed, antral washout, combined with adenotonsillectomy was the mainstay of surgical management on the basis that the tonsils and adenoids acted as reservoirs of infection, with inferior meatal antrostomy reserved for recalcitrant cases. It should always be remembered, however, that congenital abnormalities of immune and mucociliary function may present in the upper respiratory tract at a young age and these should be considered in any individual who does not improve with conservative therapy. In addition there is increasing evidence that allergy may contribute to the development of infection (Holmstrom, Lund and Scadding, 1992) and should always be adequately treated.

Endoscopic sinus surgery in the paediatric population has raised a number of concerns related to the necessity for imaging, potential complications, the possible need for subsequent general anaesthetics to perform postoperative cleaning, and suggestions that in the long term this surgery may create frontoethmoidal mucocoeles or affect facial growth. Lusk (1992) has been at the forefront of introducing functional endoscopic sinus surgery in children and has emphasized the need for great care in both patient selection and surgical conservatism. There does not appear to be any evidence of abnormal midfacial growth in children undergoing radical ethmoidal surgery such as lateral rhinotomy or craniofacial resection for benign neoplasia so it would seem unlikely that uncinectomy, opening the bulla and middle meatal antrostomy would of themselves create such problems, as research suggests that it is the cartilaginous septum and palate which are the primary determinants of growth. However, caution is certainly required in advocating this surgery and should only be undertaken by experienced surgeons familiar both with the technique and paediatric anatomy.

Conclusions

A range of operations exists for the treatment of acute and chronic rhinosinusitis; the choice will be determined by the experience and philosophical attitude of the surgeon. The importance of the ostiomeatal region in the development of infection has been recognized for a century (Caldwell, 1893) and the diagnostic role of the endoscope (and CT scan) is well established. An endoscopic approach offers many advantages over more 'conventional' operations but also requires specific training. Nor does endoscopic surgery encompass all cases of sinus inflammation and infection. Indeed, experience with an external ethmoidectomy approach is a prerequisite of endoscopic surgery should an acute orbital haematoma develop during surgery. Perhaps of greater importance is the 'renaissance in rhinology' which endoscopic surgery has generated, forcing a re-examination of the pathophysiology of rhinosinusitis, its classification, quantification and diagnosis.

References

ANAND, V. K. and PANJE, W. R. (1992) *Practical Endoscopic Sinus Surgery*. New York: McGraw-Hill

ARNES, E., ANKE, I. M. and MAIR, I. W. S. (1985) A comparison between middle and inferior meatal antrostomy in the treatment of chronic maxillary sinus infection. *Rhinology*, **23**, 65–69

BARON, S. H., DEDO, H. H. and HENRY, C. R. (1973) The mucoperiosteal flap in frontal sinus surgery. *Laryngoscope*, **83**, 1266–1280

BENNINGER, M. S., SEBEK, B. A. and LEVINE, H. L. (1989) Mucosal regeneration of the maxillary sinus after surgery. *Otolaryngology, Head and Neck Surgery*, **101**, 33–37

BJORKANDER, J., BAKE, B. and HANSON, L. A. (1984) Primary hypogammaglobulinaemia: impaired lung function and body growth with delayed diagnosis and inadequate treatment. *European Journal of Respiratory Disease*, **65**, 529–536

BOYDEN, G. L. (1952) Surgical treatment of chronic frontal sinusitis. *Annals of Otology, Rhinology and Laryngology*, **61**, 558–566

BUITER, C. T. (1988) Nasal antrostomy. *Rhinology*, **26**, 5–18

CADWELL, G. W. (1893) Diseases of the accessory sinuses of the nose and an improved method of treatment of suppuration of the maxillary antrum. *New York Medical Journal*, **58**, 526–528

CORDES, H. (1905) Bitrag zur Behandlung der chronischen Kiefleshohleneiterung. *Monatsschrift für Ohrenheilkunde*, **39**, 1

COWPER, W. (1707) In Drake, J. *Anatomy [Anthropologia Nova]*, edited by S. Smith and B. Walford, Vol. II. pp. 526–541

CUMBERWORTH, V. L., SUDDERICK, R. M. and MACKAY, I. S. (1994) Major complications of functional endoscopic sinus surgery. *Clinical Otolaryngology*, **19**, 248–253

DANIELSEN, A. (1992) Functional endoscopic sinus surgery on a day case out-patient basis. *Clinical Otolaryngology*, **17**, 473-477

DESAULT, P. J. (1798) Oeuvres chirurgicales ou expose de la doctrine et de la pratique de P. J. Desault. Vol. 1. *Maladies des parties molles*. Chez Meguignon, pp. 142–153

DESSI, P., CASTRO, F., TRIGLIA, J. M., ZANARET, M. and CANNONI, M. (1994) Difference in the height of the right and left ethmoid roofs: a possible risk factor for ethmoid surgery. *Journal of Laryngology and Otology*, (in press)

DRAF, W. (1983) *Endoscopy of the Paranasal Sinuses*. New York: Springer-Verlag

EL-KHOURY, J. and ROUVIER, P. (1992) Dacryocystorhinostomie endonasale. *Acta ORL Belgica*, **46**, 401–404

FALLOPIUS, G. (1600) Abstract Anatomica Frankfurt p. 367. Quoted in Jeanty, J. M. (1891) *De l'empyeme latent de l'antra d'Highmore*, Bordeaux

FELDMAN, C., READ, R., RUTMAN, R., JEFFREY, P., BRAIN, A., LUND, V. et al. (1992) The interaction of *Streptococcus pneumoniae* with intact human respiratory mucosa in vitro. *European Respiratory Journal*, **5** 576–583

FREEDMAN, H. M. and KERN, E. B. (1979) Complications of intranasal ethmoidectomy. *Laryngoscope*, **89**, 421–434

GASKINS, R. E. (1992) A surgical staging system for chronic sinusitis. *American Journal of Rhinology*, **6**, 5–12

GOODALE, R. L. (1945) The use of tantalum in radical frontal sinus surgery. *Annals of Otology, Rhinology and Laryngology*, **54**, 757–762

GOODALE, R. L. and MONTGOMERY, W. W. (1958) Experiences with osteoplastic anterior wall approach to the frontal sinus. *Archives of Otolaryngology*, **68**, 271–283

GOODE, R. L. (1970) An antral catheter for maxillary sinusitis. *Archives of Otolaryngology*, **91**, 302–306

HARDY, J. M. and MONTGOMERY, W. W. (1976) Osteoplastic frontal sinusotomy. *Annals of Otology, Rhinology and Laryngology*, **85**, 523–532

HARRISON, D. F. N. (1981) Surgical approach to the medial orbital wall. *Annals of Otology, Rhinology and Laryngology*, **90**, 415–419

HARRISON, D. F. N. and LUND, V. J. (1993) *Tumours of the Upper Jaw*. London: Churchill Livingstone

HASEGAWA, M., SAITO, Y., WATNABE, I. and KERN, E. B. (1979) Post-operative mucocoeles in the maxillary sinus. *Rhinology*, **17**, 253–256

HASSAB, M. and LUND, V. J. (1994) Correlation of subjective symptomatology with CT findings. *Rhinology*, (In press)

HIGHMORE, N. (1651) Corporis humani disquitio anatomica. *Hagae Comitus*, pp. 225–228

HILDING, A. C. (1932) Physiology of drainage of nasal mucous: experimental work on accessory sinuses. *American Journal of Physiology*, **100**, 644

HILDING, A. C. (1941) Experimental sinus surgery: effects of operative windows on normal sinuses. *Annals of Otology, Rhinology and Laryngology*, **50**, 379–392

HIPPOCRATES (5 BC) Works of. Translated by F. Adam *New York Aphorisms* sec. 6, no. 10, p. 251. London: Wellcome Historical Museum

HIRSCHMANN, A. (1903) Uber Endoskopie der Nase und deren Nebenhohlen. *Archiv für Laryngologie und Rhinologie*, **14**, 195–202

HOLMSTROM, M., LUND, V. J. and SCADDING, G. K. (1992) Nasal ciliary beat frequency following nasal allergen challenge. *American Journal of Rhinology*, **3**, 101–105

HORGAN, J. B. (1926) The surgical approach to the ethmoidal cell system. *Journal of Laryngology and Otology*, **41**, 510–521

HOWARTH, W. G. (1921) A radical frontal sinus operation. *Journal of Laryngology and Otology*, **38**, 341–343

HOWARTH, W. G. (1936) Some points in the technique of the fronto-ethmoidal operation. *Journal of Laryngology and Otology*, **51**, 387–390

HUNTER, J. (1835) *Collected Works*, edited by Palmer, London: Longman. Vol.ii. p. 77. London: Royal College of Surgeons

IMHOFER, R. (1910) Entfernung eines Fremdkorpers aus der Kieferhohle mit Hilfe der Endoskopie. *Zeitschrift fur Laryngologie, Rhinologie, Otologie und ihre Grenzgebeite*

JANSEN, A. (1902) Die Killian'sche Radical-Operation Chronischer Stirnhohleneiterungen. *Ohren, Nasen und Kehlkopfheilkunde*, **56**, 110–112

JONATHEN, D., LUND, V. J. and MILROY, C. (1989) Allergic aspergillus sinusitis – an overlooked diagnosis. *Journal of Laryngology and Otology*, **103**, 1181–1186

KATZENSTEIN, A. A., SALE, S. R. and GREENBERGER, P. A. (1983) Allergic aspergillus sinusitis: a newly recognised form of sinusitis. *Journal of Allergy and Clinical Immunology*, **72**, 89–93

KENNEDY, D. W. (1985) Functional endoscopic sinus surgery: technique. *Archives of Oto-Rhino-Laryngology*, **111**, 643–649

KENNEDY, D. W. (1992) Prognostic factors, outcomes and staging in ethmoid sinus surgery. *Laryngoscope*, Suppl. 57, 1–18

KENNEDY, D. W. and SHAALAN, H. (1989) Reevaluation of maxillary sinus surgery: experimental study in rabbits. *Annals of Otology, Rhinology and Larynology*, **98**, 901–906

KENNEDY, D. W., JOSEPHSON, J. S., ZINREICH, S. J., MATTOX, D. E. and GOLDSMITH, M. M. (1989) Endoscopic sinus surgery for mucoceles: a viable alternative. *Laryngoscope*, **99**, 885–895

KENNEDY, D. W., GOODSTEIN, M. L., MILLER, N. R. and ZINREICH, S. J. (1990) Endoscopic transnasal orbital decompression. *Archives of Otolaryngology, Head and Neck Surgery*, **116**, 275–282

KENNEDY, D. W., ZINREICH, S. J., ROSENBAUM, A. E. and JOHNS, M. E. (1985) Functional endoscopic sinus surgery. Theory and diagnostic evaluation. *Archives of Oto-Rhino-Laryngology*, **111**, 576–582

KENNEDY, D. W., ZINREICH, S. J., KUHN, F. SHAALAN, H., NACLERIO, R. and LOCH, E. (1987) Endoscopic middle meatal antrostomy: theory, technique and patency. *Laryngoscope*, **97** (Suppl. 43), 1–9

KILLIAN, G. (1903) Die Killian'sche Radicaloperation chronischer Stirnhohleneiterungen. *Archiv für Laryngologie und Rhinologie*, **13**, 59–88

KRAUSE, H. (1887) Instrumente rach Dr Krause. *Monatschrift für Ohrenheilkunde*, **21**, 70

LAMORIER, L. (1743) Quoted by Mickulicz, J. Sur operativen Behandlung das Empyens der Highmorshohle. *Lagenbeck's Archiv für Klinische Chirurgie*, **34**, 626–634

LAVELLE, R. J. and SPENCER HARRISON, M. (1971) Infection of the maxillary sinus: the case for the middle meatal antrostomy. *Laryngoscope*, **81**, 90–106

LAZAR, R. H., YOUNIS, R. T. and LONG, T. E. (1993) Functional endonasal sinus surgery in adults and children. *Laryngoscope*, **103**, 1–5

LEOPOLD, D. A., KELLMAN, R. M. and GOULD, L. V. (1980) Retro-orbital hematoma and proptosis associated with chronic sinus disease. *Archives of Otolaryngology*, **106**, 442–443

LEVINE, H. L. (1989) Endoscopy and the KTP/532 laser for nasal sinus disease. *Annals of Otology, Rhinology and Laryngology*, **98**, 46–51

LEVINE, H. L. (1990) Functional endoscopic sinus surgery: evaluation, surgery and follow-up of 250 patients. *Laryngoscope*, **100**, 79–84

LEVINE, S. B., GILL, A. J., LEVINSON, S. R. and COFFEY, T. K. (1990) Diagnostic nasal endoscopy and functional endoscopic sinus surgery: an update and review of complications. *Connecticut Medicine*, **55**, 574–576

LICHTWITZ, L. (1890) Recherches cliniques sur les anesthesies hysteriques des muquenses et dequelques organes des scns ct sur les zones hysterogenes des muqueses. *Bulletin de la Societe de Medecine de Paris*. Index-catalog of the Library of the Surgeon-General Office, US Army, vol. 9, Sr. 2. Washington DC: Government Printing Office

LLOYD, G. A. S., LUND, V. J. and SCADDING, G. K. (1991) Computerised tomography in the preoperative evaluation of functional endoscopic sinus surgery. *Journal of Laryngology and Otology*, **105**, 181–185

LUC, H. (1897) Une nouvelle methode operatoire pour la cure radicle et l'empyeme chronique du sinus maxillaire. *Archives internationales de laryngologie, d'otologie et de rhinologie*, **10**, 273–285

LUND, V. J. (1986) The design and function of intranasal antrostomies. *Journal of Laryngology and Otology*, **100**, 35–39

LUND, V. J., (1988) Inferior meatal antrostomy. *Journal of Laryngology and Otology*, Suppl. 15, 1–18

LUND, V. J. (1990) Surgery of the ethmoids – past, present and future. *Journal of the Royal Society of Medicine*, **83**, 377–379

LUND, V. J. (1993) The results of inferior and middle meatal antrostomy under endoscopic control. *Acta ORL Belgica*, **47**, 65–71

LUND, V. J. and MACKAY, I. S. (1993) Staging in rhinosinusitis. *Rhinology*, **31**, 183–184

LUND, V. J. and MACKAY, I. S. (1994) Outcome assessment of endoscopic sinus surgery. *Proceedings of the Royal Society of Medicine*, **87**, 70–72

LUND, V. J. and ROLFE, M. (1989) Ophthalmic considerations in fronto-ethmoidal mucocoeles. *Journal of Laryngology and Otology*, **103**, 667–669

LUND, V. J. and SCADDING, G. K. (1991) Immunologic aspects of chronic sinusitis. *Canadian Journal of Otolaryngology*, **20**, 379–381

LUND, V. J., HOLMSTROM, M. and SCADDING, G. K. (1991) Functional endoscopic sinus surgery in the management of chronic rhinosinusitis. An objective assessment. *Journal of Laryngology and Otology*, **105**, 832–835

LUSK, R. (1992) *Pediatric Sinusitis*. New York: Raven Press

LYNCH, R. C. (1921) The technique of a radical frontal sinus operation which has given me the best results. *Laryngoscope*, **31**, 1–5

MCALISTER, W. H., LUSK, R. and MUNTZ, H. R. (1989) Comparison of plain radiographs and coronal CT scan in infants and children with recurrent sinusitis. *American Journal of Radiology*, **153**, 1259–1264

MACBETH, R. G. (1954) The osteoplastic operation for chronic infection of the frontal sinus. *Journal of Laryngology and Otology*, **68**,465–477

MCDONOGH, M. and MEIRING, J. H. (1989) Endoscopic transnasal dacryocystorhinostomy. *Journal of Laryngology and Otology*, **103**, 585–587

MACKAY, I. S. (1995) Functional endoscopic sinus surgery. In: *Recent Advances in Otolaryngology*. London: Churchill Livingstone. pp. 225–241

MACKAY, I. S., STANLEY, P. and GREENSTONE, M. (1983) A nose clinic: initial results. *Journal of Laryngology and Otology*, **97**, 925–931

MCNAB JONES, R. (1986) Lavage of the sinuses. In: *Rob and Smith's Operative Surgery, Nose and Throat*, 4th edn., edited by J. C. Ballantyne and D. F. N. Harrison. London: Butterworth. p. 111

MALTZ, M. (1925) New instruments: the sinuscope. *Laryngoscope*, **35**, 805–811

MANIGLIA, A. J. (1989) Fatal and major complications secondary to nasal and sinus surgery. *Laryngoscope*, **99**, 276–283

MARAN, A. G. D., LUND, V. J., MACKAY, I. S. and WILSON, J. (1993) Endoscopic sinus surgery. *Report of Royal College of Surgeons of Edinburgh*, 15th January

MATTOX, D. E. and KENNEDY, D. W. (1990) Endoscopic management of cerebrospinal fluid leaks and cephalocoeles. *Laryngoscope*, **100**, 857–862

MEIBOMIUS, H. (1718) *De absessum interiorum natura et constitutione*. Dresden: J. J. Wincklero. p. 113

MESSERKLINGER, W. (1978) *Endoscopy of the Nose*. Baltimore: Urban & Schwarzenberg

MICKULICZ, J. (1887) Zur operativen Behandlung das Empyems der Highmorshohle. *Lagenbeck's Archiv für Klinische Chirurgie*, **34**, 626–634

MOFFATT, A. J. (1941) Postural instillation. A method of inducing local anaesthesia in the nose. *Journal of Laryngology and Otology*, **56**, 429–436

MOSHER, H. P. (1913) The applied anatomy and intranasal surgery of the ethmoidal labyrinth. *Laryngoscope*, **23**, 881–901

MOSHER, H. P. (1929) The surgical anatomy and intranasal surgery of the ethmoidal labyrinth. *Laryngoscope*, **38**, 869–901

NEGUS, V. E. (1947) The surgical treatment of chronic frontal sinusitis. *British Medical Journal*, **1**, 135–136

OGSTON, A. (1884) Trephining the frontal sinus for catarrh. *Medical Chronicles*, **1**, 235–238

OGURA, J. H., WATSON, R. K. and JURCINA, A. A. (1960) The use of a mucoperiosteal flap for reconstruction of a nasofrontal duct. *Laryngoscope*, **70**, 1229–1243

ONODI, A. (1910) *Die topographische Anatomie der Nasenhohle und ihrer Nebenhohlen*. Wurzburg: Curt Kabitzch

OSTROM, L. (1913) Ventilation rather than drainage essential for the cure of sinus disease with special notes on the antrum of Highmore. *Illinois Medical Journal*, **24**, 347–352

PAPAY, F. A., MAGGIANO, H., HASSENBUSCH, S. J., LEVINE, H. L.,

LAVERTU, P. and DOMINQUEZ, S. (1989) Rigid endoscopic repair of paranasal sinus cerebrospinal fluid fistulas. *Laryngoscope*, **99**, 1195–1201

PATTERSON, N. (1939) External operations on the frontal and ethmoidal sinuses. *Journal of Laryngology and Otology*, **54**, 235–244

READ, R., WILSON, R., RUTMAN, A., LUND, V., TODD, H. C., BRAIN, A. et al. (1991) Interaction of nontypable *Haemophilus influenzae* with human respiratory mucosa in vitro. *Journal of Infectious Disease*, **163**, 549–558

REICHERT, M. (1902) Uber eine neue Untersuchungsmethode der Oberkieferhohle mittels des Antroskops. *Berliner klinisch therapeutische Wochenschrift*, 401–408

REYNOLDS, W. V. and BRANDOW, E. C. (1975) Recent advances in microsurgery of the maxillary sinus. *Acta Otolaryngologica*, **80**, 161–166

RIEDEL, B. M. (1898) Schennke Inaug. Dissertation, Jena.

ROBINSON, P. J., EAST, C. A. and SCOTT, G. M. (1990) Recent advances in the microbiology of sinusitis and their relation to persistent ethmoidal inflammation. *American Journal of Rhinology*, **4**, 83–86

RUBIN, J. S., LUND, V. J. and SALMON, B. (1986) Fronto-ethmoidectomy in the treatment of mucoceles. *Archives of Otolaryngology*, **112**, 434–436

SARGON, F. (1908) Endoscopie directe du sinus maxillaire par les fistules. *Archives Internationales de Laryngologie*, 705–708

SCADDING, G. K., LUND, V. J., DARBY, Y. C., NAVAS-ROMERO, J., SEYMOUR, N. and TURNER, M. W. (1994) IgG subclass levels in chronic rhinosinusitis. *Rhinology*, **32**, 15–19

SCHAEFER, S. D., MANNING, S. and CLOSE, L.G. (1989) Endoscopic paranasal sinus surgery. *Laryngoscope*, **99**, 1–5

SCHAEFFER, J. P. (1920) *The Nose, Paranasal Sinuses, Nasolacrimal Passageways and Olfactory Organ in Man*. Philadelphia: Blakiston

SCHENCK, N. L. (1975) Frontal sinus disease: III experimental and clinical factors in failure of the frontal osteoplastic operation. *Laryngoscope*, **85**, 76–92

SESSIONS, R. B., ALFORD, B. R., STRATTON, C., AINSWORTH, J. and SHILL, O. (1972) Current concepts of frontal sinus surgery: an appraisal of the osteoplastic flap-fat obliteration operation. *Laryngoscope*, **82**, 918–930

SEWALL, E. C. (1935) The operative treatment of nasal sinus disease. *Annals of Otology, Rhinology and Laryngology*, **44**, 307–316

SHAPSHAY, S. M., REBEINZ, E. E. and BOHIGIAN, R. K. (1991) Holmium Yttrium Aluminum Garnet laser-assisted endoscopic sinus surgery. *Laryngoscope*, **101**, 142–149

SMITH, F. (1934) Management of chronic sinus disease. *Archives of Otolaryngology*, **19**, 158–171

SPEILBERG, W. (1922) Antroscopy of the maxillary sinus. *Laryngoscope*, **32**, 441–443

SPICER, S. (1894) The surgical treatment of chronic empyema of the antrum maxillaire. *British Medical Journal*, **2**, 1359

STAMMBERGER, H. (1984) Endoscopical diagnosis and treatment of paranasal sinus mycosis. In: *Advances in Nose and Sinus Surgery*. Dubrovnik: University of Zagreb. pp. 35–37

STAMMBERGER, H. (1985a) Endoscopic surgery for mycotic and chronic recurring sinusitis. *Annals of Otology, Rhinology and Laryngology*, Suppl., 1–11

STAMMBERGER, H. (1985b) Endoscopic endonasal surgery – new concepts in the treatment of recurring sinusitis. Part I. Anatomical and pathophysiological considerations. *Otolaryngology, Head and Neck Surgery*, **94**, 143–147

STAMMBERGER, H. (1985c) Endoscopic endonasal surgery –

new concepts in the treatment of recurring sinusitis. Part II. Surgical technique. *Otolaryngology, Head and Neck Surgery*, **94**, 143–147

STAMMBERGER, H. (1991) *Functional Endoscopic Sinus Surgery*. Philadelphia: BC Decker

STAMMBERGER, H. and POSAWETZ, W. (1990) Functional endoscopic sinus surgery: concept, indications and results of the Messerklinger technique. *European Archives of Otorhinolaryngology*, **240**, 63–76

STAMMBERGER, H. and WOLF, G. (1988) Headaches and sinus disease: the endoscopic approach. *Annals of Otology, Rhinology and Laryngology*, **97** (suppl. 134), 3–23

STAMMBERGER, H., ZINREICH, S. J., KOPP, W., KENNEDY, D. W., JOHNS, M. E. and ROSENBAUM, A. E. (1987) Zur operativen behandlung der chronisch-rezidivierenden sinusitis Caldwell-Luc versus funktionelle endoskopische technik. *HNO*, **35**, 93–105

STANKIEWICZ, J. A. (1987) Complications of endoscopic intranasal ethmoidectomy. *Laryngoscope*, **97**, 1270–1273

STANKIEWICZ, J. (1989) Complications in endoscopic intranasal ethmoidectomy. *Laryngoscope*, **99**, 686–690

STANKIEWICZ, J. A. (1991) Cerebrospinal fluid fistula and endoscopic sinus surgery. *Laryngoscope*, **101**, 250–256

WARD, P. H. and BAUKNIGHT, S. (1973) A serious complication of the osteoplastic flap. *Archives of Otolaryngology*, **98**, 389–390

WATSON, D. J. and GRIFFITHS, M. V. (1988) The safety and efficiency of intra-nasal ethomoidectomy. *Journal of Laryngology and Otology*, **102**, 802–804

WAXMAN, J. E., SPECTOR, J. G., SALE, S. R. and KATZENSTEIN, A. A. (1987) Allergic aspergillus sinusitis: concepts in diagnosis

and treatment of a new clinical entity. *Laryngoscope*, **97**, 261–266

WELLS, S. (1870) Abscess of the frontal sinus. *Lancet*, i, 694–695

WIGAND, M. E. (1981) Transnasal ethmoidectomy under endoscopic control. *Rhinology*, **19**, 7–15

WIGAND, M. E. (1990) *Endoscopic Surgery of the Paranasal Sinuses and Anterior Skull Base*. Stuttgart: Georg Thieme Verlag

WIGAND, M. E. and HOSEMANN, W. G. (1991) Results of endoscopic surgery of the paranasal sinuses and anterior skull base. *Journal of Otolaryngology*, **20**, 385–390

WOLF, G., ANDERHUBER, H. and KUHN, F. (1993) Development of the paranasal sinuses in children: implications for paranasal sinus surgery. *Annals of Otology, Rhinology and Laryngology*, **102**, 705–711

WRIGHT, J. (1914) *A History of Laryngology and Rhinology*. Index-catalog of the Library of the Surgeon General Office, US Army, vol. 21. ser.2. Washington, DC: Government Printing Office

YAMAGUCHI, N., ARAI, S., MITANI, H. and UCHIDA, Y. (1991) Endoscopic endonasal technique of the blowout fracture of the medial orbital wall. *Operative Techniques in Otolaryngology, Head and Neck Surgery*, **94**, 257–259

ZINREICH, S. J., KENNEDY, D. W., ROSENBAUM, A. E., GAYLER, B. W., KUMAR, A. J. and STAMMBERGER, H. (1987) Paranasal sinuses: CT imaging requirements for endoscopic surgery. *Radiology*, **163**, 769–775

ZUCKERKANDL, E. (1893) *Normale und Pathologische Anatomie der Nasenhohle und Interpneumatischen Anhange*. Leipzig: W. Braumuller

13

The complications of sinusitis

V. J. Lund

In a society used to the immediate dispensing of a broad-spectrum antibiotic at the merest suggestion of sinusitis, it is difficult always to appreciate the potential dangers of sinus infection. Before antibiotics were freely available, sinusitis frequently resulted in complications from which the patient succumbed and the radical approach to sinus surgery at the beginning of this century reflects these concerns.

Fortunately these severe complications are now a rarity in most developed countries but when they occur, they are frequently undertreated and are associated with a significant morbidity and mortality which has not substantially altered in 20 years. This failure to treat adequately may be due to an underestimation of the problem on the part of the patient and clinician alike or may result from a masking of symptoms by antibiotics, often taken in subtherapeutic doses as apparent clinical improvement occurs.

Surgical anatomy

The anatomy of this area is already covered in detail (Volume 1, Chapter 5 and Chapter 12, this volume) but a few points are worthy of emphasis.

Routes of spread

Local

The majority of complications are associated with acute bacterial infection where natural dehiscences and weaknesses of the surrounding bone are exploited, with local extension of disease usually when natural drainage routes are blocked by the inflammation. While sclerosis of adjacent bone is often encountered in chronic sinus infection, massive osteolysis can accompany acute sinusitis when there is outflow obstruction which effectively represents an abscess with bony walls. As a consequence of the development of the sinuses frontal sinusitis does not occur in early childhood, though complicated ethmoiditis can arise rapidly from an ostensibly 'ordinary cold' in young children.

Specific areas of weakness are found in the lamina papyracea which is naturally exquisitely thin and may be dehiscent in the very young and old resulting in a variety of orbital complications (Mills and Kartush, 1985). Similarly the infraorbital canal represents an area of weakness in the orbital floor, though the distribution of orbital abscesses suggests that these result more usually from ethmoiditis and frontal infection than from the maxillary sinus. Collections of infection may be within the bony orbit, but may lie external or internal to the orbital periosteum. Sometimes, infection is described as 'preseptal' indicating that it lies superficial to the orbital septum. This structure is a thin broad connective tissue sheet extending from the orbital margin into the lids. Laterally it fuses with the lateral palpebral ligament, medially it splits around the lacrimal sac, and forms the medial palpebral ligament. Local spread may also occur due to the associated thrombophlebitis, particularly through the diploic veins (of Breschet) of the frontal bone, or from the sphenoid, affecting the bone itself and spreading into the adjacent cranial fossa. Significantly the venous connections between the sinuses and the orbit have no valves (Batson, 1936; Avery, 1953; Chandler, Langenbrunner and Stevens, 1970), allowing free communication of infection.

The roots of the second premolar and first molar are intimately related to the floor of the maxillary sinus and in some individuals in direct contact with the mucosa of the sinus. This provides a two-way route for spread of infection and a dental problem should always be suspected when an isolated maxillary sinusitis is encountered, particularly if associated with pain and swelling of the cheek.

Distant

Most complications of sinusitis arise in adjacent structures but rarely distant spread may occur as part of a generalized septicaemia.

Patient attributes

There is usually little to indicate why an individual who has had many previous uneventful viral upper respiratory tract infections should suddenly develop a complicated sinusitis. These complications appear more commonly in the young but generally occur spontaneously in otherwise fit and healthy individuals. Occasionally the complication may be part of an overwhelming infection in a severely immunocompromised patient, e.g. in AIDS or leukaemia, but more frequently immune deficiency presents either with lower respiratory tract infection or in the milder subclass deficiencies with recurrent acute or chronic sinusitis. The incidence of gross hypogammaglobulinaemia is low in the general population (1–2/50 000) though IgG subclass deficiencies may be more common than previously realized (Scadding *et al.*, 1994). However, they are rarely of relevance to the acute complicated case.

Similarly, congenital and acquired abnormalities of the mucociliary clearance mechanisms and allergy (Lund and Scadding, 1991) may contribute to chronic infection but are rarely implicated in an acute complication.

While a number of studies have considered the importance of local anatomical variation in the development of chronic sinusitis (Zinreich *et al.*, 1987; Lloyd, Lund and Scadding, 1991), there are insufficient data to know whether these are responsible for progression to a complication of infection.

Pathogen attributes

The majority of sinus infections probably begin with a viral upper respiratory tract infection. Occasionally these may progress to a serious generalized viraemia, and more specifically an encephalitis, but this is exceptional.

There are few good bacteriological studies of acute complicated sinusitis, largely due to therapeutic interventions being undertaken 'out-of-hours' or because high doses of intravenous antibiotics have already been administered. The range of bacteria found in complicated sinusitis (Table 13.1) does not differ markedly from that in uncomplicated forms, with *Streptococcus pneumoniae* and *Haemophilus influenzae* being commonly found. However, many others are

Table 13.1 Bacteriology of complications of sinusitis

Orbital

Aerobes
  Staphylococcus aureus
  Haemophilus influenzae
  Streptococcus pneumoniae
  Moraxella catarrhalis
  Streptococcus milleri
  Streptococcus pyogenes
Anaerobes

Intracranial

Aerobes
  Staphylococcus aureus
  Streptococcus pneumoniae
  Haemophilus influenzae
  Pseudomonas aeruginosa
  Streptococcus spp.
    β haemolytic
    non-*β* haemolytic
  Klebsiella spp.
Anaerobes

encountered, sometimes acting as co-pathogens, e.g. *Moraxella catarrhalis* or as part of a mixed flora, e.g. anaerobes. It is thought by some that anaerobes may be the primary causative agent in brain abscess (Idriss, Gutman and Kronfol, 1978; Brook *et al.*, 1980; Maniglia *et al.*, 1989). However, in many series, *Staphylococcus aureus* is the most frequent finding, acting as a particularly aggressive organism and it should never be dismissed as a contaminant under these circumstances (Moloney, Badham and McRae, 1987; Maniglia *et al.*, 1989; Swift and Charlton, 1990; Clayman *et al.*, 1991). It is the commonest organism in extradural abscesses.

Fungal sinusitis is relatively uncommon in its invasive form. This can occur in otherwise healthy individuals but in its fulminating form is usually associated with severe immune deficiency or other debilitating disease such as diabetes mellitus or tuberculosis. The *Aspergillus* species and *Rhizopus oryzae* (mucormycosis) are the most commonly implicated agents.

Efficacy of treatment

Patient compliance in taking the prescribed oral antibiotic may play a part in some cases, but often in the young, the complication develops very rapidly, even before treatment is sought.

Poor controls on prescribing of antibiotics in certain parts of the world have also led to marked bacterial resistance, particularly with *Staphylococcus* and with beta-lactamase production by *Haemophilus* and *Moraxella*, which may render some common broad-spectrum antibiotics less effective (Lusk, 1992a). In these circumstances a 5- or 7-day oral course of treatment may be wholly or partially ineffective.

Despite all of the above, it is remarkable how rarely sinus infections do progress and indeed it has been suggested that the majority would resolve spontaneously without any treatment.

Management of complications

The complications associated with sinusitis may be broadly divided into acute or chronic, and local or distant (Table 13.2). The local acute complications are by far the more common and more serious, and may be considered as orbital, intracranial and bony.

Orbital

In the preantibiotic era, 17–20% of patients with orbital cellulitis died of meningitis (Gamble, 1933) or had permanent visual loss (Jarrett and Gutman, 1969). Orbital complications of sinusitis most frequently affect the young with 85% under 20 (Moloney, Badham and McRae, 1987) and 50% or more being under 6 years of age (Hawkins and Clark, 1977; Fearon, Edmonds and Bird, 1979). The complications are thus most frequently due to an ethmoiditis

Table 13.2 Complications of sinusitis

Acute
Local
　Orbital
　　preseptal cellulitis
　　orbital cellulitis without abscess
　　orbital cellulitis with sub- or extraperiosteal abscess
　　orbital cellulitis with intraperiosteal abscess
　　cavernous sinus thrombosis
　Intracranial
　　abscess
　　　extradural
　　　subdural
　　　intracerebral
　　meningitis
　　encephalitis
　　cavernous or sagittal sinus thrombosis
　Bony
　　osteitis/osteomyelitis (Pott's puffy tumour)
　Dental
Distant
　Toxic shock syndrome

Chronic
Mucocoele/pyocoele

Associated diseases
? Otitis media, adenotonsillitis, bronchiectasis

in the absence of frontal sinus development (Chandler, Langenbrunner and Stevens, 1970; Schramm, Myers and Kennerdell, 1978; Wald, 1983; Moloney, Badham and McRae, 1987; Swift and Charlton, 1990). In adults the frontal sinus is frequently responsible, though acute sphenoiditis can also have a direct effect on the optic nerve and cavernous sinus in individuals with a dehiscent intervening lateral sphenoidal wall. Curiously, the left orbit has consistently been shown to be more frequently affected (Gamble, 1933; Gellady, Shulman and Ayoub, 1978; Schramm, Myers and Kennerdell, 1978; Guindi, 1983; Weizman and Mussaffi, 1986; Moloney, Badham and McRae, 1987).

The incidence of orbital complications secondary to sinusitis has been reported at between 21 and 90% (Chandler, Langenbrunner and Stevens, 1970; Schramm, Myers and Kennerdell, 1978; Weiss *et al.*, 1983; Goodwin, 1985) but does not appear to have altered during the last 20 years (Moloney, Badham and McRae, 1987; Swift and Charlton, 1990). The frequency appears to be higher during the winter and spring (Haynes and Cramblett, 1967; Welsh and Welsh, 1974; Guindi, 1983; Swift and Charlton, 1990; Skedros *et al.*, 1993).

In 1937, Hubert classified the orbital complications of sinusitis into five groups:

1 Inflammatory oedema of the eyelids with or without oedema of orbital contents
2 Subperiosteal abscess with
　a oedema of the lids or
　b spread of pus to the lids
3 Abscess of orbital tissues
4 Mild to severe orbital cellulitis with phlebitis of ophthalmic veins
5 Cavernous sinus thrombosis.

A similar classification in adults was devised by Smith and Spencer in 1948 but they emphasized that the distinctions were often blurred. Chandler, Langenbrunner and Stevens modified this classification in 1970 which is widely accepted (Figure 13.1).

1 Preseptal cellulitis – characterized by oedema of the lids without tenderness, visual loss or limitation of extraocular motility (Figure 13.2)
2 Orbital cellulitis, without abscess formation – characterized by diffuse oedema of the adipose tissues (Figure 13.3)
3 Orbital cellulitis with subperiosteal (extraperiosteal) abscess. There is displacement of the globe which, if severe, may limit extraocular movement and be associated with visual loss (Figure 13.4).
4 Orbital cellulitis with intraperiosteal abscess. The displacement of the globe is severe, with obvious limitation of extraocular movement and visual loss due to optic neuropathy in up to 13% of cases (Weiss *et al.*, 1983)
5 Cavernous sinus thrombosis.

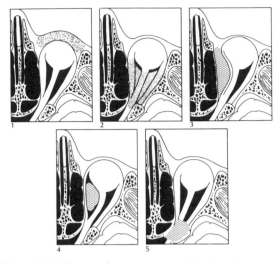

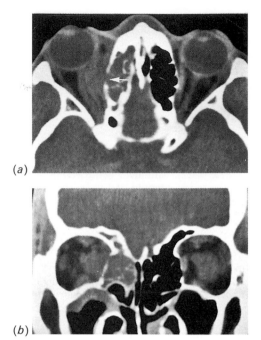

Figure 13.1 Diagram showing various orbital complications on axial projection (after Lusk, 1992b). 1: Preseptal inflammation; 2: orbital cellulitis; 3: orbital cellulitis with subperiosteal (extraperiosteal) abscess; 4: orbital cellulitis with intraperiosteal abscess; 5: cavernous sinus thrombosis.

(*a*)

(*b*)

Figure 13.4 (*a*) Axial and (*b*) coronal CT scan showing ethmoiditis with associated extraperiosteal orbital abscess

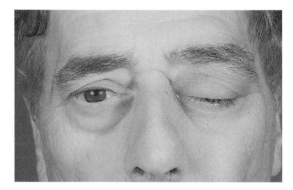

Figure 13.2 Mild orbital cellulitis

With the exception of preseptal cellulitis, all other forms of the acute orbit are associated with significant pain, tenderness and displacement of the globe.

Preseptal cellulitis is a not infrequent accompaniment to sinusitis and although the globe is completely unaffected, should be treated seriously as it presages a potentially more dangerous complication.

As *orbital cellulitis* increases, genuine proptosis of the globe occurs and this can be difficult to distinguish from the oedema of the lids. The proptosis will be exaggerated by a specific collection of pus which is most often *sub-* or *extra-periosteal*. Pus readily collects between the sinus and orbit, stripping the periosteum from the adjacent lamina papyracea. The position of the abscess will determine the angle of displacement, usually combining a degree of axial proptosis with lateral and inferior displacement. The movements of the globe may be restricted by the presence of the mass and/or oedema of the ocular structures. Visual loss will depend upon the extent and the speed with which displacement develops. Colour vision is often impaired first, with the patient unable to distinguish red from brown and blue from black. Once vision is lost, it is exceptional for it to return even after surgical and medical decompression. If infection affects the posterior ethmoids containing an Onodi cell, the optic nerve may be particularly vulnerable.

Occasionally, and less seriously, a *preseptal abscess* forms in the upper lid which may discharge through a fistula.

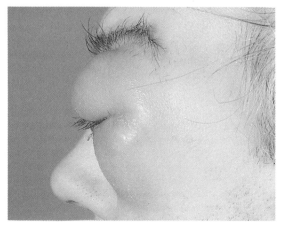

Figure 13.3 Severe orbital cellulitis

An even more serious consequence of orbital cellulitis is the development of an *intraperiosteal abscess* which leads to rapid fixation of extraocular muscles and internal ophthalmoplegia of the globe with fixation of the pupil and visual deterioration. Additional cranial nerves may be affected as an 'orbital apex syndrome' develops with paraesthesia in the distribution of the ophthalmic and maxillary divisions of the trigeminal.

In *cavernous sinus thrombosis*, thrombophlebitis extends posteriorly from the orbit, and can cross the basilar venous plexus to affect the opposite side and thence spreads intracranially. It is generally associated with posterior ethmoiditis or sphenoiditis and carries a serious morbidity, often with bilateral blindness and mortality. This is a complication predominantly of the young, with two-thirds under 20 years (Shahin, Gullane and Dayal, 1987). The patient will complain of headache and painful paraesthesia in the distribution of the trigeminal nerve. Thereafter, the other cranial nerves related to the cavernous sinus may be involved (II–VI), affecting extraocular movements and resulting in permanent ophthalmoplegia. The cause for this may be masked by the local effects of intraperiosteal oedema. The sudden development of bilateral orbital signs should alert the clinician to this complication. Prior to antibiotics, cavernous sinus thrombosis carried a 50% mortality which nevertheless still stands at a significant 10–27% (Fearon, Edmonds and Bird, 1979; Lew, Southwick and Montgomery, 1983).

Management of orbital complications

When faced with a patient with an orbital complication, the diagnosis of an underlying sinusitis may already have been made but, notwithstanding this, a careful history of past and recent events, including medication and other medical history is taken. A general otorhinolaryngological examination will obviously include anterior and posterior rhinoscopy and whenever possible rigid endoscopy of the nose. This should be done after applying adequate local anaesthesia and decongestants which may in themselves prove therapeutic. This may simply reveal inflammation and oedema of the middle meatus but it may be possible to take bacteriological specimens and may also indicate other pathology such as sinonasal malignancy.

Examination of the eye should concentrate on assessing displacement of the globe as distinct from oedema of the lids, ocular movement and most importantly visual acuity. Ideally this should be done with the aid of an ophthalmic colleague, but as for the imaging, when faced with a patient who is already losing vision, surgical decompression should not be delayed if clinically indicated. Clearly, a CT scan can be of considerable advantage in determining the location of an abscess but should only be obtained if the

clinical situation is stable. Furthermore, regular checks of visual acuity must continue thereafter, and during any clinical investigation however uncomfortable it may be for the patient to have the swollen lids opened. As a general rule, generalized oedema of the orbit results in symmetrical axial proptosis, whereas specific collections produce displacement away from that quadrant. Similarly, asymmetric restriction of movement will suggest a localized, extraperiosteal collection. Severe proptosis will lead to chemosis.

Changes in visual acuity must be distinguished from diplopia due to restricted muscle movement or the mass action of the abscess and the blurring of conjunctivitis. Ideally it should be assessed using a pinhole. Optic neuropathy due to compression of the nerve, its dural sheath or its blood supply, is accompanied by a relative afferent pupillary defect. The patient reports that the image is darker when looking only through the affected eye. The compressed nerve fails to transmit light impulses as readily as a normal nerve. This produces a small amount of pupillary dilatation when a torch is moved from the normal eye to the abnormal eye. Although in chronic conditions such as a mucocoele, the globe will tolerate up to 2 cm of displacement when it occurs over a long period, any rapid compression of the central retinal arteries and ophthalmic arteries has an immediate effect on vision. Oedema of the optic disc and retinal vein engorgement is only evident if compression occurs close to where the nerve leaves the globe so fundal changes are often absent. Although there is a number of case reports in the literature of vision returning (Kerkenezov, 1955; Leeson, 1959; Harley and Guerier, 1978), animal experiments and clinical experience suggests that compression must be relieved within 100 minutes if vision is to be restored (Anderson and Edwards, 1980; Hayreh and Weingeist, 1980). In addition to compression, the local effects of inflammation can also result in optic nerve damage. A general neurological examination is also mandatory particularly to exclude cavernous sinus thrombosis and bearing in mind that multiple complications occur in 20% of such individuals. The patients are often unwell, pyrexial and have a neutrophil leucocytosis.

Unless there is only the mildest preseptal cellulitis which has not already been treated with broad-spectrum antibiotics, patients should be admitted to hospital for observation and given intravenous antibiotics. This should include agents which cover the common sinus pathogens, including the beta-lactam producers and anaerobes, e.g. cefuroxime and metronidazole or amoxycillin/clavulanate. This should be combined with intranasal decongestants and analgesics. It would seem that the younger the patient, the more likely that medical therapy alone will resolve matters (Lusk, 1992b). However, if there is any evidence of visual loss, surgical decompression should be performed forthwith as it represents a genuine surgical emergency. Asymmetric displacement and limitation of extraocular movement will strongly indicate an extraperiosteal abscess.

In the first instance a simple antral washout may improve the situation but a formal surgical drainage under general anaesthetic is to be preferred. An endoscopic approach has been advocated by some authors, but unless one is very experienced with this technique and fully cogniscent of the extent of the problem, an external approach via a modified Lynch-Howarth incision is preferable. This allows complete decompression of the orbit, drainage of the frontoethmosphenoid complex and of any orbital collection, be it extraperiosteal, preseptal or intraperiosteal. This approach may be combined with a middle meatal antrostomy performed endoscopically. Although trephination of the frontal sinus could alternatively be performed in the first instance, a formal decompression offers the most reliable solution. If there is no specific contraindication, parenteral steroids (8–12 mg dexamethasone in an adult) may be helpful pre- or peroperatively, when vision is compromised.

The number of patients requiring surgical intervention varies from 12 to 98% in the literature (Welsh and Welsh, 1974; Hawkins and Clark, 1977; Noel, Clarke and Peacocke, 1981; Schramm, Curtin and Kennerdell, 1982) but this reflects different patient populations and referral patterns.

If there is no obvious danger to vision, a response to the intravenous antibiotics can be awaited over the succeeding 24 hours during which a CT scan can be obtained (Schramm, Myers and Kennerdell, 1978). Sinus X-rays may be of use in confirming opacification of the frontal or maxillary sinus with associated bone loss but have little value in localizing infection in relation to the orbit (Moseley, 1991). If a CT scan is performed, attention should also be paid to the adjacent anterior cranial fossa where covert collections may form. Indeed it is advisable to perform a scan in any individual who has had an orbital complication secondary to sinusitis within the succeeding 2 months if there are any persistent symptoms, e.g. of headache or malaise. Although it is unusual for patients with orbital complications to have clinical signs of meningitis, a CT scan should be performed prior to lumbar puncture to eliminate the possibility of an intracranial abscess. MRI is less useful for orbital complications than CT unless a more detailed intracranial examination is also required.

An emergency CT scan is required when cavernous sinus thrombosis is suspected and management includes high-dose intravenous antibiotics with specific anti-staphylococcal activity which is a common pathogen in sphenoiditis (Lusk, 1992b), combined with surgical drainage.

Long-term sequelae of orbital complications

In addition to permanent visual loss and ophthalmoplegia, the cornea may become anaesthetic or permanently damaged due to exposure keratitis and ulceration (Duke-Elder and McFaul, 1974). Other ocular changes include infarction of the sclera, choroid and retina (El Shewy, 1973), uveitis, choroiditis and glaucoma. Rupture of the globe and iris prolapse have also been described due to increased intraorbital pressure (Forstot and Ellis, 1979).

Intracranial (Figure 13.5)

It is difficult to obtain an accurate incidence of intracranial complications associated with sinusitis. They are less common than orbital complications, but the two can coexist and a covert intracranial problem should always be considered in any patient with an orbital complication. They occur most commonly in adolescents and young adults (Zellers and Donowitz, 1987; Parker *et al.*, 1989), mainly in males (Kaufman, Litman and Miller, 1983; Johnson *et al.*, 1988; Clayman *et al.*, 1991). It has been suggested that the diploic system is at peak vascularity in adolescence (Kaplan, 1976) but there is no explanation for the male preponderance.

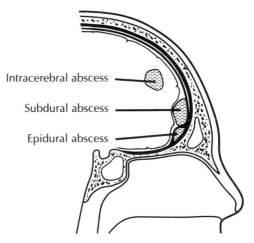

Figure 13.5 Diagram showing positions of intracranial abscesses (after Lusk, 1992b)

They may be divided into abscesses – extradural (epidural), subdural, intracerebral – meningitis/encephalitis, and cavernous or superior sagittal sinus thrombosis.

Nearly two-thirds of brain abscesses are secondary to infections in the ears and paranasal sinuses (Bradley, Manning and Shaw, 1984; Harrington, 1984; Maniglia *et al.*, 1989) of which the sinuses are now becoming the commonest source (Snell, 1978; Bradley and Shaw, 1983; Johnson *et al.*, 1988; Macdonald, Findlay and Tator, 1988; Hoyt and Fisher, 1991) (Table 13.3).

Table 13.3 Incidence of intracranial complications with sinusitis

Study	%	Country
Snell (1978)	24	Canada
Yang (1979)	0.5	China
Morgan and Morrison (1980)	9.0	USA
Bradley and Shaw (1983)	15.7	England
Clayman *et al.* (1991)	3.7	USA

After Lusk, 1992b

Intracranial abscesses are most commonly found subdurally, followed by a frontal lobe abscess (Figure 13.6). They commence as a cerebritis which localizes with necrosis and liquefaction within a capsule (Maniglia *et al.*, 1980). Once the process of septic thrombophlebitis is initiated, multiple abscesses may form, both in number and site and there may be associated *thrombosis of the cavernous* or (more rarely) *superior sagittal sinuses*. Twelve of the 19 cases reported by Maniglia *et al.* (1989) had multiple intracranial complications. Intracranial abscesses are relatively uncommon in infants, generally affecting individuals over 10 years of age (Zellers and Donowitz, 1987; Johnson *et al.*, 1988). Their presentation may be acute or chronic. In the acute phase, an abscess in the frontal region gives few symptoms and signs until a large size is reached (Liston, Walikerle and Robinson, 1979) and those few features may be masked by other problems, e.g. orbital complications,

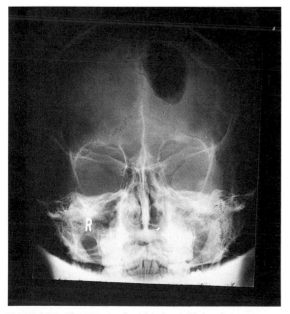

Figure 13.6 Plain X-ray showing frontal lobe abscess in child with orbital cellulitis secondary to ethmoiditis

while in the longer term, the subliminal symptoms of a chronic brain abscess may be ignored.

Fever, a leucocytosis and headache may not immediately alert the clinician and may be the only symptoms of an extradural abscess. A subdural or intracerebral abscess may only be suspected when the patient develops seizures, nuchal rigidity or focal neurological signs. Papilloedema, nausea, vomiting and decreased consciousness due to raised intracranial pressure may take some time to develop (Nager, 1966; Bradley, Manning and Shaw, 1984; Harrington, 1984).

Meningitis tends to be associated with acute sphenoiditis, either due to direct venous spread or because of parameningeal inflammation of the cavernous sinus. Symptoms for meningitis can be similar to those of an abscess.

Management of intracranial complications

It is necessary to entertain a high index of suspicion, combined with a careful history and full neurological examination. If there is any suspicion of an abscess, a CT scan (or MRI) should be obtained urgently prior to proceeding to lumbar puncture to reduce the risk of coning. CT with contrast has been the imaging of choice (Rotheram and Kessler, 1978; Zimmerman and Bilaniuk, 1980; Carter, Bankoff and Fisk, 1983; Moseley and Kendal, 1984; Oliveira, Reimao and Diament, 1984; Johnson *et al.*, 1988; Dietrich *et al.*, 1989) to demonstrate localized intracranial infection but, if available, MRI offers an excellent alternative as it will define very small collections (Weingarten *et al.*, 1989) and demonstrate more generalized cerebritis. The benefit of lumbar puncture, given that an abscess is more likely than meningitis, is outweighed by the attendant risks, until imaging has clarified matters.

Intravenous antibiotics must be given in high-doses, selected to cross the blood–brain barrier and to cover the common sinus pathogens. Cefuroxime and metronidazole are a reasonable combination though other authors have suggested chloramphenicol and oxacillin, or a combination of methicillin, cefotaxime and metronidazole. The course of treatment should be given for 4–6 weeks (Johnson *et al.*, 1988; Parker *et al.*, 1989) with serial CT scanning used to chart progress. In the presence of a localized collection of pus, drainage is almost always required. Medical management alone is only successful when there is disseminated infection or the abscess is small (Whelan and Hilal, 1980; Rennels, Woodward and Robinson, 1983; Johnson *et al.*, 1988). The role of steroids is rather controversial as while they reduce inflammation, they may also interfere with antibiotic penetration (Maniglia *et al.*, 1989).

Surgery should aim at treating both the complication and the underlying sinusitis. It should be possible to drain an extradural abscess via the approach to the frontal sinuses but otherwise neurosurgical assistance will usually be required. Simple burr holes may be adequate if the collection can be accurately located (Kaufman, Litman and Miller, 1983), but if there is any doubt or with multiple abscesses, a formal craniotomy is preferred. In subdural empyema, the mortality rate has been reported as three times higher with burr holes than with craniotomy (Bannister and Willaims, 1981).

Again it is worth emphasizing the need for a follow-up CT scan in any individual with a severe frontal sinusitis, especially if complicated by orbital spread if there is any clinical suspicion, however slight, of a covert frontal abscess (Maniglia *et al.*, 1989).

Long-term sequelae of intracranial complications

Despite antibiotics and improved diagnostic imaging, the mortality from intracranial complications is still between 15 and 43% (Bradley, Manning and Shaw, 1984; Kahn and Griebel, 1984; Oliveira, Reimao and Diament, 1984; Maniglia *et al.*, 1989), and increases with age (Bradley, Manning and Shaw, 1984; Rosenbaum and Cunha, 1989). Multiple subdural abscesses with associated cortical thrombophlebitis carry the worst prognosis, with three out of seven succumbing in Maniglia *et al's.* series (1989). Another 40% will have some permanent disability (Bradley, Manning and Shaw, 1984). This includes convulsions in 7.5% and hemiparesis in 2–17% (Bradley, Manning and Shaw, 1984; Clayman *et al.*, 1991). Understandably, the earlier the medical and surgical intervention, the better the likely outcome.

Bony complications of sinusitis

The term 'Pott's puffy tumour' has been used to describe this complication of frontal sinusitis in which the overlying frontal bone becomes involved, following its description in 1760 by Sir Percival Pott. The frontal bone is diploic bone with a marrow cavity and thus is capable of developing osteomyelitis. Both the anterior and posterior walls may be affected. Infection may spread anteriorly onto the forehead or posteriorly, to form a subdural abscess.

There is typically fluctuant swelling over the forehead, though it is not necessarily particularly painful (Figure 13.7). *Staphylococcus aureus*, streptococci and anaerobes are the major causative agents and CT scanning should be performed to establish whether concomitant intracranial problems exist.

Although intravenous broad-spectrum antibiotics should be given, surgical intervention is invariably required (Feder, Cates and Cementina, 1987) usually via a bilateral coronal or spectacle incision. In addition to drainage of the pus, the affected bone is debrided. The cosmetic defect can be dealt with at a later date when infection has completely settled, using bone grafts or a variety of exogenous materials. The antibiotics are the same as those given for other sinus complications,

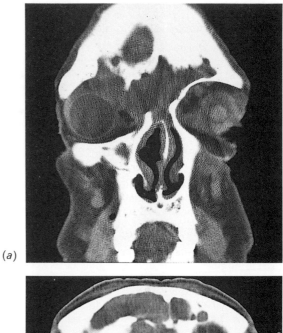

(a)

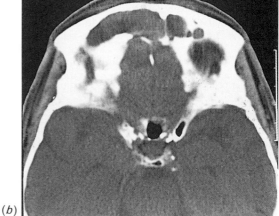

(b)

Figure 13.7 Frontoethmoidal mucocoele (*a*) Coronal CT scan showing opacification of the frontal sinuses with erosion of the supraorbital rim. (*b*) Axial CT scan of same patient showing erosion of the posterior frontal sinus wall

though they may be modified by subsequent microbiology. Treatment should continue for at least 4–6 weeks as antibiotic penetration into bone is notoriously poor.

Dental

The close proximity of the second premolar and molars to the floor of the maxillary sinus means that acute sinusitis may produce dental pain which may confuse the diagnosis and, conversely, a dental abcess may be erroneously mistaken for sinusitis. The latter is usually associated with significant swelling of the gum and overlying cheek which is rarely encountered in all but the most severe complicated cases of maxillary infection. Occasionally, the two conditions may coexist.

Systemic

Toxic shock syndrome

This condition which was described by Todd, Fishaut and Kapral in 1978, is a rare but potentially fatal complication of sinus infection, frequently associated with *Staphylococcus aureus*. The condition can arise from any focus of staphylococcal infection and has been reported with the streptococcus group of organisms (Gallo and Fontanarosa, 1990). Sinusitis may be the source of this condition in both adults (Gallo and Fontanarosa, 1990) and children (Griffith and Perkin, 1988) and should be considered if toxic shock develops. Symptoms include fever, hypotension, rash with desquamation and multisystem failure.

Chronic complications of sinusitis

Frontoethmoidal mucocoeles (Figure 13.7)

The role of sinusitis in the development of sinus mucocoeles is uncertain (Lund, 1987). However, sinus infection or its surgical treatment does precede presentation with a frontoethmoidal mucocoele in 25% (Figure 13.8). A pyocoele forms when a mucocoele becomes secondarily infected (Figure 13.9). Where a positive culture was obtained in a personal series of 125 mucocoeles and pyocoeles, *Staphylococcus aureus*, *Haemophilus influenzae* and *Streptococcus pneumoniae* were the commonest pathogens.

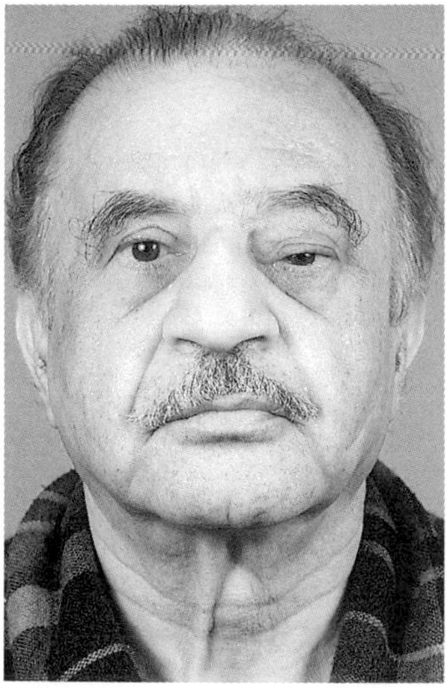

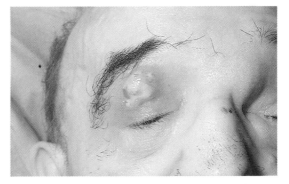

Figure 13.8 Typical displacement of the globe in a frontoethmoidal mucocoele

The optic nerve can tolerate considerable stretching with up to 20 mm of axial proptosis when it occurs over a long period of time, but when further displacement occurs rapidly due to acute infection,

Figure 13.9 Patient with pyocoele, discharging fistula through upper lid and erosion of anterior table of frontal bone

vision is rapidly compromised. As for other orbital abscesses and with the same provisos surgical decompression under intravenous antibiotic cover should be undertaken.

Other respiratory tract conditions

In the absence of a specific problem with mucociliary clearance (e.g. primary ciliary dyskinesia, cystic fibrosis) or immune deficiency, it is difficult to assess the interdependence of sinusitis, otitis media, adenotonsillitis and lower respiratory tract infections. That an interrelationship exists is supported by clinical experience but whether this belies some subtle local or systemic susceptibility is uncertain.

References

ANDERSON, R. L. and EDWARDS, J. J. (1980) Bilateral visual loss after blepharoplasty. *Annals of Plastic Surgery*, **5**, 288–292

AVERY, L. B. (1953) The sense organs. In: *Morris Human Anatomy*, edited by J. P. Schaeffer. New York: Blakiston, pp. 1152–1153

BANNISTER, G. and WILLIAMS, B. (1981) Treatment of subdural empyema. *Journal of Neurosurgery*, **55**, 82–88

BATSON, O. V. (1936) Relationship of the eye to the paranasal sinuses. *Archives of Ophthalmology*, **16**, 322–323

BRADLEY, P. J. and SHAW, M. D. (1983) Three decades of brain abscess on Merseyside. *Journal of the Royal College of Surgeons*, **28**, 223–228

BRADLEY, P. J., MANNING, K. P. and SHAW, M. D. (1984) Brain abscess secondary to paranasal sinusitis. *Journal of Laryngology and Otology*, **98**, 719–725

BROOK, I., FRIEDMAN, E. M., RODRIGUEZ, W. J. and CONTRONI, G. (1980) Complications of sinusitis in children. *Pediatrics*, **66**, 568–572

CARTER, B. L., BANKOFF, M. S. and FISK, J. D. (1983) Computed tomographic detection of sinusitis responsible for intracranial and extracranial infections. *Radiology*, **147**, 739–742

CHANDLER, J. R., LANGENBRUNNER, D. J. and STEVENS, E. R. (1970) The pathogenesis of orbital complications in acute sinusitis. *Laryngoscope*, **80**, 1414–1428

CLAYMAN, G. L., ADAMS, G. L., PAUGH, D. R. and KOOPMANN, C. F. JR (1991) Intracranial complications of paranasal sinusitis. A combined institutional review. *Laryngoscope*, **101**, 234–239

DIETRICH, U., FELDGES, A., NAU, H. E. and LOHR, E. (1989) Epidural abscess following frontal sinusitis – demonstration of communication by epidural contrast medium and coronal computerized tomography. *Computerized Medical Imaging and Graphics*, **13**, 351–354

DUKE-ELDER, S. and MCFAUL, P. A. (1974) *System of Ophthalmology*, vol 13. London: Kimpton. pp. 859–889

EL SHEWY, T. M. (1973) Acute infarction of the choroid and retina – a complication of orbital cellulitis. *British Journal of Ophthalmology*, **57**, 204–205

FEARON, B., EDMONDS, B. and BIRD, R. (1979) Orbital facial complications of sinusitis in children. *Laryngoscope*, **89**, 947–953

FEDER, H. M. JR, CATES, K. L. and CEMENTINA, A. M. (1987) Pott's puffy tumor: a serious occult infection. *Pediatrics*, **79**, 625–629

FORSTOT, S. L. and ELLIS, P. P. (1979) Nontraumatic rupture of the globe secondary to orbital cellulitis. *American Journal of Ophthalmology*, **88**, 262–264

GALLO, U. E. and FONTANAROSA, P. B. (1990) Toxic streptococcal syndrome. *Annals of Emergency Medicine*, **19**, 1332–1334

GAMBLE, R. C. (1933) Acute inflammation of the orbit in children. *Archives of Ophthalmology*, **10**, 483–497

GELLADY, A. M., SHULMAN, S. T. and AYOUB, E. M. (1978) Periorbital and orbital cellulitis in children. *Pediatrics*, **61**, 272–277

GOODWIN, W. J. JR (1985) Orbital complications of ethmoiditis. *Otolaryngologic Clinics of North America*, **18**, 139–147

GRIFFITH, J. A. and PERKIN, R. M. (1988) Toxic shock syndrome and sinusitis – a hidden site of infection. *Western Journal of Medicine*, **148**, 580–581

GUINDI, G. M. (1983) Acute orbital cellulitis: a multidisciplinary emergency. *British Journal of Oral and Maxillofacial Surgery*, **21**, 261–267

HARLEY, M. J. and GUERIER, T. H. (1978) Orbital cellulitis related to an influenza A virus epidemic. *British Medical Journal*, **2**, 13–14

HARRINGTON, P. C. (1984) Complications of sinusitis. *Ear, Nose and Throat Journal*, **63**, 163–171

HAWKINS, D. B. and CLARK, R. W. (1977) Orbital involvement in acute sinusitis. Lessons from 24 childhood patients. *Clinical Pediatrics (Philadelphia)*, **16**, 464–471

HAYNES, R. E. and CRAMBLETT, H. G. (1967) Acute ethmoiditis. Its relationship to orbital cellulitis. *American Journal of Diseases of Childhood*, **114**, 261–267

HAYREH, S. S. and WEINGEIST, T. A. (1980) Experimental occlusion of the central artery of the retina. IV: Retinal tolerance time to acute ischaemia. *British Journal of Ophthalmology*, **64**, 818–825

HOYT, D. J. and FISHER, S. R. (1991) Otolaryngologic management of patients with subdural empyema. *Laryngoscope*, **101**, 20–24

HUBERT, L. (1937) Orbital infections due to nasal sinusitis. *New York State Journal of Medicine*, **37**, 1559–1564

IDRISS, Z. H., GUTMAN, L. T. and KRONFOL, N. M. (1978) Brain abscesses in infants and children: current status of clinical findings, management and prognosis. *Clinical Pediatrics (Philadelphia)*, **17**, 738–740

JARRETT, W. H. and GUTMAN, F. A. (1969) Ocular complications of infection in the paranasal sinuses. *Archives of Ophthalmology*, **98**, 2004–2006

JOHNSON, D. L., MARKLE, B. M., WIEDERMANN, B. L. and HANAHAN, L. (1988) Treatment of intracranial abscesses associated with sinusitis in children and adolescents. *Journal of Pediatrics*, **113**, 15–23

KAHN, M. and GRIEBEL, R. (1984) Subdural empyema: a retrospective study of 15 patients. *Canadian Journal of Surgery*, **27**, 283–288

KAPLAN, R. (1976) Neurological complications of infections of the head and neck. *Otolaryngologic Clinics of North America*, **9**, 729–734

KAUFMAN, D. M., LITMAN, N. and MILLER, M. H. (1983) Sinusitis: induced subdural empyema. *Neurology*, **33**, 123

KERKENEZOV, N. (1955) Acute non-specific infections of the orbit with a report of three cases. *Medical Journal of Australia*, **2**, 293–295

LEESON, P. (1959) A case of cellulitis secondary to suppurative pansinusitis: Jacksonian epilepsy: drainage of the sinuses: recovery. *Journal of Laryngology and Otology*, **73**, 392–395

LEW, D., SOUTHWICK, F. S. and MONTGOMERY, W. W. (1983) Sphenoid sinusitis: a review of 30 cases. *New England Journal of Medicine*, **309**, 1149–1154

LISTON, E. D., WALIKERLE, J. F. and ROBINSON, W. (1979) Intracranial abscess with behavioral changes. *Archives of Otolaryngology*, **105**, 343–346

LLOYD, G. A. S., LUND, V. J. and SCADDING, G. K. (1991) Computerised tomography in the preoperative evaluation of functional endoscopic sinus surgery. *Journal of Laryngology and Otology*, **105**, 181–185

LUND, V. J. (1987) Anatomical considerations in the aetiology of fronto-ethmoidal mucocoeles. *Rhinology*, **25**, 83–88

LUND, V. J. and SCADDING, G. K. (1991) Immunologic aspects of chronic sinusitis. *Canadian Journal of Otolaryngology*, **20**, 379–381

LUSK, R. P. (1992) *Pediatric Sinusitis*. New York: Raven Press. (a) p. 71; (b) p. 127–146

MACDONALD, R. L., FINDLAY, J. M. and TATOR, C. H. (1988) Sphenoethmoid sinusitis complicated by cavernous sinus thrombosis and pontocerebellar infarction. *Canadian Journal of Neurologic Sciences*, **15**, 310–313

MANIGLIA, A. J., VAN BUREN, J., BRUCE, W., BELLUCCI, R. J. and HOFFMAN, S. (1980) Intracranial abscesses secondary to ear and paranasal sinus infections. *Otolaryngology, Head and Neck Surgery*, **88**, 670–680

MANIGLIA, A. J., GOODWIN, W. J., ARNOLD, J. E. and GANZ, E. (1989) Intracranial abscesses secondary to nasal, sinus and orbital infections in adults and children. *Archives of Otolaryngology – Head and Neck Surgery*, **115**, 1424–1429

MILLS, R. P. and KARTUSH, J. M. (1985) Orbital wall thickness and the spread of infection from the paranasal sinuses. *Clinical Otolaryngology*, **10**, 209–216

MOLONEY, J. R., BADHAM, N. J. and MCRAE, A. (1987) The acute orbit. Preseptal (periorbital) cellulitis, subperiosteal abscess and orbital cellulitis due to sinusitis. *Journal of Laryngology and Otology*, **12** (Suppl.), 1–18

MORGAN, P. R. and MORRISON, W. V. (1980) Complications of frontal and ethmoid sinusitis. *Laryngoscope*, **90**, 661–666

MOSELEY, I. (1991) The plain radiograph in ophthalmology: a wasteful and potentially dangerous anachronism. *Journal of the Royal Society of Medicine*, **84**, 76–80

MOSELEY, I. F. and KENDAL, B. E. (1984) Radiology of intracranial empyemas with specific reference to computed tomography. *Neuroradiology*, **26**, 333–345

NAGER, G. T. (1966) Mastoid and paranasal sinus infections and their relation to the central nervous system. *Clinical Neurosurgery*, **14**, 288–313

NOEL, L. P., CLARKE, W. N. and PEACOCKE, R. A. (1981) Periorbital and orbital cellulitis in childhood. *Canadian Journal of Ophthalmology*, **16**, 178–180

OLIVEIRA, T. D., REIMAO, R. and DIAMENT, A. J. (1984) Intracranial abscesses in infancy and childhood: report of 40 cases. *Arquivos de Neuro-psiquiatria*, **42**, 195–202

PARKER, G. S., TAMI, T. A., WILSON, J. F. and FETTER, T. W. (1989) Intracranial complications of sinusitis. *Southern Medical Journal*, **82**, 563–569

POTT, P. (1760) *Observations on the Nature and Consequences of Wounds and Contusions of the Head*. London: Hitch & Howes. pp. 53–58

RENNELS, M. B., WOODWARD, C. L. and ROBINSON, W. L. (1983) Medical cure of apparent brain abscesses. *Pediatrics*, **72**, 220–224

ROSENBAUM, G. S. and CUNHA, B. A. (1989) Subdural empyema complication frontal and ethmoid sinusitis. *Heart and Lung*, **18**, 199–202

ROTHERAM, E. B. JR and KESSLER, L. A. (1978) Use of computerized tomography in nonsurgical management of brain abscess. *Archives of Neurology*, **36**, 25–26

SCADDING, G. K., LUND, V. J., DARBY, Y. C., NAVAS-ROMERO, J., SEYMOUR, N. and TURNER, M. W. (1994) IgG subclass levels in chronic rhinosinusitis. *Rhinology*, **32**, 15–19

SCHRAMM, V. L. JR., MYERS, E. N. and KENNERDELL, J. S. (1978) Orbital complications of acute sinusitis: evaluation, management and outcome. *ORL*, **86**, 221–230

SCHRAMM, V. L. JR, CURTIN, H. D. and KENNERDELL, J. S. (1982) Evaluation of orbital cellulitis and results of treatment. *Laryngoscope*, **92**, 732–738

SHAHIN, J., CULLANE, P. J. and DAYAL, V. S. (1987) Orbital complications of acute sinusitis. *Journal of Otolaryngology*, **16**, 23–27

SKEDROS, D. G., HADDAD, J., BLUESTONE, C. D. and CURTIN, H. D. (1993) Subperiosteal orbital abscess in children: diagnosis, microbiology and management. *Laryngoscope*, **103**, 28–32

SMITH, A. T. and SPENCER, J. F. (1948) Orbital complications resulting from lesions of the sinuses. *Annals of Otology, Rhinology and Laryngology*, **57**, 5–27

SNELL, G. E. (1978) Sinogenic and otogenic brain abscess. *Journal of Otolaryngology*, **7**, 289–296

SWIFT, A. C. and CHARLTON, G. (1990) Sinusitis and the acute orbit in children. *Journal of Laryngology and Otology*, **104**, 213–216

TODD, J., FISHAUT, M. and KAPRAL, F. (1978) Toxic shock syndrome associated with phage group-1 staphylococci. *Lancet*, ii, 1116–1118

WALD, E. R. (1983) Acute sinusitis and orbital complications in children. *American Journal of Otolaryngology*, **4**, 424–427

WEINGARTEN, K., ZIMMERMAN, R. D., BECKER, R. D., HEIER, L. A., HAIMES, A. B. and DECK, M. D. (1989) Subdural and epidural empyemas: MR imaging. *American Journal of Radiology*, **152**, 615–621

WEISS, A., FRIENDLY, D., EGLIN, K., CHANG, M. and GOLD, B. (1983) Bacterial periorbital and orbital cellulitis in childhood. *Ophthalmology*, **90**, 195–203

WEIZMAN, Z. and MUSSAFI, H. (1986) Ethmoiditis-associated periorbital cellulitis. *International Journal of Pediatric Otorhinolaryngology*, **11**, 147–151

WELSH, L. W. and WELSH, J. J. (1974) Orbital complications of sinus diseases. *Laryngoscope*, **84**, 848–856

WHELAN, M. A. and HILAL, S. K. (1980) Computed tomography as a guide in the diagnosis and follow-up of brain abscess. *Radiology*, **135**, 663–671

YANG, S-Y. (1979) Brain abscess. Review of 400 cases. *Journal of Neurosurgery*, **55**, 794–799

ZELLERS, T. M. and DONOWITZ, L. G. (1987) Brain abscess and ethmoid sinusitis presenting as periorbital cellulitis in a two-month-old infant. *Pediatric Infectitious Diseases Journal*, **6**, 213–215

ZIMMERMAN, R. A. and BILANIUK, L. T. (1980) CT of orbital infection and its cerebral complications. *American Journal of Radiology*, **134**, 45–50

ZINREICH, S. J., KENNEDY, D. W., ROSENBAUM, A. E., GAYLER, B. W., KUMAR, A. J. and STAMMBERGER, H. (1987) Paranasal sinuses: CT imaging requirements for endoscopic surgery. *Radiology*, **163**, 769–775

14

Cerebrospinal fluid rhinorrhoea

C. A. Milford

Definition

Leakage of cerebrospinal fluid (CSF) from the nose is a symptom of failed containment of spinal fluid to its subarachnoid compartment. It indicates a communication with the subarachnoid space and, therefore, an opening of arachnoid, dura and bone to permit exit of the CSF to the nose. The origin of the CSF may be from any of the cranial fossae, i.e. anterior, middle or posterior. This may occur from the anterior cranial fossa through the frontal, sphenoidal or ethmoidal sinuses or directly through the cribriform plate. CSF from the middle fossa may enter the nose either directly through the sphenoid sinus or indirectly from the mastoid air cells/middle ear through the eustachian tube (CSF otorhinorrhoea). Escape of CSF from the posterior fossa into the nose again may rarely occur directly via the sphenoid or more commonly indirectly via the mastoid air cells/middle ear through the eustachian tube (Figure 14.1). Although the actual loss of CSF itself is of no particular consequence, a persistent dural fistula represents a persistent hazard for a potentially fatal purulent meningitis and death complicates most cases of unrecognized CSF rhinorrhoea (Chandler, 1983). Persistent CSF rhinorrhoea is therefore an absolute indication for the surgical repair of the leak.

Historical background

Leakage of CSF from the confines of the skull into the nose has long been a matter of concern. The earliest theories held that a normal communication existed between the spinal fluid space and the nose. Indeed, in the second century AD, Galen theorized that CSF was periodically purged by way of pituitary and ethmoid regions into the nose. Until the seventeenth century it was believed that there was a normal free communication between the brain and the nose. The first recorded instance of CSF rhinorrhoea is thought to be a case described by Willis in 1676 (MacDonald, 1945), in which clear fluid was drained from the patient's nose. The first comprehensive description of a CSF leak is credited to Miller who, in 1826, described finding, at necropsy, a fistula between the nasal cavity and subarachnoid space in a hydrocephalic child who had suffered an intermittent clear nasal discharge. The first series of cases in the English literature was published in 1899 by St Clair Thompson in a summary of his findings on 20 patients. He included a chemical analysis of CSF and suggested diagnostic criteria for differentiating CSF from other conditions in which a clear fluid may be discharged from the nose. He was the first to use the term 'rhinorrhoea' for nasal CSF discharge.

Pathophysiology

The factors responsible for CSF fistulae involve a disruption of the arachnoid and dura, coupled with an osseous defect, and a CSF pressure gradient that is either continuously or intermittently greater than the healing tensile strength of the disrupted tissue. This eventually causes separation of the dural fibres and CSF leakage (Calcaterra, 1980). It is not difficult to appreciate how this may happen after trauma, but it is more difficult to account for this in non-traumatic cases of CSF rhinorrhoea. Postulated mechanisms for CSF escape generally begin with increased intracranial pressure (ICP). Raised ICP, even of a transient nature, could start a leak if the potential pathways are present. This may be the case even if there is no evidence of increased intracranial pressure, because the leak may act as a safety valve. Raised ICP,

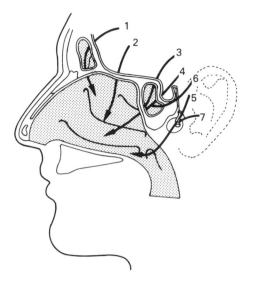

Anterior cranial fossa via   1 Frontal sinus
                              2 Ethmoid sinus/cribriform plate
                              3 Sphenoid sinus

Middle cranial fossa via   4 Sphenoid sinus
                              5 Mastoid air cells/middle ear and
                                eustachian tube

Posterior cranial fossa via   6 Sphenoid sinus
                              7 Mastoid air cells/middle ear and
                                eustachian tube

Figure 14.1 Pathways of CSF leakage into the nose

however, may not even be necessary for the development of spontaneous CSF rhinorrhoea. It has been noted that the onset of non-traumatic CSF rhinorrhoea usually occurs in adults, which coincides with the attainment of the highest levels of normal CSF pressure, an increase from 40 mm in infants to approximately 140 mm in the adult. In addition, the normal CSF pressure is positive in many positions of the head and is subject to recurring fluctuations, averaging 80 mm CSF fluid every few seconds. The normal arterial and respiratory pulse waves also affect CSF pressure. It is believed that the deep excavations of the cranial vault occupied by arachnoid granulations are produced by the normal CSF pressure pulse. In Ommaya's theory of focal atrophy (see below), he suggested that the normal contents of the cribriform plate or sella turcica areas can become reduced in bulk, possibly because of ischaemia. The empty space becomes a pouch filled with CSF. The normal pressure pulse causes this pouch to exert a focal and continually erosive effect, analogous to the creation of the cranial vault excavations, and this can possibly lead to a CSF fistula (Beckhardt, Setzen and Carras, 1991).

Theories for non-traumatic leaks in the anterior cranial fossa include focal atrophy, rupture of the arachnoid sleeves passing through the cribriform plate with olfactory nerve filaments, and persistence of an embryonic olfactory lumen (Ommaya, 1964).

Aetiology

Ommaya *et al.* (1968) are responsible for establishing the most widely used classification regarding aetiology, dividing the causes into traumatic and non-traumatic (spontaneous). The traumatic group is further divided into acute and delayed, while the non-traumatic group is divided into high and normal intracranial pressure groups (Table 14.1). This classification is by no means perfect (as the author admits) as the aetiological classes are not mutually exclusive in so far as the mechanics of the CSF leakage are concerned, i.e. it is possible that in certain cases of delayed traumatic CSF leakage the precipitating cause

Table 14.1 Causes of CSF rhinorrhoea

Traumatic
  Accidental
    Acute
    Delayed
  Iatrogenic
    Acute
    Delayed

Non-traumatic
  High pressure
    Tumours
      Direct
      Indirect
    Hydrocephalus
  Normal pressure
    Congenital anomalies
    Focal atrophy
      Olfactory
      Sellar
    Osteomyelitic erosion
    Idiopathic

for the rhinorrhoea may be analogous to mechanisms producing non-traumatic leaks. Approximately 80% of all cases of CSF rhinorrhoea are secondary to head trauma with an associated skull base fracture, 16% are the result of operations in the nasal/paranasal cavities and skull base. Only 3–4% are considered non-traumatic or spontaneous (Beckhardt, Setzen and Carras, 1991).

Traumatic

The true incidence of traumatic CSF leaks is not known, although it has been estimated that they complicate 2% of all head injuries and 5% of fractures of the skull base, most of which occur through the anterior cranial fossa (Calcaterra, 1980). Trauma to the floor of the anterior cranial fossa must have disruption of the arachnoid, a tear in the dura, and a fracture of bone (as well as a tear through the periosteum and mucosa) to result in a fistula. The bone of the anterior skull is thin with densely adherent dura and hence fractures here often result in dural tears. The most common location of anterior fistulae is the region of the fovea ethmoidalis (roof of the ethmoids) and the posterior frontal sinus wall, followed by the cribriform plate and the sphenoid sinus (Park, Strelzow and Friedman, 1983). The 'T'-shaped mass of the crista galli and cribriform plate is strong and moves as a unit. Thus in trauma it is more likely to see a fracture in the medial fovea ethmoidalis (Morley and Hetherington, 1957). The cribriform area is a more common location for atraumatic fistulae through the olfactory tracts.

Middle cranial fossa fractures are less common injuries that can cause leakage to the nose via the sphenoid sinus (lateral extensions of the sinus may underlie the middle cranial fossa, and both congenital and traumatic leaks may occur from this site) or eustachian tube.

CSF rhinorrhoea may also occur from the posterior fossa in fracture of the clivus allowing CSF into the sphenoid sinus, and fracture of the petrous temporal bone allowing fluid to enter the mastoid air cell system and hence the eustachian tube (in the presence of an intact tympanic membrane).

Post-traumatic CSF rhinorrhoea is immediate in the majority of cases. When delayed it appears within 3 months in 95% of cases (Shugar *et al.*, 1981), although it has been known to occur as long as 20 years after trauma (Krauss, 1962). The pathophysiology of these delayed cases is not well understood. It has been suggested that, at the time of injury, oedema and inflammation can temporarily obstruct the flow of CSF. As this resolves in the first week after injury, 70% of fistulae have already manifested themselves (Marentette and Valentino, 1991). In delayed fistulae, resorption of bone and soft tissues in the fracture site probably occurs secondary to the disrupted blood supply. This gradually weakens the pia arachnoid seal, until an elevation of intracranial pressure initiates a leak.

Leakage of CSF after skull base surgery is a fairly common occurrence. It may follow any type of skull base procedure, although it occurs most commonly after procedures disturbing the roof of a sinus (e.g. excision of a sinus neoplasm), intradural procedures that extend into a sinus (e.g. excision of a meningocoele), procedures in and around the ear that include dissection in the subarachnoid space (e.g. excision of an acoustic neuroma), and trans-sphenoidal hypophysectomies. Endoscopic ethmoid surgery for chronic sinus disease is being performed with increasing frequency and CSF leak is a significant potential complication of this surgery (Wigand, 1981; Stankiewicz, 1987). It seems likely, therefore, that iatrogenic trauma may become an increasingly frequent cause of CSF rhinorrhoea.

Non-traumatic

Non-traumatic CSF rhinorrhoea is uncommon. As recently as 1969, fewer than 150 cases had been reported in the literature (Brisman, Hughes and Mount, 1969). Forty-five per cent of cases are high pressure leaks and 55% of cases are normal pressure leaks (Shugar *et al.*, 1981). Most of the non-traumatic cases occur in adults in the fourth decade of life with females outnumbering males 2:1. It may present after an episode of sneezing, coughing or a minor upper respiratory tract infection. The initial onset is insidious, often mistaken for a feature of rhinitis (Brockbank, Veitch and Thomson, 1989).

High pressure leaks

The 'high pressure' fistulae are encountered in the cribriform area in 75% of cases (Ommaya, 1976). This is indicative of its fragility and unique anatomy in which a prolongation of the subarachnoid space follows the olfactory filaments. The leak functions as a safety valve alleviating the increased intracranial pressure. Eighty-four per cent of high pressure leaks are associated with slow-growing intracranial tumours and 16% associated with hydrocephalus (Shugar *et al.*, 1981). Pituitary neoplasms are the most common type of intracranial tumour found, followed by a variety of posterior fossa lesions. The important point to be noted is that direct invasion of the skull base is not the usual mechanism of the leak (Ommaya, 1964). This is emphasized by Cushing's series (Henderson, 1939) in which only 2.4% of pituitary tumours extended to the nasopharynx and none of these were complicated by a CSF leak.

As in this high pressure group the leakage of CSF is usually acting as a real safety valve, closure of the leak will invariably worsen the patient's condition if the causative lesion is not treated.

Normal pressure leaks

The normal pressure fistulae are most often located in the cribriform area and the sella turcica, but can sometimes be identified in the middle cranial fossa. Ninety per cent of cases are thought to originate from potential and/or congenital pathways and 10% are due to direct erosion of the skull base by tumour or infection (Shugar *et al.*, 1981).

The potential pathways include the prolongation of the subarachnoid space along the olfactory nerves and stalk of the hypophysis. Minor degrees of maldevelopment of the cribriform plate or the diaphragma sella may allow further extension of the subarachnoid space through the foramina of the cribriform plate or around the hypophysis (empty sella). The former is a much more common experience accounting for the majority of normal pressure leaks, whereas only 14 cases associated with an empty sella had been described by 1981 (Shugar *et al.*, 1981). Congenital osseous defects in the skull base can occur in conjunction with a meningoencephalocoele and are extremely rare causes of CSF leakage in adult life.

Non-traumatic normal pressure CSF rhinorrhoea can occasionally originate from the mastoid or middle ear. It is most commonly seen in younger patients and may occur via congenital defects in the tegmen or through and around the stapes in cases of Mondini's dysplasia (Weider, Geurkink and Saunders, 1985).

Direct erosion of the skull base by tumour or infection may produce a CSF leak. As mentioned above, intracranial neoplasms very rarely produce a leak by this mechanism. However, osteomas of the frontoethmoid region have this potential, as do nasopharyngeal angiofibroma and nasopharyngeal carcinoma, rarely. Osteomyelitic erosion of the skull base due to local sinus infection has been reported as a rare cause of CSF rhinorrhoea (MacDonald, 1945).

Diagnosis

The diagnosis of a dural fistula in the acute stage of trauma is not difficult. On the other hand the diagnosis of delayed traumatic or non-traumatic fistulae is more frequently delayed because of their more varied presentation.

The evaluation of a patient suspected of having CSF rhinorrhoea should first confirm the presence of the leak (i.e. confirm that the fluid is CSF), secondly demonstrate the cause whenever possible, and thirdly identify the site of the leak if surgical repair is necessary. Diagnostic difficulties are common. If the amount of CSF escaping through the nose is small, it may be difficult to distinguish it from serous nasal secretion. Exact localization of the fistula is extremely difficult, even in the presence of profuse rhinorrhoea.

Confirm the presence of a leak

History

In cases of trauma (both head injury and surgical), any persistent rhinorrhoea should be considered to be CSF until proven otherwise. The possibility of delayed dural fistulae should be kept in mind in all patients who, at one time, have sustained either facial or cranial trauma. Cases of spontaneous CSF rhinorrhoea may escape diagnosis until they develop the complications associated with dural fistulae. A patient who has had repeated attacks of meningitis, especially the pneumococcal type, should be regarded as having a dural defect with CSF leakage to the upper airway until proven otherwise, even though there is no demonstrable fluid drainage from the nose (McCoy, 1963).

The patient with CSF rhinorrhoea will usually, although not necessarily, present with unilateral, clear nasal discharge which may be persistent or intermittent. They may note a salty taste and bending the head forward usually will increase the rate of flow (as will the Valsalva manoeuvre or compression of both jugular veins).

Headache (not associated with meningitis) that is caused by either high or low CSF pressure can accompany CSF fistulae. Low pressure headache is caused when the leak allows sufficient CSF to escape in a normal pressure situation. The headache is relieved by reclining or straining, thereby returning the intracranial pressure to normal levels. In high pressure headaches, the pain is relieved by the rhinorrhoea. This headache is caused by increased intracranial pressure and should alert the clinician to the possibility of concomitant hydrocephalus.

Anosmia may be noted, which suggests a cribriform plate fracture with olfactory tract trauma.

Fistulae caused by space-occupying lesions will vary in their presentation according to the localization of the lesion, while CSF otorhinorrhoea may be associated with audiovestibular symptoms.

Examination

Physical examination is usually unremarkable except for the presence of rhinorrhoea. Positional change or jugular compression can increase the flow and help confirm the diagnosis. The reservoir sign is a well known physical finding used to elicit rhinorrhoea. After being supine for some time, the patient is brought to an upright position with the neck flexed. A sudden rush of clear fluid is indicative of CSF fistulae. It is a useful method for collecting fluid for biochemical analysis.

Classically the handkerchief test (fluid associated with rhinitis contains mucus which stiffens the handkerchief while CSF does not) and halo sign (when the CSF rhinorrhoea is blood stained it dries out with a central blood stain surrounded by a clear ring) have been described as confirmatory tests regarding the presence of CSF.

Use of nasal endoscopes would now be considered mandatory in the examination of the patient suspected of having CSF rhinorrhoea. Used alone or in conjunction with intrathecal fluorescein (as in methods for localization), it may help confirm the presence of a leak as well as its localization. If the CSF 'rhinorrhoea' is in fact CSF otorhinorrhoea then the CSF in the middle ear may simulate a middle ear effusion with an associated conductive hearing loss. In the event of the leak being related to a fracture through the labyrinthine capsule, there may be an associated sensorineural hearing loss and lower motor neuron facial palsy. Nasal endoscopy under these circumstances may identify the CSF escaping into the postnasal space via the eustachian tube orifice.

Biochemistry/immunochemistry

Glucose concentration

Various chemical tests, such as the determination of glucose, protein and electrolytes in the fluid have been advocated for the differentiation between CSF and other secretions. However, contamination of CSF with nasal secretions, blood, saliva, tears etc. renders a diagnosis of CSF leak invalid.

Glucose oxidase–impregnated test strips have been shown to be unreliable, because lacrimal gland secretions and nasal mucus have reducing substances that may cause a positive reaction with glucose concentrations as low as 5 mg/dl (0.28 mmol/l) (Calcaterra, 1980). A negative test, however, virtually rules out CSF as the tested fluid (Marentette and Valentino, 1991).

One of the main criteria for identification of the discharge is based on laboratory quantitative glucose determination. A concentration of 30 mg/dl (1.67 mmol/l) of glucose is considered confirmatory of CSF, if the patient has normal blood glucose levels (active meningitis can lower CSF glucose concentration and therefore confound the results of quantitative glucose analysis). However, *if the CSF is contaminated by blood then the test is invalid*.

β2-Transferrin

In the routine protein electrophoresis of serum, only one transferrin band is seen in the β1-fraction. Two electrophoretically different transferrins can be found in the electrophoresis of the CSF proteins: the β1-fraction of normal transferrin and a second band of transferrin, in the β2-fraction. This β2-fraction is pathognomonic for CSF (Meurman *et al.*, 1979).

The assay is carried out first by performing normal agar gel electrophoresis. After electrophoresis a cellulose acetate strip containing antitransferrin serum is applied at the β-area. If the sample contains CSF, stained immunoprecipitates appear both in the β1- and the β2- zones.

Generally 5–7 ml of fluid are needed for the electrophoresis of CSF. However, in this immunochemical identification only about 50 μl are needed. Moderate contamination with the other body fluids does not invalidate the method. The detection of β2-transferrin can clearly demonstrate whether CSF leakage exists or not.

In the majority of hospitals in the UK this assay is not available routinely. In order for it to be provided the interested clinician needs to approach the clinical chemistry department concerned.

If doubt persists, the ultimate proof is the finding in the rhinorrhoea of a label introduced into the CSF, as in the methods for localization.

Demonstrate the cause

Over half the cases of non-traumatic rhinorrhoea are high pressure leaks, and the majority of these are related to intracranial tumours. CT and MRI are obviously important investigations to exclude this possible cause of non-traumatic leaks.

Localization of the leak

The clinical finding of CSF rhinorrhoea represents only the site of exiting CSF; the origin of the fistula is not deduced easily from the clinical examination. Accurate definition of the leakage site is undoubtedly the most important factor in successful treatment of this problem. Finding the site may be complicated because the leak may be profuse and obscure the studies, or may be intermittent and not present at the time of evaluation. Dandy (1944) wrote 50 years ago, 'disclosure of the fistulous tract may be exceedingly difficult, perhaps even impossible'. Despite all the advances in imaging techniques this statement is still largely true.

Radiology

Radiology plays a key role in the management of this condition. It may help confirm the presence of the CSF leak and may identify any underlying cause (see above). Finally, radiology may determine the anatomical site, side and size of the fistula and thereby assist in planning the surgical approach.

A variety of radiological techniques has been used to localize the leakage site. In the majority of these bone defects, air–fluid levels and erosions are used to identify the possible site.

Plain films may be useful in demonstrating pneumocephalus or air–fluid levels. Fractures in the skull base with fluid in an adjacent sinus are suggestive of a fistula. If pneumocephalus is present following craniofacial trauma (Figure 14.2), an intradural-extracranial communication also must have been present. This may be a transient tract, but CSF fistula also can accompany this finding.

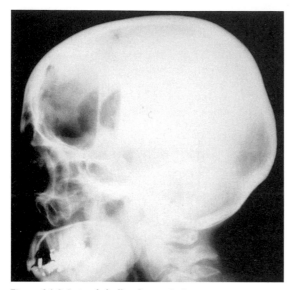

Figure 14.2 Lateral skull radiograph showing pneumocephalus following craniofacial trauma

CT scanning may be extremely helpful, and the importance of thorough thin section axial and coronal cuts on a high resolution machine cannot be overemphasized. The CT scan has become a sensitive method for detecting skull base fractures and CSF fistulae, as well as pneumocephalus (Marentette and Valentino, 1991). In evaluating anterior cranial fossa leaks coronal CT scans are most helpful. On coronal scanning, detailed information can be gathered about the integrity of the cribriform plate, the fovea ethmoidalis, the planum sphenoidale, the floor of the frontal sinus, the pituitary fossa and orbital roof. The frontal, ethmoid and sphenoid sinuses can be examined for evidence of fluid collection (Figure 14.3). Tolley, Lloyd and Williams (1991) have shown, in their series of non-traumatic CSF rhinorrhoea, that all patients showed deviation of their crista galli (a radiological sign hitherto unreported).

Axial CT scans examine the anterior and posterior tables of the frontal sinus, together with the extension of linear fractures into the frontal sinuses, the medial orbital walls, and the perpendicular plate of the ethmoid.

Investigation in all non-traumatic cases should include CT views of the anterior, middle and posterior cranial fossae (inclusive of the inner ears) as well as

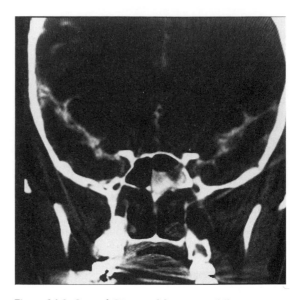

Figure 14.3 Coronal CT scan of the sinuses (following injection of intrathecal contrast) in a patient with CSF rhinorrhoea showing contrast within the sphenoid sinus. (Supplied by Dr P. Anslow, Consultant Neuroradiologist, Radcliffe Infirmary, Oxford)

an intracranial CT to exclude the possibility of tumour or hydrocephalus.

Metrizamide CT cisternography has been shown to be the most useful and reliable method for identifying and localizing CSF leaks, but only if there is actual leakage of CSF from the cranial cavity at the time of the radiological studies.

Visualization of metrizamide passing through a bony defect is certainly irrefutable evidence of a CSF leak. In addition, the combination of a bony defect with extracranial metrizamide adjacent to the bony defect adequately defines the site of the CSF leakage. The presence of extracranial metrizamide within one sinus or in one focal area at the base of the skull does not precisely delineate the site of CSF leakage. However, it does localize the site of CSF leakage to a specific area at the skull base, and thereby provides valuable information for the surgeon planning the repair (Figure 14.4).

Metrizamide CT cisternography is best performed in the position of maximal leakage, although elevation of intracranial pressure by the Valsalva manoeuvre or infusion of saline intrathecally may be used to increase the leakage and demonstrate the fistula. Numerous studies have shown success rates varying between 22% and 100% with metrizamide CT cisternography for fistula localization (Chow, Goodman and Mafee, 1989). Mamo *et al.* (1982) had a success rate of only 22% but none of the patients studied had an active leak at the time of the study. Manelfe *et al.* (1982), however, achieved a success rate of 83%

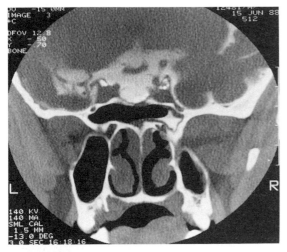

Figure 14.4 CT cisternogram in the coronal plane showing contrast in an empty sella. The bony floor of the sella is deficient and contrast can be seen in the lateral part of the sphenoid sinus on the right. (Supplied by Dr J. Byrne, Consultant Neuroradiologist, Radcliffe Infirmary, Oxford)

where all patients had active leaks at the time of the study. Naidich and Moran (1980) reported a 100% success rate in identifying the site of the CSF leakage when CSF pressure was artificially increased in order to convert an inactive leak into an active leak. It would therefore seem that metrizamide CT cisternography is more helpful in localizing the site of CSF leakage in patients with active leaks.

Recently Byrne *et al.* (1990) have combined CT cisternography with digital subtraction of fluoroscopy images. They feel that the dynamic view provided by digital subtraction cisternography allows more confident demonstration of CSF fistulae, particularly in larger defects associated with postoperative rhinorrhoea. It gives information additional to that available from CT cisternography alone including the demonstration of multiple fistulae. There is a minimal morbidity associated with the use of metrizamide; the most frequent symptom consisting of a mild headache. However, there have been reports of neurotoxicity and metrizamide has now been replaced by the next generation of iodine-based contrast media such as Iohexol.

MRI is generally not used in the investigation of CSF rhinorrhoea, because it is not as effective as CT in demonstrating bone windows, which is necessary in trying to localize the site of leakage. However, Di Chiro *et al.* (1986) have used MRI after cisternal introduction of gadolinium to demonstrate the site of CSF rhinorrhoea in dogs. MRI would offer obvious advantages, such as lack of exposure to ionizing radiation, if this technique could eventually be adopted in man.

Isotope studies

In the case of inactive, intermittent, small or questionable CSF leaks, metrizamide or Iohexol CT cisternography still may not reveal the leak. Radionuclide cisternography has been more effective in identifying the presence of the leaks, although often not giving precise anatomical localization. Indium 111-DPTA is now generally used for this purpose (Park, Strelzow and Friedman, 1983). Its reduced half-life (2.8 days) and much lower radiation absorption combined with higher quality images and lower neurotoxicity are its chief advantages; however it is very sensitive and frequently results in overly positive scans of little localizing benefit. Localization may be improved by introducing pledgets into the different regions of the nose and examining these with a gamma counter.

Intrathecal dyes

An intrathecal dye (indigo-carmine) was used as early as 1933 to assist in localizing CSF leaks (Fox, 1933). This method of study fell into disrepute owing to several reports of neural complications. More recently Messerklinger (1972) has described the combination of intrathecal fluorescein (which stains the CSF a bright yellow-green colour) and nasal endoscopes to diagnose anterior cranial fossa leaks (both preoperatively and intraoperatively).

This technique has been elegantly described by Stammberger (1992). Through a lumbar puncture, 1 ml of CSF is withdrawn and 1 ml of 5% sodium fluorescein is injected intrathecally. Subsequently, the patient is kept in the prone position with the head slightly lower than the rest of the body. This allows the dye to be distributed throughout the entire dural space, since it has a higher specific gravity than CSF.

If there is a large CSF fistula, occasionally bright yellowish-green CSF can be seen dripping from the nose within a few minutes after the injection. The patient is then placed in the supine position for endoscopic examination. The nose is sprayed with a topical anaesthetic and vasoconstritor (4% lignocaine with 1:1000 adrenaline) and the endoscopic examination can begin after a minute using a 4 mm 30° endoscope. If the fluorescein test is strongly positive, white light will show the stained CSF clearly and allow it to be followed back to its source. At the least, the examiner can determine whether the leak originates in the lamina cribrosa, the anterior or posterior ethmoid, or the sphenoid. In a lateral skull base fracture with an associated CSF otorhinorrhoea it may be possible to identify CSF leaking into the nasopharynx from the eustachian tube orifice (especially during swallowing).

If the CSF fistula is small and there is only a small leak of CSF at the time of the study, it may be difficult to recognize the leak. In such cases the use of a blue light source is helpful to display the fluorescence of the CSF-fluorescein mixture. Even minimal traces of CSF appear under blue light as a bright whitish-green streak, while simple nasal secretions remain colourless and do not fluoresce. This blue light technique is extremely sensitive and is positive up to a dilution of 1:10 million. In the event of a negative fluorescein test, it can prove useful to place small Merocel sponges into the nose for 6 hours. These sponges absorb the nasal secretions and can then be examined under blue light.

Complications from intrathecal fluorescein are infrequent (Reck and Wissen-Siegert, 1984) and it would seem likely that with increasing experience this will become the method of choice in localizing CSF leaks.

Management

The importance of close cooperation between neurosurgeon, neuroradiologist and otolaryngologist cannot be overemphasized. An interdisciplinary team approach to this difficult problem offers the patient the best chance of a successful outcome.

The management of CSF rhinorrhoea is controversial but can be divided into a medical and surgical philosophy. The most appropriate treatment choice depends upon several factors including the severity and extent of the injury, the aetiology, and the anatomical site of the CSF leak (Park, Strelzow and Friedman, 1983).

Medical (conservative) treatment

In the acute CSF leak an initial trial of conservative treatment should be considered (especially as the majority of acute traumatic fistulae will seal spontaneously). This involves bed rest in the 'head-up' position. The patient is advised to avoid coughing, sneezing, nose blowing and straining due to physical activity. Different medications may be used to reduce the spinal fluid production rate (acetazolamide, frusemide) but are probably minimally effective. Most effective in decreasing intracranial CSF pressures is the repeated removal of CSF fluid via repeat lumbar taps or an indwelling lumbar subarachnoid drain. This modality allows the dural tears to approximate each other inducing healing by primary intention of the CSF fistula. Opponents of this approach suggest that an indwelling lumbar drain can increase the risk of meningitis and many would not use it without covering the patient with antibiotics. The place of prophylactic antibiotics (when not using a drain) is still controversial and their use has been both condoned (Lewin, 1954; Leech and Paterson, 1973) and condemned (Hoff, Brewin and U, 1976). The proponents of this practice argue that the CSF is exposed to potentially pathogenic microorganisms of the upper airway, and antibiotics might prevent the development of meningitis. The opponents of the practice argue that prophylactic antibiotics expose the patient to potentially resistant organisms and a more serious infection. In a recent review of the English language literature, prophylactic antibiotics were found not to provide protection against development of meningitis in patients with CSF leaks (Rathore, 1991). A large controlled prospective study is needed to address this management issue.

If non-operative treatment has failed after 10–14 days, or if the leak recurs or is chronic, the problem of localization and surgical treatment must be addressed.

Surgical treatment

This not only involves closure of the fistula but also removing the cause in the case of non-traumatic leaks. This will involve surgery to deal with the underlying intracranial neoplasm or the underlying hydrocephalus, i.e. CSF shunt procedures.

Operative approaches for closure of the fistula are divided into intracranial (intradural and extradural) and extracranial. The choice of procedure (or combination of procedures) depends on the preoperative localization of the fistula. Poor localization demands wide exposure, whereas, with precise localization, a more limited procedure is adequate. A high recurrence rate (20% according to Myers and Sataloff, 1984) may be anticipated whichever route is chosen, although more recently Persky *et al.* (1991) have claimed an initial success rate of 86% for extracranial approaches. The place of an indwelling subarachnoid lumbar drain in the postoperative period is not clear but would seem to be a reasonable option in the hope of improving the success rate for this type of surgery.

Intracranial

Dandy documented the first successful intracranial repair of a CSF fistula in 1926. A craniotomy through the frontal, parietal or temporal region (depending upon the site of the leak) exposes the floor of one or more cranial fossae. The approach may be either intradural or extradural, although the former is preferred (Ommaya, 1976). Once the subarachnoid dehiscence has been identified, its intradural repair with sutures permits a watertight seal. It is described as having the advantages of direct visualization of the dural tear, inspection and treatment of adjacent cortex, and a better chance at tamponading a leak in the face of increased intracranial pressure. It involves greater morbidity, brain retraction and frequent loss of olfaction (in surgery of the anterior cranial fossa) in comparison to the extracranial approaches, but is the procedure of choice in the case of non-identifiable CSF leaks, i.e. leaks that cannot be localized pre-operatively.

Extracranial

When the site of the fistula can be localized, an extracranial approach can be considered. Since Dohlman in 1948 and Hirsch in 1952 first described the extracranial approaches to CSF rhinorrhoea, Montgomery (1966, 1973) has developed and publicized these techniques widely and his mono-graph is still the definitive work on the subject. The particular technique adopted is dependent upon the site, size and nature of the leak. It is now accepted (at least by otolaryngologists!) that an extracranial ap-proach offers a reasonable chance of success with minimal morbidity and mortality. Hubbard *et al.* (1985) reviewed the experience of the Mayo Clinic over a 10-year period and concluded that crani-otomy should be used only after failure of these extracranial approaches.

Leakage of CSF through the frontal sinus

Repair of a CSF leak via the posterior wall of the frontal sinus may be made via the anterior osteoplas-tic flap procedure using either the eyebrow or coronal incision. It is important to ensure that the entire mucous membrane lining of the frontal sinus is re-moved and this can be accomplished by removing the inner cortical lining of the sinus with a rotating cutting burr. Subcutaneous fat is harvested and used to fill the sinus completely. Fascia lata may also be used to repair a defect in the dura of the frontal lobe if required.

Leakage of CSF through the cribriform plate and roof of ethmoid

CSF leakage via this route may be repaired via an external ethmoidectomy approach. All the ethmoid cells are cleared up to the level of the cribriform plate and the middle turbinate is removed to facilitate exposure.

The septomucosal flap used to repair a fistula via the cribriform plate and roof of the ethmoid is based posteriorly. The superior incision extends along the anteroposterior dimension of the superior nasal septum at the junction of the septum and the olfac-tory slit. This incision is carried as far anteriorly as possible. The lower incision is approximately 1.5 cm below, and parallel to, the superior incision. The anterior incision merely connects the anterior aspect of the superior and inferior mucosal incisions. The septomucosal flap is rotated 90° so as to cover the point of leakage and adjacent dura of the olfactory and ethmoid regions.

Leakage of CSF through the sphenoid sinus

Hirsch (1952) was the first to use a septal flap for repair of CSF leakage via the sphenoid sinus. A complete external ethmoidectomy is carried out ini-tially as described above. A septal mucosal flap must be fashioned prior to entering the sphenoid sinus, for the mucosa covering its anterior wall makes up the base of this flap. The flap is based at the inferior margin of the front face of the sphenoid sinus (as opposed to the posterior base of the flap used for cribriform plate/ethmoid fistulae). After the mucosal flap has been carefully elevated and reflected into the nasopharynx, the anterior wall of the sphenoid sinus is removed. Usually it is necessary to remove the intersphenoid septum and a small portion of the posterior aspect of the nasal septum in order to provide wide exposure of the sphenoid sinus complex. The mucosal lining of the sphenoid sinuses is re-moved and the septal mucosal flap is placed over the point of leakage. If the dural defect is large it may be plugged with fat or fascia lata before the septal mu-cosal flap is placed.

A trans-septal approach may also be used but visibility is restricted and does not offer the versatility of the transethmoid approach described above.

Leakage of CSF through the mastoid and middle ear

CSF leakage via the mastoid or middle ear can be successfully stopped by obliterative techniques as almost all the dura surrounding the petrous bone can be approached extracranially from below. Robson *et al.* (1989) described the use of pedicled sternomas-toid muscle and in larger leaks a free fat graft may be employed. The dura surrounding the defect is widely exposed so that the flap or graft can be packed tightly against the point of leakage. The mastoid incision is tightly closed in layers without drainage.

In all of the extracranial repair techniques de-scribed above, there is evidence to suggest that the use of fibrin glue, by its adhesive sealing properties, enhances the results of repair of CSF fistulae (Nishi-hira and McCaffrey, 1988).

Endoscopic repair of CSF fistulae

More recently endoscopic closure of minor CSF leaks occurring during ethmoidectomy has been reported by Wigand (1981), Papay *et al.* (1989) and Stankie-wicz (1989). CSF leak is a significant potential compli-cation of endoscopic ethmoidectomy and immediate endoscopic repair of such leaks should be considered by any surgeon performing endoscopic nasal surgery if a CSF rhinorrhoea is discovered intraoperatively. Delayed onset CSF leaks which are visible endoscopi-cally are also amenable to endoscopic repair.

All authors describe slightly different techniques

but all stress the importance of identifying the defect accurately. The mucosa is elevated from the surrounding bone and the abdominal fat or musculofascial graft (temporalis fascia, fascia lata) is 'tucked in' above the bony skull base where possible, i.e the intracranial side is supported. Muscle or mucoperiosteum (from the nasal septum) is then placed over the defect and the edges are tucked under the mucosal edges around the defect. The use of tissue glue or microfibrillar collagen help secure it and further support is provided by the use of Gelfoam packing. The application of endoscopic techniques to intranasal closure of CSF leaks has a number of advantages over conventional methods (Mattox and Kennedy, 1990) including:

1 Excellent field of vision, allowing exact localization of the leak
2 The ability precisely to clean mucosa from the bony defect without significantly increasing the size of the defect
3 Accurate position of the graft material over the defect.

Summary (Figure 14.5)

Unfortunately, a review of the literature regarding CSF rhinorrhoea and its management poses more questions than it answers. The most important of these are:

1 Having made the diagnosis, should treatment be conservative or surgical?
2 If conservative treatment is adopted, how long does one continue before resorting to surgery?
3 What is the place of prophylactic antibiotics?
4 If surgical treatment is felt appropriate, should an intracranial of extracranial approach be used?
5 What is the place of lumbar drainage in surgical treatment?

Individual cases have to be judged on their own merits and, in the future, prospective randomized trials may provide the answers to some of the above questions. For the moment, the sequential algorithm in Figure 14.5 shows a simplified approach to this difficult management problem.

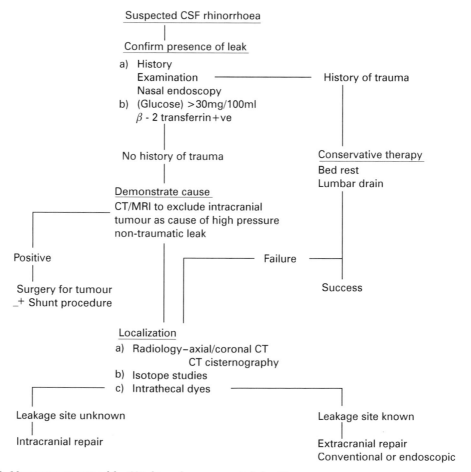

Figure 14.5   Management protocol for CSF rhinorrhoea: sequential algorithm

References

BECKHARDT, R. N., SETZEN, M., and CARRAS, R. (1991) Primary spontaneous cerebrospinal fluid rhinorrhea. *Otolaryngology – Head and Neck Surgery*, **104**, 425–432

BRISMAN, R., HUGHES, J. E. O. and MOUNT, L. A. (1969) Cerebrospinal fluid rhinorrhoea and the empty sella. *Journal of Neurosurgery*, **31**, 538–543

BROCKBANK, M. J., VEITCH, D. Y. and THOMSON, H. G. (1989) Cerebrospinal fluid in the rhinitis clinic. *Journal of Laryngology and Otology*, **103**, 281–283

BYRNE, J. V., INGRAM, C. E., MACVICAR, D., SULLIVAN, F. M. and UTTLEY, D. (1990) Digital subtraction cisternography: a new approach to fistula localisation in cerebrospinal fluid rhinorrhoea. *Journal of Neurology, Neurosurgery and Psychiatry*, **53**, 1072–1075

CALCATERRA, C. T. (1980) Extracranial surgical repair of cerebrospinal fluid rhinorrhoea. *Annals of Otology, Rhinology and Laryngology*, **89**, 108–116

CHANDLER, J. R. (1983) Traumatic cerebrospinal fluid leakage. *Otolaryngologic Clinics of North America*, **16**, 623–632

CHOW, S. M., GOODMAN, D. and MAFEE, M. F. (1989) Evaluation of CSF rhinorrhoea by computerized tomography with metrizamide. *Otolaryngology – Head and Neck Surgery*, **100**, 99–105

DANDY, W. E. (1926) Pneumocephalus (intracranial pneumatocele or aerocele). *Archives of Surgery*, **12**, 949–982

DANDY, W. E. (1944) Treatment of rhinorrhea and otorrhea. *Archives of Surgery*, **49**, 75–85

DI CHIRO, G., GIRTON, M. E., FRANK, J. A., DIETZ, M. J., GANSOW, O. A., WRIGHT, D. C. et al. (1986) Cerebrospinal fluid rhinorrhoea:depiction with MR cisternography in dogs. *Radiology*, **160**, 221–222

DOHLMAN, G. (1948) Spontaneous cerebrospinal fluid rhinorrhea. Case operated by rhinologic methods. *Acta Otolaryngologica*, (Suppl.) **67**, 20–23

FOX, N. (1933) Cure in a case of cerebrospinal rhinorrhea. *Archives of Otolaryngology*, **17**, 85–86

HENDERSON, W. R. (1939) Pituitary adenomata: follow-up study of surgical results in 338 cases (Dr Harry Cushing's series). *British Journal of Surgery*, **26**, 811–921

HIRSCH, O. (1952) Successful closure of cerebrosinal fluid rhinorrhea by endonasal surgery. *Archives of Otolaryngology*, **56**, 1–12

HOFF, J. T., BREWIN, A. and U, H. S. (1976) Antibiotics for basilar skull fractures. *Journal of Neurosurgery*, **44**, 649

HUBBARD, J. L., MCDONALD, T. J., PEARSON, B. W. and LAWS, E. R. (1985) Spontaneous cerebrospinal fluid rhinorrhoea; evolving concepts in diagnosis and surgical management based on the Mayo Clinic experience from 1970 through 1981. *Neurosurgery*, **16**, 314–323

KRAUSS, H. (1962) Schadelverletgungen mit Eroffnung der Nebenhohlen. *Journal of the International College of Surgeons*, **38**, 373–376

LEECH, P. J. and PATERSON, A. (1973) Conservative and operative management for cerebrospinal fluid leakage after closed head injury. *Lancet*, i, 1011–1016

LEWIN, W. (1954) Cerebrospinal fluid rhinorrhoea in closed head injuries. *British Journal of Surgery*, **42**, 1–8

MCCOY, G. (1963) Cerebrospinal rhinorrhea: a comprehensive review and a definition of the responsibility of the rhinologist in diagnosis and treatment. *Laryngoscope*, **73**, 1125–1157

MACDONALD, R. (1945) The occurrence of spontaneous cerebrospinal rhinorrhoea in the literature, the experience of the writer, and other diplomats of the American Boards of Otolaryngology and Neurosurgeons. *Laryngoscope*, **55**, 552–586

MAMO, L., COPHIGNON, J., REY, A. and THUREL, C. (1982) A new radionuclide method for the diagnosis of posttraumatic cerebrospinal fistulas – a study of 308 cases. *Journal of Neurosurgery*, **57**, 92–98

MANELFE, C., CELLERIER, P., SOBEL, D., PREVOST, C. and BONET, A. (1982) Cerebrospinal fluid rhinorrhea: evaluation with metrizamide cisternography. *American Journal of Radiology*, **138**, 471–476

MARENTETTE, L. J. and VALENTINO, J. (1991) Traumatic anterior fossa cerebrospinal fluid fistulae and craniofacial considerations. *Otolaryngologic Clinics of North America*, **24**, 151–163

MATTOX, D. E. and KENNEDY, D. W. (1990) Endoscopic management of cerebrospinal fluid leaks and cephaloceles. *Laryngoscope*, **100**, 857–862

MESSERKLINGER, W. (1972) Nasendoscopie: Nachweis, Lokalisation und Defferentialdiagnose der Nasalen Liquorrhoe. *HNO; Wegweiser für die Fachaerztliche Praxis (Berlin)*, **20**, 268–270

MEURMAN, O. H., IRJALA, K., SUONPAA, J. and LAURENT, B. (1979) A new method for the identification of cerebrospinal fluid leakage. *Acta Otolaryngologica*, **87**, 366–369

MILLER, C. (1826) Case of hydrocephalus chronicus with some unusual symptoms and appearances on dissection. *Transactions of the Medical-Chirurgical Society of Edinburgh*, **2**, 243–248

MONTGOMERY, W. W. (1966) Surgery for cerebrospinal fluid rhinorrhea and otorrhea. *Archives of Otolaryngology*, **84**, 538–550

MONTGOMERY, W. W. (1973) Cerebrospinal fluid rhinorrhea. *Otolaryngologic Clinics of North America*, **6**, 757–771

MORLEY, T. P. and HETHERINGTON, R. F. (1957) Traumatic CSF rinorrhoea and otorrhoea, pneumocephalus and meningitis, *Surgery, Gynecology and Obstetrics*, **104**, 88–98

MYERS, D. L. and SATALOFF, R. T. (1984) Spinal fluid leakage after skull base surgical procedures. *Otolaryngologic Clinics of North America*, **17**, 601–612

NAIDICH, T. P. and MORAN, C. J. (1980) Precise anatomic localisation of atraumatic sphenoethmoidal fluid rhinorrhea by metrizamide CT cisternography. *Journal of Neurosurgery*, **53**, 222–228

NISHIHIRA, S. and MCCAFFREY, T. V. (1988) The use of fibrin glue for the repair of experimental CSF rhinorrhea. *Laryngoscope*, **98**, 625–627

OMMAYA, A. K. (1964) Cerebrospinal fluid rhinorrhea. *Neurology*, **14**, 106–113

OMMAYA, A. K. (1976) Spinal fluid fistulae. *Clinical Neurosurgery*, **23**, 363–392

OMMAYA, A. K., DI CHIRO, G., BALDWIN, M. and PENNYBACKER, J. B. (1968) Non-traumatic cerebrospinal fluid rhinorrhea. *Journal of Neurology, Neurosurgery and Psychiatry*, **31**, 214–225

PAPAY, F. A., MAGGIANO, H., DOMINQUEZ, S., HASSENBUSCH, S. J., LEVINE, H. L. and LAVERTU, P. (1989) Rigid endoscopic repair of paranasal sinus cerebrospinal fluid fistulas. *Laryngoscope*, **99**, 1195–1201

PARK, J., STRELZOW, V. V. and FRIEDMAN, W. H. (1983) Current management of cerebrospinal fluid rhinorrhea. *Laryngoscope*, **93**, 1294–1300

PERSKY, M. S., ROTHSTEIN, S. G., BREDA, S. D., COHEN, N. L., COOPER, P. and RANSOHOFF, J. (1991) Extracranial repair of cerebrospinal fluid otorhinorrhea. *Laryngoscope*, **101**, 134–136

RATHORE, M. H. (1991) Do prophylactic antibiotics prevent meningitis after basilar skull fracture? *Pediatric Infectious Disease Journal*, **10**, 87–88

RECK, R. and WISSEN-SIEGERT, I. (1984) Ergebnisse der Fluoreszein-Asenendoskopie bei der Diagnositic der Rhinoliquorrho. *Laryngologie, Rhinologie, Otologie*, **63**, 353–355

ROBSON, A. K., CLARKE, P. M., DILKES, M. and MAW, A. R. (1989) Transmastoid extracranial repair of CSF leaks following acoustic neuroma resection. *Journal of Laryngology and Otology*, **103**, 842–844

SHUGAR, J. M. A., SOM, P. M., EISMAN, W. and BILLER, H. F. (1981) Non-traumatic cerebrospinal fluid rhinorrhea. *Laryngoscope*, **91**, 114–119

STAMMBERGER, H. (1992) *Atlas of Functional Endoscopic Sinus Surgery*. New York: Decker

STANKIEWICZ, J. (1987) Complications of intranasal endoscopic ethmoidectomy. *Laryngoscope*, **97**, 1270–1273

STANKIEWICZ, J. (1989) Complications in endoscopic intranasal ethmoidectomy: an update. *Laryngoscope*, **99**, 686–690

ST CLAIR THOMPSON (1899) *The Cerebrospinal Fluid: Its Spontaneous Escape from the Nose with Observations of its Composition and Function in Human Subjects*. London: Cassell

TOLLEY, N. S., LLOYD, G. A. S. and WILLIAMS, H. O. L. (1991) Radiological study of primary spontaneous CSF rhinorrhoea. *Journal of Laryngology and Otology*, **105**, 274–277

WEIDER, D. J., GEURKINK, N. A. and SAUNDERS, R. L. (1985) Spontaneous cerebrospinal fluid rhinorrhea. *American Journal of Otology*, **6**, 416–422

WIGAND, M. E. (1981) Transnasal ethmoidectomy under endoscopic control. *Rhinology*, **19**, 7–15

15

The upper airways and their relation to the respiratory system

J. Paul Dilworth and David M. Mitchell

It is common for diseases of the nose and paranasal sinuses (rhinosinusitis), larynx, pharynx and of the lower respiratory tract to occur together and this chapter is concerned with conditions where this association is important. In the first section we discuss general aspects of inflammatory disease of the upper airways and their relationship to chest diseases. Infectious causes of rhinosinusitis are frequently associated with lower respiratory disease and are discussed in this chapter. Mechanical obstruction to the upper respiratory tract, autonomic imbalance, and hormonal causes have few respiratory manifestations and are dealt with elsewhere. The major importance of allergic rhinitis demands a section on its own (in Chapter 6), although the relationship between allergic rhinitis and asthma is discussed further in this chapter.

The presence of rhinosinusitis should always prompt the search for disease of the lower respiratory tract. It is useful to take a respiratory history with reference to cough, sputum production, haemoptysis, wheeze and breathlessness. Inquiry about atopic symptoms, smoking and occupational history is useful. A chest X-ray and spirometry will frequently be helpful and further respiratory assessment performed if indicated.

This chapter starts with a general approach to the assessment of the lower respiratory tract in the context of upper airway disease, including interpretation of pulmonary function tests. This is followed by a discussion of defence mechanisms of the respiratory tract. Further sections discuss the upper and lower respiratory tract in bronchiectasis, cystic fibrosis, tuberculosis, AIDS, granulomatous conditions and also the relationship between asthma and allergic rhinitis. The aetiology of rhinosinusitis is given in Table 15.1.

Table 15.1 Aetiology of rhinosinusitis

1 Allergy (seasonal, perennial, occupational)
2 Infection
   Acute
   Chronic
      specific (bacterial, fungal, etc.)
      non-specific (secondary to host defence deficiency)
3 Mechanical (anatomical variant, trauma, tumour, foreign body)
4 Other (e.g. autonomic imbalance, hormonal, granulomatous

An approach to assessment of the lower respiratory tract

Many symptoms and some physical signs are shared between diseases that originate in the upper and lower respiratory tract and it is important that those seeing referrals with these symptoms should consider a complete differential diagnosis for both systems as the two are strongly interlinked. Initially, a way to assess the lower respiratory tract is presented in the context of upper airway disease.

Symptoms

The cardinal symptoms of lower respiratory tract disease are cough, sputum, haemoptysis, breathlessness, wheeze and chest pain. Many of these may also be present with upper respiratory tract problems.

Cough is abnormal when persistent. It is initiated by irritant receptors in the respiratory tract especially in the pharynx, larynx, trachea and bifurcations of major airways. In the presence of a foreign body or excess secretions, by expelling materials it aids mucociliary clearance in maintaining patency of the airway. It may be stimulated by sputum production, smoke, odours and cold air. It may be present for weeks after a viral infection, with a postnasal drip and with bronchial carcinoma. Nocturnal cough is common in asthma, pulmonary oedema and acid reflux. A full list of causes is given in Table 15.2.

Sputum is generally removed by mucociliary clearance and when in excess this is assisted by cough. The amount and degree of purulence should be recorded. Large amounts may indicate bronchiectasis or occasionally an alveolar cell carcinoma. It may be mucoid as in chronic bronchitis, yellow with inflammation or infection or green with infection. Expectoration of plugs may suggest asthma. In asthma, sputum may be discoloured in the absence of infection.

Haemoptysis is always a significant symptom which requires investigations although quite frequently no cause is found. Patients may be unclear as to whether blood has been genuinely coughed up or produced from the upper respiratory tract and mouth or even vomited. The commonest serious causes from the lower respiratory tract are carcinoma, infection (including aspergilloma, tuberculosis, abscess and bronchiectasis), pulmonary embolism, pulmonary oedema, alveolar haemorrhage syndromes (include systemic lupus erythematosus, Wegener's granulomatosis and other forms of pulmonary vasculitis), trauma, vascular abnormalities and bleeding diathesis (includes haematological disorders and anticoagulant therapy). Investigations required include a chest X-ray and in those over 40 years of age, particularly in smokers, bronchoscopy should always be considered even in the presence of a normal chest X-ray. In the absence of a lower respiratory tract cause, the upper respiratory tract should be carefully examined.

Breathlessness has a wide differential diagnosis. The speed of onset of breathlessness often gives an indication of the cause (Figure 15.1). Diurnal variation suggests asthma or left ventricular failure. An assessment of current and previous exercise tolerance will help in determining the cause and severity. Orthopnoea and paroxysmal nocturnal dyspnoea will help to identify patients with pulmonary oedema, reversible airflow limitation or occasionally suggest acid reflux or obstructive sleep apnoea. Obstruction of the trachea or larynx by tumour or a foreign body may present as breathlessness with stridor and can be assessed by pulmonary function tests and CT scanning.

Wheeze is common in patients with airflow limitation but it may also occur in left ventricular failure (cardiac asthma). Inspiratory wheeze may indicate laryngeal, tracheal or main bronchial narrowing and these patients may be misdiagnosed as having asthma initially.

Chest pain may originate from cardiac, gastrointestinal, respiratory or musculoskeletal causes. The pain of tracheitis associated with an upper respiratory tract viral illness is a raw retrosternal pain worse on deep inspiration.

In addition to these primary symptoms, a full smoking and occupational history are important. It is useful to enquire about atopy, medications being taken or previously taken, symptoms suggestive of respiratory failure (e.g. morning headache or ankle swelling), or of obstructive sleep apnoea (e.g. daytime sleepiness, loud snoring and apnoeas). Finally, systemic symptoms indicating weight loss and fever may be helpful in diagnosis.

Table 15.2 Causes of persistent cough

Cause	Clinical feature
Viral bronchial infection	Cough can persist for many weeks but does resolve eventually
Nasal and sinus infection/inflammation/allergy	Cough follows infection or exposure to allergens. Postnasal drip is common
Chronic bronchitis/smoking	Usually seen in smokers. When patients stop smoking the cough ceases
Bronchiectasis	Productive of sputum, often purulent. May be positional
Tuberculosis	Often with history of weight loss and fever
Asthma/bronchial hyperreactivity	Worse at night, on exercise or following exposure to allergen, cold air, dusts etc
Bronchial carcinoma/carcinoid/benign bronchial neoplasms	Cough that becomes worse than usual in a smoker. Occasionally a new symptom
Repeated bronchial aspiration	Oesophageal disorders, neurological disease affecting swallowing
History of inhaled foreign body	Relatively common in children. History of inhaled body frequently missed or not present
Gastro-oesophageal reflux	Responds to H_2 antagonists
Pulmonary fibrosis	Patients usually breathless, cough is dry
Drug induced	ACE inhibitors, beta-blockers
Psychogenic	Patient otherwise well. No cough at night or when distracted. No response to cough suppressants or other specific treatments

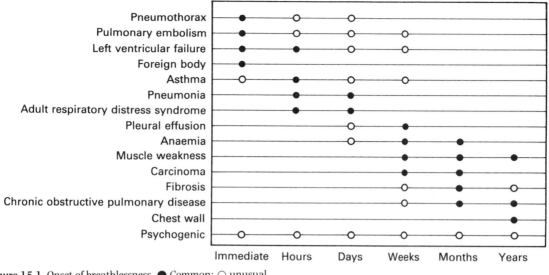

Figure 15.1 Onset of breathlessness. ● Common; ○ unusual

Examination and investigation

All patients presenting with upper and lower respiratory tract symptoms should have an examination of the chest and a summary and checklist is given in Table 15.3.

Investigation of a patient with respiratory tract disease may include a full blood count, to assess anaemia and polycythemia, and a white cell count (elevated neutrophil count suggests bacterial infection, lymphocyte elevation suggests viral infection). Erythrocyte sedimentation rate and C-reactive protein, if abnormal, confirm the presence of inflammatory disease and can be used as a marker of progression or response to treatment. Oxygen saturation or arterial blood gas measurements are used to assess for the presence of respiratory failure. Examination of sputum for eosinophils, microbiology, acid fast bacilli and malignant cells may be clinically indicated. An ECG may indicate right ventricular hypertrophy secondary to pulmonary hypertension as a result of a wide spectrum of severe chronic lung diseases.

In patients with lower respiratory tract symptoms, perhaps the most useful investigations are a chest X-ray and lung function tests. The former may give useful information on the presence of bronchial carcinoma, or hyperinflation (airflow limitation), infections including tuberculosis, pneumonia or bronchiectasis and presence of interstitial lung disease.

Pulmonary function testing

Routine pulmonary function tests provide useful information on the state of the airways, the lung volumes and gas transfer. Upper respiratory tract conditions such as large airway obstruction due to tumours can be identified as well as an assessment made of lower respiratory tract disease, such as asthma, bronchiectasis, sarcoid and AIDS.

As airways bifurcate from the carina downwards the cross-sectional area increases thus progressively minimizing the effect of pathologically decreased size on airway resistance. Hence, in health, the upper airway contributes almost all the resistance to airflow. In chronic obstructive pulmonary disease the total airway resistance becomes significant only when very substantial damage has occurred and so tests only become abnormal in late stage disease. Tests of airway function are therefore particularly sensitive for picking up large obstructive lesions in the upper airways.

Airways

Peak expiratory flow (PEF) – a simple measure of maximum rate of airflow with sudden expiration. This is especially useful for measuring trends in airflow limitation and is routinely used for the diagnosis and monitoring of therapeutic response in asthma.

Spirometry – FEV_1 (forced expiratory volume in one second) and FVC (forced vital capacity) measures volume exhaled versus time (Figure 15.2a). It helps

Table 15.3 Examination of the respiratory system

Inspection	Nicotine Cyanosis Hypercapnoea (bounding pulse) Clubbing Breathing pattern and rate Cough Stridor Jugular venous pressure (JVP) Chest wall (scoliosis, ribs/sternum, scars/veins, accessory muscles, abdominal and sternal movements)
Palpation	Expansion (> 5 cm) Lymphadenopathy Subcutaneous emphysema Tracheal displacement Apex beat Vocal fremitus
Percussion	
Auscultation	Vesicular v bronchial (bronchial breathing is a harsh high frequency sound similar to that heard over the larynx) Vocal resonance ('99') and whispering pectoriloquy ('1, 2, 3') Aegophony ('bleating' heard over upper limit of effusion)
Wheeze	Not significant if heard during forced expiration Usually indicates obstruction; (asthma/bronchitis). Occasionally in fibrosing alveolitis (squawk) and extrinsic allergic alveolitis. If only on inspiration may suggest emphysema
Crackles	Due to opening of abnormally closed bronchioles Early inspiration in diffuse airway obstruction Present on late inspiration in fibrosis Late/pan inspiratory in fibrosis, oedema or consolidation and bronchiectasis, expiratory in emphysema
Rub	Inspiratory and expiratory or same time in each cycle

Summary of signs in consolidation, collapse and pleural effusion

	Mediastinal shift	Movements	Percussion note	Breath sounds	Other
Consolidation	○	↓	↓	↓	Bronchial breathing Increased vocal resonanance and whispering pectoriloquy
Collapse	○/→	↓	↓	○/↓	Often few signs
Pleural effusion	←/○	↓	↓↓	↓↓	Axillary dullness Aegophony over upper border

to distinguish between obstructive (Figure 15.2*b*) and restrictive (Figure 15.2*c*) lung disease. In airflow obstruction, reversibility testing is helpful and if greater than 15% suggests asthma.

The flow volume loop is better than simple spirometry in assessing early obstructive airways disease and large airway (e.g. tracheal or laryngeal) obstruction (Figure 15.3). In fixed extrathoracic obstruction (e.g. carcinoma or thyroid goitre), there is a plateau on both the inspiratory and expiratory curves (Figure 15.3*a*). In variable large airways obstruction, when extrathoracic (e.g. vocal cord paralysis), there is an inspiratory plateau (Figure 15.3*b*) and when intrathoracic an inspiratory plateau (Figure 15.3*c*).

If a flow volume curve is not available the ratio between peak expiratory flow and the FEV_1 provides a useful guide to the presence of upper airways obstruction. Normally this ratio is greater than 10; a ratio of less than 10 suggests severe upper airway obstruction.

Lung volumes

Lung volumes can be measured by the helium dilution technique or by total body plethysmography. The measurements are total lung capacity (TLC = total volume of gas in the lungs), residual volume (RV = volume of gas remaining after maximum expiration), vital capacity (VC = volume of gas expired from total lung capacity to residual volume) and functional residual capacity (FRC = volume of

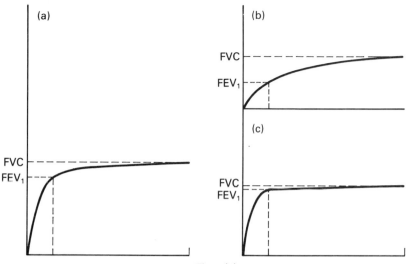

Figure 15.2 Typical spirograms demonstrating (*a*) normal, (*b*) obstructive and (*c*) restrictive pattern in parenchymal disease

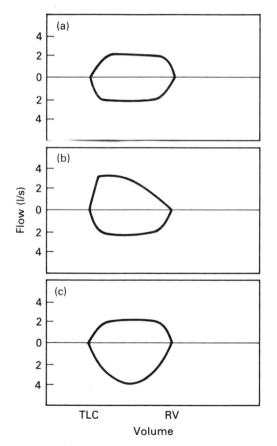

Figure 15.3 Flow-volume loops. (*a*) Fixed extrathoracic obstruction; (*b*) variable extrathoracic obstruction; (*c*) intrathoracic obstruction. TLC: Total lung capacity; RV: residual volume

gas in the lung at resting state, i.e. end of expiration during tidal breathing).

Total lung capacity is the most useful of these measurements clinically and may be elevated in chronic obstructive pulmonary disease, emphysema and asthma and is reduced in restrictive lung disease such as fibrosing alveolitis.

Gas transfer measurements

This measures the rate of transfer of gas from the alveolus to pulmonary capillaries and is recorded as the transfer factor (TLCO) or the diffusion coefficient (KCO) which is the transfer factor divided by accessible lung volume (alveolar volume) to give a measurement of gas transfer efficiency per unit volume of lung. Increased transfer factor and diffusion coefficient are found in polycythemia, pulmonary haemorrhage and left to right intracardiac shunts (e.g. atrial septal defect). A diminished transfer factor and normal diffusion coefficient can occur in asthma, sarcoid, pneumonectomy and pulmonary oedema. The combination of a diminished transfer factor with elevated diffusion coefficient occurs in respiratory muscle, chest wall or pleural disease. In most other respiratory conditions both measurements are diminished. As well as providing supportive evidence for diagnosis of organic lung disease, these measurements are used for prognosis and to monitor response to treatment in several conditions.

Defence mechanisms of the respiratory tract

Both the upper and lower respiratory tract are continually exposed to gases and airborne particles and the importance of host defence mechanisms is vital. Physical barriers, clearance systems and cellular or humoral immune processes combine to protect lungs from damage and infection (Table 15.4) (Friedman *et al.*, 1977). Where abnormalities of these mechanisms occur, pathology may first present to the otolaryngologist and later serious bronchopulmonary involvement may occur. It is therefore important that the otolaryngologist has an understanding of these mechanisms and can diagnose them before lung damage occurs. Total clearance of inhaled particles (i.e. mucociliary, cough and all other mechanisms) can be assessed by various radiographic techniques (Friedman *et al.*, 1977; Del Donno *et al.*, 1988), but these have little clinical use. Early lung clearance of particles within hours is by mucociliary clearance and cough but late alveolar clearance proceeds over days and months via phagocytosis by alveolar macrophages.

Table 15.4 System of defences of the respiratory tract

Local (resident) mechanisms
1   Non-specific
    Reflexes (cough, sneeze)
    Mucociliary clearance
    Epithelial integrity and lining fluid
    Antimicrobial substances (e.g. lysozyme)
    Pulmonary macrophage

2   Specific
    Immunoglobulin (secretory IgA, IgE)
    Lymphocytes

Systemic (recruited) mechanisms
1   Non-specific
    Serum factors (e.g. opsonins, complement)
    Granulocyte phagocytosis
    Mononuclear phagocytosis

2   Specific
    Serum immunoglobulins (IgA, IgG, IgM, IgE)
    Lymphocytes

Physical defences

Larger particles are cleared mainly by physical mechanisms in the upper respiratory tract which acts as a physical filter and also warms inspired air (Proctor, 1977). The principal defence mechanism for both the upper and lower respiratory tracts is mucociliary clearance. Cough acts as an additional mechanism to maintain patency of the lower airway in the presence of excess secretions; a role played by sneeze in the upper respiratory tract (Schlesinger, Gurman and Lippmann, 1982).

Mucociliary

Mucociliary clearance (Pavia, 1984a) is the predominant clearance mechanism for the airways of the upper and lower respiratory tracts as far as the sixteenth bronchial division. Over the anterior portion of the inferior and middle turbinates and below the larynx where most inhaled dusts are deposited clearance is towards the mouth, in the nose and oropharynx it is away from the mouth. The saccharin test is a reproducible and simple test of nasal mucociliary clearance which generally also reflects lung mucociliary clearance. A 0.5 cm particle of saccharin is placed 1 cm behind the anterior border of the inferior turbinate. It is important not to place it too far anteriorly as clearance here is forwards. The time for a sweet taste to be reported in the posterior nasopharynx is noted. Patients must sit with the head flexed about 10° to avoid the particle falling back and should not eat, drink, sniff or cough. Their ability to taste saccharin in the first place should be determined. A normal time is less than 30 minutes (Stanley *et al.*, 1984).

The two components of the mucociliary escalator are the ciliated cells and the secretions above them. Cilia beat in a coordinated fashion with a ciliary beat frequency of 12–14 beats per second, independent of nervous control but strongly influenced by local factors and by disease processes. Assessment of ciliary function can be made by nasal or bronchial brushings classifying the proportion of motile and immotile cilia. Ciliary beat frequency may also be measured directly by photometry. Mucus secretion from goblet cells is under complex chemical and vagal control (American Review of Respiratory Disease, 1987; Jany and Basbaum, 1991; Leff, 1988). Mucus is a viscoelastic liquid and consists of glycoproteins 2%, water 95%, immunoglobulins, lysozyme and lactoferrin 1% and inorganic salts 1% (Lopez–Vidriero, 1984). In the nose there are also contributions from seromucous and lacrimal glands. Lung clearance is determined largely by activity of the cilia and mucus. The daily volume of transported mucus in health is approximately 10 ml but may rise to 300 ml in an exacerbation of chronic obstructive pulmonary disease (Pavia, Bateman and Clarke, 1984).

Mucociliary clearance varies in different physiological situations (Del Donno *et al.*, 1988). It diminishes with age (Pavia, 1984a), in sleep (Bateman, Pavia and Clarke, 1978) and with cigarette smoke (Camner, 1980). Beta-two agonists (Pavia, 1984b) may improve mucociliary clearance. Pathological suppression of mucociliary clearance may be congenital (cystic fibrosis, primary ciliary dyskinesia) or acquired (Young's syndrome, asthma, viral and bacterial infection, cigarette smoke, drugs). In cystic fibrosis there is a defect in ion transport of chloride and sodium (Cole, 1984; Dor *et al.*, 1985) giving rise to viscous mucus that is difficult to clear and underlies the predisposition to infection. Primary ciliary dyskinesia (Greenstone *et al.*, 1988) is an autosomal recessive condition with incomplete penetrance with a disordered ciliary ultrastructure giving rise to poorly coordinated beating. Chronic bronchial infection and sinusitis are usual; bronchiectasis is common and situs inversus (Kartagener's) occurs in 50%. Young's syndrome (Handelsman *et al.*, 1984) is an acquired defect with azoospermia, sinusitis and bronchiectasis of unknown aetiology, although it may be associated with Pink's disease (mercury poisoning in infancy). Ciliary function is normal but respiratory secretions are abnormally viscid (Wilson and Cole, 1988). Severe asthma (Dulfano and Luk, 1982; Wilson, 1988), virus infection (Wilson *et al.*, 1987a) and bacterial infection (Wilson and Cole, 1988), cigarette smoking (Stanley *et al.*, 1986) and drugs (e.g. lignocaine) may all cause secondary ciliary dyskinesia where the cilia are intrinsically normal but beating is slowed or uncoordinated. In bacterial infection, bacterial products have been shown to be the cause of this by destroying coordinated beating (Figure 15.4). Normal function after epithelial damage takes up to 6 weeks to return to normal.

Nasal polyps may occur with primary ciliary dyskinesia in between 13 and 40% of cases (Pedersen and Mygind, 1982; Levison *et al.*, 1983; Greenstone *et al.*, 1985). If polyps do not respond to topical corticosteroids, they will require surgical removal. Glue ear is another common finding in primary ciliary dyskinesia. Insertion of grommets was without success in four out of 16 patients reviewed by Greenstone *et al.*

(1985). The ears continued to discharge through the ventilation tube until it was either removed or extruded. Since there is no likelihood of primary ciliary dyskinesia resolving, insertion of ventilation tubes should be resisted unless the hearing loss is considerable and persistent in which case it may be worth considering inserting a grommet in one ear, leaving the other ear dry which can be fitted with a hearing aid if necessary. Fortunately hearing loss in most cases does not seem severe. For many patients with primary mucociliary clearance problems their otological and rhinological symptoms present little more than an inconvenience and a medical regimen is often sufficient. In some, surgery to improve drainage is required. Early referral for chest management is essential.

Cough

The importance of cough in maintaining patency of the tracheobronchial tree in the presence of excess secretions has been clearly demonstrated (Leith, 1977; Pucelle *et al.*, 1980; Pavia, Agnew and Clarke, 1986). In this situation it may account for removal of up to 50% of inhaled particles. However, in patients without excess secretions it plays little or no part in mucus clearance. Cough is a reflex initiated by stimulation of afferent airway receptors in the larynx and upper airways. The role of each type of afferent receptor remains unclear (Karlsson, Sant'Ambrigio and Widdicombe, 1988). Afferent impulses travel in branches of the superior laryngeal nerve and vagus

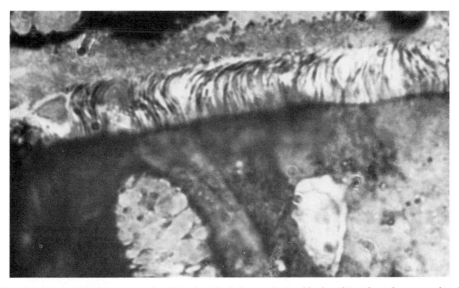

Figure 15.4 Light micrograph of a portion of a ciliated epithelial strip obtained by brushing the inferior nasal turbinate and used for determining nasal ciliary beat frequency. It shows a thick mucus layer overlying cilia in thin periciliary fluid above the epithelial cells (magnification × 2000; prepared by Andrew Rutman)

to the cough centre in the midbrain where efferent nerves emanate to produce coordinated contraction of the respiratory musculature. A brief inspiration is followed by glottic closure and abrupt rise in pleural pressures up to 100 mmHg due to expiratory muscle contraction. Glottic opening is then accompanied by an expiratory flow of up to 12 m/s. Shearing forces are produced with expectoration of excess secretions. Sneezing, sniffing and blowing of the nose perform an equivalent function and are also of importance only in the present of excess secretions.

Cellular and humoral defences

The upper and lower respiratory tract also share similar cellular and humoral defence mechanisms. In immunodeficiency states pathology may present first to the otolaryngologist and later with serious bronchopulmonary involvement. It is, therefore, essential that the otolaryngologist has an understanding of these mechanisms and can diagnose them before lung damage occurs.

Immunoglobulins

In contrast to plasma, IgA is the predominant immunoglobulin in the respiratory tract in health with less IgG and IgM being present. Most IgA is produced locally from B lymphocytes in the lymphoid tissue (bronchus associated lymphoid tissue; BALT) in the respiratory tract. IgA is present as two subclasses, IgA1 and IgA2, and is usually found as a dimer, i.e. two molecules conjoined. IgG is divided into four subclasses (Barnett, 1986).

The function of IgA is only partly understood but the dimeric form is capable of preventing epithelial cell binding by bacteria and viruses. IgA can enhance macrophage phagocytosis (Richards and Gauldie, 1985) and act synergistically with IgG in stimulating antibody dependent cell mediated cytotoxicity (Shen and Fanger, 1981). Some insight can be gained from study of patients with isolated IgA deficiency (the most common immune defect occurring in 1:700 live births). Some patients have an increased incidence of upper and lower respiratory tract infection but many have few respiratory symptoms (Ammon and Hong, 1971; Koistinen, 1975). However, a normal secretory IgA can be present in the respiratory tract with plasma IgA deficiency and also IgM may compensate by replacing IgA in these patients (Brandtzaeg, Fellanges and Gjeruldsen, 1968). Hence local IgA deficiency is rare and in subjects with systemic IgA deficiency local compensatory mechanisms may be adequate to prevent disease. IgA deficiency may be associated with IgG2 deficiency making it amenable to treatment by immunoglobulin replacement therapy.

The protective effects of IgG are dependent upon each subclass. IgG1 and 2 can activate the classic complement pathway. Macrophages bind IgG3 and 4. IgG concentration is higher in the lower airways and alveoli but the precise role remains to be determined. Recurrent infections occur with IgG deficiency states especially in those with deficiency of IgG2 or IgG4 (Oxelius, 1974) or in those with deficiency of IgG2 or IgG3 in association with IgA deficiency (Bjorkander, Bake and Oxelius, 1985). IgG2 deficiency seems to be particularly important in protection against capsulated bacteria such as *Streptococcus pneumoniae* and *Haemophilus influenzae*.

IgM is the most effective complement fixing immunoglobulin but its role in protecting the lung from infection is uncertain. IgD is found in small amounts and its role is undetermined. IgE binds to mast cells and releases active mediators of allergic inflammation. This may have a role in defence against metazoal parasites.

Most forms of immune deficiency may be congenital or acquired. Neutropaenia may be secondary to leukaemia or chemotherapy; functional neutrophil defects occur in uraemia, alcoholism etc. These patients may be prone to bacterial infection. T lymphocyte defects occur with immunosuppressants after organ transplantation, AIDS, lymphoma, after chemotherapy, thymic aplasia, purine metabolism defects, and severe combined immunodeficiency disease. Viral, mycobacterial and parasitic infection may occur. Immunoglobulin deficiency occurs in multiple myeloma, chronic lymphatic leukaemia, nephrotic syndrome and various inherited syndromes.

In general there are three principal presentations of infection to the otolaryngologist and chest physician in patients with immunodeficiency which cause problems in diagnosis and management: first, acute overwhelming infection usually in patients with profound immunodeficiency (e.g. panhypoglobulinaemia, AIDS); second, recurrent acute episodes with apparently normal periods in between; and third, the patient with chronic purulent bronchial disease (usually bronchiectasis) which is associated with upper respiratory tract symptoms and frank purulent sinusitis.

In one series, nine of 250 patients presenting with upper respiratory tract symptoms were found to have an immunodeficiency (Mackay *et al.*, 1983). Symptoms included (recurrent) acute or acute on chronic infection with mucopurulent rhinorrhoea, hyperaemic and swollen mucous membranes and purulent postnasal drip. Infections were also present at other sites such as ears or skin.

Early recognition and treatment of these diseases may prevent later severe and irreversible lung damage. Conditions in which IgG and IgM are low and are producing significant clinical conditions are treated with intravenous immunoglobulin infusions which have now replaced painful intramuscular injections (Chapel, 1994). The decision to embark on this therapy has to be carefully considered because of cost, inconvenience to the patient and side effects of the therapy. Infusions are given at 2–4 weekly intervals and are usually well tolerated (Chapel, 1994). There is a low incidence of anaphylactic reactions especially in those with IgA deficiency but the first few infusions should be given under careful medical observation. Immunoglobulin preparations are expensive and time consuming to give so that a useful reduction in the frequency of exacerbations or chronic symptoms should have been demonstrated before life-long treatment is recommended. Selective IgA deficiency is not treatable at present, but coexisting IgG subclass estimation should be performed and treated if deficiency is present.

Cellular defences

Phagocytic cells play a major role in defences and include alveolar macrophages with a primary scavenging role and blood polymorphonuclear leucocytes and monocytes providing a secondary backup role once inflammation is established. The alveolar macrophage is motile and found in the alveoli and lower airways. In addition to phagocytosis and cell killing, it secretes numerous products, has a role in antigen presentation and tissue remodelling (du Bois, 1985). The neutrophil represents less than 2% of cells from lung lavage in health but much higher numbers in disease. During the process of phagocytosis, tissue oxygen radicals and enzymes may leak out of the cell and the process therefore has the ability both to protect and damage lung tissue (Movat, 1985). Many lymphoid cells are also found in the respiratory tract, both B and T lymphocytes being present (Bienenstock, 1984).

Other defences

Transferrin and lactoferrin bind iron which is required by *H. influenzae* and other bacterial organisms for proliferation. Lysozyme attacks the carbohydrate polymers that comprise the external membrane of bacteria. Many proteins from the complement system have been found in respiratory secretions (Toews and Vial, 1984). Most are probably derived by diffusion from plasma during secondary inflammation. Their importance is highlighted by the effect of deficiency of individual components. Deficiency of C2 is the most common in man; few patients have recurrent infections although there is an increased risk of septicaemia. This suggests that the classic pathway is important in removal of bacteria from vascular spaces but less important in the lung. Some patients with C3 deficiency have recurrent infection in upper and lower respiratory tracts with many organisms including *Strep. pneumoniae* and *H. influenzae* (Toews and Vial, 1984). Numerous cytokines are secreted by cells of the immune system with the ability to activate

other cells (Stockley *et al.*, 1988); these include interleukins, interferons, tumour necrosis factor and chemotaxins. Finally the lung produces several inhibitors of proteolytic enzymes which act as a protective layer to reduce lung damage.

Many patients with an unusual susceptibility to respiratory tract infections have no physical abnormality or immunodeficiency demonstrable by current techniques but significant advances continue to be made in basic research and many of these patients may eventually be shown to have a genetic susceptibility being manifested by a diminution in the effectiveness of these mechanisms.

Bronchiectasis

Bronchiectasis is a condition of abnormally and permanently damaged and dilated large airways (Reid, 1950), and is clinically associated with chronic expectoration of often large quantities of purulent or mucopurulent sputum. Haemoptysis is quite common and sputum is occasionally foul smelling. As the definition of bronchiectasis is an anatomical term, the diagnosis strictly speaking, relies on an imaging technique, such as high resolution CT scanning or bronchography – procedures which require justification. This problem has led to the condition being underdiagnosed as mild and moderate disease produce less severe symptoms which may be confused with other conditions such as chronic bronchitis or recurrent acute bronchitis.

Pathogenesis

In bronchiectasis, the airway wall becomes damaged by the direct effects of microorganisms and the host inflammatory response to them. This may occur if natural resolution is prevented by partial obstruction of the airway (e.g. inhaled foreign body, stricture, previous bronchial inflammatory damage, carcinoma), abnormalities of mucus (e.g. cystic fibrosis) or mucociliary clearance (e.g. Kartagener's syndrome). This has led to the concept of the 'vicious circle' (Figure 15.5) where what should be a self-limiting process is perpetuated and leads to bronchiectasis (Cole, 1984; Lapa E Silva *et al.*, 1989). For example, an initial insult such as a viral infection or a genetic defect such as primary ciliary dyskinesia or cystic fibrosis compromises mucociliary clearance. The result is that microorganisms cannot be cleared leading to further damage to mucociliary clearance. Microbial colonization increases, inflammation persists and increases with progressive damage to host tissue and further microbial colonization. Microbes can directly damage host defence by inhibiting ciliary function (Wilson, Roberts and Cole, 1985; Wilson *et al.*, 1986, 1989; Steinfort *et al.*, 1989) (see Figure 15.4), producing direct damage to epithelium, inhibiting

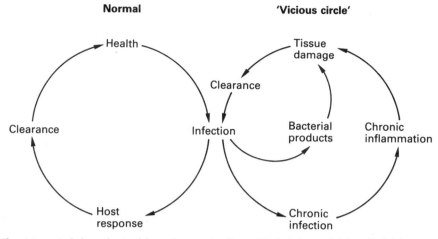

Figure 15.5 The vicious circle hypothesis of the pathogenesis of bronchiectasis (amended from P. Cole)

transport in damaged epithelial cells (Strutts *et al.*, 1986) and producing stasis of secretions (Somerville *et al.*, 1988). Evidence that tissue damage is produced by the host's own inflammatory response can be demonstrated by injection of indium-111 labelled granulocytes, where 50% of circulating granulocytes penetrate directly into the bronchial lumen of patients with severe bronchiectasis (Currie *et al.*, 1987).

Bronchiectasis is the final common pathway for a number of disease processes. Seventy per cent of cases are idiopathic, although there may be a genetic predisposition as yet undetermined, but deficiencies of antiproteases may be important (Kalsheker *et al.*, 1987). Other known causes are listed in Table 15.5. Conditions associated with bronchiectasis include rheumatoid arthritis, ulcerative colitis, male and possibly female infertility (primary ciliary dyskinesia, cystic fibrosis, Young's syndrome), alpha-1-antitrypsin deficiency and yellow nail syndrome (recurrent pleural effusions and dystrophic nails).

Diagnosis

The diagnosis of bronchiectasis should be considered with a history of persistent purulent sputum production with or without recurrent haemoptysis, with recurrent haemoptysis alone or with episodic fever, malaise and pleuritic pain with or without sputum. Examination findings may reveal local or bilateral crackles, wheeze, or finger clubbing. Sputum should be cultured and the quantity estimated. Baseline lung function to determine physiological deficit, and a chest X-ray should be performed (Figure 15.6). High resolution CT scanning should be considered if the diagnosis is in doubt and to determine the location and extent of abnormal bronchial anatomy (Figure 15.7). The cause of the bronchiectasis may be clear from the history (e.g.

Table 15.5 Causes of bronchiectasis

Idiopathic (?antiprotease deficiency)
Congenital (deficiencies of bronchial wall cartilage, e.g. William-Campbell syndrome)
Secondary to bronchial obstruction (carcinoma, foreign body)
Bronchial damage due to inhalation/aspiration
Secondary to granulomatous or fibrotic processes
Allergic bronchopulmonary aspergillosis
Post-transplantation of lung
Immunodeficiency
Mucociliary clearance defects (primary and secondary ciliary dyskinesia, Young's syndrome and cystic fibrosis)
Post severe infection (e.g. measles, chicken pox, respiratory syncytial virus etc)
Bronchopulmonary dysplasia (post adult respiratory distress syndrome)

aspiration). Immunoglobulins should be measured to detect hypogammaglobulinaemia; estimation of IgG, IgA, IgM and IgG subclasses (especially IgG2 and IgG4 deficiency which are associated with an increased risk of infection); skin tests to detect immediate hypersensitivity to *Aspergillus* and measurement of *Aspergillus* precipitins to detect allergic bronchopulmonary aspergillosis, sweat tests and an assessment of mucociliary clearance will be helpful. Where there is no obvious cause patients may identify a viral illness as the trigger factor, although the precise role of this is uncertain.

Treatment

Management consists of treatment of the primary cause, if this can be identified (e.g. immunoglobulin

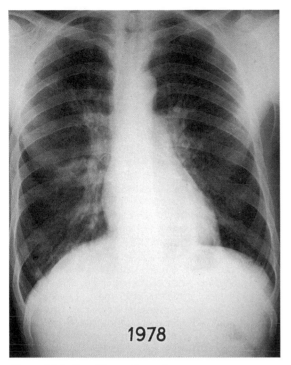

1978

Figure 15.6 Chest X-ray of bronchiectasis

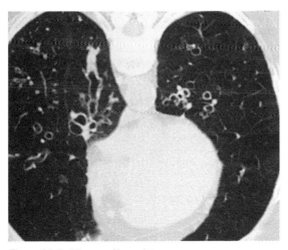

Figure 15.7 CT scan of bronchiectasis

replacement). Physiotherapy remains the cornerstone of treatment and should be performed once or twice daily even if little expectoration is present. Bronchodilators may be of benefit if there is reversible airflow obstruction and inhaled corticosteroids may be of benefit. High doses of appropriate antibiotics may be required to treat exacerbations and courses of lengthy duration are often necessary. The choice of antibiotic may be guided by sensitivities, if available, otherwise second generation oral cephalosporins (e.g. cefaclor), quinolones (e.g. ciprofloxacin) or broad-spectrum penicillins, either amoxicillin or beta-lactamase resistant penicillins such as amoxicillin/clavulanic acid combination, may be used either as a single course or on a continuous rotational basis with other antibiotics. Troublesome symptomatic disease which is very localized and which cannot be controlled medically may occasionally require surgical resection. Recurrent or profound haemoptysis can sometimes be treated successfully by bronchial artery embolization. Lung transplantation for end-stage disease remains an option.

Upper respiratory tract disease in bronchiectasis

Eighty per cent of bronchiectasis patients also have upper respiratory tract symptoms and over one-third have frank chronic purulent rhinosinusitis. Postnasal drip is the commonest symptom and nasal secretions can be either mucoid, mucopurulent after virus infections, or persistently purulent. One-third of patients have persistent chronic purulent sinus sepsis and in many this has resulted in previous upper airway surgical procedures. Ear symptoms are common ranging from serous otitis media (which is almost invariably present in patients with primary ciliary dyskinesia and maybe associated with hearing loss) (Greenstone *et al.*, 1985) to purulent otitis with a discharge. Symptoms of intermittent eustachian tube obstruction are common.

On examination there may be mucopus visible on the posterior pharyngeal wall and in cases of bronchiectasis due to ciliary dyskinesia a stagnant pool of unmoving pus seen on the floor of the nostril is almost pathognomonic. Sinus radiographs show mucosal thickening, sometimes with a fluid level and there may be the appearance of previous sinus surgery on examination and on radiography. CT scanning of the sinuses gives more reliable information.

Rhinosinusitis may be treated by installation of local intranasal corticosteroid drops in the head down and forward position (Chalton *et al.*, 1985; Wilson *et al.*, 1987b) to enable gravity-assisted access of the drops, to the ostiomeatal complex and ethmoid sinuses twice a day for a minimum of 2 minutes on each occasion. It may be useful to use corticosteroid drops combined with topical antibiotics (Sykes *et al.*, 1986) but if so these should be stopped if sense of smell or taste becomes impaired by the action of the antibiotic on the olfactory nerve. Following a short course of such drops improvement may be obtained by using a suitable local corticosteroid nasal spray. Systemic antibiotics may be required in severe cases, but without local therapy they may be ineffective as nasal clearance is re-established best by local therapy. Should medical treatment be unsuccessful or unmaintainable, surgery may be required to ensure drainage.

Cystic fibrosis

Cystic fibrosis results in bronchiectasis but the problems involved are specialized so that it merits individual comment. It is a disease characterized by chronic bronchopulmonary infection, often accompanied by airflow obstruction, malabsorption, failure to thrive and a high sweat sodium concentration. Survival has improved since 1938 (Anderson, 1938) when 80% died in the first year of life to 1990 when the average age of death in the UK was 27 years (British Paediatric Working Party on cystic fibrosis, 1988). There are about 6000 patients with cystic fibrosis currently in the UK.

Pathogenesis

Cystic fibrosis is the most common congenital cause of bronchiectasis and is inherited as an autosomal recessive disease. It is due to a gene mutation. The gene responsible produces a protein called the cystic fibrosis transmembrane regulator (CFTR) which functions as a chloride channel and is regulated by cyclic AMP (Anderson *et al.*, 1991). The essential abnormality (Knowles, Gat and Brucher, 1981) is an increased electrical potential across the airway epithelium (cystic fibrosis > 35 mV, normal < 30 mV). There is chloride impermeability of the luminal surface of the airway epithelial cells and sodium transport through airway epithelium is increased leading to a relative deficiency of water in the airway secretions. Hence, there is a combination of chloride impermeability and excess sodium and water transport from the airway lumen. The lungs and upper airways become colonized by microorganisms which cause most of the damage to the bronchial wall and surrounding lung.

Diagnosis

Most patients are diagnosed in the first year of life by sweat tests, a high sweat sodium confirming the diagnosis (Gapp Conference Report, 1975). There are cases of inappropriate over-diagnosis and two sweat tests should usually be performed to confirm the diagnosis. In adolescents and adults sweat sodium is higher and the test less reliable (Kuzembo and Healey, 1983). Measuring the potential difference across the respiratory epithelium may be helpful (Alton *et al.*, 1990) but invalid in the presence of upper respiratory tract infections and nasal polyps. In difficult cases, genetic analysis can be performed.

Clinical features (Table 15.6)

Pulmonary function, in so far as it can be assessed, is usually normal at birth and may remain so for many years. However, by the age of 5 years, 63% of cases will have respiratory disease and this is almost universal by the age of 21 (Penleth *et al.*, 1987). The chronic pulmonary infection and bacterial colonization lead to neutrophil recruitment to the lung. Neutrophil elastase which is produced and released leads to further damage resulting in severe bronchiectasis and then to respiratory failure. The bacteria most commonly isolated are *Pseudomonas aeruginosa*, *Staphylococcus aureus* and *Haemophilus influenzae* (Penleth *et al.*, 1987). Symptoms are of increasing sputum production, haemoptysis and progressive breathlessness. Chest signs vary but clubbing is usual. The chest radiograph shows increasing abnormalities initially with thickening of the bronchial walls, particularly in the upper zones. Later ill-defined nodular shadows appear with scattered areas of atelectasis and increasing signs of pulmonary hypertension. Lung function tests gradually deteriorate and measurement of the FEV_1 is a good indicator of prognosis. Later in the disease, in addition to respiratory failure, spontaneous pneumothorax, massive haemoptysis and allergic bronchopulmonary aspergillosis, are important complications.

Table 15.6 Features suggestive of a diagnosis of cystic fibrosis

Major criteria	Minor criteria
Bronchopulmonary infection	Nasal polyps
Failure to thrive	Meconium ileus equivalent*
Malabsorption	Rectal prolapse
Meconium ileus	Intussusception
Family history	Biliary cirrhosis*
Azoospermia*	Pancreatitis*
	Peptic ulcer*
	Diabetes mellitus*
	Pneumothorax*

* More common in adolescents and adults than children

Hayfever is present in 15% of adults with cystic fibrosis and eczema in 5%. Immediate type hypersensitivity (Moss, 1983) is increased with over 60% of patients having positive skin prick tests and 40% raised IgE levels. This is possibly due to increased allergen penetration through damaged respiratory epithelium. Eighty-five per cent of patients have gastrointestinal problems with steatorrhoea due to defective production of pancreatic enzymes (Shwachman, 1975; Zenkler–Monro, 1983) and this is treated with replacement enzymes and an appropriate nutritional diet. Distal intestinal obstruction also occurs (meconium ileus equivalent). Diabetes mellitus occurs in approximately 10% with onset generally after the age of 15 years (Finkelstein *et al.*, 1988). Amyloid arthropathy, vasculitis, cirrhosis with portal hypertension and male infertility also occur. The psychosocial aspects of cystic fibrosis care are very important (Pinkton *et al.*, 1985). Poor physical condition, late development of secondary sexual characteristics, multiple hospital admissions, difficulty finding employment and male infertility may all require counselling. End-stage disease may be particularly difficult to manage in these young patients. It has been recently recognized that *Pseudomonas cepacia* is an important pathogen in cystic fibrosis patients, often antibiotic resistant and person-to-person transmission has been reported (Lipiema *et al.*, 1990). Hence many centres operate a policy of segregation between those cystic fibrosis patients colonized and those not colonized with this organism.

Management

The cornerstone of treatment for cystic fibrosis patients, as with any bronchiectatic patient, is physiotherapy, at least twice daily, and comprises forced expiration techniques (a huff combined with periods of relaxation and controlled breathing) and postural drainage (Pryor *et al.*, 1978; Hodson and Gascol, 1993). Antibiotics as required, either orally or intravenously, should be used promptly for exacerbations. Bronchodilators and corticosteroids have an important role in some patients. Meticulous attention to intensive management has been the principal reason for increased survival. Some centres advocate aggressive routine use of intravenous antibiotics and this policy may slow the rate of deterioration in lung function.

Upper respiratory tract disease in cystic fibrosis

Most referrals to the otolaryngological department will have been already diagnosed but a few patients will present with otolaryngological problems in whom the diagnosis of cystic fibrosis has not been suspected and the presence of sinus and nasal symptoms in children should prompt consideration of cystic fibrosis.

Radiological studies of the sinuses of cystic fibrosis patients with plain radiography and especially with coronal CT or MRI scanning reveal a very high incidence of abnormalities. There is usually opacification of the antra and ethmoid sinuses and failure of pneumatization of the frontal sinuses (Umetsu *et al.*, 1990). Occasionally an ethmoid mucocoele or pyocoele is present. Maxillary sinus opacification is almost universal. Despite these widespread radiological abnormalities there are only a few patients with cystic fibrosis who have severe clinical symptoms of sinusitis and plain sinus radiographs have little role

in management. Older patients may complain of headaches and symptoms of nasal congestion.

Nasal polyposis occurs in 6–36% of patients with cystic fibrosis most frequently between the age of 4 and 12 years (Capero *et al.*, 1987; Tos, 1990) though it may also be common in adults (Kerrebijn, Poublon and Overbeek, 1992). They are frequently multiple and bilateral and recur frequently. Allergy and infection are probably involved in the aetiology and the histology of the polyps is the same as in patients without cystic fibrosis.

The presence of pulmonary artery hypertension and, when severe, dilatation of the pulmonary trunk in late cystic fibrosis may very occasionally lead to recurrent laryngeal nerve palsy and hoarseness (Zitsch and Riley, 1987). Change in viscosity of saliva occurs but is rarely of clinical significance. The incidence of secretory otitis media or glue ear is no higher than in individuals without cystic fibrosis (Forman *et al.*, 1979; Crocket *et al.*, 1987). Likewise, acute suppurative otitis media and eustachian tube problems are no commoner. Sensorineural hearing loss is more frequently secondary to antibiotic therapy with aminogycosides and careful monitoring is necessary.

Treatment

Management of sinus disease is essentially the same as that for patients without cystic fibrosis. Appropriate antibiotics after nasopharyngeal sampling will be required for nasal and sinus infection. Mucosal thickening and minor polyposis can be treated with intranasal steroids. Surgery should generally be kept to a minimum except for occasional removal of obstructing polyps (David, 1986). Treatment on the basis of abnormal radiology should be avoided and guided by clinical features.

Where surgery is required to avoid the complications of obstructing polyps there are differing views on the extent (Tos, 1990). Kerribijn, Poublon and Overbeek (1992) recommended initial simple polypectomy or antral irrigation followed by intranasal steroids and frequent nasal irrigation and then endoscopic surgery if there is a recurrence, again followed by topical steroids and further irrigations. If there is still significant recurrence endoscopic sinus surgery and occasionally more radical surgery may be justified (Duplechain, White and Muller, 1991).

Asthma

The majority of patients with asthma will have upper respiratory tract symptoms at some time, especially rhinitis. Many aspects of allergic rhinitis are dealt with in depth in Chapter 6.

Although allergy is frequently involved, the precise cause of these diseases is still uncertain. Any theory of the pathogenesis of asthma must explain an abnormal degree of airway hyperresponsiveness which is an exaggerated bronchoconstrictor response to a variety of inhaled stimuli. However, asthma involves more than spasm of airway smooth muscle. Patients dying from asthma have oedematous and chronically inflamed airways full of tenacious mucus and exudate containing many inflammatory cells. These features have implications for treatment with anti-inflammatory agents as well as bronchodilators.

In children, asthma is the commonest form of chronic respiratory disease. Over 20% of children will wheeze at some time though in most this is mild and in at least 50% of these individuals symptoms will entirely resolve with adolescence. In most, the onset is before 7 years and those with onset before 2 years are more likely to have chronic asthma. Up to 10% of adults will have asthma at some time.

Diagnosis is straightforward in a subject who describes wheeze, with or without breathlessness or cough, especially if symptoms occur at night, on waking or on exertion. To confirm the diagnosis or where there is doubt other investigations will be necessary.

Measurement of peak expiratory flow by the patient at home for a few weeks and FEV_1/FVC with post-bronchodilator reversibility testing at the time of consultation are useful in confirming the diagnosis. These tests may be normal if the asthma is in remission or very mild. Small degrees of airflow limitation may be revealed on a flow volume loop during expiration or by a prolonged forced expiratory time. Occasionally an exercise test to provoke bronchospasm or measurements to demonstrate increased bronchial reactivity to histamine or methacholine may be necessary. A common diagnostic problem is the smoker with airflow obstruction and limited reversibility on routine investigations. In these individuals a 2-week trial of oral or high dose inhaled corticosteroids may demonstrate reversibility of airflow obstruction confirming a diagnosis of asthma rather than chronic bronchitis. A further problem in diagnosis relates to children with 'wheezy bronchitis' who may in fact have asthma. Skin prick tests are positive in greater than 90% of young asthmatics but also in 20–30% of the general population. If there is an occupational element to the asthma, the basic symptoms are the same but initially, at least, the symptoms are often worse in the evening and at night and improve at the weekend, reflecting the pathogenesis via the late bronchoconstrictor response.

Management increasingly centres on patient education, monitoring of peak flows at home and self-management plans. House dust mite and allergen avoidance have a useful role though obsessional advice may be counterproductive. Drug therapy is divided into bronchodilator drugs (beta-2 agonists, antimuscarinic agents and methylxanthenes) and prophylactic drugs (corticosteroids, sodium cromoglycate and occasionally other immunosuppressants). All patients who have symptoms several times a week should be on an inhaled steroid. Assessment of the appropriate inhaler device and inhaler technique are essential.

Asthma and the upper respiratory tract
(Table 15.7)

Rhinitis

There are many similarities between asthma and rhinitis and some important differences. Rhinitis is even more common than asthma, especially in adolescents and young adults. Like asthma its prevalence has increased (Broder *et al.*, 1974; Mygind, 1977; Aberg, 1989) and it was virtually unknown before the Industrial Revolution (Emanuel, 1988). Pollutants and dietary changes have been implicated in this increased incidence (Saarinen *et al.*, 1979; Lynch *et al.*, 1984; Ownby, 1990). Rhinitis occurs in 75% of patients with allergic asthma and the focus is often on the asthma so that the rhinitis may be neglected. Prevalence of asthma in those with rhinitis is only 20% (Smith, 1983). In patients with both conditions onset may be with either condition (Pedersen and Weeke, 1983).

Table 15.7 Epidemiology of allergic disorders

Disorder	Frequency (%)	
Seasonal allergic rhinitis	21	of the general population
Non-seasonal allergic rhinitis	5	
Asthma	5	
Chronic urticaria	4	
Nasal polyps in asthma	7	
Nasal polyps in rhinitis	2	
Nasal polyps in aspirin intolerance	36	

Patients with allergic rhinitis but with no respiratory symptoms have increased bronchial reactivity to methacholine (Ramsdal *et al.*, 1985; Bakke, Baste and Gulsvik, 1991), although usually less so than asthmatics. In seasonal allergic rhinitis there is a slight increase in functional residual capacity and the volume of trapped gas during the hay fever season (Svenonius *et al.*, 1982), perhaps reflecting subclinical bronchospasm. A partial beta-adrenergic blockade similar to that seen in asthma, is found in patients with allergic rhinitis which may account for these abnormalities (Townley, Trafari and Szerturanyi, 1967). A mild degree of beta-adrenergic hyper-responsiveness in patients with allergic rhinitis could cause a readily reversible increase in resting bronchial tone without asthmatic symptoms. It is frequently possible to obtain bronchoconstriction in patients with allergic rhinitis when allergic challenge is given. However, late asthmatic reactions in response to an allergic challenge is much more frequent in asthmatics than rhinitic patients (Stevens and Van

Vever, 1989). Approximately 26% of students with allergic rhinitis develop asthma compared with 1.3% of students without allergic rhinitis (Hagy and Settefane, 1976). Why some atopic patients develop asthma and others develop rhinitis is unclear. Recent work (Townley, 1984) suggests that although patients with allergic rhinitis and no symptoms of asthma often show a 20% decrease in FEV_1 with low concentrations of methacholine, they reach a plateau response with increasing dosages without a further fall in FEV_1. Only 5% show a high positive response without plateau and these subjects may be at greater risk of developing asthma. The nasal mucosa is subject to a greater allergen load than the bronchial surface. Allergic manifestations, although reflecting the different anatomical and histological structure of the nasal and bronchial mucosa, tend to parallel each other; both are suppressed by steroid preparations, whereas the nasal mucosa is more susceptible to antihistamine treatment than beta-2 agonists when compared to the bronchial mucosa.

Sinusitis

Infection of the paranasal sinuses can complicate rhinitis and nasal polyps. It has been suggested that there is an association between sinusitis and asthma (Slavin, 1988). Stimulation of nerves in an infected sinus may result in a parasympathetic stimulation to the bronchial tree and in smooth muscle contraction. Indeed the treatment of acute or chronic sinusitis has been found to improve asthmatic episodes in certain cases (Slavis, 1982).

Aspirin-induced asthma

On the basis of history, 1.7–5.6% of asthmatics have aspirin sensitivity but, on challenge studies, this figure may rise to up to 20% (Dor et al., 1985). It only rarely occurs in children (Fischer et al., 1983). Most patients with aspirin sensitivity are sensitive to other non-steroidal analgesics. The pathogenesis, although unknown, may be related to prostaglandin metabolism (Spector, Morris and Selner, 1981; Stevenson et al., 1984). Classically there is an association between late onset asthma, absence of atopy, aspirin-induced asthma and nasal polyps but this is not universal (Slepian, Matthews and McLean, 1985). Usually the asthma has been present for some time before the aspirin sensitivity is recognized. In its most acute form, aspirin may provoke life-threatening asthma attacks. In most cases the diagnosis is clear but, if there is a doubt or if there is a necessity to continue a non-steroidal anti-inflammatory agent, then carefully controlled challenge testing may be justified.

Management generally consists of that for any asthmatic. A salicylate-free diet may be appropriate in a few cases. Occasionally desensitization can be attempted although this tends to improve nasal symptoms much more than the asthma (Pleskow et al., 1982; Fischer et al., 1983; Stevenson et al., 1984).

AIDS and the upper airway

Since the first clinical descriptions in 1979, a vast amount of clinical data has accumulated regarding the numerous opportunist infections which characterize AIDS, the last clinical stage of chronic infection with the human immunodeficiency virus (HIV) (Murray, Garay and Hopewell, 1987). This retrovirus, occurs in two distinct subtypes: HIV 1 which causes most of the disease seen in Western Europe and the USA and HIV 2 which causes disease predominantly in Western Africa. The virus principally affects the CD4 helper T lymphocyte, but other cells are also infected. The CD4 + lymphocyte is the cell responsible for the initiation of nearly all immunological responses to pathogens and following infection by HIV there is a gradual attrition of the CD4 cell population. The exact mechanism of the immunopathology remains a matter of investigation but in the course of HIV disease there is a gradual reduction in the numbers of CD4 cells circulating in the peripheral blood and indeed routine clinical measurement of the CD4 cell count has become a surrogate marker for disease progression (Rosenberg and Fauci, 1989). Various complications of HIV disease correlate quite closely with the CD4 cell count which is used clinically to determine when antiretroviral therapy with zidovudine should be instituted and when prophylactic antimicrobial agents, e.g. to prevent Pneumocystis carinii pneumonia, should be introduced (Hirsch and D'Aquila, 1993). The predominant abnormality in immune function, in HIV infection, is seen in cell-mediated immune events which particularly protect against intracellular parasites (e.g. viruses, protozoa and mycobacteria), although all arms of the immune systems are affected and failure of antibody-mediated immune responses is also present. In particular, low levels of immunoglobulin G subclass 2 are seen (normally protective against capsulated bacteria). The generalized immune defect also prevents appropriate antibody responses to neoantigens. There may also be disturbances of IgE production and regulation with increased IgE levels being reported in some patients with HIV infection. This may be relevant to reports of recrudescence of asthma during HIV disease and some of the sinus disease seen.

The main pulmonary complications of AIDS are listed in Table 15.8. Pneumocystis carinii pneumonia prior to widespread use of prophylaxis with co-trimoxazole or other agents, was the index diagnosis in 60% of AIDS cases and occurred in up to 80% during some part of the natural history. It remains the most common serious opportunistic lung infection. Bacterial pneumonia due to pyogenic organisms is also common in HIV infected individuals as is mycobacterial infection due to both tuberculosis and atypical

Table 15.8 Common pulmonary complications of AIDS

Pneumocystis carinii pneumonia
Bacterial pneumonia
   Streptococcus pneumoniae
   Haemophilus influenzae
   Moraxella catarrhalis
   Staphylococcus aureus
   Pseudomonas aeruginosa
   Legionella pneumoniae
Mycobacterial infection
   Tuberculosis
M. avium intracellulare
Cytomegalovirus infection
Kaposi's sarcoma

organisms, in particular *Mycobacterium avium intracellulare*. Cytomegalovirus is frequently cultured from lung samples in AIDS cases but is thought not to be an important cause of pneumonia. Of the secondary neoplastic disease seen in HIV, Kaposi's sarcoma is by far the most common problem in the lung, although there may well be an increased incidence of bronchogenic carcinoma and lymphoma within the lung (Murray, Garay and Hopewell, 1987).

As the upper and lower respiratory tracts are contiguous it is hardly surprising that many of the diseases affecting the lower respiratory tract also affect the upper respiratory tract, but there are some interesting differences as well. For example, *Pneumocystis carinii* pneumonia is almost exclusively an alveolar disease, the parasite rarely spreading elsewhere. On the other hand, there are certain problems affecting the oropharynx and upper respiratory tract that rarely spread to the lung. Oropharyngeal candidiasis is almost universal in AIDS patients at some stage and can cause painful pharyngitis. The majority of AIDS patients require continuous antifungal therapy for this condition. The presence of oral candidiasis in a young person should trigger enquiry regarding HIV unless there is an obvious alternate cause such as use of high dose topical steroid therapy for asthma. Candidiasis in HIV infection can also produce oesophageal lesions with painful dysphagia. Good response to appropriate antifungal agents such as fluconazole is to be expected. The white striated lesions along the edge of the tongue which characterize oral hairy leucoplakia may be seen in the mouths of HIV-infected individuals. The aetiology of these lesions remains undetermined. Unlike plaques of candidiasis they cannot easily be dislodged with a spatula. Deep penetrating painful ulceration of the tongue, fauces, tonsils or pharynx may result in disabling symptoms including dysphagia and produce a diagnostic problem. These often require biopsy for definitive diagnosis but usually respond to appropriate antiviral therapy with acyclovir for herpes simplex infection or ganciclovir or foscarnet for cytomegalovirus infection.

Respiratory tract infections

Infections due to pyogenic bacteria are more common in HIV-infected individuals than in normals. The most commonly isolated organisms are *Streptococcus pneumoniae*, *Haemophilus influenzae*, *Staphylococcus aureus*, *Pseudomonas aeruginosa* and other Gram-negative organisms, *Moraxella catarrhalis*, *Legionella* and various anaerobic organisms. Severe staphylococcal infection and Gram-negative infection tend to occur towards the later stages of AIDS (Murray, Garay and Hopewell, 1987). All these organisms can cause severe life-threatening pneumonia as well as acute and chronic bronchitis and acute and chronic sinusitis.

Intravenous drug users with HIV infection have a particular tendency to develop severe pneumococcal infection and some authorities recommend that HIV-infected individuals should be immunized with polyvalent pneumococcal polysaccharide vaccine. Upper respiratory tract infections including colds, sore throats and episodes of sinusitis are more common among HIV-positive than HIV-negative patients, the peak incidence being during the winter months.

Sinusitis

The incidence of sinusitis in HIV-positive individuals has been reported as between 7% and 68% depending on the clinical and radiological criteria used (Sample, Lenahan and Secwonska, 1989; Zurco *et al.*, 1992; Godofsky *et al.*, 1992). *Streptococcus pneumoniae* and *Haemophilus influenzae* are the most frequently isolated organisms followed by the other organisms listed in Table 15.8 (Godofsky *et al.*, 1992). More infrequently non-bacterial pathogens may cause sinusitis (Greenberg, Fischl and Bergen, 1985; Meiteles and Lucente, 1990). These include *Cryptococcus neoformans*, *Alternaria* and *Acanthamoeba castellani* (Gonzalez, Gould and Dickinson, 1986; Choi, Lawson and Buttore, 1988). Cytomegalovirus has also been reported to cause sinusitis with good response clinically to ganciclovir (Brillhart, Gathe and Piot, 1991).

The clinical features resemble sinusitis in non-HIV infected individuals with fever, frontal headache, nasal congestion, periorbital or maxillary area pain and postnasal drip predominating, often associated with respiratory symptoms of cough and sputum production. Where pain predominates, the differential diagnosis should include meningitis or encephalitis, in particular toxoplasma encephalitis or cryptococcal meningitis. Purulent postnasal discharge and lymphoid hypertrophy may be evident in the posterior oropharynx. Because of the underlying immune defect, symptoms tend to be chronic and recurrent and disease tends to be diffuse and bilateral, the majority having unilateral or bilateral maxillary sinus involvement, ethmoid disease being next most common (Godofsky *et al.*, 1992; Zurco *et al.*, 1992).

Standard plain radiographs of the sinuses are of diagnostic value, particularly if air fluid levels are observed or opacification, but CT or MRI provide better images and greater diagnostic sensitivity (Godofsky *et al.*, 1992). Nasal endoscopy and maxillary antral puncture however remain the gold standard for diagnosis.

As with lower tract respiratory disease there is a tendency to relapse and to chronicity, but otherwise the treatment of sinusitis in HIV-positive patients follows the principles of treatment of sinusitis generally, with appropriate antibacterial agents, decongestants and expectorants. As *Streptococcus pneumoniae* and *Haemophilus influenzae* are the most common pathogens, broad spectrum antibiotics such as amoxycillin or co-trimoxazole are appropriate, but given the frequent resistance of *H. influenzae* to amoxycillin, amoxycillin/clavulanic acid combination or an oral second generation cephalosporin, such as cefuroxime should be considered. In view of the tendency to relapse, a 3-week course of treatment is recommended and the use of decongestants is often symptomatically useful. If *Staphylococcus* is isolated, flucloxacillin is appropriate. If Gram-negative organisms are present, ciprofloxacin should be considered and clindamycin is useful for anaerobic infections (Meiteles and Lucente, 1990). For chronic antibiotic resistant disease, surgical drainage should be considered.

Kaposi's sarcoma

Kaposi's sarcoma is the most common of the secondary neoplasms complicating HIV infection and is a multicentric vascular neoplastic condition. The precise aetiology remains undetermined but the oropharynx, upper airway and lung are frequently involved. Indeed the first signs of the disease often arise as purpuric, relatively well circumscribed, circular or oval lesions on the hard palate. Kaposi's sarcoma is particularly common in individuals whose risk factors for acquiring HIV was via homosexual or bisexual lifestyle (40%), whereas it is very rarely seen in HIV-positive haemophiliacs, raising the possibility that it may be due to a co-pathogen only present in certain transmission routes for HIV. The predominant sites of involvement are the skin and lymph nodes but the hard palate, buccal mucosa, pharynx and upper airway may also be involved and produce symptoms due to obstruction, secondary infection and bleeding (Greenberg, Fischl and Bergen, 1985). Symptomatic response to local radiotherapy or intralesional injection with vincristine is usually excellent, but as the condition is usually widely disseminated palliation with combination chemotherapy is normally required and over 60% can expect good relief of symptoms with intravenous vincristine and bleomycin and more recently with liposomal doxorubicin (Laubenstein, Kregel and Odajnyk, 1984).

Sarcoidosis in the upper respiratory tract

Sarcoidosis is a chronic granulomatous disease of undetermined aetiology, although some evidence suggests that it might be related to mycobacterial infection in that some recent studies have shown evidence of the presence of mycobacterial DNA in sarcoid tissue detected by the polymerase chain reaction. Sarcoidosis may either be asymptomatic and an incidental finding on a chest X-ray or can present with various quite typical clinical patterns that are easy to recognize, 80% of patients having pulmonary involvement. In the remaining 20% manifestations are protean and virtually any organ system can be involved. It is a condition with a relatively benign prognosis, up to 80% can expect a spontaneous remission. However, 20% develop chronic disease (Mitchell and Scadding, 1974).

The diagnosis is based on typical histological features on biopsy from affected organs, or a positive Kveim reaction. The exclusion of other granulomatous diseases, such as tuberculosis, is required. Further support for the diagnosis can be obtained by finding an elevated serum angiotensin converting enzyme or a typical appearance on gallium scan with uptake of gallium in the lungs, the parotid and the lacrimal glands.

The upper respiratory tract can become involved and this is more frequently seen in women than in men. In reported series the incidence is variable but overall, 6% of all sarcoid cases have upper respiratory tract involvement (Scadding and Mitchell, 1985). Involvement of the upper respiratory tract occurs, particularly in those with chronic disease and associated bone and skin involvement, and also in the aggressive form of sarcoidosis frequently seen in individuals of Afro-Caribbean origin, where troublesome upper airway symptoms may be present due to nasal obstruction and polyp formation. The most commonly affected site is the nasal mucosa, in particular the inferior turbinates and the adjacent septum. The paranasal sinuses, pharynx, soft palate, epiglottis and larynx are less frequently involved (Neville, Mills and Jash, 1976). Histologically a nasal granulomatosis is found and the differential diagnosis in the absence of obvious sarcoidosis at other sites includes tuberculosis, leprosy and Wegener's granulomatosis. Of those with nasal mucosa involvement approximately 50% will have additional lupus pernio, a characteristic violaceous infiltration and induration of the nasal skin and surrounding soft tissues which frequently involves the nasal vestibule and mucosa also (Neville, Mills and Jash, 1976; Selroos and Niemisto, 1977). Upper airway obstruction may be manifested by overt nasal obstruction with or without discharge and crusting and blood-stained discharge or frank epistaxis. On examination there is frequently thickening of the nasal mucosa, particularly over the inferior turbinates, and occasionally minute yellow nodules may be observed on the nasal mucosa. Septal perforation has been reported (Godofsky *et al.*, 1992).

Other sites in the upper airways are less frequently involved. The sinuses may be involved as evidenced radiologically by mucosal thickening, but only occasionally are symptoms produced. Olfactory nerve involvement is rare but may result in loss of smell. In the nasopharynx, polypoid soft tissue hypertrophy may be observed radiologically or may produce symptoms of obstruction. The tonsils tend to be involved histologically rather than produce symptoms. Involvement of the palate has been reported and all parts of the larynx can be affected but more frequently the epiglottis and epiglottic folds. The trachea is involved only rarely. As with other sites, the treatment indicated for severe disease is systemic corticosteroids and satisfactory remission is normally achieved. Local treatment with topical steroids is variably successful and surgical procedures to relieve obstruction should only be resorted to following an adequate trial of systemic steroid therapy (Scadding and Mitchell, 1985).

Tuberculosis involving the upper airway

Tuberculosis involving the upper airway is only occasionally seen nowadays. Overall, the incidence of tuberculosis in the UK has been falling over the last 40 years with a slight increase in incidence over the last 5 years. This increase is thought to be due to factors other than the appearance of HIV disease. In the general population, tuberculosis remains a rare condition and involvement of the upper respiratory tract is unusual unless there is extensive pulmonary disease present (Watson, 1991). Generally, lesions due to tuberculosis seen in the upper respiratory tract will be ulcerative in nature, often associated with pain. In contrast, tuberculosis may present with cervical lymphadenopathy, particularly among individuals from the Indian subcontinent (Medical Research Council and Chest Diseases Unit, 1987). Indeed the commonest site of non-respiratory tuberculosis, since the eradication of bovine tuberculosis is tuberculous lymphadenitis. In the pharynx tuberculosis may be seen as ulcerating lesions normally associated with marked pain and dysphagia. Laryngeal tuberculosis, very common and fatal in the last century, is now uncommon. An awareness of its continued existence is necessary for clinically the laryngeal lesion may resemble carcinoma and the diagnosis of tuberculous laryngitis may be overlooked. Extensive pulmonary tuberculosis is not always present and hoarseness with minimal pulmonary involvement may be the presentation of tuberculosis.

Conclusions

This chapter has attempted to focus on the relationship between the upper and lower respiratory tract and the disease processes which affect them both. This account is not complete as more detailed discussions of allergic disease, asthma, rhinosinusitis and vasculitis are given in other chapters in this book.

References

ABERG, N. (1989) Asthma and allergic rhinitis in Swedish conscripts. *Clinical and Experimental Allergy*, **19**, 59–63

ALTON, E. W., CURRY, D., LOGAN–SINCLAIR, R., WARNER, J. O., HODSON, M. E. and GEDDES, D. M. (1990) Nasal potential difference – a clinical diagnostic test for cystic fibrosis. *European Respiratory Journal*, **38**, 922–926

AMERICAN REVIEW OF RESPIRATORY DISEASE (1987) The role of neuropeptides in regulating airway function. 2nd Transatlantic Airway Conference. *American Review of Respiratory Disease*, **136**, no. 6, part 2

AMMON, A. J. and HONG, R. (1971) Selective IgA deficiency: Presentation of 30 cases and a review of the literature. *Medicine (Baltimore)*, **50**, 223–237

ANDERSON, D. H. (1938) Cystic fibrosis of the pancreas and its relation to coeliac disease. A clinical and pathological study. *American Journal Diseases of Children*, **56**, 344–399

ANDERSON, M. P., RICH, D. P., GREGORY, R. J., SMITH, A. E. and WELSH, M. J. (1991) Generation cyclic AMP activated chloride currents by expression of CFTR. *Science*, **251**, 679–682

BAKKE, P. S., BASTE, V. and GULSVIK, A. (1991) Bronchial responsiveness in a Norwegian community. *American Review of Respiratory Diseases*, **143**, 17–22

BARNETT, D. (1986) Immunoglobulins in the lung. *Thorax*, **41**, 337–344

BATEMAN, J. R. M., PAVIA, D. and CLARKE, S. W. (1978) The retention of lung secretions during the night in normal subjects. *Clinical Science and Molecular Medicine*, **55**, 523–527

BIENENSTOCK, J. S. (ed.) (1984) Bronchus associated lymphoid tissue. In: *Immunology of the Lung and Upper Respiratory Tract*. New York: McGraw-Hill Book Company. pp. 96–119

BJORKANDER, J., BAKE, B., OXELIUS, V.-A. and HANSON, L. A. (1985) Impaired lung function in patients with IgA deficiency and low levels of IgG2 or IgG3. *New England Journal of Medicine*, **313**, 720–724

BRITISH PAEDIATRIC ASSOCIATION WORKING PARTY ON CYSTIC FIBROSIS (1988) Cystic fibrosis in the UK 1977–1985, an improving picture. *British Medical Journal*, **297**, 1599–1602

BRANDTZAEG, P., FELLANGER, I. and GJERULDSEN, S. T. (1968) Immunoglobulin M: local synthesis and selective secretion in patients with immunoglobulin A deficiency. *Science*, **160**, 789–799

BRILLHART, T., GATHE, J. and PIOT, D. (1991) Symptomatic cytomegalovirus rhinosinusitis in patients with AIDS (abstract MB 2182). *Proceedings of the 7th International Conference on AIDS*. Florence, Italy. 227

BRODER, I., HIGGINS, M. W., MATTHEWS, K. P. and KEELER, J. B. (1974) Epidemiology of asthma and allergic rhinitis in a total community. Tecumseh, Michigan 3: Second survey of the community. *Journal of Allergy and Clinical Immunology*, **53**, 127–138

CAMNER, P. (1980) Clearance of particles from the human tracheobronchial tree. *Clinical Science*, **59**, 79–84

CAPERO, R., SMITH, R. J., CATLIN, F. I., BRESLER, K. L., FRURUTA,

G. T. and SHANDEORA, K. C. (1987) Cystic fibrosis and otolaryngological perspective. *Journal of Otolaryngology– Head and Neck Surgery*, **87**, 356–360

CHALTON, R., WILSON, R., MACKAY, I. and COLE, P. J. (1985) Double-blind placebo controlled trial of betamethasone nasal drops for nasal polyposis. *British Medical Journal*, **295**, 788–794

CHAPEL, H. M. (1994) Consensus panel for the diagnosis and management of primary antibody deficiencies. *British Medical Journal*, **308**, 581–585

CHOI, S. S., LAWSON, W., and BUTTORE, N. A. (1988) Cryptococcal sinusitis: A case report and review of the literature. *Otolaryngology – Head and Neck Surgery*, **99**, 414–418

COLE, P. J. (1984) A new look at the pathogenesis and management of persistent bronchial sepsis: a vicious circle hypothesis and logical therapeutic connotation. In: *Strategies for the Management of Chronic Bronchial Sepsis*, edited by R. J. Davis. Oxford: The Medicine Publishing Foundation

CROCKET, D. M., MCGILL, T. J., HEALY, G. B., FRIEDMAN, E. M. and SALKELD, L. J. (1987) Nasal and paranasal sinus surgery in children with cystic fibrosis. *Annals of Otology, Rhinology and Laryngology*, **96**, 367–372

CURRIE, D. C., SAVARYMUTU, S. H., PETERS, A. M., NEEDHAM, S. G., GEORGE, P., DHILLON, D. P. *et al.* (1987) Indium 111 labelled granulocyte accumulation in respiratory tract of patients with bronchiectasis. *Lancet*, **i**, 1335–1338

DAVID, T. J. (1986) Nasal polyposis, opaque paranasal sinuses and usually normal hearing: the otorhinolaryngological features of cystic fibrosis. *Journal of the Royal Society of Medicine*, **79** (suppl. 12), 23–26

DUBOIS, R. M. (1985) The alveolar macrophage. *Thorax*, **40**, 321–327

DEL DONNO, M., PAVIA, D., AGNEW, J. E., LOPEZ-VIDRIERO, M. T. and CLARKE, S. W. (1988) Variability and reproducibility in the measurement of tracheobronchial clearance in healthy subjects and patients with different obstructive lung diseases. *European Respiratory Journal*, **1**, 613–619

DOR, P. J., VERVLOET, D., BALDOCCHI, G. and CHARPIN, J. (1985) Aspirin intolerance and asthma induction of tolerance and long term monitoring. *Clinical Allergy*, **15**, 37–45

DULFANO, M. J. and LUK, C. K. (1982) Sputum and ciliary inhibition in asthma. *Thorax*, **37**, 646–651

DUPLECHAIN, J. K., WHITE, J. A. and MULLER, R. H. (1991) Paediatric sinusitis. The role of endoscopic sinus surgery in cystic fibrosis and other forms of sinonasal disease *Archieves of Otolaryngology – Head and Neck Surgery*, **117**, 422–426

EMANUEL, M. B. (1988) Hay fever, a post industrial revolution epidemic: a history of its growth during the 19th century. *Clinical Allergy*, **18**, 295–304

FINKELSTEIN, S. M., VIALINSKI, C. L., ELLIOT, G. R., WARWICK, W. J., BARBOSA, J., SHU-CHEN, W. *et al.* (1988) Diabetes mellitus associated with cystic fibrosis. *Journal of Paediatrics*, **112**, 373–377

FISCHER, T. J., GUILFOILE, T. D., KESARWALA, H. H., WIRART, J. G., KEARNS, G. L., GARTSIDE, P. S. *et al.* (1983) Adverse pulmonary responses to aspirin and acetaminophen in chronic childhood asthma. *Paediatrics*, **71**, 313–319

FORMAN, F. B., ABRAMSON, A. L., GORVOY, J. D. and STEIN, T. (1979) Cystic fibrosis and hearing loss. *Archives of Otolaryngology*, **105**, 338–342

FRIEDMAN, M., STOTT, F. D., POOLE, D. O., DEUGHOTY, R., CHAPMAN, G. A., WATSON, H. *et al.* (1977) A new roentgenographic method for estimating mucous velocity in airways. *American Review of Respiratory Diseases*, **115**, 67–72

GAPP CONFERENCE REPORT (1975) *Problems of Sweat Testing.* Atlanta, Georgia; Cystic Fibrosis Foundation

GODOFSKY, E. W., ZINREICH, J., ARMSTRONG, M., LESLIE, J. M. and WEWIBEL, C. S. (1992) Sinusitis in HIV-1 infected patients: a clinical and radiographic review. *American Journal of Medicine*, **93**, 163–170

GONZALEZ, M. M., GOULD, E. and DICKINSON, G. (1986) Acquired, immunodeficiency syndrome assocaited with *Acanthamoeba* infection and other opportunist organisms. *Archives of Pathology and Laboratory Medicine*, **110**, 749–751

GREENBERG, J. E., FISCHL, M. A. and BERGEN, J. R. (1985) Upper airway obstruction secondary to acquired immunodeficiency syndrome-related Kaposi's sarcoma. *Chest*, **88**, 638–640

GREENSTONE, M., RUTMAN, A., DEWAR, A., MACKAY, I. and COLE, P. (1988) Primary ciliary dyskinesa: cytological and clinical features. *Quarterly Journal of Medicine*, **233**, 405–430

GREENSTONE, M., STANLEY, P., COLE, P. J. and MACKAY, I. (1985) Upper airway manifestations of primary ciliary dyskinesia. *Journal of Laryngology and Otology*, **99**, 985–991

HAGY, G. W. AND SETTEFANE, G. A. (1976) Risk factors for developing asthma and allergic rhinitis: a 7 year follow-up study of college students. *Journal of Allergy and Clinical Immunology* **58**, 330–336

HANDELSMAN, P. J., CONWAY, A. J., BOYLAN, A. M. and TURTLE, J. R. (1984) Youngs syndrome. Obstructive azoospermia and chronic sinopulmonary infections. *New England Journal of Medicine*, **310**, 3–9

HIRSCH, M. S. and D'AQUILA, R. T. (1993) Therapy for human immunodeficiency virus. *New England Journal of Medicine*, **328**, 1686–1695

HODSON, M. E. and GASCOL, D. V. (1993) Cystic fibrosis London therapy. In: *Physiotherapy in Cystic Fibrosis*, edited by M. E. Hodson. London: Bailliere Tindall

JANY, J. and BASBAUM, C. B. (1991) Modification of mucin gene expression in airway disease. *American Review of Respiratory Diseases*, **144**, s. 38–41

KALSHEKER, N. A., HODSON, I. J., WALTERS, J. L., WHITE, J. P., MORRISON, H. M. and STOCKLEY, R. A. (1987) Deoxyribonucleic acid (DNA) polymorphism of the alpha-1 antitripsin gene in chronic lung disease. *British Medical Journal*, **296**, 1511

KARLSSON, J. A., SANT'AMBRIGIO, G. and WIDDICOMBE, J. (1988) Afferent neural pathways in cough and reflux bronchoconstriction. *Journal of Applied Physiology*, **65**, 1007–1023

KERREBIJN, J. D. F., POUBLON, R. M. L. and OVERBEEK, S. E. (1992) Nasal and paranasal disease in adults, cystic fibrosis patients. *European Respiratory Journal*, **5**, 1239–1242

KNOWLES, M., GAT, C. J. T. and BRUCHER, R. (1981) Increased electric difference across respiratory epithelial in cystic fibrosis. *New England Journal of Medicine*, **305**, 1489–1493

KOISTINEN, J. (1975) Selective IgA deficiency in blood donors. *Vox Sanguis*, **29**, 192–196

KUZEMKO, J. A. and HEALEY, A. F. (1983) Diagnostic methods and screening. In: *Cystic Fibrosis*, edited by M. E. Hodson, A. Normal and J. C. Batton. London: Bailliere Tindall. Ch. 2

LAPA E SILVA, J. R., GUERREIRO, D., NOBLE, B., POULTER, L. W. and COLE, P. J. (1989) Immunology of experimental bronchiectasis. *American Journal of Respiration and Cell Molecular Biology*, **1**, 297–302

LAUBENSTEIN, L. J., KREGEL, R. L. and ODAJNYK, C. (1984)

Treatment of epidemic Kaposi's sarcoma with etoposide or a combination of doxirubicin, bleomycin and vinblastine. *Journal of Clinical Oncology*, **2**, 1115–1124

LEFF, A. R. (1988) Endogenous regulation of bronchomotor tone. *American Review of Respiratory Diseases* **137**, 1198–1216

LEITH, D. E. (1977) Cough. In: *Respiratory Diffuse Mechanism* Part II, edited by J. D. Brain, D. F. Proctor and L. M. Reid. New York: Marcel Decker. p. 545

LEVISON, J., MINDROFF, C. M., CHOU, J., TURNER, J. A., STURGESS, J. M., and STRINGER, D. A. (1983) Pathophysiology of the ciliary motility syndrome. *European Journal of Respiratory Diseases*, **64** (suppl. 127), 102–116

LIPIEMA, J. J., DASSON, S. E., NIELSEN, D. W., STERN, R. C. and STEELE, T. L. (1990) Person to person transmission of *Pseudomonas cepacia* between patients with cystic fibrosis. *Lancet*, ii, 1094–1096

LOPEZ-VIDRIERO, M. T. (1984) Lung secretions. In: *Aerosols and the Lung*, edited by S. W. Clarke and D. Pavia. London: Butterworths. pp. 19–36

LYNCH, N. R., MEDOUZE, L., DE PRISCO-FUENMAYOR, M. C., VERDE, O., LOPEZ, R. I. and MALAVE, C. (1984) Incidence of atopic disease in a helminthiasis. *Journal of Allergy and Clinical Immunology*, **73**, 229–233

MACKAY, I., STANLEY, P., GREENSTONE, M., HOLMES, P, and COLE, P., (1983) A nose clinic; initial results. *Journal of Laryngology and Otology*, **97**, 925–931

MEDICAL RESEARCH COUNCIL AND CHEST DISEASES UNIT (1987) National Survey of Tuberculosis Notifications in England and Wales in 1983: characteristics of disease. *Tubercle*, **68**, 19–32

MEITELES, L. Z. and LUCENTE, F. E. (1990) Sinus and nasal manifestations of the acquired immunodeficiency deficiency syndrome. *Ear Nose and Throat Journal*, **69**, 454–459

MITCHELL, D. M. and SCADDING, J. G. (1974) Sarcoidosis. State of the art. *American Review of Respiratory Disease*, **110**, 774–802

MOSS, R. B. (1983) Immunology of cystic fibrosis immunity, immunodeficiency and hypersensitivity. *Text book of Cystic Fibrosis*, edited by J. D. Lloyd Still. Bristol: John Wright. pp. 109–125

MOVAT, H. Z. (1985) *The Inflammatory Reaction*. Amsterdam: Elsevier. pp. 229–247

MURRAY, J. F., GARAY, S. M. and HOPEWELL, P. C. (1987) NHLBI workshop summary: Pulmonary complications of the acquired immunodeficiency syndrome. An update. *American Review of Respiratory Disease*, **135**, 504–509

MYGIND, N. (1979) *Nasal Allergy*, 2nd edn. Oxford: Blackwell Scientific Publications. p. 219

NEVILLE, E., MILLS, R. G. S. and JASH, D. G. (1976) Sarcoidosis of the upper respiratory tract and its association with lupus pernio. *Thorax*, **31**, 660–664

OWNBY, D. R. (1990) Environmental factors versus genetic determinants of childhood inhalant allergies. *Journal of Allergy and Clinical Immunology*, **86**, 279–287

OXELIUS, V.-A. (1974) Chronic infections in a family with hereditary deficiency of IgG2 and IgG4. *Clinical and Experimental Immunology*, **17**, 19–27

PAVIA, D. (1984a) Lung mucociliary clearance. In *Aerosols and the Lung*, edited by S. W. Clarke and D. Pavia. London: Butterworths. pp. 127–148

PAVIA, D. (1984b) Effects of pharmacologic agents on the clearance of airway secretions. *Seminars in Respiratory Medicine*, **5**, 345–367

PAVIA, D., AGNEW, J. E. and CLARKE, S. W. (1986) Cough and mucociliary clearance. *Bulletin Europeen de Physiopathologie Respiratoire*, **23** (Suppl. 10), 41–45

PAVIA, D., BATEMAN, J. R. M. and CLARKE, S. W. (1980) Deposition and clearance of inhaled particles. *Bulletin Europeen de Physiopathologie Respiratoire*, **16**, 335–341

PEDERSEN, M. and RYGIND, N. (1982) Rhinitis, sinusitis and other media in Kartagener's Syndrome (primary ciliary dyskinesia). *Clinical Otolaryngology*, **7**, 373–380

PEDERSEN, P. A. and WEEKE, E. R. (1983) Asthma and allergic rhinitis in the same patients. *Clinical Allergy*, **38**, 25–29

PENLETH, A. R. L., WISE A., MEIRS, M. B., HODSON, M. E. and BATTON, J. C. (1987) Cystic fibrosis in adolescence and adults. *Thorax*, **42**, 526–532

PINKTON, P., TRAUER, T., DUNCAN, F., HODSON, M. E. and BATTON, J. C. (1985) Cystic fibrosis in adult life. A study of coping patterns. *Lancet*, ii, 761–763

PLESKOW, W. W., STEVENSON, D. D., MATHISON, D. A., SIMON, R. A., SIMON, M. and ZEIGER, R. S. (1982) Aspirin desensitization in aspirin sensitive asthmatic patients: Clinical manifestations and characterization of the refractory period. *Journal of Allergy and Clinical Immunology*, **69**, 11–17

PROCTOR, D. F. (1977) The upper airways. II The larynx and trachea. *American Review of Respiratory Diseases* **115**, 315–342

PRYOR, J. A., WEBB, B. A., HODSON, M. E. and BATTON, J. C. (1979) Evaluation of the forced expiration technique as an adjunct to postural drainage in the treatment of cystic fibrosis. *British Medical Journal*, **2**, 417–418

PUCHELLE, E., ZAHM, J. M., GERARD, F., BERTRAND, A., POLU, J. M., AUG, F. *et al.* (1980) Mucociliary transport in vivo and in vitro. Relations to sputum properties in chronic bronchitis. *European Journal of Respiratory Diseases*, **61**, 254–264

RAMSDAL, E. H., MORRIS, M. M., ROBERTS, R. S. and HARGREAVE F. E. (1985) A symptomatic bronchial hyperresponsiveness in rhinitis. *Journal of Allergy and Clinical Immunology*, **75**, 573–577

REID, L. M. (1950) Reduction in bronchial subdivision in bronchiectasis. *Thorax*, **5**, 233–237

RICHARDS, C. D. and GAULDIE, J. (1985) IgA mediated phagocytosis by mouse alveolar macrophages. *American Review of Respiratory Diseases*, **132**, 82–85

ROSENBERG, Z. F. and FAUCI, A. S. (1989) The immunopathogenesis of HIV infection. *Advances in Immunology*, **47**, 377–431

SAARINEN, U. M., KAJOSSARI, M., BACKMAN, A. and SIIMES, M. A. (1979) Prolonged breast-feeding as prophylaxis for atopic disease. *Lancet*, ii, 163–166

SAMPLE, S., LENAHAN, G. A. and SECWONSKA, M. M. (1989) Allergic diseases and sinusitis in acquired immune deficiency syndrome. *Journal of Allergy and Clinical Immunology*, **83**, 190

SCADDING, J. G. and MITCHELL, D. M. (1985) *Sarcoidosis of the Upper Respiratory Tract*, 2nd edn. London: Chapman and Hall. pp. 290–301

SCHLESINGER, R. C., GURMAN, J. L and LIPPMANN, M. (1982) Particle deposition within bronchial airways. *Annals of Occupational Hygene*, **26**, 47–53

SELROOS, O. and NIEMISTO, M. (1977) Sarcoidosis of the nose. *Scandinavian Journal of Respiratory Disease*, **58**, 57–62

SHEN, L. and FANGER, M. W. (1981) IgA antibodies synergise with IgG in promoting ADCC by human polymorphonuclear cells, moncytes and lymphocytes. *Cell Immunology*, **59**, 75–81

SHWACHMAN, M. (1975) Gastro-intestinal manifestations of cystic fibrosis. *Pediatric Clinics of North America*, **22**, 787–805

SLAVIN, R. G. (1988) Sinusitis in adults and its relation to allergic rhinitis, asthma, and nasal polyps. *Journal of Allergy and Clinical Immunology*, **82**, 950–956

SLAVIS, R. G. (1982) Relationship of nasal disease and sinusitis to bronchial asthma. *American Allergy*, **49**, 76–80

SLEPIAN, I. K., MATTHEWS, K. P. and MCLEAN, J. A. (1985) Aspirin-sensitive asthma. *Chest*, **87**, 386–392

SMITH, I. M. (1983) Epidemiology and natural history of asthma, allergic rhinitis and allergic dermatitis (eczema). In: *Allergy: Principles and Practice*, 2nd edn., edited by E. Middleton Jr, C. E. Reed and E. F. Ellis. St Louis: CV Mosby Company. pp. 771–804

SOMERVILLE, M., RICHARDSON, P. S., TAYLOR, G. W., WILSON, R. W. and COLE, P. J. (1988) Chloroform extract of *Pseudomonas aeruginosa* stimulates mucus output into cat trachea in vivo. *American Review of Respiratory Disease*, **137**, 172–178

SPECTOR, S. L., MORRIS, H. G. and SELNER, J. C. (1981) Clinical responses and serum prostaglandin levels in aspirin idiosyncracy. *Chest*, **80**, 676–673

STANLEY, P., MACMILLAN, L., GREENSTONE, M., MACKAY, I. and COLE, P. J. (1984) Efficacy of a saccharin test for screening to detect abnormal mucociliary clearance. *British Journal of Diseases of the Chest*, **78**, 62–65

STANLEY, P. J., WILSON, R., GREENSTONE, M. A., MACWILLIAM, L. and COLE, P. J. (1986) Effect of cigarette smoking on nasal mucociliary clearance and ciliary beat frequency. *Thorax*, **41**, 519–523

STEINFORT, C., WILSON, R., MITCHELL, T., FELDMAN, C., RUTMAN, A., TODD, H. *et al.* (1989) The effect of *Streptococcus pneumoniae* on human respiratory epithelium in vitro. *Infection and Immunology*, **57**, 2006–2014

STEVENS, W. J. and VAN VEVER, H. P. (1989) Frequency and intensity of late asthmatic reactions after bronchial allergen challenge in asthma and rhinitis. *Allergy*, **44**, 471–476

STEVENSON, D. D., PLESKOW, W. W., SIMON, R. A., MATHISON, D. A., LUMY, W. R. and SCHATZ, M. (1984) Aspirin sensitive rhinosinusitis asthma: a double blind crossover study of treatment with aspirin. *Journal of Allergy and Clinical Immunology*, **73**, 500–506

STOCKLEY, R. A., SHAW, J., HILL, S. L. and BURNETT, D. (1988) Neutrophil chemotaxis in bronchiectasis: a study of peripheral cells and lung secretions. *Clinical Science*, **74**, 625–630

STRUTTS, K. J., SCHWAB, J. H., CHEN, M. G., KNOWLES M. R. and BOUCHER, R. C. (1986) Effects of *Pseudomonas aeruginosa* on bronchial epithelial ion transport. *American Review of Respiratory Disease*, **134**, 17–21

SVENONIUS, E., ARBORELIUS, M. J. R., KAUTTO, R. and LILJA, B. (1982) Lung function studies in children with allergic rhinitis. *Allergy*, **37**, 87–92

SYKES, D., WILSON, R., CHAN, K. L., MACKAY, I. S. and COLE, P. J. (1986) Relative importance of antibiotic and improved clearance in topical treatment of chronic mucopurulent rhinosinusitis. A controlled study. *Lancet*, ii, 359–360

TOEWS, G. B. and VIAL, W. C. (1984) The role of C5 in polymorphonuclear leukocyte recruitment in response to *Streptococcus pneumoniae*. *American Review of Respiratory Diseases*, **129**, 82–86

TOS, M. (1990) Cystic fibrosis (muco-viscidosis). In: *Diseases of the Nose and Sinuses*, vol II, edited by G. M. English. Philadelphia: Lipincott. p. 11

TOWNLEY, R. G. (1984) Allergic rhinitis and airway reactivity to medications. In: *Rhinitis*, edited by G. A. Settipane. Providence, Rhode Island: New England and Regional Allergy Proceedings

TOWNLEY, R. G., TRAFARI, I. L. and SZERTURANYI, A. (1967) Sensitization to anaphylaxis and to some of its pharmacological mediators by blockage of the beta adrenergic receptors. *Allergy*, **39**, 177

UMETSU, D. J., MOSS, R. B., KING, V. V. and LEWISTON, N. J. (1990) Sinus disease in patients with severe cystic fibrosis: relation to pulmonary exacerbation. *Lancet*, i, 1077–1078

WATSON, J. M. (1991) Tuberculosis in perspective. *Communicable Disease Report*, **1**, R129–132

WILSON, R. (1988) Secondary ciliary dysfunction. *Clinical Science*, **75**, 113–120

WILSON, R. and COLE, P. J. (1988) The effect of bacterial products on ciliary function. *American Review of Respiratory Diseases* **138**, 549–553

WILSON, R., ROBERTS, D. and COLE, P. J. (1985) Effects of bacterial products on human ciliary function in vitro. *Thorax*, **40**, 125–131

WILSON, R., PITT, T., RUTMAN, A., ROBERTS, D. and COLE, P. J. (1986) *Haemophilus influenzae* and *Haemophilus parainfluenzae*, slow and disorganise the beating of human cilia in vitro. *Clinical Science*, **70**, 26P

WILSON, R., ALTON, E., RUTMAN, A., HIGGINS, P., AL NAHIB, W., GEDDES, D. H. (1987a) Upper respiratory tract viral infection and mucociliary clearance. *European Journal of Respiratory Diseases* **70**, 272–278

WILSON, R., SYKES, D., CHAN, K. L., COLE, P. J. and MACKAY, I. S. (1987b) Effect of head position on the efficacy of topical treatment of chronic mucupurulent rhinosinusitis. *Thorax*, **42**, 631–632

WILSON, R., SYKES, D. A., WATSON, D., RUTMAN, A., TAYLOR, G. W. and COLE, P. J. (1988) Measurement of *Pseudomonas aeruginosa*, phenazine pigments in sputum and assessment of their contribution to sputum sol toxicity for respiratory epithelium. *Infection and Immunology*, **56**, 2515–2521

WILSON, R., MUNTO, N., HASTIE, A. and COLE P. J. (1989) *Pseudomonas aeruginosa* produces low molecular weight molecules which damage human respiratory epithelium in vitro and slow mucociliary transport in the guinea pig trachea in vitro. *Chest*, **95**, 214S

ZENKLER-MONRO, P. L. (1983) Gastro-intestinal disease in adults. In: *Cystic Fibrosis*, edited by J. D. Lloyd Still. London: Bailliere Tindall. Ch. 8

ZITSCH, R. P. and RILEY, J. S. (1987) Vocal cord paralysis associated with cystic fibrosis. *Annals of Otology, Rhinology and Laryngology*, **96**, 680–683

ZURCO, J. J., FEURESTEIN, I. M., LEBOVICS, R. and LANE, A. C. (1992) Sinusitis in HIV-1 infection. *American Journal of Medicine*, **93**, 157–162

16

Fractures of the facial skeleton

Michael Gleeson

Aetiology

Fractures of the nose, mandible and middle third of the facial skeleton are most commonly the result of road traffic accidents, attempted suicide or physical combat (Hagan and Huelke, 1961; van Hoof, Merkx and Stekelenburg, 1977; Starkhammar and Olofsson, 1982; Brook and Wood, 1983). In recent years the introduction of compulsory seat belt legislation has decreased the incidence of these injuries in the UK (Price, 1983; Steele and Little, 1983). In children, falls, accidents while playing and sports injuries are the major causes of facial fractures (Fortunato, Fielding and Guernsey, 1982). The possibility of non-accidental injury should never be overlooked (Rowe, 1969; Hall, 1972). Fractures resulting from complicated dental extractions and pathological lesions of the jaws are seen in all age groups.

Primary care of maxillofacial injuries

Maxillofacial fractures can endanger the airway and are frequently associated with brain damage (Hoffman, 1976). Although a patient with a fracture of the middle third presents an alarmingly dramatic picture the first considerations are to:

1 Ensure an adequate *airway*, while maintaining alignment of the neck in case there is an unstable cervical spine injury
2 Assess and establish *breathing* so that ventilation is effective
3 Maintain the *circulation* and control sources of blood loss
4 Assess the level of consciousness and neurological *dysfunction*
5 Carefully *expose* the patient to identify all other injuries.

Detailed examination and definitive treatment of the facial injury must take second place to these requirements (Gentleman *et al.*, 1993).

The establishment of a safe airway and effective ventilation is the most essential primary measure to prevent hypoxia and retention of carbon dioxide, as these are the most important factors in the development of post-traumatic cerebral oedema and damage.

The need for endotracheal intubation should be carefully considered in both the conscious and comatose patient. Posterior displacement of the tongue secondary to mandibular fractures, or posteroinferior displacement of the maxilla with middle third injuries, directly compromises the airway. It may be necessary to reduce a middle third fracture immediately by hooking the fingers of one hand around the posterior margin of the patient's hard palate and pulling the displaced jaw forward. Even those patients with a good airway initially may deteriorate to a very critical state as oropharyngeal oedema develops. Paradoxical chest movement due to a flail segment is a further indication for primary intubation. In conscious patients the loss of voice, dysphagia, surgical emphysema of the neck and pain on palpation of the thyroid cartilages suggests a fracture of the larynx. Increasing stridor with these symptoms and signs is a mandate for immediate tracheostomy.

Haemorrhage into the airway from either the nose or mouth can be torrential. It usually ceases spontaneously but must be controlled by nasal packs, balloons, catheters, sutures or arterial ligation. Super-selective arteriography and embolization is very effective and indicated in severe late onset bleeds (Mehrotra *et al.*, 1984). Shock is rarely the result of haemorrhage from a facial fracture and, when present, is likely to be due to rupture of abdominal viscera, intrathoracic injury, fractures of the limbs or extensive soft tissue lacerations. The source of blood loss must be recognized, controlled and replaced appropriately and promptly, otherwise hypotension further compromises the patient's cerebral state.

Only after such complications have been controlled should assessment of the head injury be undertaken. The level of consciousness is the most useful criterion and it is imperative that the initial level is recorded. Regularly repeated accurate documentation of spontaneous speech, response to command and reaction to painful stimuli provides a clinically useful scale (Figure 16.1) which reflects improvement or deterioration of the cerebral state (Teasdale and Jennet, 1974). Alcohol is frequently a factor in the acquisition of these injuries and it should be remembered that it may be contributing to the depression of the level of consciousness. Facial swelling may make examination of the eyes exceptionally difficult. However, pupil size and reaction to light must be recorded. Dilatation of a pupil at some interval after injury is highly suggestive of an ipsilateral expanding supratentorial lesion. Urgent reduction of pressure by either medical or surgical means is essential in such cases (Garfield,

1972). Sadly, burr holes placed by inexperienced personnel rarely save a life. All too often they either miss the haematoma, which in any case may be intradural, or just lose valuable time during which the patient could be transferred to a neurosurgical unit. Subdural pressure monitoring is a sophisticated method of detecting changes in intracranial pressure before the traditional clinical signs develop. It is available in nearly all neurosurgical centres and facilitates patient management.

Absence of limb movements in an acute head injury indicates primary cerebral damage. Such patients will have a diminished level of consciousness. The presence of a mono-, para- or quadriplegia in a relatively alert patient is highly suggestive of a plexus or cord lesion for which immediate immobilization should be instituted.

The cranium must be palpated very carefully to detect depressed fractures. Scalp lacerations are a possible source of intracranial infection and should never be probed in case the venous sinuses are damaged. Lacerations can be satisfactorily managed by irrigation with saline and dry dressings. Cerebrospinal fluid rhinorrhoea and otorrhoea may be present and,

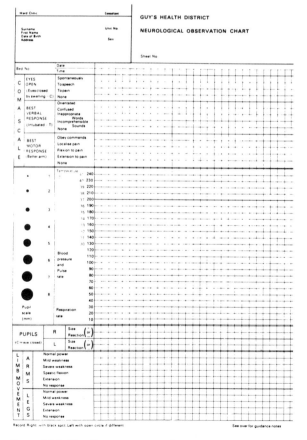

Figure 16.1 The Glasgow coma scale

in the acute situation, can be very difficult to detect, especially when mixed with blood. It may be distinguished at this stage by comparing the discharge with blood escaping from other sites. As the blood flow diminishes due to clotting the escape of cerebrospinal fluid becomes more obvious. If present, prophylactic antibiotics should be administered. Nasal intubation should be avoided, when possible, if the cerebrospinal fluid leak is from the nose.

Tetanus prophylaxis should be administered to any patient who has either not been immunized or received a reinforcement dose of adsorbed vaccine within 10 years of the accident; 0.5 ml adsorbed tetanus toxoid intramuscularly is the recommended booster dose for those immunized more than 10 years before their injury. Those patients who have never been immunized should receive a full three dose course of vaccine. Both categories of patient should also be given 250 IU of human antitetanic globulin but at a different site. Those with severely contaminated or devitalized wounds should also be given prophylactic treatment regardless of their immune status. It should be remembered that patients with impaired immunity, e.g. HIV, are increasingly common in today's society. They may not respond to tetanus vaccine and must receive antitetanus immunoglobulin (Department of Health, 1992).

Clinical examination of facial injuries

There is rarely any urgent need to reduce and fix facial fractures. Indeed the optimal time for definitive treatment is between the fifth and eighth days posttrauma. This allows sufficient time to assess the fracture, make splints if required and improve the general medical condition of the patient. Some complications, such as orbital haematoma, require urgent treatment and even if initially absent may develop before or after reduction. The clinical condition of the patient on admission can preclude full radiological examination and unavoidably some emergency room films lack sufficient definition. There is therefore no substitute for careful clinical extra- and intraoral examination. The following is an accepted approach to the clinical examination of these injuries.

Eyes

On admission look for penetrating injuries, corneal abrasions, dislocation of the lens and lacerations involving the lacrimal apparatus. Inspect any subconjunctival haemorrhage and determine its posterior limit. In the conscious patient, check the visual acuity, the discs for signs of retinal damage and ischaemia, light reflexes, external eye movements and direction of maximal diplopia if present. An assessment of ocular level should be made by comparing the position of the pupils.

Lack of patient cooperation and periorbital oedema limits the accuracy of the ophthalmic examination. Only gross displacements of the globe will be obvious initially. As oedema subsides such deformities become more evident. In patients with diplopia a forced duction test may then be appropriate to determine the presence of significantly herniated orbital contents (Figure 16.2). Avulsion of the medial canthal ligament produces an abnormal slant of the palpebral fissure. In such injuries lateral traction of the eyelid fails to produce tension at the medial canthus.

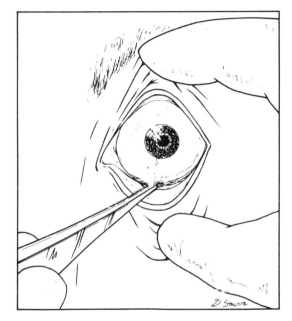

Figure 16.2 The forced duction test. After application of local anaesthetic to the conjunctiva the inferior rectus muscle is grasped with forceps. Limitation of upward rotation indicates herniation of the orbital contents through the orbital floor

Nose

It is often not possible to make an accurate assessment of an isolated nasal injury until all soft tissue swelling has subsided. Though this may take 5–7 days, it is essential to establish at the outset whether or not there is a septal haematoma, as it would require immediate drainage. This is particularly important in children for whom there is an increased incidence of this complication with nasal trauma and even more significant implications for future nasal growth (Stucker, Bryarly and Shockley, 1984). While some degree of nasal obstruction is experienced with all injuries to the nose, it is often more complete when a septal haematoma is present. In these cases, the septum is diffusely swollen and usually plum coloured, though sometimes not discoloured at all. A diagnostic incision should be made under local anaesthesia if any doubt exists. As stated earlier, a haematoma should be completely evacuated and adequate drainage established by making a generous hemitransfixion incision, aspirating the clot and inserting a small rubber drain. The mucoperichondrial flaps are then firmly apposed to the septal cartilage by antibiotic impregnated packs. This is an unpleasant procedure and is best performed under general anaesthetic. Systemic antibiotics should be prescribed for a minimum period of 1 week to reduce the risk of a septal abscess.

Failure to recognize and evacuate a significant septal haematoma results in a thickened septum at best and cartilage necrosis with subsequent saddle deformity of the nasal septum at worst. When pain increases and nasal obstruction persists for days after the initial injury, with or without pyrexia, abscess formation within a septal haematoma should be suspected. Extensive cartilage necrosis often results and must be minimized by urgent drainage and systemic antibiotic therapy.

The nose should also be carefully inspected for obvious external deformity in terms of its projection or lateral deviation. Displacement of the nasal bones may be palpable. Clots should be carefully removed from the nostrils by gentle suction and, with the aid of topical vasoconstriction (0.5% ephedrine or 5% cocaine), abnormalities of the septal anatomy should be recorded and an assessment made of whether these represent new or old injuries. The importance of making an adequate and accurate record of the initial nasal injuries cannot be emphasized too strongly as most are the result of an assault and many are the subject of subsequent litigation.

Two further, less obvious, features should be considered if only to be excluded. Cerebrospinal fluid rhinorrhoea may accompany minor facial trauma and is not solely a consequence of serious nasal and middle third injuries. Leaks can be intermittent and may only be shown by tipping the patient head and face down. Second, unilateral epistaxis in the absence of a direct nasal injury suggests a fracture involving the maxillary antrum.

Middle third of the face

The face should be inspected with particular attention to the distribution of oedema and ecchymoses. Disproportionate lengthening secondary to posterior displacement of Le Fort fractures, although masked by swelling in the acute phase, becomes apparent during the first week as the oedema subsides. The occlusion should be checked as posterior displacement of the maxilla also causes the molars to gag the bite open anteriorly. The bony contour of the face should be

palpated to detect step deformities and surgical emphysema. Sensory testing to determine the distribution of any deficit and evaluation of facial nerve function must be recorded.

Mandible

The bony outline of the lower jaw should be felt for step deformity. Careful observation of the symmetry of jaw movement on opening, while placing the little finger of each hand in the patient's external auditory canals, ascertains temporomandibular joint function. In addition, there is often bleeding from the ears in patients with damaged temporomandibular joints. Any sensory deficit of the lower lip should be noted.

Mucosa and dentition

The state of the dentition is partcularly relevant to the management of these injuries. Missing or fractured teeth should be recorded as they may have been inhaled or dislodged into the soft tissues. The health of the residual teeth is also important in planning methods of fixation. A general inspection of the dental arches for asymmetry is essential. Segments of the dental arches should be gently manipulated to elicit any abnormal mobility or crepitus. The occlusion is frequently subtly or grossly deranged, but may need expert dental assessment for its detection. Blood-stained saliva is a further indication of a fracture which is compound into the oral cavity. The mucosa should be examined for lacerations and haematomas of the buccal and lingual sulci, and of the palate. If the patient is edentulous, the dentures can be of immense assistance, even if broken. They should be obtained or retrieved and any missing fragments accounted for.

Signs of mandibular fractures
Body, angle and symphysis fractures

1 Step deformity palpable externally or intraorally
2 Asymmetry of the lower dental arch and derangement of the occlusion
3 Pain, paradoxical movement and crepitus on distraction of the fractured segments
4 Haematomas in the buccal sulcus or floor of the mouth
5 Blood-stained saliva
6 Anaesthesia in the distribution of the mental nerve.

Condylar neck fractures

1 Tenderness over the temporomandibular joint
2 Trismus

3 Deviation of the jaw towards the injured side on opening the mouth

4 Inability to move the mandible to the side opposite the injury

5 Deviation of the jaw to the fractured side at rest with anterior open bite secondary to gagging of the occlusion on the molar teeth in fracture dislocation

6 Symmetrical anterior open bite in bilateral fractures of the necks of the condyles.

Signs of middle third fractures

These injuries are classified into central and lateral (zygomatic complex) types, although in clinical practice these are frequently combined.

Central middle third fractures

1 Epistaxis
2 Circumorbital ecchymosis (panda facies)
3 Facial oedema
4 Surgical emphysema
5 Lengthening of the face
6 Oral respiration
7 Infraorbital nerve sensory deficit
8 Anterior open bite (Le Fort 2 and 3)
9 Haematoma at the junction of the hard and soft palate
10 Floating palate and teeth (Le Fort 1).

Lateral middle third (zygomatic complex) fractures

Many of the features seen in fractures of the central middle third are present also in the lateral variety, e.g. circumorbital ecchymosis, facial oedema and surgical emphysema. In addition the following may be seen:

1 Subconjunctival ecchymosis
2 Proptosis
3 Alteration of the ocular level
4 Increase in interpupillary distance
5 Limitation or absence of external eye movements
6 Diminished visual acuity
7 Step deformity of the orbital margin
8 Epiphora
9 Limitation of mandibular movement with depressed arch fractures
10 Flattening of the cheek
11 Step deformity of the zygomatic buttress on intraoral examination
12 Haematoma of the buccal sulcus
13 Infraorbital nerve deficit.

Radiological evaluation of maxillofacial fractures

All patients must have chest, cervical spine and supine lateral skull radiographs taken. In this way significant chest and spinal fractures will be recognized at the outset. Their treatment may take precedence over further radiographical examination or contraindicate the neck extension required for other facial views. Fluid levels in the sinuses are a common finding and usually represent blood, but when associated with air within the cranium indicate the presence of a cerebrospinal fluid leak which might otherwise be unrecognized.

In each case a standard facial series should be taken. The entire mandible can be demonstrated by a 10° posteroanterior view, an orthopantomogram or panellipse and lower occlusal films. The facial bones are best seen with a 30° occipitomental, a 30° anteroposterior (Townes) and submentovertical views, while the orbits are more clearly projected on a 45° occipitomental radiograph. Further films and projections may be necessary after this screen, e.g. orbital tomograms and temporomandibular joint films.

Fracture lines are seen more clearly with computerized tomography and this is indicated for all severe injuries. This technique has the further advantage of aiding the assessment of cerebral damage. The only relatively minor drawback of this method of examination is that it must await establishment of a secure airway.

Radiological evaluation of an isolated, simple, nasal fracture is unnecessary and rarely helpful. Suture lines and vascular markings are constantly misinterpreted as fractures both by radiologists and physicians. As a result, the patient may become convinced that his injury is more serious than in fact it is and then futile and unwarranted surgical intervention may be undertaken.

Principles of treatment

The general principles of management of fractures of the long bones apply equally to the facial skeleton. The fractured segments must be accurately reduced, securely immobilized and maintained free of infection for a period of time sufficient to allow bony union.

Facial fractures differ to some extent from others in that nearly all are compound, either directly into the mouth, nose, paranasal sinuses or indirectly into the mouth through the periodontal ligament. In the case of fractures of the jaw, it may not be in the best interests of the patient to effect closure by extraction of those teeth involved in the fracture, as their continued presence may be required for fixation or for guidance of the jaws into a functional position. Experience has shown that this compromise between potential infection and accurate reduction is acceptable.

The viability of small fractured segments of the nose and jaws is far better than elsewhere in the body. In general they should be retained as their preservation aids the restoration of facial contours and sequestrum formation is uncommon.

Both closed and open techniques of reduction are practised. All methods usually aim to fix the fractured part to the nearest superior structure in continuity with the base of the skull. Precise restoration of the occlusion registers the correct functional position of the jaws and the dentition forms an additional splint. The period of fixation is exceedingly variable and depends on such factors as age of the patient, site of fracture, degree of initial displacement, stability of reduction, etc. It can be as short as 24 hours if used merely to relieve pain but is usually 7 days for a simple nasal fracture, 10 days for a condylar fracture and 6 weeks for angle or body fractures of the mandible and Le Fort fractures.

Fractures of the nose

Surgical anatomy

Several patterns of nasal fracture are recognized and the extent of the injury sustained by the patient is largely determined by the force and direction of the blow (Schultz and DeVillers, 1974; Courtiss, 1978; Harrison 1979; Stranc and Robertson, 1979). Some classifications of these injuries have been unnecessarily cumbersome. From a clinical standpoint, it is probably more useful to divide nasal fractures into three broad categories which characterize progressive degrees of damage sustained with increased force, each category demanding a different method of treatment (Murray, 1989).

Class 1 fractures

The depressed nasal fracture is the simplest form of a class 1 fracture. Relatively little force is required to fracture the nasal bones. It has been estimated that as little as 25–75 pounds per square inch (173–518 kPa) is all that is necessary (Nahum, 1975). The fracture lines run parallel to the dorsum of the nose and nasomaxillary suture, joining at the point where the nasal bone becomes thicker, approximately two-thirds of the way along its length (Figure 16.3). The fractured segment usually regains its position as it is attached along its lower border to the upper lateral cartilage which gives it some recoil. The nasal septum is not involved in this particular injury, but is in a more severe variant in which both nasal bones are fractured. On the side of the blow, the fracture line runs parallel to the nasomaxillary suture, while on the contralateral side the fracture runs parallel to the dorsum and just below it. They connect across the

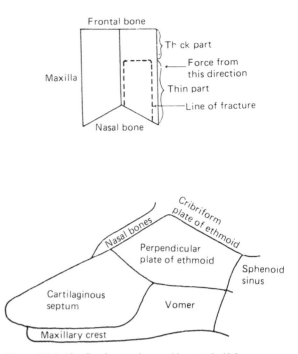

Figure 16.3 The distal part of a nasal bone is half the thickness of the proximal part. When it fractures the nose is apparently deviated but the impression of deviation is optical. It is important to recognize this injury. The edges of the stable segment can often be palpated. (Courtesy of Professor A. G. D. Maran)

dorsum at the point of thickening of the nasal bones. The cartilaginous septum, which is attached to the dorsum, is fractured approximately 0.5 cm below the dorsum and this may extend posteriorly into the perpendicular plate of the ethmoid and on to the skull base. This fracture is named after Chevallet who first described it.

Class 1 fractures do not cause gross lateral displacement of the nasal bones, though a persistently depressed fragment can give that illusion. Often they are barely perceptible unless the depressed fragment fails to recoil into its original postion because of impaction beneath the residual nasal bone. In children these fractures may be of the 'greenstick' variety and a significant nasal deformity subsequently develops at puberty when nasal growth accelerates (Persig and Lehmann, 1975).

Class 2 fractures

These fractures cause significant cosmetic deformity as in addition to the nasal bones they also involve the frontal process of the maxilla and septal structures (Figure 16.4). From the clinical standpoint, there are

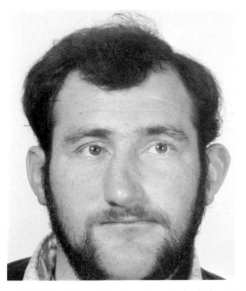

Figure 16.4 Class 2 nasal fracture showing high deviation of the nasal skeleton. (Courtesy of Professor A. G. D. Maran)

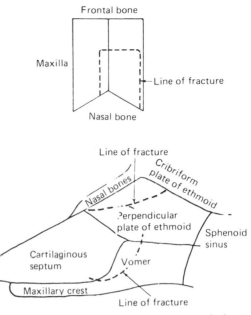

Figure 16.5 A class 2 nasal fracture involves the thicker proximal portion of the nasal bone. It results in true deviation and also fracture of the perpendicular plate of the ethmoid and quadrilateral cartilage. (Courtesy of Professor A. G. D. Maran)

two important reasons for recognizing this category of injury. First, both the septum and nasal bones will need to be reduced in order to obtain a cosmetically acceptable result. Second, although the nose will have absorbed considerable energy, the ethmoid labyrinth and adjacent orbital structures should be intact.

The precise deformity is determined by the direction of the blow. A frontal impact may comminute the nasal bones and cause gross flattening and widening of the dorsum, while a lateral blow of similar magnitude is likely to produce a high deviation of the nasal skeleton. The perpendicular plate of the ethmoid is inevitably involved in a septal fracture which is characteristically C-shaped. The fracture begins just beneath the nasal tip in the quadrilateral cartilage. It extends posteriorly and caudally through the perpendicular plate of the ethmoid to the anterior border of the vomer at which point it runs forward through the lower part of the perpendicular plate of the ethmoid into the inferior part of the quadrilateral cartilage (Figure 16.5). Although often thought to be merely a dislocation of the quadrilateral cartilage from the maxillary crest, it is in fact a fracture and has been called after Jarjavay.

Class 3 fractures

Class 3 fractures are the most severe nasal injuries encountered and are usually caused by high velocity trauma. In the past they have been known by a variety of terms which include ethmoid fracture, naso-orbital fracture and nasoethmoid fracture. More recently, the term naso-orbitoethmoid fracture has become popular and reflects the clinical importance of the orbital component of these injuries.

Two categories of naso-orbitoethmoid fractures have been recognized (Raveh *et al.*, 1992) and both are often acquired in association with a Le Fort fracture. The anterior skull base, posterior wall of the frontal sinus and optic canal remain intact in the first type in which the external butresses of the nose give way and the ethmoid labyrinth collapses or telescopes on itself (Figure 16.6*a*, *b*). As a consequence, the perpendicular plate of the ethmoid is rotated and the quadrilateral cartilage is pulled backwards. This movement imparts a classical, pig-like, appearance to the patient, whose nose is foreshortened and saddled with the nostrils facing forwards (Figure 16.7). The space between the eyes is also increased (telecanthus) and may be exaggerated still further by disruption of the medial canthal ligament from the crest of the lacrimal bone.

In the second type of naso-orbitoethmoid fracture, there is disruption of the posterior frontal sinus wall, multiple fractures of the roof of the ethmoid and orbit sometimes extending as far back as the sphenoid and parasellar regions (Figure 16.8). The dura is extremely adherent to the roof of the ethmoid and, consequently, multiple dural tears, cerebrospinal fluid leaks, pneumocranium and cerebral herniation often complicate this type of injury.

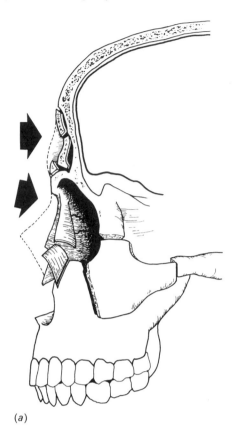

(a)

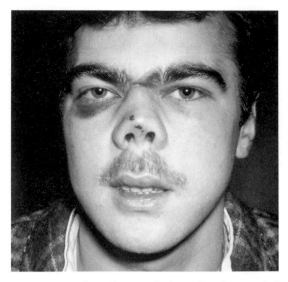

Figure 16.7 A class 3 fracture: the bones have been pushed back under the frontal bones and into the space created by a comminuted ethmoid labyrinth. The patient's nostrils become prominent. (Courtesy of Professor A. G. D. Maran)

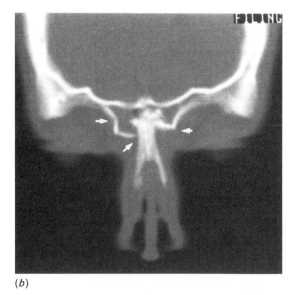

(b)

Figure 16.6 (a) Type 1 naso-orbitoethmoid fracture. The ethmoid labyrinth has collapsed and the nose telescoped. Despite this the skull base is largely intact. (b) Coronal CT scan of type 1 naso-orbitoethmoid fracture (arrows). Note that the anterior skull base has remained intact

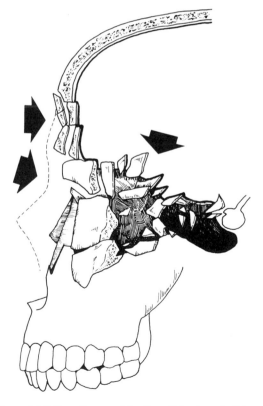

Figure 16.8 Type 2 naso-orbitoethmoid fracture. In this fracture there is disruption of the posterior frontal sinus wall and multiple fractures of the anterior cranial base

Management of nasal fractures

A significant number of patients referred to otolaryngology clinics with a *fractured nose* either do not have one at all, or it is not significantly displaced and does not need to be reduced. Most of these patients have some oedema which distorts their appearance and makes breathing through their nose difficult. As stated before, they must be well documented in case there is subsequent litigation (Illum, 1991). A second examination a week later is prudent for those cases where there is doubt about the degree of underlying displacement. Often, reassurance that there has been no significant damage and the prescription of vasoconstrictor drops to improve nasal airflow are all that are necessary.

Great care has to be taken to distinguish between recently acquired and old deformities. Sadly, nasal trauma is a frequent event for some patients. They present with an acute injury superimposed on a long-standing gross deviation of the nasal bones and septum. These patients are not materially helped by treatment and are better counselled that a definitive septorhinoplasty would be more appropriate at a later phase in their life. The same advice is appropriate for contact sportsmen.

Class 1 fractures

Reduction of these fractures is preferably undertaken when the overlying oedema has subsided and before significant fixation of the bone fragments has taken place. In adults this is usually 5–7 days after the injury and a little sooner in children. While this would seem to offer considerable latitude for the otolaryngologist, all can be lost by delayed referral by accident and emergency department staff. An interval of 2 weeks between the injury and evaluation in an outpatient clinic may be just sufficient to commit that patient to require osteotomies for reduction.

Most class 1 fractures can be manipulated and reduced as effectively with local anaesthesia as general anaesthesia. For this purpose, local anaesthetic is infiltrated around the nasal dorsum and the mucosa sprayed or painted with 5% cocaine. Nearly all patients find this method of anaesthesia perfectly adequate and acceptable (Cook *et al.*, 1990; Owen, Parker and Watson, 1992). Digital pressure may be all that is necessary to reduce the deformity. In some, where the fractured segment has become impacted, Walsham's forceps or an elevator may have to be applied. These instruments can cause considerable damage to the nasal mucosa and provoke brisk haemorrhage. A nasal pack left in place for a period of 3 days helps to maintain the reduction and may need to be reinforced by an external splint if the reduction is particularly unstable.

Class 2 fractures

Closed reduction of this type of fracture rarely gives a satisfactory result as the final postion of the nasal dorsum reflects the deformity of the underlying septum (Harrison, 1979; Murray and Maran, 1984; Murray, 1989; Verwoerd, 1992). At least 50% of these fractures remain displaced because of overlapping segments of the fractured perpendicular plate of the ethmoid or septal cartilage which are not repositioned by closed reduction. Closed manipulation of the nasal bones should be accompanied by an open reduction of the septal deformity (Figure 16.9). Through a Killians incision, the mucoperichondrium is elevated on both sides of the septal cartilage and the overlapping parts of the nasal septum are elevated. The bony/cartilaginous junction is disrupted and a narrow vertical strip of cartilage is removed from just beneath the nasal bones to the maxillary crest. The realigned nasal septum is maintained by a nasal pack or quilting with a 4/0 plain catgut suture and the nasal bones by a plaster of Paris splint. Packs, when used, can be removed after 3 days and the splint at a week.

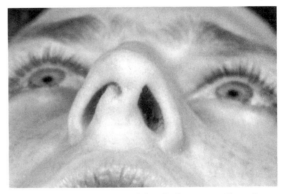

Figure 16.9 'Dislocated' caudal end of septum. When the caudal end presents in one nostril it either represents a Chevallet or a Jarjavay fracture further back. (Courtesy of Professor A. G. D. Maran)

Class 3 fractures

Most class 3 (naso-orbitoethmoid) fractures should be treated by open reduction and internal fixation. The major problem is that even if the nasal bones can be easily distracted from the skull base, the adjacent structures which normally support them, such as the frontal bone and medial wall of the orbit, have also been comminuted and are unstable. It is, therefore, one of the primary aims of treatment to reconstruct and stabilize the anterior table of frontal bone so that other parts of the nasal skeleton can derive support from it. In the past the reduced frontonasal complex would be supported by transnasal wires tied externally over either silicon or lead plates and the comminuted medial orbital wall left to reattach and reorganize itself (Figure 16.10).

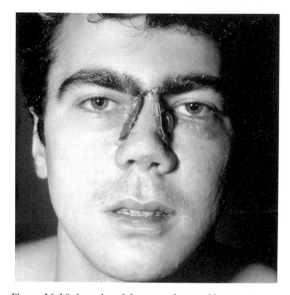

Figure 16.10 In a class 3 fracture, the nasal bones are pulled forwards and stopped from slipping back by wire slings. The wires are supported by lead plates. (Courtesy of Professor A. G. D. Maran)

The recent development of miniplate systems has had a huge impact on the management of these fractures (Weerda and Siegert, 1990). With these plates, it has been possible to reconstruct comminuted fragments of bone to a high degree of accuracy and even replace the medial orbital wall with split rib bone grafts. For this, it is essential to have good exposure which can usually be provided by a combination of coronal and medial canthal incisions. Sometimes access is aided by extension of a skin laceration. A sequence of surgical steps has been identified by Ellis (1993) which should be considered, though not necessarily all required, in every case. These include:

1 Provision of adequate surgical exposure to provide an unobstructed view of all components of the fracture
2 Identification of the medial canthal ligament. This is very rarely avulsed and is usually attached to a large fragment of bone. Once identified, the ligament should be reattached or secured to avoid subsequent telecanthus
3 Reduction and reconstruction of the medial orbital rim. This is often still best achieved by transnasal, 26-gauge, wires. If plates are used for this purpose, they should be as thin as possible otherwise they are conspicuous when the tissues have healed

4 Reconstruction of the medial orbital wall and floor with bone grafts
5 Transnasal canthopexy for those cases where canthal displacement persists despite reattachment of medial canthal ligament
6 Realignment of the nasal septum
7 Augmentation of the nasal dorsum and/or columella with bone grafts
8 Accurate soft tissue readaptation should be encouraged with splints so that post-surgical thickening is avoided.

Results and complications of management

Cosmesis and nasal function

It is sad to reflect that, despite the frequency of this injury, the most common complication is an unsatisfactory cosmetic result. Most substantive series report poor results in a large proportion of patients (Mayell, 1973; Harrison, 1979; Dickson and Sharpe, 1986; Illum, 1986). Changes in the shape of the nose attributable to the fracture may continue to develop for several years after the incident, e.g. saddling and hump formation. Some degree of stenosis may also become apparent over time and require surgical treatment. Factors which contribute to an unsatisfactory cosmetic result include the degree of initial displacement, delay in reduction, inappropriate surgical technique and previous nasal trauma.

Conventional medial and lateral osteotomies should not be used on nasal bones that have healed after trauma. This technique usually produces an irregular fracture running along the old fracture line. Mackay (1986) advocated a triple osteotomy technique for this group of patients. He employs complete medial, intermediate and lateral osteotomies which effectively shatter the nasal bones and render them completely manipulable. After realignment, the nose is packed and splinted in its new postion (Figure 16.11).

Orbital complications

Telecanthus can be acquired despite every effort at initial reduction. Further attempts can be made to reattach or tension the medial canthal ligament. Alternatively, correction of any flattening of the nasal dorsum or augmenting its height has the effect of diminishing the apparent deformity. Epiphora secondary to a damaged lacrimal duct is an infrequent complication which can usually be resolved by a dacryocystorhinostomy.

Cerebrospinal fluid leaks

CSF rhinorrhoea is common immediately after naso-orbitoethmoid fractures and initial treatment is

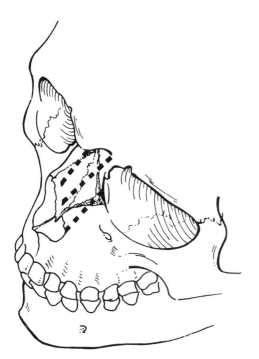

Figure 16.11 The triple osteotomy: the nasal bone will fracture along these three lines – allowing easy repositioning. (Courtesy of Professor A. G. D. Maran)

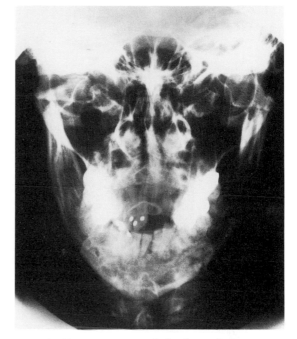

Figure 16.12 Posteroanterior skull radiograph showing bilateral subcondylar fractures together with a fracture of the body of the mandible in the left canine region. (Dr Beeching's case)

discussed later in this chapter. The vast majority stop after reduction and fixation of the fracture. Any leak that persists for more than 2 weeks after the initial injury should be considered for formal repair. Though meningitis is relatively uncommon in these patients, they are at constant risk of developing it. Symptoms suggestive of incipient meningitis should be taken very seriously in this group of patients.

Fractures of the mandible
Surgical anatomy

There are several patterns and combinations of fractures recognized in the mandible. Each is determined by the magnitude of the impact, the direction of the blow, the age of the patient, state of his jaws and condition of his dentition (Hodgson, 1967; Huelke and Harger, 1969). Stability or displacement of the fragments is determined mainly by the action of the attached musculature and the plane of the fracture line.

The weakest part of the mandible is the subcondylar region and it is therefore the most common site to fracture (Figure 16.12). The angle, often weakened by the presence of unerupted third molars, is the next most frequent region (Figure 16.13), followed by the body, lateral chin and symphysis (Table 16.1).

Single and multiple fractures occur with equal frequency (Hagan and Huelke, 1961). The most usual combinations of mandibular fractures are bilateral subcondylar fractures (see Figure 16.12), fractures of the body and opposite angle and fractures of the body with the contralateral condyle. Bilateral body (Figure 16.14), bilateral angle and comminuted fractures are comparatively rare.

The subcondylar region is protected by the zygomatic arch and is therefore usually fractured as the result of an indirect force delivered either to the chin or contralateral mandibular body. Such fractures are rarely grossly displaced. Anteromedial rotation of the condyle secondary to the pull of the attached lateral pterygoid muscle is usual. Fracture dislocations of the joint posteriorly and centrally into the middle cranial fossa are also occasionally seen (Lindahl, 1977).

Displacement of angle fractures is determined by two factors. First the masseter, medial pterygoid and temporalis muscles pull the posterior segment medially upward and forward. The second factor is the direction of the fracture line in the vertical and horizontal planes. Fractures running forward from lingual to buccal resist medial displacement of the posterior fragment and are called *vertically favourable*. Those running in the opposite direction are more easily displaced lingually and are therefore *vertically*

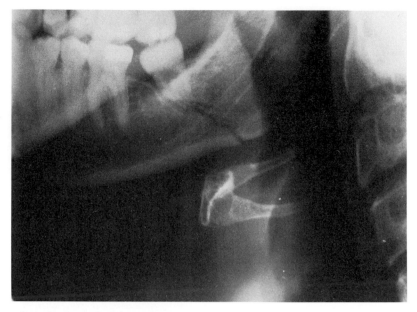

Figure 16.13 Oblique lateral radiograph of the mandible showing a fracture of the angle passing through the molar tooth socket. (Dr Beeching's case)

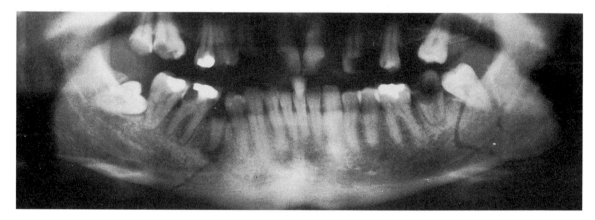

Figure 16.14 Panellipse radiograph of the mandible showing bilateral mandibular body fractures. The fracture on the right passes through a periapical cyst and the fracture on the left through a tooth socket. (Dr Beeching's case)

Table 16.1 Regional distribution (%) of mandibular fractures

	Nakamura and Gross (1973) (n = 91)	van Hoof, Merckx and Stekelenburg (1977) (n = 797)	Hagan and Huelke (1961) (n = 319)
Angle	24.3	14.0	20.5
Body	27.1	10.0	21.2
Condyle	19.6	47.0	36.3
Coronoid	1.0	0.7	2.1
Dentoalveolar	1.9		2.8
Ramus	4.7	1.2	2.2
Lateral chin/symphysis	21.4	27.1	14.9
	100.0	100.0	100.0

unfavourable (Figure 16.15). Similarly, fractures which run from the superior border of the mandible forward to the inferior margin resist upward displacement and are termed *horizontally unfavourable* (Figures 16.16 and 16.17). In patients with third molar teeth the fracture line invariably runs through either the socket or crypt.

Body fractures are mainly sustained in the first molar or canine regions. Like all fractures through tooth-bearing areas they are usually compound into the mouth. The tendency of the posterior fragment to upward displacement is counteracted, to some extent,

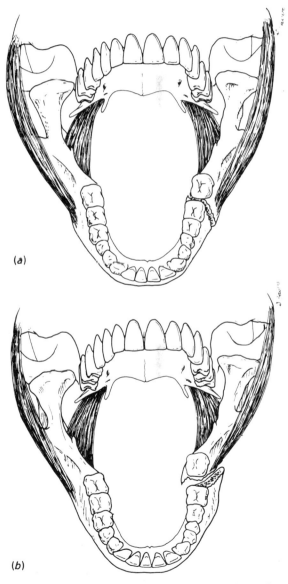

Figure 16.15 (*a*) Vertically favourable fracture of the angle of the mandible. (*b*) Vertically unfavourable fracture of the angle of the mandible

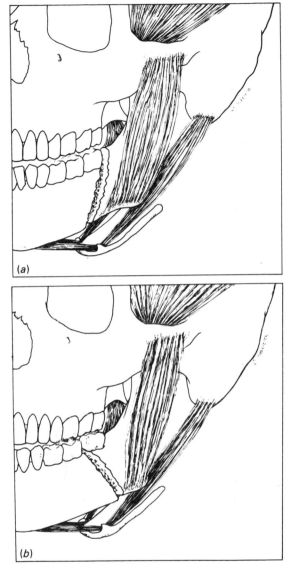

Figure 16.16 (*a*) Horizontally favourable fracture of the angle of the mandible. (*b*) Horizontally unfavourable fracture of the angle of the mandible

by the attachment of the mylohyoid muscle. However, the action of this muscle encourages medial displacement of the posterior fragment.

Displacement of anterior fractures is governed by the extrinsic muscles of the tongue. The part of the mandible bearing the genial tubercles is pulled lingual to the other. Fractures of the ramus and coronoid process are stabilized by the splinting action of the masseter and medial pterygoid muscles and therefore minimally displaced. Conversely, multiple or comminuted fractures are usually grossly displaced.

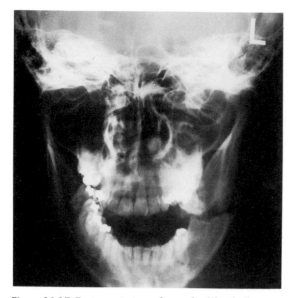

Figure 16.17 Posteroanterior radiograph of the skull showing an unfavourable fracture of the mandible through the lower molar tooth socket. The posterior segment has been displaced superiorly and medially. (Dr Beeching's case)

Closed reduction techniques

Intermaxillary fixation

There are several modifications of interdental wiring techniques, termed intermaxillary fixation. In a cooperative, dentate patient wiring can be undertaken under local anaesthesia. This method of fixation has much to commend it. Simplicity apart, of most significance is the fact that the conscious patient has control of his airway throughout the procedure and is less likely to vomit in the immediate postoperative period.

Method

Soft, 0.35 mm and 0.5 mm diameter stainless steel wire is work hardened by stretching a further 10% of its length. Small loops are made in the wire and fixed to groups of teeth in both jaws by encircling the free ends of the wires around the necks of the teeth before twisting their ends together in a clockwise fashion. The smaller diameter wire is used for the anterior teeth and the larger diameter wire on posterior teeth. These anchorage points are subsequently linked and bound tightly together by elastic or wire so that the dentition comes together in centric occlusion (Figure 16.18).

In the partially dentate patient, preformed arch bars or sectional silver cap splints can be used to link the dentition into a functional unit. Intermaxillary fixation is then applied by means of wire or elastic bands. In the immediate postoperative period intermaxillary fixation is safer with elastic bands than

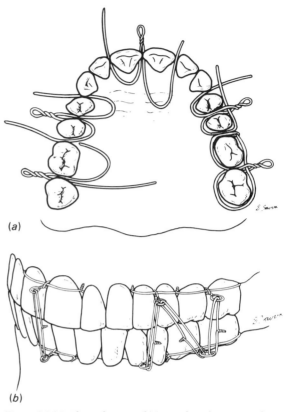

Figure 16.18 The technique of (*a*) interdental wiring and (*b*) establishing intermaxillary fixation

wire as they can be cut or removed faster and more easily in the event of airway obstruction.

The addition of cleats to the dentures of an edentulous patient makes these highly suitable as splints to hold the mandible and maxilla together in the correct relationship. These Gunning-type splints are retained by peralveolar wiring through the maxilla and circumferential wires around the mandible. Placement of the wires is effected by the use of an awl (Figure 16.19).

The above methods of fixation are only applicable to fractures of the tooth-bearing parts of the mandible. They will not provide adequate immobilization for fractures of the condyle, ramus or for some unfavourable fractures of the angle or posterior body. In these instances other methods of fixation should be employed.

External pin fixation

External pin fixation still finds favour in particular situations. It can be employed to advantage in cases with combined fractures of both the mandible and maxilla, those with gross comminution or bone loss, e.g. pathological fractures, gun shot wounds and in patients with atrophic edentulous jaws or osteomyelitis.

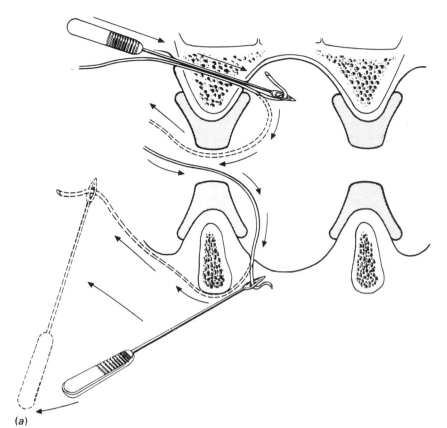

(a)

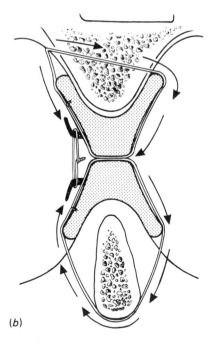

(b)

Figure 16.19 The technique of wiring Gunning splints

Method

Pairs of pins linked by cross struts are screwed into the main fragments of the mandible. These are then connected and secured by a universal joint bar assembly so that the fragments are maintained in the correct relationship.

The biphase appliance is a modification of external pin fixation. Specially designed screws, with threads at both ends, are inserted into the bone fragments and connected by a temporary metal bar. A permanent plastic connector is fashioned from cold cure acrylic resin, adapted over the free ends of the pins and secured by nuts (Figure 16.20). This system is tolerated extremely well by the tissues for prolonged periods. It is therefore particularly useful for patients in whom bone grafting is required, particularly for avulsive trauma and resection of malignant tissue.

Open reduction techniques

Transosseous wiring

Direct transosseous wiring is a satisfactory and simple method of fixation. It has particular advantages in controlling the edentulous posterior fragment, comminuted fractures which are compound externally and in multiple fractures for stabilizing the lower border of the mandible.

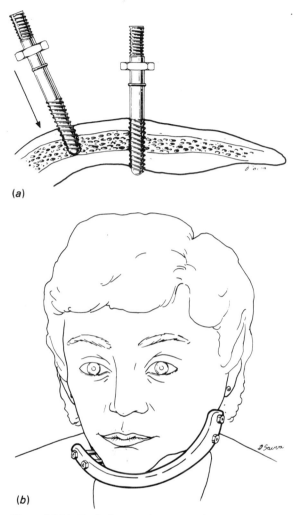

(a)

(b)

Figure 16.20 The biphase appliance. (*a*) The screws for the biphase must grip both plates of the mandible. (*b*) The pairs of screws are linked by an acrylic bar

Method

Holes are drilled with a no. 6 rose-head burr either side of the fracture line, taking great care not to damage either the marginal branch of the facial nerve in gaining access to the mandible or the inferior dental nerve when drilling the holes. Stainless steel wire, 0.5 mm in diameter, is passed through these holes and tightened to approximate the fractured segments. The reduction can be further secured by a second wire inserted through the same drill holes but tied in a figure-of-eight across the lower border (Figure 16.21).

In the past every method of plating and pinning familiar to orthopaedic surgeons has been employed to stabilize fractures of the jaws, e.g. Kirschner wires (Vero, 1968), Steinmann's pins, titanium mesh, titanium plates (Battersby, 1967; Frost, El-Attar and

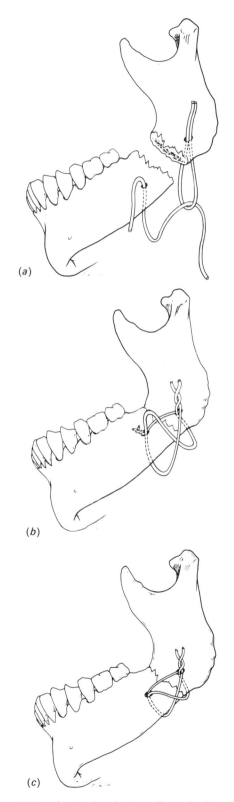

(a)

(b)

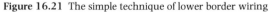

(c)

Figure 16.21 The simple technique of lower border wiring

Moos, 1983), nylon straps and bone staples (Williams, 1985). Although available in most hospitals, and therefore convenient for use, they have all been superseded by the development of bone plates. The degree of fixation achieved by these methods is unrivalled (Figures 16.22 and 16.23). Furthermore, reduction and fixation accelerate and materially alter the histological pattern of bone healing (Becker, 1974; Champy *et al.*, 1978).

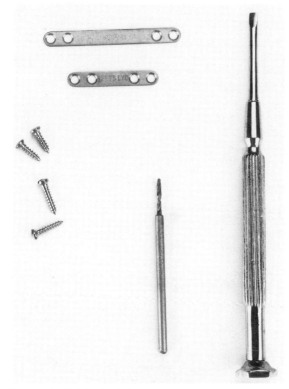

Figure 16.22 A basic plating set

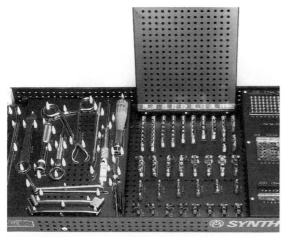

Figure 16.23 A complex compression plating set

Bone plates

The plates are available in several lengths ranging from 3 cm to 7 cm and in either stainless steel or titanium. In one end of some types of plate there is a circular fixation hole by which one side of the fracture is secured with screws. At the other end is an oblong hole and an eccentrically countersunk compression hole. The insertion and tightening of a screw in the compression hole forces the fragments together along the plane determined by the screw in the oblong hole. This compression facility is not essential and simple plates are probably equally effective. It is most essential that plates and screws of identical metals are used and not mixed, otherwise an electrolytic action can take place and the plates become weakened. No other form of fixation is normally required, but it has been found beneficial by some to place the jaws in intermaxillary fixation until the soft tissues have healed.

Oblique fractures are not always suitable for compression plating. In such cases compression can be achieved with lag screws which engage the lingual plate through a buccally prepared hole. Tightening the screws draws the fragments together. Neither compression plates nor lag screws need to be removed unless they become infected.

Plates are particularly useful when prolonged immobilization of the jaws would be better avoided in such patients as epileptics, the aged and in body fractures associated with fractures around the temporomandibular joint. Plating is only contraindicated in cases with gross contamination or wounds that will not close.

Management of condylar neck fractures

Fortunately, the degree of displacement is not significant in the majority. The ultimate aim is to produce a functional result either by creation of a pseudoarthrosis or bony reunion of the condyle. Much controversy exists over the correct method of treatment. The fragments can be plated or wired directly but this is not a simple procedure and places the main trunk of the facial nerve at considerable risk of surgical trauma. However, intermaxillary fixation for 10 days is usually sufficient to establish a functional jaw relationship. This makes the patient more comfortable while local muscle spasm and pain subside and is followed by graduated mobilization of the joint.

Fractures of the middle third

Central middle third

Surgical anatomy

These injuries are usually the result of a blow to the front of the face. It is traditional to divide them into alveolar and Le Fort 1, 2, and 3, as most follow these lines of weakness (Le Fort, 1901). This division is of considerable practical significance as it establishes the precise level from which the fractured segment can be suspended and to which structures it may be secured.

Alveolar

This is a fracture through the alveolar process only. It may or may not contain teeth.

Le Fort 1 (Guerin)

This type of fracture runs above the floor of the nasal cavity, through the nasal septum, maxillary sinuses and inferior parts of the medial and lateral pterygoid plates (Figure 16.24).

Le Fort 2

This is a fracture which runs from the floor of the maxillary sinuses superiorly to the infraorbital margin, through the zygomaticomaxillary suture. In the orbit it passes across the lacrimal bone to the nasion. The infraorbital nerve is often damaged by involvement in this fracture (Figures 16.25 and 16.26).

Le Fort 3

This represents a disconnection of the facial skeleton from the cranial base. The fracture traverses the medial wall of the orbit to the superior orbital fissure and exits across the greater wing of the sphen-

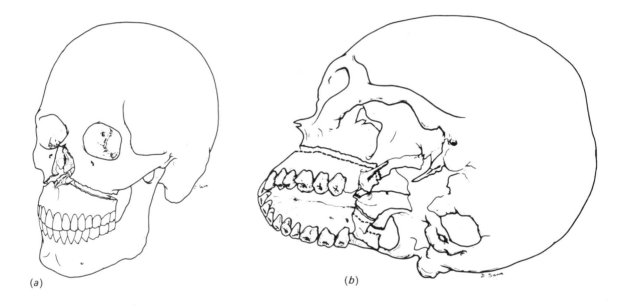

(a)

(b)

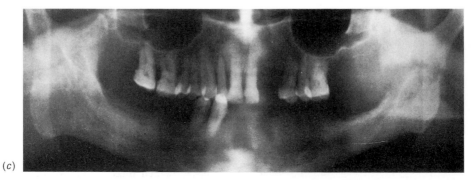

(c)

Figure 16.24 (*a*) and (*b*) Le Fort 1 fracture lines. (*c*) Panellipse radiograph of bilateral Le Fort 1 fractures together with bilateral fractures of the mandibular ramus. (Dr Beeching's case)

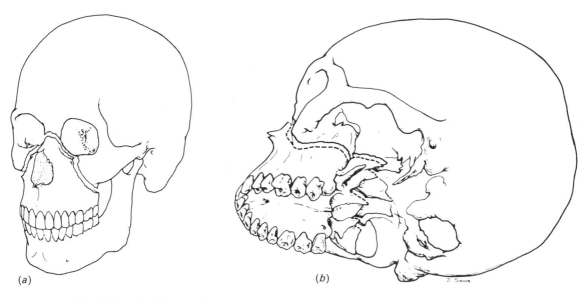

Figure 16.25 (*a*) and (*b*) Le Fort 2 fracture lines

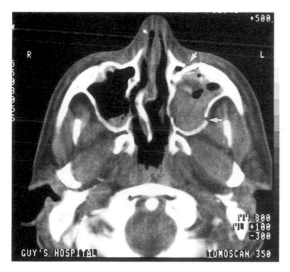

Figure 16.26 CT scan showing fractures (arrow)

oid and zygomatic bone to the zygomaticofrontal suture. Posteriorly it runs inferior to the optic foramen, across the lesser wing of the sphenoid to the pterygomaxillary fissure and sphenopalatine foramen. The arch of the zygoma is also broken (Figure 16.27).

Displacement of all these fractures is the result of the initial impact and tends to be backwards and downwards along the base of the skull. This imparts a characteristic dish face deformity to the patient. All are compound to the nose or paranasal sinuses and some breach the dura. A few are associated with a paramedian split of the palate.

External fixation techniques

External frames tend to be bulky and unsightly. They interfere with the patient's visual field and sleep and cannot be used if there is a possibility that a craniotomy will be required or if the patient is likely to have an epileptic fit. External fixation has therefore diminished in popularity since the advent of plating systems which overcome these problems. It is, however, still occasionally used for fractures with gross anteroposterior instability, e.g. combined Le Fort and condylar fractures. In these circumstances it usually complements other open methods of fixation.

Disimpaction and reduction of the maxilla may require some force. Either Walsham's or Rowe's forceps can be used to grip the maxillary segment, one blade being placed in the nose and the other on the palate (Figure 16.28). The maxilla is then gently rocked laterally and forward into its correct position. Occasionally it is impacted behind a fractured malar bone and is quite impossible to reposition until the latter has been reduced. The mandibular dentition is the most accurate guide to the correct, functional position of the maxilla on the cranial base, assuming that the mandible itself is or has been rendered intact. Intermaxillary fixation is therefore applied after reduction of the maxilla in these cases.

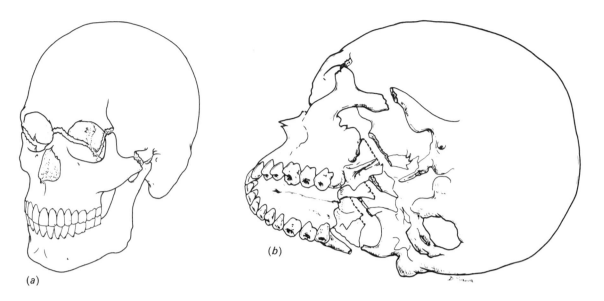

Figure 16.27 (*a*) and (*b*) Le Fort 3 fracture lines

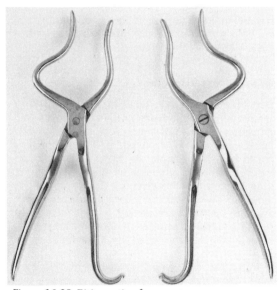

Figure 16.28 Disimpaction forceps

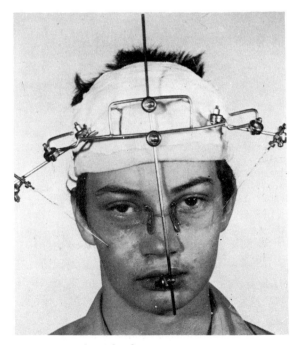

Figure 16.29 Plaster head cap

The first type of external fixation used was that of a plaster head cap and metal outrigger (Figure 16.29). It had several disadvantages, not the least of which were instability and patient discomfort. It has been superseded by designs incorporating skeletal pins, e.g. Box frame (Figure 16.30) Levant frame (Figure 16.31) and Royal Berkshire halo (Levant, Gardner-Berry and Snow. 1969; Mackenzie and Ray, 1970; Levant, Cook and MacFarlane, 1973; Georgiade *et al.*, 1981). All these devices provide a stable frame attached to the cranium at several points. The maxillary alveolar ridge or dentition is then firmly attached to this frame. These frames are simple to apply using Toller or Moule skeletal pins and universal joints, though care has to be taken to avoid electrolytic action between dissimilar metals by the

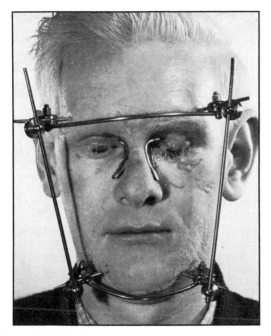

Figure 16.30 The Box frame

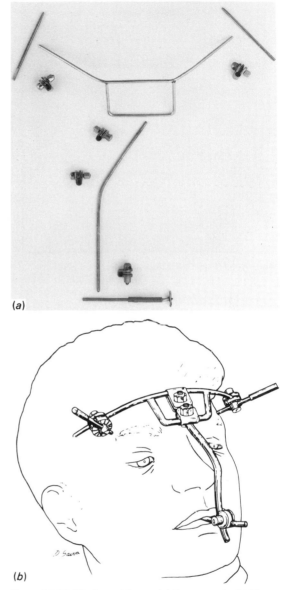

(a)

(b)

Figure 16.31 The Levant frame. (*a*) Components. (*b*) The frame *in situ*

placement of insulation at junctions bathed in saliva. They are comfortable and well tolerated by the patient.

Facial transfixion is rarely used today, although it is simple and effective. It is particularly suited to Le Fort 2 fractures in which the zygomatic complex is intact and for those cases where external frames are contraindicated due to skull fracture. Remarkable stability can be achieved by driving a Kirschner wire through the zygomatic bone, across the facial skeleton in a plane inferior and parallel to the inferior orbital rim to exit via the opposite zygoma. The ends are protected by corks or trimmed short (Figure 16.32). No anaesthesia is required for their removal (Vero, 1968).

Internal skeletal fixation

The simplest method of fixation is that of internal wire suspension (Adams, 1942; Kufner, 1970). The fractured maxillary segment may be suspended from various points of the craniofacial skeleton which depend only on the level of the fracture, e.g. zygomatic arches, orbital rims, forehead, pyriform apertures (Figures 16.33 and 16.34). Thus a Le Fort 3 may only be suspended from the frontal bone, whereas a Le Fort 1 can be suspended from any of the above points. This form of suspension is not ideal as it may exert a backward force on the fractured segment and thus encourage the relapse of the dis-

placement. To avoid this, modifications using steel implants have been developed (Stoll, Schilli and Joos, 1983).

Direct wiring can be used as easily for maxillary fractures as for those of the mandible. It permits accurate alignment of the reduced fragments through simple surgical approaches. The technique is identical to that used in the mandible and similarly the wires need not be removed. Miniaturized compression plates serve exactly the same purpose and are far superior to wiring in terms of stability.

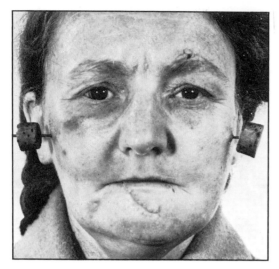

Figure 16.32 Facial transfixion by Kirschner wire

Lateral middle third (zygomatic complex)

Surgical anatomy

The body and processes of the zygomatic bone constitute the lateral middle third. Blows to this part of the face are common and may cause either a depressed fracture of the entire zygomatic bone or a fracture of the arch.

Depressed fractures of the zygomatic bone are sometimes called tripod fractures because the bone breaks in three places – frontozygomatic suture, the infra-orbital rim and the zygomatic buttress (Figure 16.35). These fractures are classified according to their rotation about vertical and horizontal axes. The vertical axis runs between the frontozygomatic suture and the first molar tooth, while the horizontal axis is in the plane of the zygomatic arch. Fractures may therefore be rotated medially or laterally about these planes. In severe injuries the bone is dislocated or comminuted and, in all, there is disruption of the orbital floor.

Two factors govern the degree and type of displacement. First the direction and site of the impact relative to the axes of the zygomatic bone and second, the pull of the masseter and integrity of the facial attachments.

The arch tends to break at its weakest point which lies just posterior to the zygomaticotemporal suture. Displacement is usually in a medial direction and can produce trismus by interfering with the coronoid process and temporalis muscle. If the temporalis and masseteric fascia is disrupted the arch tends to collapse inferiorly (Figure 16.36).

Blows to this aspect of the facial skeleton do not always break the zygomatic bone. A sudden impact with the globe may cause fracture of the orbital floor alone, producing a 'blow-out'. The external eye movements are then frequently restricted by herniation or incarceration of the orbital contents through this defect.

Management

Many fractures of the zygomatic complex will not require reduction (Rowe, 1985). Indeed, there is a very real risk of iatrogenic blindness following treatment

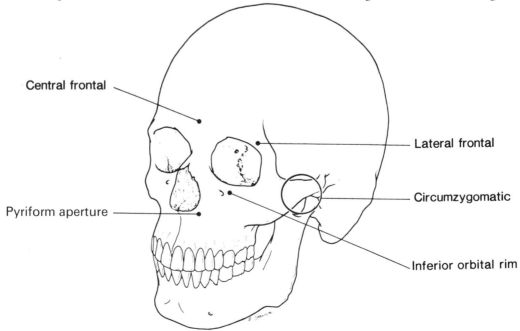

Figure 16.33 Sites for internal suspension of Le Fort fractures

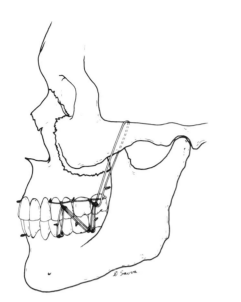

Figure 16.34 Le Fort 2 fracture being suspended by circum-zygomatic wires; note the posterior pull of the wires

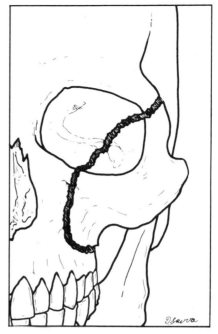

Figure 16.35 The malar fracture lines

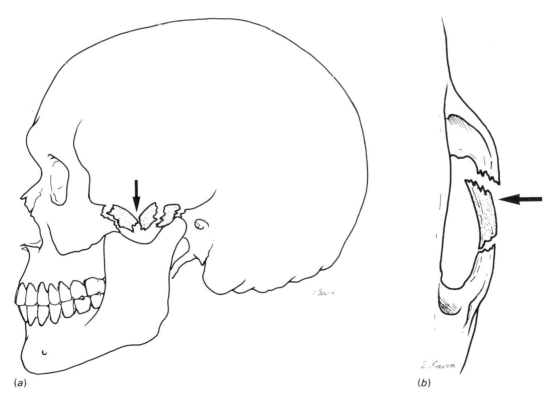

(a)

(b)

Figure 16.36 (*a*) An unstable inferiorly displaced fracture of the zygomatic arch. (*b*) A stable depressed fracture of the zygomatic arch

which should be considered in all those with minimal deformity and impaired vision on the contralateral side (Ord, 1981).

Some patterns of fracture are likely to be stable immediately after reduction, e.g. medially displaced fractures of the arch, fractures rotated about the vertical axis. Others are unstable and require additional fixation, e.g. inferiorly displaced arch fractures and fractures rotated about the horizontal axis. Stability after reduction depends to a great extent on the integrity of the periosteum covering the bone and that of its facial and muscular attachments.

Unlike other facial fractures, reduction of the zygomatic complex can only be performed by open techniques. The restitutional force can be applied in either a direct or indirect fashion. The classical method is that described by Gillies, Kilner and Stone (1927) using the temporal fossa approach. A skin incision is made just behind the hair line anterosuperior to the pinna. The incision is developed through the temporal fascia so that an elevator of the Bristow type can be passed deep to it on the surface of the temporalis muscle to lie behind the body of the zygomatic bone. Controlled elevation can then be applied to the bone which usually snaps back into place. Great care should be taken to avoid undue pressure on the parietal bone in this manoeuvre. The Rowe elevator avoids this by incorporating a hinged lifting arm of the same length as the elevator. Furthermore, the precise location of the tip of the elevator can be gauged by the position of the lifting handle relative to the orbit (Figure 16.37). This is also the preferred

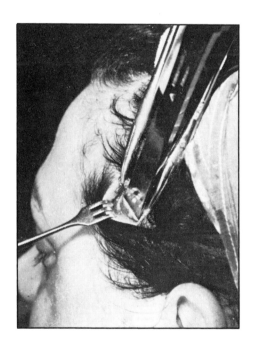

(a)

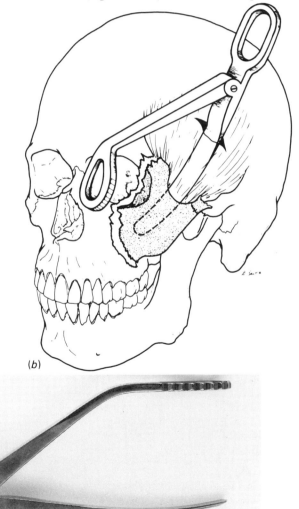

(b)

(c)

Figure 16.37 Gillies' method for the reduction of malar fractures. (*a*) The elevator passes deep to the temporal fascia. The incision must be high in the hair, never over the arch. (*b*) Mode of application of elevator. (*c*) Rowe's elevator

method for the reduction of a medially displaced fracture of the arch.

Elevation of the body of the zygoma has also been described through a direct, transcutaneous approach using a hook (Poswillo, 1976) and through the buccal sulcus using a periosteal elevator (Balasubramaniam, 1967; Quinn, 1977). Temporary fixation may be applied either by packing the maxillary antrum with bismuth-iodine-paraffin paste gauze through a Caldwell-Luc approach, by a silicone wedge supporting the lateral antral wall (Gorman, 1979) or a Foley catheter inserted through an intranasal antrostomy.

Fractures found to be unstable following reduction need to be wired or plated using a direct approach. Stabilization across both the frontozygomatic suture and the infraorbital margin is then obtained. The zygomatic arch can be reassembled in a similar fashion, but it is also wise to darn the periosteum of the arch to the temporalis fascia in order to prevent subsequent inferior relapse.

In a few cases the floor of the orbit together with some of the orbital contents collapses into the antrum. This produces severe limitation of the movement of the globe and permanent alteration of its position. This so-called 'orbital blow-out' fracture, may be an isolated injury or the result of a direct blow to the eye ball itself. More commonly, herniation of the orbital contents into the maxillary antrum is part of a Le Fort 2, 3 or zygomatic complex fracture.

The decision to intervene operatively can be very difficult, as minor degrees of blow-out are not always attended by subsequent diplopia and nearly all orbital injuries cause diplopia in the acute phase (Crumley *et al.*, 1977; Steidler, Cook and Reade, 1980). It is sensible to explore and provide support for the orbital floor during the acute phase in some circumstances, e.g. gross herniation of orbital contents. Certainly it adds little to the procedure of transosseous wiring of the orbital rim and similarly an antral pack can serve the dual role of providing temporary fixation for a tripod fracture while reducing the blow-out. In other cases, it is better to adopt a conservative approach by observing eye movements at regular intervals until it becomes clear that fixation or limitation of movement has developed (van Herk and Hovinga, 1973; Bartkowski and Krystkowa, 1982). In cases where doubt exists the antrum can be opened to inspect the defect. Fibreoptic inspection using a sinuscope is a simpler way to obtain the same information (Westphal and Kreidler, 1977).

There is a wide choice of methods for repairing the orbital floor or medial wall. Transconjunctival and subciliary approaches are described and both have their advocates (Tessier, 1973; Converse *et al.*, 1973; Wray *et al.*, 1977). The inexperienced may find that the transconjunctival route gives them inadequate access and that a lateral canthotomy is required. The

operative field is rarely a problem with the subciliary route, although postoperative ectropion, either transient or permanent, can follow. In most, gentle freeing of the incarcerated contents together with reduction of the malar fracture will suffice. More significant deficiencies need to be grafted with bone or supported by Silastic (Figure 16.38). Occasionally these may need to be supported by an antral pack.

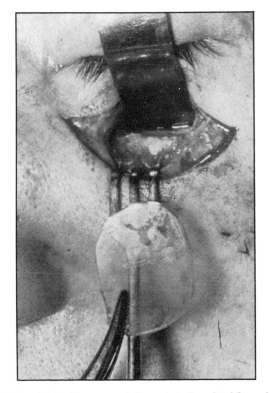

Figure 16.38 Placement of silicone into the orbital floor of a 'blow-out' fracture

It is essential that the retinal blood vessels, visual acuity or pupillary reflexes are carefully monitored in the immediate postoperative period as the central retinal artery may be compromised by retrobulbar haemorrhage. Immediate evacuation of haematoma must be undertaken if the sight is to be preserved. The clinical signs of this painful complication are increasing proptosis and intraocular pressure, and afferent pupillary defect, pallor of the optic disc and diminishing visual acuity.

Postoperative care

Careful nursing attention should be paid to oral hygiene. The nursing staff must swab the mouth three times a day with saline or diluted hydrogen peroxide followed by aqueous chlorhexidine (Corsodyl mouth-wash). A hygienist should visit regularly to attend to local inflammation of the gingivae. The intermaxil-lary fixation needs to be regularly checked, wires or bands replaced as necessary and their free ends care-fully buried between the teeth or protected with wax so that they do not traumatize the soft tissues. In due course damaged teeth, having served their purpose of fixation, require restoration or removal and missing teeth may need to be replaced.

Cerebrospinal fluid rhinorrhoea

Cerebrospinal fluid rhinorrhoea is classified into aetiological categories under two main subdivisions, traumatic and non-traumatic (Ommaya *et al.*, 1968) (Table 16.2). Most cases are produced by accidental or iatrogenic trauma. Non-traumatic cerebrospinal fluid rhinorrhoea is important to consider and recog-nize but rare.

Table 16.2 Classification of cerebrospinal fluid rhinorrhoea

1 Traumatic
      Accidental (acute or delayed)
      Iatrogenic (acute or delayed)
2 Non-traumatic
      High pressure
          tumours (direct or indirect)
          hydrocephalus (obstructive or communicating)
      Normal pressure
          congenital anomalies
          focal atrophy
          osteomyelitic erosion

From Ommaya *et al.*, 1968

It has been reported that between 2% and 9% of head injuries are complicated by cerebrospinal fluid rhinorrhoea and, in those with fractures involving the paranasal sinuses, this incidence increases to 25% (Lewin, 1954; Raaf, 1967; Charles and Snell, 1979). Most of these involve the anterior cranial fossa and allow cerebrospinal fluid to leak through the cribriform plate or roof of the ethmoids where the dura is attached firmly and easily torn. In others the cerebrospinal fluid passes through a breach in the posterior wall of the frontal sinus (Calcaterra, 1980).

Cerebrospinal fluid leaks from fracture or congeni-tal defects of the temporal bone may also present as rhinorrhoea if the tympanic membrane is intact. The cerebrospinal fluid then escapes via the eustachian tube into the nasopharynx. Non-traumatic cerebro-spinal fluid rhinorrhoea is usually secondary to intra-cranial tumour or hydrocephalus (Ommaya, 1964).

Pituitary tumours are the most common neoplasm to produce a leak but cases associated with nasopha-ryngeal carcinomas and acoustic neuromas have been reported. Despite local disease, e.g. pituitary adenomas, which might be expected to predispose to leakage from the sphenoid sinus, this entity is rare. Almost all fistulae arise in the anterior cranial fossa (Kaufman, 1969). Escape of cerebrospinal fluid from the middle cranial fossa directly to the nose may result from the persistence of the craniopharyngeal canals (Lowman, Robinson and McAllister, 1966; Hooper, 1971). Leakage from this area is more often a complication of trans-sphenoidal surgery, the im-plantation of yttrium seeds (Bateman, 1966) or sec-ondary to tumour erosion (Norsa, 1953).

Symptoms

Nasal discharge is the most prominent symptom. It may be provoked or increased by physical work or change in posture. Some patients are aware of a persistent salty taste in their mouths and others may be troubled by a continuous headache secondary to low pressure.

Diagnosis and localization

Cerebrospinal fluid is usually clear with a specific gravity of 1.004–1.008. Unlike other pure nasal secre-tions it contains glucose. The clinical diagnosis de-pends on the measurement of the glucose content which must be undertaken carefully to ensure that the result is consistent with concurrently drawn lumbar cerebrospinal fluid. Glucose oxidase papers (Clinistix) are not reliable for this purpose (Gadeholt, 1964). Examination of the nose and nasopharynx with a flexible nasopharyngoscope may help localize the side from which cerebrospinal fluid is leaking (von Haacke and Croft, 1983). It is usually necessary to introduce markers or dyes, e.g. indigo carmine, methylene blue, fluorescein (Kirchner and Proud, 1960) or radioactive tracers into the lumbar theca and then, subsequently, to measure their relative concentrations in patties placed at the sinus ostea in ostea in the lateral wall of the nose. Aseptic meningitis has been reported following these procedures.

Plain radiographs are seldom helpful in localizing the origin of cerebrospinal fluid rhinorrhoea, al-though polytomography will often demonstrate the defect either directly or indirectly through changes in the adjacent paranasal sinuses or their linings (Charles and Snell, 1979). High resolution CT scan-ning is very useful in traumatic cases and even more so for the investigation of non-traumatic cases where an underlying tumour or hydrocephalus must be found or excluded (von Haacke and Croft, 1983). It should be remembered that cerebrospinal fluid rhinor-rhoea in association with congenital malformations may be arising from multiple sites. The correction of these cases is frequently problematic.

Treatment

The majority of traumatic cerebrospinal fluid leaks heal without surgical intervention. Until the leak ceases the patient is at a significant risk of developing pneumococcal meningitis. All should be given adequate antibiotic prophylaxis, instructed to avoid nose blowing and kept quietly in hospital. For adults, orally administered penicillin 500 mg four times daily and sulphadimidine 500 mg four times daily provide adequate antibiotic cover. Leech and Paterson (1973) considered that repair should be undertaken if the cerebrospinal fluid rhinorrhoea persisted for longer than 7 days as the protection afforded by long-term antibiotic prophylaxis dimished after that period. Earlier repair offers no better protection against meningitis and carries with it the morbidity of a surgical procedure to close a defect that may heal spontaneously.

The first successful intradural repair, using autogenous fascia lata, was reported by Dandy in 1926. Until recently, variations of this technique were accepted as the standard approach to this problem. It is now recognized that craniotomy is attended by a significant morbidity, usually followed by anosmia and not universally successful, failure rates of up to 27% being reported (Ray and Bergland, 1967; Calcaterra, 1980).

The extracranial approach to repair a defect of the cribriform plate was reported by Dohlman in 1948. Leaks from the frontal sinus, cribriform plate and sphenoid sinus may be tackled by an external ethmoidectomy or endoscopic endonasal approach using fascia or a mucosal flap from the nasal septum as described by Hirsch in 1952.

The trans-septal route employed for hypophysectomy may also be used to control cerebrospinal fluid rhinorrhoea from this region (Calcaterra and Rand, 1976). This has the advantage of avoiding any facial incision and allows the sphenoid to be packed with fascia and a free muscle graft without any open communication with the nasal cavity. In all these cases lumbar cerebrospinal fluid drainage is advisable for a few days postoperatively in order to maintain a constant low pressure on the closure.

It is thought that high pressure leaks act as a safety valve limiting the potential damage of persistent raised intracranial pressure. The repair of these should, therefore, only be undertaken after the cause of the high pressure has been dealt with or a suitable shunt inserted.

Facial asymmetry

No face is perfectly symmetrical. A degree of facial asymmetry adds character and sometimes enhances an individual's appearance. The rapid development of asymmetrical features is a common presentation of neoplastic, cystic and inflammatory lesions of both the facial skeleton and soft tissues. It is alarming for patients and on occasion prompts them to consult a surgeon at a relatively early stage, even before the onset of pain, anaesthesia or functional deficits. Other asymmetries, frequently subtle at the outset, continue to develop for a more prolonged period of time, sometimes spanning several decades. These conditions are usually genetic disorders or malformations. It is therefore reasonable to outline these disorders on a chronological basis according to the age at which they first manifest, detailing only those not dealt with elsewhere in the text.

Facial asymmetry of childhood

Dental infections, paranasal sinus sepsis and viral parotitis are the most common causes of acute facial asymmetry in this age group. The diagnosis of these conditions is rarely problematic.

First and second branchial arch syndromes

A wide spectrum of deformities is seen in patients with these syndromes. They are thought to be caused by a haemorrhage arising in the anastomosis which precedes the formation of the stapedial arterial stem (Poswillo, 1973). A number of synonyms have therefore been applied to these conditions, e.g. necrotic facial dysplasia, otomandibular dysostosis, craniofacial microsomia, lateral facial dysplasia and hemifacial microsomia.

Although almost invariably unilateral in presentation some bilateral cases have been recorded. Even in these there is considerable difference in expression between the two sides. The most common abnormalities are hypoplasia of the external and middle ear, mandibular ramus and condyle, zygoma, muscles of mastication and facial expression, parotid gland and occasionally the facial nerve. These defects often appear mild at birth but progress to severe asymmetrical deformities with growth. Some are amenable to surgical correction (Murray, Kaban and Mulliken, 1984).

A number of recognized syndromes exists in which branchial arch dysplasia is but one component. Most of these syndromes are symmetrical.

Goldenhar's syndrome

This consists of hemifacial microsomia, clefts of the lips and palate, epibulbar dermoids, vertebral, cardiac and renal abnormalities. A few of these patients are mentally retarded. The degree of expression is variable and the mode of inheritance far from clear.

Hemifacial hypertrophy (Curtois' syndrome, Steiner's syndrome)

There is no recognized basis for this deformity which affects both the hard and soft tissues of the face and jaws. In some there may be total body hemihypertrophy, while in others the enlargement is limited to the face. The degree of distortion is very variable. In some it is mild while in others it is monstrous. Nearly all are evident at birth, become accentuated at puberty and stabilize when active growth stops.

Klippel-Trenaunay-Weber syndrome (angio-osteohypertrophy syndrome)

In this condition facial hemihypertrophy is seen in association with a segmentally distributed angiomatous naevus, most commonly in the second trigeminal dermatome.

Facial asymmetry secondary to osteomyelitis or trauma to the temporomandibular joint

This is a rare cause of progressive facial asymmetry which is secondary to ankylosis of the temporomandibular joint and retardation in growth of the mandible (Souyris, Moncarz and Rey, 1983). Infection may spread to the joint from localized osteomyelitis of the jaw, severe middle ear infection or follow a generalized septicaemia. In the past this was most often seen after scarlet fever, typhoid, pneumonia, influenza and measles.

Facial asymmetry of adolescence

Fibrous dysplasia

In this condition areas of bone are replaced by fibrous tissue and become enlarged. These lesions may be monostotic or polyostotic. The polyostotic variety tends to be unilateral in distribution. Enlargement of the facial bones is painless, usually noticed in adolescence and continues after somatic growth has ceased. These lesions may cause derangement of the dentition, protrusion of the eyes, obliteration of the sinuses and nasal passages. Foraminal encroachment can result in deafness and blindness. When the long bones are affected they become bowed and sometimes fracture repeatedly.

Polyostotic fibrous dysplasia when associated with cutaneous pigmentation and endocrine disorders is known as Albright's syndrome. The degree of pigmentation is proportional to the extent of bone involvement. Precocious puberty is the most frequently associated endocrine disorder but hyperthyroidism, diabetes mellitus and acromegaly have all been recorded. Skeletal growth in these children is rapid, but as the epiphyses tend to fuse early the resulting adult stature is short.

Progressive hemifacial atrophy (Parry-Rhomberg syndrome)

Unilateral progressive wasting of some or all of the facial tissues in this uncommon condition commences in the second decade. Atrophy of the subcutaneous fat and muscle proceeds together with underdevelopment of the facial bones. In some, intracerebral calcification has been seen and is thought to be associated with haemangiomas. Reflex asymmetry, impaired sensory function and optic atrophy may also be present.

Neurofibromatosis (von Recklinghausen's disease)

This disease is transmitted in an autosomal dominant fashion but rarely becomes clinically obvious before puberty. The tumours in this condition are usually multiple, smooth, and rounded, and may attain a considerable size, thereby producing craniofacial distortion. Any cutaneous, visceral or cranial nerve can be affected. Cutaneous pigmentation, café-au-lait spots, is present in these patients. Later sarcomatous change in the neurofibromas is well recognized.

Cysts of the jaws

Many types of cysts arise within the jaws. Some emanate from odontogenic tissue, e.g. primordial, dentigerous and periodontal cysts. Others develop from sequestrated fissural epithelium, e.g. globulomaxillary and median cysts. Although swelling limited to the jaws, displacement of adjacent teeth, infection or fracture is the most common mode of presentation, some may achieve considerable proportions so slowly and symptomatically that facial asymmetry is the first sign.

Facial asymmetry of adult life

In this age group, facial asymmetries are more usually the result of sinus mucocoeles, osteomyelitis, benign salivary tumours or tumours of the jaws. In this later category ameloblastoma, Ewing's tumour, osteosarcoma and fibrosarcoma should be considered as they afflict a younger age group than other oral neoplasms.

Facial asymmetry of old age

Malignant salivary tumours, sinus neoplasms and carcinomas of the oral cavity are the predominant causes of facial asymmetry. These conditions produce asymmetry of the face relatively rapidly and are described elsewhere.

Paget's disease (osteitis deformans)

The bony enlargement seen in this disease is not always symmetrical. The facial bones are frequently affected early in the clinical course which may extend for decades. Foraminal encroachment may produce deafness and blindness. Sarcomatous change in the affected bones is a well recognized late complication of this disorder.

References

ADAMS, W. M. (1942) Internal wire fixation of facial fractures. *Surgery*, **12**, 523–540

BALASUBRAMANIAM, S. (1967) Intra-oral approach for reduction of malar fractures. *British Journal of Surgery* **4**, 189–191

BARTOWSKI, S. B. and KRYSTKOWA, K. M. (1982) Blow-out fracture of the orbit. Diagnostic and therapeutic considerations, and results in 90 patients treated. *Journal of Maxillo-facial Surgery*, **10**, 155–164

BATEMAN, G. H. (1966) Experiences with CSF rhinorrhoea arising from the pituitary fossa. *Proceedings of the Royal Society of Medicine*, **59**, 169–174

BATTERSBY, T. G. (1967) Plating of mandibular fractures. *British Journal of Oral Surgery*, **4**, 194–201

BECKER, R. (1974) Stable compression plate fixation of mandibular fractures. *British Journal of Oral Surgery*, **12**, 13–23

BROOK, I. M. and WOOD, N. (1983) Aetiology and incidence of facial fractures in adults. *International Journal of Oral Surgery*, **12**, 293–298

CALCATERRA, T. C. (1980) Extracranial surgical repair of cerebrospinal rhinorrhoea. *Annals of Otology, Rhinology and Laryngology*, **89**, 108–116

CALCATERRA, T. C. and RAND, R. W. (1976) Current adjuncts in surgery of the sphenoid sinus. *Laryngoscope*, **86**, 1692–1698

CHAMPY, M., LODDE, J. P., JAEGER, J. H. and MUSTER, D. (1978) Mandibular osteosynthesis by miniaturised screwed plates via a buccal approach. *Journal of Maxillo-facial Surgery*, **6**, 14–21

CHARLES, D. A. and SNELL, D. (1979) Cerebrospinal fluid rhinorrhoea. *Laryngoscope*, **89**, 822–826

CONVERSE, J. M., FIRMIN, F., WOOD-SMITH, D. and FRIEDLAND, J. A. (1973) The conjunctival approach in orbital fractures. *Plastic and Reconstructive Surgery*, **52**, 656–657

COOK, J. A., MCRAE, R. D., IRVING, R. M. and DOWIE, L. N. (1990) A randomized comparison of manipulation of the fractured nose under local and general anaesthesia. *Clinical Otolaryngology*, **15**, 343–346

CRUMLEY, R. L., LEIBSOHN, J., KRAUSE, C. J. and BURTON, T. C. (1977) Fractures of the orbital floor. *Laryngoscope*, **87**, 934–947

COURTISS, E. H. (1978) Septorhinoplasty of the traumatically deformed nose. *Annals of Plastic Surgery*, **1**, 443–449

DANDY, W. D. (1926) Pneumocephalus (intracranial pneumocele or aerocele). *Archives of Surgery*, **12**, 949–982

DEPARTMENT OF HEALTH, WELSH OFFICE, SCOTTISH OFFICE HOME AND HEALTH DEPARTMENT, DHSS NORTHERN IRELAND (1992) *Immunisation against Infectious Diseases.* London: HMSO

DICKSON, M. G. and SHARPE, D. T. (1986) A prospective study of nasal fractures. *Journal of Laryngology and Otology*, **100**, 543–551

DOHLMAN, G. (1948) Spontaneous cerebrospinal rhinorrhoea. *Acta Otolaryngologica Supplementum*, **67**, 20–23

ELLIS, E. (1993) Sequencing treatment for naso-orbito-ethmoid fractures. *Journal of Oral and Maxillofacial Surgery*, **51**, 543–558

FORTUNATO, M. A., FIELDING, A. F. and GUERNSEY, L. H. (1982) Facial bone fractures in children. *Oral Surgery*, **53**, 225–230

FROST, D. E., EL-ATTAR, A. and MOOS, K. F. (1983) Evaluation of metacarpal bone plates in the mandibular fracture. *British Journal of Oral Surgery*, **21**, 214–221

GADEHOLT, H. (1964) The reaction of glucose-oxidase test paper in normal nasal secretion. *Acta Otolaryngologica*, **58**, 271–272

GARFIELD, J. (1972) Deterorating head injuries. *British Journal of Hospital Medicine*, **8**, 262–266

GENTLEMAN, D., DEARDEN, M., MIDGLEY, S. and MACLEAN, D. (1993) Guidelines for resuscitation and transfer of patients with serious head injury. *British Medical Journal*, **307**, 547–552

GEORGIADE, N., GEORGIADE, G., SERAFIN, D. and RIEFKOHL, R. (1981) Twenty-five year evaluation of external halo fixation for severe maxillofacial injuries. *Plastic and Reconstructive Surgery*, **68**, 444–447

GILLIES, H.D., KILNER, T. P. and STONE, D. (1927) Fractures of the malar zygomatic compound. *British Journal of Surgery*, **14**, 651–656

GORMAN, J. M. (1979) Malar fractures: silicone wedge stabilisation. *British Journal of Oral Surgery*, **17**, 244–247

HAGAN, E. H. and HUELKE, D. F. (1961) An analysis of 319 case reports of mandibular fractures. *Journal of Oral Surgery*, **19**, 93–104

HALL, R. K. (1972) Injuries of the face and jaws in children. *International Journal of Oral Surgery*, **1**, 65–75

HARRISON, D. H. (1979) Nasal injuries; their pathogenesis and treatment. *British Journal of Plastic Surgery*, **32**, 57–64

HIRSCH, O. (1952) Successful closure of cerebrospinal fluid rhinorrhoea by endonasal surgery. *Archives of Otolaryngology*, **56**, 1–13

HODGSON, V. R. (1967) Tolerance of the facial bones to impact. *American Journal of Anatomy*, **120**, 113–122

HOFFMAN, E. (1976) Mortality and morbidity following road accidents. *Annals of the Royal College of Surgeons of England*, **58**, 233–240

HOOPER, A. C. (1971) Sphenoidal defects – a possible source of cerebrospinal fluid rhinorrhoea. *Journal of Neurology, Neurosurgery and Psychiatry*, **34**, 739–742

HUELKE, D. F. and HARGER, J. H. (1969) Maxillofacial injuries: their nature and mechanisms of production. *Journal of Oral Surgery*, **27**, 451–460

ILLUM, P. (1986) Long term results after treatment of nasal fractures. *Journal of Laryngology and Otology*, **100**, 273–277

ILLUM, P. (1991) Legal aspects in nasal fractures. *Rhinology*, **29**, 263–266

KAUFMAN, H. H. (1969) Non-traumatic cerebrospinal rhinorrhoea. *Archives of Neurology*, **21**, 59–65

KIRCHNER, F. R. and PROUD, G. O. (1960) Method for identification and localization of CSF rhinorrhoea and otorrhoea. *Laryngoscope*, **70**, 921–930

KUFNER, J. (1970) A method of craniofacial suspension. *Journal of Oral Surgery*, **28**, 260–262

LE FORT, R. (1901) Etude experimentale sur les fractures de la machoire superieure. *Revue Chirurgical*, 23, 8

LEECH, P. J. and PATERSON, A. (1973) Conservative and operative management for cerebrospinal fluid leakage after closed head injury. *Lancet*, i, 1013–1016

LEVANT, B. A., COOK, R. M. and MACFARLANE, W. I. (1973) Experience with the Levant frame for cranio-maxillary fixation. *British Journal of Oral Surgery*, 11, 30–35

LEVANT, B. A., GARDNER-BERRY, B. and SNOW, R. S. (1969) An improved cranio-maxillary fixation. *British Journal of Plastic Surgery*, 22, 288–290

LEWIN, W. (1954) Cerebrospinal fluid rhinorrhoea in closed head injuries. *British Journal of Surgery*, 42, 1–18

LINDAHL, L. (1977) Condylar fractures of the mandible. *International Journal of Surgery*, 6, 12–21

LOWMAN, R., ROBINSON, F. and MCALLISTER, W. B. (1966) The craniopharyngeal canal. *Acta Radiologica Diagnosis*, 5, 41–54

MACKAY, I. S. (1986) The deviated nose. *Facial Plastic Surgery*, 3, 253–266

MACKENZIE, D. L. and RAY, K. R. (1970) The Royal Berkshire Hospital 'halo'. *British Journal of Oral Surgery*, 8, 27–31

MAYELL, M. J. (1973) Nasal fractures. *Journal of the Royal College of Surgeons of Edinburgh*, 18, 31–36

MEHROTRA, O. N., BROWN, G. E., WIDDOWSON, W. P. and WILSON, J. P. (1984) Arteriography and selective embolisation in the control of life-threatening haemorrhage following facial fractures. *British Journal of Plastic Surgery*, 37, 482–485

MURRAY, J. A. M. (1989) Management of septal deviation with nasal fractures. *Facial Plastic Surgery*, 6, 88–94

MURRAY, J. A. M. and MARAN, A. G. D. (1984) Open v closed reduction of the fractured nose. *Archives of Otolaryngology*, 110, 797–802

MURRAY, J. E., KABAN, L. B. and MULLIKEN, J. B. (1984) Analysis and treatment of hemifacial microsomia. *Plastic and Reconstructive Surgery*, 74, 186–199

NAHUM, A. M. (1975) The biomechanics of maxillofacial trauma. *Clinical Plastic Surgery*, 2, 59–64

NAKAMURA, T. and GROSS, C. W. (1973) Facial fractures. Analysis of five years of experience. *Archives of Otolaryngology*, 97, 288–290

NORSA, L. (1953) Cerebrospinal rhinorrhoea with pituitary tumours. *Neurology*, 3, 864–868

OMMAYA, A. K. (1964) Cerebrospinal fluid rhinorrhoea, *Neurology*, 3, 864–868

OMMAYA, A. K., DI CHIRO, G. L., BALDWIN, M. and PENNY-BACKER, J. B. (1968) Non-traumatic cerebrospinal fluid rhinorrhoea. *Journal of Neurology, Neurosurgery and Psychiatry*, 31, 214–225

ORD, R. A. (1981) Post-operative retrobulbar haemorrhage and blindness complicating trauma surgery. *British Journal of Oral Surgery*, 19, 202–207

OWEN, G. O., PARKER, A. J. and WATSON, D. J. (1992) Fractured-nose reduction under local anaesthesia. Is it acceptable to the patient? *Rhinology*, 30, 89–96

PERSIG, W. and LEHMANN, I. (1975) The influence of trauma on the growing septal cartilage. *Rhinology*, 13, 39–46

POSWILLO, D. (1973) The pathogenesis of the first and second branchial arch syndrome. *Oral Surgery*, 35, 302–328

POSWILLO, D. (1976) Reduction of the fractured malar by a traction hook. *British Journal of Oral Surgery*, 14, 76–79

PRICE, J. D. (1983) Facial fractures and seat belts. *British Dental Journal*, 155, 112

QUINN, J. H. (1977) Lateral coronoid approach to intraoral

reduction of fractures of the zygomatic arch. *Journal of Oral Surgery*, 35, 321–322

RAAF, J. (1967) Post-traumatic cerebrospinal fluid leaks. *Archives of Surgery*, 35, 321–322

RAVEH, J., LAEDRACH, K., VUILLEMIN, T. and ZINGG, M. (1992) Management of combined frontonaso-orbital/skull base fractures and telecanthus in 355 cases. *Archives of Otolaryngology – Head and Neck Surgery*, 118, 605–614

RAY, B. S. and BERGLAND, R. M. (1967) Cerebrospinal fluid fistula: clinical aspects, techniques of localisation and methods of close. *Journal of Neurosurgery*, 30, 399–405

ROWE, N. L. (1969) Fractures of the jaws in children. *Journal of Oral Surgery*, 27, 497–507

ROWE, N. L. (1985) Fractures of the zygomatic complex and orbit. In: *Maxillofacial Injuries*, edited by N. L. Rowe and J. Ll. Williams. Edinburgh: Churchill Livingstone. pp. 435–537

SCHULTZ, R. C. and DE VILLERS, Y. T. (1974) Nasal fractures. *Journal of Trauma*, 15, 319–327

SOUYRIS, F., MONCARZ, V. and REY, P. (1983) Facial asymmetry of developmental etiology. *Oral Surgery*, 56, 113–124

STARKHAMMAR, H. and OLOFSSON, J. (1982) Facial fractures: a review of 922 cases with special reference to the incidence and aetiology. *Clinical Otolaryngology*, 7, 405–409

STEELE, R. J. and LITTLE, K. (1983) Effect of seat belt legislation. *Lancet*, ii, 341

STEIDLER, N. E., COOK, R. M. and READE, P. C. (1980) Residual complications in patients with major middle third fractures. *International Journal of Oral Surgery*, 9, 259–266

STOLL, P., SCHILLI, W. and JOOS, U. (1983) The stabilization of midface-fractures in the vertical dimension. *Journal of Maxillo-facial Surgery*, 11, 248–251

STRANC, M. F. and ROBERTSON, G. A. (1979) A classification of injuries of the nasal skeleton. *Annals of Plastic Surgery*, 2, 468–474

STUCKER, F. J., BRYARLY, R. C. and SHOCKLEY, W. W. (1984) Management of nasal trauma in children. *Archives of Otolaryngology*, 110, 190–192

TEASDALE, G. and JENNET, B. (1974) Assessment of coma and impaired consciousness. A practical scale. *Lancet*, ii, 81

TESSIER, P. (1973) The conjunctival approach to the orbital floor and maxilla in congenital malformation and trauma. *Journal of Maxillo-facial Surgery*, 1, 3–8

VAN HERK, W. and HOVINGA, J. (1973) Choice of treatment of orbital floor fractures as part of facial fractures. *Journal of Oral Surgery*, 31, 600–603

VAN HOOF, R. F., MERKX, C. A. and STEKELENBURG, E. C. (1977) The different pattern of fractures of the facial skeleton in four European countries. *International Journal of Oral Surgery*, 6, 3–11

VERO, D. (1968) Jaw injuries. Use of Kirschner wires to supplement fixation. *British Journal of Oral Surgery*, 6, 18–30

VERWOERD, C. D. A. (1992) Present day treatment of nasal fractures: closed versus open reduction. *Facial Plastic Surgery*, 8, 220–223

VON HAACKE, N. P. and CROFT, C. B. (1983) Cerebrospinal fluid rhinorrhoea and otorrhoea: extracranial repair. *Clinical Otolaryngology*, 8, 317–327

WEERDA, H. and SIEGERT, R. (1990) Stable fixation of the nasal complex. *Facial Plastic Surgery*, 7, 185–188

WESTPHAL, D. and KREIDLER, J. (1977) Sinuscopy for the diagnosis of blow-out fractures. *Journal of Maxillo-facial Surgery*, 5, 180–183

WILLIAMS, L. LL. (1985) Mandibular fractures: treatment by open reduction and direct skeletal fixation. In: *Maxillofacial Injuries*, edited by N. L. Rowe and L. Ll. Williams. London: Churchill Livingstone. pp. 332–335

WRAY, R. C., HOLTMANN, B. L., RIBAUDO, J. M., KEITER, J. and WEEKS, P. M. (1977) A comparison of conjunctival and subciliary incisions for orbital fractures. *British Journal of Plastic Surgery*, **30**, 142–145

17

Rhinoplasty

T. R. Bull and I. S. Mackay

A knowledge of nasal plastic surgery is necessary for otolaryngologists as variations in the external nasal shape are frequently linked with septal deformities. Correction of the airway associated with rhinoplasty forms a considerable part of nasal surgery.

In recent decades, a standard technique for rhinoplasty has evolved. The surgical steps present little technical difficulty, but their correct application is far from easy and rhinoplasty is a branch of surgery where errors related to lack of judgement are very obvious. Septoplasty aims to reposition the septum to the midline with minimal exclsion of the cartilaginous and bony components.

In almost all cases, correction of the septum can be combined with rhinoplasty in one operation. When the septal or external nasal deformity is gross, however, the patient should be warned that two steps may be necessary. A surgical anachronism is a standard submucosal resection to be followed at a later date by a rhinoplasty. A standard surgical step in rhinoplasty involves some degree of separation of the upper lateral cartilages from the septum. With inadequate support in the midline following removal of the septal cartilage, the division of the upper laterals from the remaining septum is likely to result in collapse of the nasal dorsum with saddling of the nose (Figure 17.1). A rhinoplasty after a standard submucosal resection is, therefore, compromised and a satisfactory result may not be achieved.

Analysis and selection of patients

A sense of aesthetics and common sense are necessary qualities to combine with sound surgical technique if satisfactory rhinoplasty results are to be achieved with minimal postoperative problems. The main cause of patient dissatisfaction following rhino-

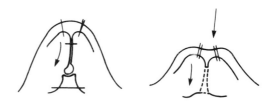

Figure 17.1 Excision of septal cartilage and bone of the maxillary crest, if combined with partial or total separation of the upper lateral cartilage from the septum, predisposes to collapse of the nasal dorsum

plasty is a failure of the surgeon to understand the patient's wishes. It is important for the patient to have a clear and realistic idea of the limitations of surgery. Good preoperative photographs arc essential and the changes possible with surgery can be demonstrated to the patient on the photographs. Photographs also give the surgeon an excellent concept of the changes which can be achieved and the correct surgical steps which must be applied (Figure 17.2). In postoperative analysis, photographs once again are extremely helpful.

The surgical approach to rhinoplasty should be influenced by the sex of the patient. In the female, one is operating for 'beauty'; in the male, the common complaint about the nose is that it gives rise to ridicule and comment and the operation is to eliminate these unsettling factors. Also, in the male, rhinoplasty may be carried out if a change in a particular racial appearance is required. Occasions, however, in which 'beauty' is involved for males are obviously less common.

In a male, particularly, a complaint about nasal deformity may be the presenting symptom of a profound psychiatric disturbance. It is important to

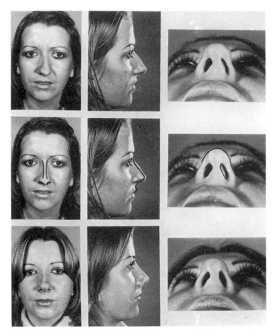

Figure 17.2 Good photographs are essential for pre- and postoperative rhinoplasty assessment. The preoperative photographs enable the surgeon to give a realistic idea to the patient of the changes possible, and lines drawn on these photographs are helpful

detect these disturbed personalities in the preoperative assessment. Eight surgeons have been killed by disenchanted and mentally disturbed patients after rhinoplasty. The well-adjusted patient is invariably specific in the dislike about the shape of the nose. A complaint that the nose is too large, deviated or has a hump, which links with the examination findings, is usually a clearcut case for rhinoplasty without psychological problems. The disturbed patient, however, is non-specific and evasive in the complaints about the nasal shape. A preoperative psychiatric assessment is necessary for those in whom the surgeon is doubtful about the patient's exact wishes and motives.

Care must be taken not to 'over-operate': the changes with rhinoplasty should be definite but subtle in most cases, and over-dramatic change may well predispose to a surgical or 'operated' appearance.

The age of the patient also has specific relevance for rhinoplasty. It is usually not advisable to operate under the age of 15 or 16 years, for the septum and the nasal bones may continue to grow or the shape continue to change. In older patients, a less radical alteration should be the aim. A gross nasal reduction in the more elderly not only tends to appear unnatural, but the elasticity of the skin is less and may not 'take up', leaving folds over the dorsum of the nose.

The height of the patient is another factor to be considered before rhinoplasty, in that a small nose may well be suitable for a small patient but frequently, and particularly in the male, a small nose on a tall patient – especially if the nasal tip is overrotated – looks unnatural.

The moderate nasal deformity is probably the easiest to correct. In correcting a minimal deformity, extreme accuracy is necessary to achieve the desired result. Gross nasal deformity, which appears to present as an easy surgical challenge, may also be difficult. A natural-looking nose following a gross nasal reduction is not easy to achieve.

Finally, it is important to assess the nasal skin texture before rhinoplasty. With thick skin, changes or reductions made in the underlying cartilage and bone are not so obvious when the thick 'blanket' of skin is redraped. In thin skin, however, minimal change is apparent and any irregularity or asymmetry in reduction may present an obvious deformity. Telangiectasia of the skin may also be more obvious after a rhinoplasty and tethering of the skin to the bone or cartilage is more common with thin, ageing or atrophic skin.

Surgical anatomy of the nose

Approximately one-third of the supporting structure of the nose is made up of bone, the remaining two-thirds being cartilaginous. This may, however, vary considerably.

The bony skeleton

The two nasal bones project from the nasal process of the frontal bone superiorly and from the frontal process of the maxilla laterally. These bones are supported in the midline by bony nasal septum – the perpendicular plate of the ethmoid which is continuous with the vomer inferiorly and the cartilaginous septum anteriorly (Figure 17.3) The nasion is the depression of the profile at the root of the nose where the nasal bones meet the bossed glabella of the frontal bones (Figure 17.4).

The floor of the nose is formed posteriorly by the palatine bone and anteriorly by the maxilla. These paired structures both fuse in the midline to form a crest which supports the bony and cartilaginous septum. Anteriorly, the crest of the maxilla protrudes forwards as the nasal spine. If this projects too far, it can make the nasolabial angle more obtuse and give the appearance of a tethered and short upper lip.

Cartilages of the nose

The mid-third of the nose is formed by the cartilaginous septum and the paired upper lateral nasal cartilages (Figure 17.5). The upper laterals are triangular

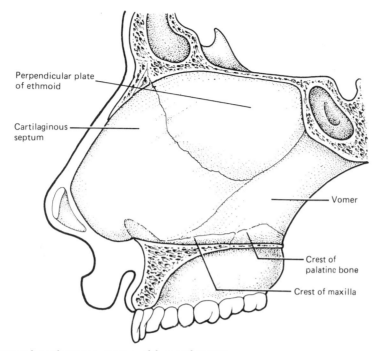

Figure 17.3 The bony and cartilaginous anatomy of the nasal septum

in shape and are overlapped superiorly by the nasal bones and frontal process of the maxilla and overlapped inferiorly by the lower lateral nasal cartilages; the groove thus formed is known as the limen nasi and is the landmark for the 'intercartilaginous incision'. It is important to note that the upper laterals lie below the nasal bones superiorly, and it is easy to disarticulate these structures when attempting to elevate the skin and periosteum overlying the nasal bones, leading to an unsightly deformity.

The lower lateral nasal cartilages are also known as the alar cartilages and form the lower third of the

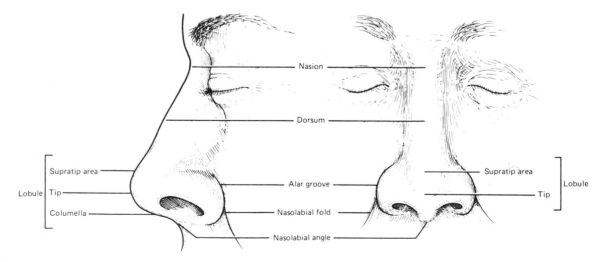

Figure 17.4 Surface anatomy of the nose

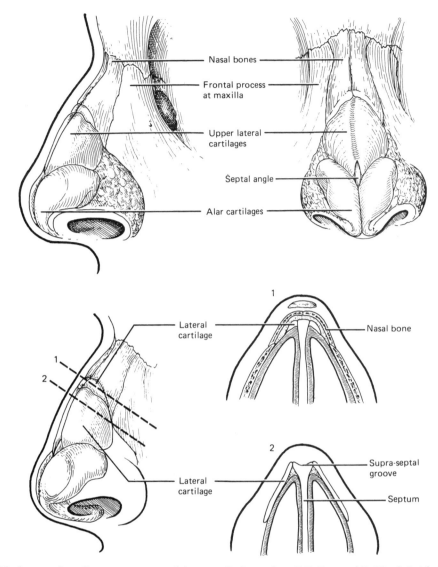

Figure 17.5 The bony and cartilaginous anatomy of the nose. (Redrawn from T. D. Rees and D. Wood–Smith, 1973, *Cosmetic Facial Surgery*, Philadelphia: W. B. Saunders)

nose. These two cartilages are made up of a medial crus, which forms the columella, and a lateral crus, which provides the framework for the tip of the nose, preventing alar collapse on inspiration.

The lower margin of the lateral crus does not follow up the margin of the nostril but ascends away from it as it travels laterally, that is the margin of the lower lateral cartilages may be 1 cm from the margin of the nostril laterally, but only 1 mm distance medially. The fact that these two margins do not run parallel is of utmost importance surgically, whether attempting to follow the rim of the cartilage for a 'rim incision' or perhaps, even more significantly,

when leaving 3–4 mm of cartilage undisturbed in a 'cartilage-splitting incision'.

The highest point of the lower lateral cartilage is referred to as the dome. This is usually at the junction of the medial and lateral crus but may, on occasions, be at a variable distance along the lateral crus. A 'facet' is found in most patients lying between the columella and lateral rim of the nostril. This facet is also referred to as the 'soft triangle'; it is not backed by cartilage and surgical interference at this point should be avoided as postoperative notching may occur which is impossible to correct.

Lying between the upper and lower lateral cartilages are several variable cartilages referred to collectively as the sesamoid cartilages.

The columella is formed by the caudal end of the septum, the nasal spine and the medial crura of the lower lateral cartilages. The nasolabial angle is that angle formed between the lip and the columella and is normally about 90° in males and a little greater in females.

Muscles of the nose

The procerus can be considered as a continuation of the frontalis muscle (Figure 17.6). Contraction of this muscle shortens the nose, pulling it upwards. Many surgeons in the past have removed a small portion of the procerus in an attempt to deepen the frontonasal angle. Since this is usually replaced by scar tissue, it is seldom helpful. Laterally, the alar fibres of the nasalis and levator labii superioris shorten the nose and dilate the nostrils while the transverse fibres of the nasalis muscle compress and contract the nostril. Inferiorly, the paired depressor septi nasi muscles pass from the bone of the maxilla above the incisor teeth to the septum and alar cartilages and depress the tip of the nose. In some patients, excessive activity of this muscle can cause the tip of the nose to move excessively while talking and division of this muscle may prevent this. Other facial muscles have an indirect effect on movement of the nose. All these muscles are innervated by the VIIth cranial nerve.

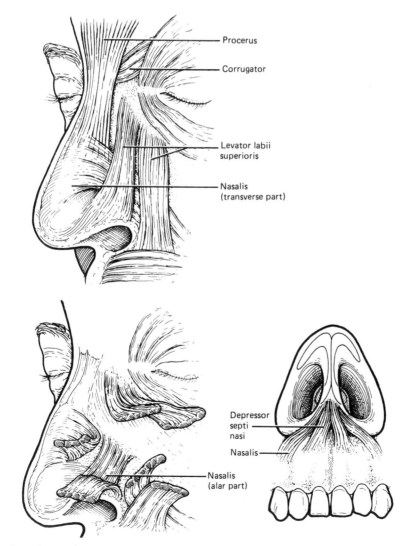

Figure 17.6 Muscles acting on the nose

Anaesthesia

In the majority of cases, the authors prefer to undertake surgery under general anaesthesia with the airway protected by a cuffed endotracheal tube and bleeding controlled by both topical application and infiltration with a vasoconstrictor. If this is undertaken in a careful and thorough manner as described below, bleeding is minimal. Controlled hypotensive anaesthesia results in excellent operating conditions, but involves risks over and above a standard anaesthetic.

If a general anaesthetic is to be given, the patient will need to be admitted a reasonable period prior to surgery. A full history must be taken and thorough general examination undertaken, together with any relevant preoperative investigations to ensure that there are no contraindications to general anaesthesia.

The patient must have nothing to eat or drink for a minimum of 4 hours preoperatively and is premedicated in the usual way. As the nose is to be infiltrated with vasoconstrictors, the anaesthetists may wish to avoid halothane and use a β-blocking agent, provided this is not contraindicated, e.g. by asthma. The patient is intubated with a cuffed endotracheal tube which is inflated and the pharynx then packed with moist ribbon gauze. It is important to ensure that the tube is firmly fixed in the midline with strapping to avoid any asymmetry of the face. The patient should be monitored with an electrocardiographic (ECG) recorder throughout.

The patient should be placed on the operating table in the supine position with the head on a head-ring and the table rotated to about 15–30° in the head-up position. The operating lights are then arranged with one directly above and a satellite directed at the nose from the foot of the table (Figure 17.7). A headlight or fibreoptically illuminated instruments will also be required, particularly if any septal work is required.

In addition to topical application of vasoconstrictors to the nasal mucous membrances, the nose may be injected with 1% lignocaine containing 1:80 000 adrenalin. Care must be exercised while undertaking this, with a small bleb injected at a time, using a maximum of 6 ml. The following sites should be injected:

1 Between the upper and lower lateral cartilages
2 Along the nasal dorsum
3 Laterally, towards the infraorbital nerve
4 Along the site of the lateral osteotomy
5 The columella
6 The lower margin of the lower lateral cartilages.

It is important to wait about 10 minutes for the vasoconstrictors to have maximum effect.

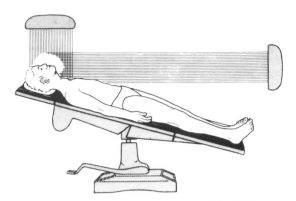

Figure 17.7 Patient in head-up position with headlight arranged directly above and a satellite directed at the nose from foot of the table

The osteocartilaginous vault

A prominent dorsal nasal hump is the commonest cause of patient dissatisfaction with the appearance of their nose. In theory, the steps taken to 'dehump' and 'infracture' the nose are not difficult; nonetheless, it is all too easy for the final result to be 'unfavourable'.

A secondary hump or 'pollybeak' will result from inadequate removal, of cartilage in the supratip region (Figure 17.8), while excessive removal of bony hump, particularly in males, can produce a most unsatisfactory appearance and incomplete lateral osteotomies may prevent proper infracture of the nasal bones, leading to an 'open-roof' deformity.

How much hump to remove? This is a question which cannot easily be answered as it will depend on the thickness of the skin, the amount of cartilaginous hump relative to bony hump, the width of the hump and angulation of the tip of the nose, as well as the inclination of the nasofrontal angle. The aim, however, should be to reduce the nose in harmony with the remaining facial features, remembering that it is always better to remove too little than too much.

There is much debate as to whether it is better to reduce the hump before the tip or remodel the tip before the hump. Those in favour of undertaking tip-plasty first will argue that one cannot judge how far to reduce the hump until the tip has been corrected; on the other hand, it can be argued that the degree of tip modification will depend on the new profile following correction of the osteocartilaginous vault. Another point in favour of the profile alignment first, is that this requires the introduction of relatively large and cumbersome saws and osteotomes which may more easily damage the lower lateral cartilage or tear the delicate flaps in the vestibular skin following tip-plasty. Those in favour of leaving the bony work until last will also argue that this causes most bleeding and should not be done until all the finer work is complete. The authors have no special preference,

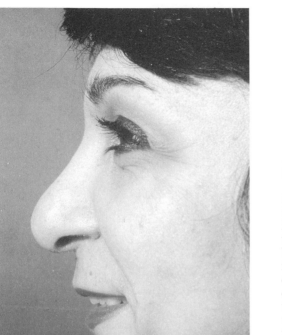

Figure 17.8 Pollybeak deformity due to inadequate removal of cartilage in the supratip region

although they tend to undertake profile correction first, followed by tip-plasty except possibly in those cases with a short columella, where *projection* of the tip can be seen to be the main aim following which little, if any, hump reduction is required (Figure 17.9).

The first step after suitably arranging the patient in the head-up position, cleaning the nose and infiltrating with vasoconstrictors, will be to trim the vibrissae of the nasal vestibule as these not only get in the way of surgery but also tend to cake with blood clot afterwards, causing discomfort.

An incision is made along the sulcus formed by the lower lateral cartilage overlapping the upper lateral cartilage – the limen nasi. This intercartilaginous incision is continued medially to become continuous with the transfixion incision which separates the columella from the caudal border of the septum. Some surgeons will include a small sliver of cartilage in the columella (high transfixion incision) to prevent contracture of the scar pulling the tip of the nose downwards, contributing to a 'pollybeak'.

A 'hemitransfixion incision' is a contradiction in terms and may relate to two quite separate procedures: either a short incision which completely trans-

kes the columella but extends only a short distance own towards the nasal spine, or an incision which oes not completely transfix the columella since the ncision may be made on the right but not extend nrough to the left, while still being complete because exposes the whole of the caudal end of the septum. he former incision is thought by some to reduce the kelihood of a pollybeak deformity due to scar contracure pulling down on the tip of the nose. The latter is articularly useful where extensive septal work is to e undertaken, and the surgeon will find it easier to levate the mucosa if one side remains intact to act as a retractor.

The skin overlying the upper lateral cartilages is then elevated up to and a little beyond the osteocartilaginous junction of the nasal bones and upper lateral nasal cartilages. One then attempts to elevate the skin and periosteum overlying the nasal bones, being careful not to disarticulate the upper laterals from the undersurface of the pyriform aperture. The elevation is continued up towards the glabella. Lateral elevations should not be continued too far, particularly if multiple osteotomies are to be undertaken when the comminuted fractured bones will rely on the overlying skin and underlying mucosa to splint them in position. If multiple osteotomies are not required, the elevation may be continued a little more laterally; wider elevation may be helpful in 'redraping' the skin if a radical reduction is to be undertaken.

The upper lateral nasal cartilages are then divided from the nasal septum, keeping as close as possible to the nasal septum to prevent the formation of a 'T-shaped' structure which may be difficult to lower at a later stage. Occasionally, patients may have a 'V-shaped' deformity where the upper lateral nasal cartilages and nasal septum join, which can be confusing unless the problem is recognized.

The upper lateral nasal cartilages and septum are then lowered, each by the same amount, up to the nasal bones using Foman scissors and the hump reduction completed with an osteotome or chisel. The bony and cartilaginous hump can then be removed with a large artery forceps, but should always be pushed further into the nose prior to withdrawal to detach any adhesions remaining between mucous membrane, periosteum and bone.

An alternative method is to lower the osteocartilaginous hump using a Bull's nasal saw which has a single fine blade, allowing the operator to remove even a small hump and a rounded blunt end to prevent damage to the overlying skin.

The nasal bones can be reduced further with a rasp, although cartilage must be removed with a scalpel or scissors. Once a satisfactory profile has been achieved, the lateral walls of the nose will need to be infractured to close the flat 'open' bridge. In order to achieve this, lateral and medial osteotomies will be required. If these are curved in towards each

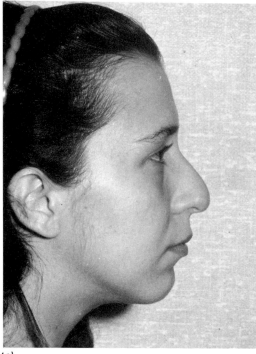

(a)

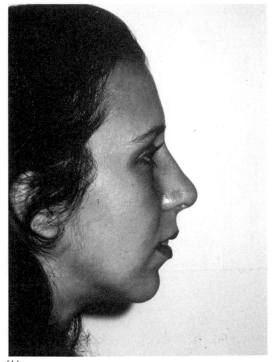

(b)

Figure 17.9 (*a*) Pre- and (*b*) postoperative photographs of patient with a short columella where projection of the tip is the main aim following which little, if any, hump reduction will be required

other, these may suffice; if not, a superior osteotomy may be additionally required.

The techniques for undertaking the lateral osteotomy differ greatly. Few surgeons now use the saw as this requires elevation of a tunnel of skin and periosteum laterally along the line of the proposed osteotomy, which leads to marked swelling postoperatively, is laborious, and may cause bone dust which can become infected. A small 2–3 mm osteotome may be introduced intranasally at the lateral aspect of the pyriform aperture, via a sublabial incision or through a tiny stab incision directly through the skin. Whichever method is used, it is important that this osteotomy should be as low as possible to prevent a 'step' deformity which can often be felt and may be seen postoperatively. Once the osteotomies have been performed, the nasal bones can be infractured.

The height of the septum and lower lateral cartilages should then be rechecked. Ideally, the upper laterals and septum should be lowered equally. It is preferable to remove a little too much cartilage from the supratip region rather than too little as a secondary hump or 'pollybeak' deformity is the commonest cause of secondary revision although, in some cases, this may well result from hypertrophic scar tissue rather than inadequate removal of cartilage.

Reducing the caudal end of the septum will not, in itself, shorten the nose – to achieve this will require surgery to the lower lateral cartilages or tip-plasty in addition to often minimal reduction of the septum. Excessive removal of caudal septal cartilage simply results in columellar retraction or an excessively obtuse nasolabial angle (Figure 17.10).

Nasal tip rhinoplasty

In the early days of rhinoplasty, the finer surgery of the nasal tip was relatively ignored and more attention was given to the steps of hump removal and nasal bone infracture with lowering of the septum and upper lateral cartilages. In the last two decades, more thought and more elaborate techniques for the alar cartilages have been developed. Finer, more subtle and predictable changes in nasal tip anatomy can be achieved. Nonetheless, the more elaborate tip techniques have the disadvantages of producing more problems with tip asymmetries and deformities if wrongly applied or incorrectly carried out. Nasal tip deformities, furthermore, are probably more conspicuous than any other site on the nose or face (Figure 17.11).

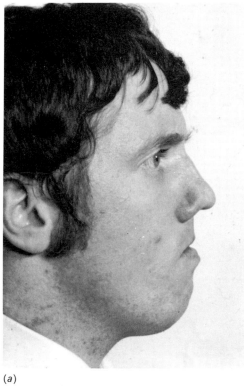

(a)

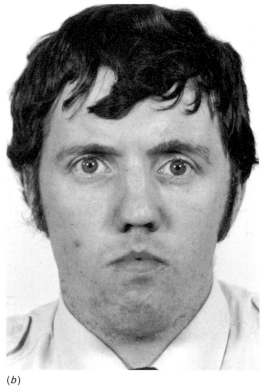

(b)

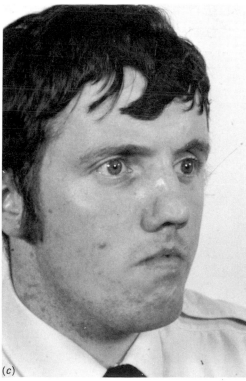

(c)

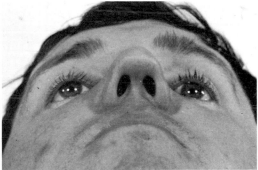

(d)

Figure 17.10 Excessive removal of the caudal end of the septum does not shorten the nose but results in columella retraction

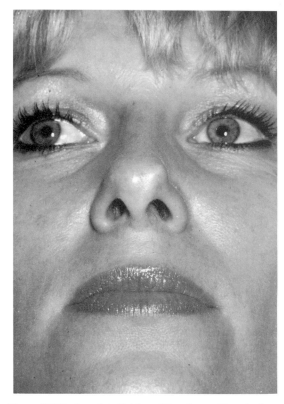

Figure 17.11 Complete division of the alar cartilage in the division of the dome will give rise to obvious tip asymmetry particularly if the division is asymmetrical and the cartilage is 'strong' with thin overlying skin

One of the more common problems in the nasal tip is a bulbosity or fullness over the upper or cephalic aspect of the alar cartilages. Excision of the cephalic aspect of the alar cartilage not only achieves narrowing of this area, but makes some rotation of the nasal tip possible by a 'visoring' of the caudal rim of the alar cartilage into the cephalic defect (Figure 17.12).

Access to the cephalic portion of the alar cartilage is commonly achieved by a retrograde dissection via the intercartilaginous incision. With this approach, however, it is not easy to achieve an accurate and symmetrical excision of cartilage and a cartilage-splitting incision and delivery of the cephalic portion of the cartilage is preferred (Figure 17.13). Whichever approach or technique is applied to the cartilage, it is important to preserve the underlying vestibular skin. If an excess of vestibular skin is excised, pinching and alar collapse may follow. This problem, unsatisfactory from the point of view of both airway and cosmesis, is also probable if there is a failure to preserve a sufficient rim of alar cartilage to support the lateral wall of the nose. About 3–4 mm of carti-

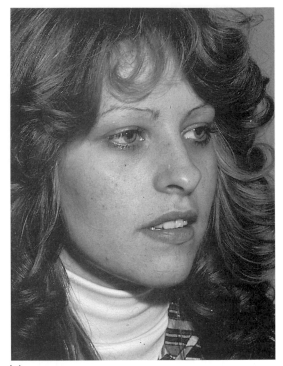

(a)

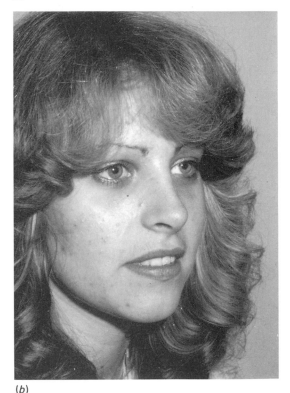

(b)

Figure 17.12 Narrowing and rotation of tip achieved by excision of the cephalic aspect of the alar cartilage

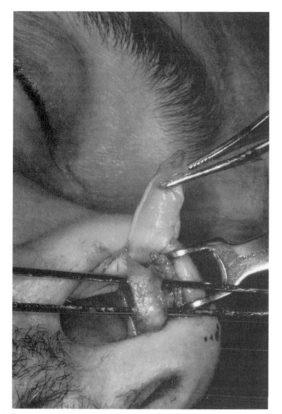

17.13 Cartilage-splitting alar cartilage incision with delivery of the caudal aspect of the cartilage

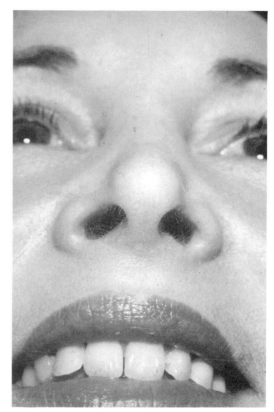

Figure 17.14 'Knock-kneed' tip deformity due to excessive removal of vestibular skin and lower lateral cartilage

lage are necessary to maintain the alae in a lateral position and prevent this collapse, but in a thin-walled nose with thin skin and rather lax cartilage, more lateral crus may be necessary. The texture of the skin and cartilage, therefore, may well determine the probability of this lateral alar collapse; with relatively thick skin and strong cartilage, a rim of 2 mm will suffice for support. If, however, skin and cartilage are removed from the lateral wall of the vestibule and removed to excess, then the pinching or 'knock-kneed' tip deformity will result (Figure 17.14). It is also important to excise equal portions of alar cartilage from each side to preserve tip symmetry and this is particularly necessary when the overlying skin is thin and the underlying cartilage is relatively strong and resilient.

Although the cartilage-splitting incision allows delivery of the upper aspect of the alar cartilage, this approach will not suffice when more radical changes are needed in tip anatomy. A rim incision with complete delivery of cartilage is necessary in these cases.

The rim of the alar cartilage does not follow the margin of the nasal vestibule. The alar cartilage is placed obliquely and although, medially, the medial crus forms the rim of the vestibule, the lateral crus is up to 5 mm or more above the margin of the nostril. The rim incision and full delivery of the alar cartilage is necessary to correct bifid or flat nasal tip deformities. It is also necessary if lengthening of the columella is needed, and may be required to reduce a marked tip projection. Any radical change in tip anatomy which may be needed in such gross deformities as the cleft-nose nasal tip, also require a full delivery of the nasal cartilages. The rim incision and delivery of the alar cartilage gives an almost complete exposure of the lateral crus, the dome and the medial crus of the cartilage. If the cephalic half or two-thirds of the alar cartilage is removed (with preservation of vestibular skin), rotation or visoring of the remaining rim of cartilage achieves marked tip rotation. In most instances, it is better to avoid dividing the lower lateral cartilage at the dome or elsewhere for, although incision of cartilage in itself will alter tip anatomy as the crura spring apart, irregularity or sharp edges will result. This problem is particularly likely with resilient cartilage underlying thin skin. Symmetry of any cartilage incision or excision and the avoidance of any sharp edges is, therefore, important in these cases. It may be necessary however, to divide the alar cartilages separating the lateral and medial crus completely from one another to increase tip projection. In the technique described by Goldman (1965) – which is one of the better established techniques for increasing tip projection – the alar cartilages are divided lateral to the dome; the medial crura, plus the medial portion of the lateral crura are then sutured back-to-back (Figure 17.15). Cartilage grafts and struts are also advocated for insertion between the medial crura and are another way to increase tip projection and lengthen the columella. Sheen (1978) advocated the case of cartilage grafts to give increased tip projection and a more pleasing tip anatomy. These grafts certainly have a proven place in revision rhinoplasty. In these cases, an excess of cartilage has almost certainly been excised at a previous operation or operations and replaced with fibrous tissue. Cartilage replacement is often clearly needed. Shield grafts are easily secured via an external rhinoplasty approach as described below.

An additional tip sculpture technique which has gained popularity over the past two decades is the transdomal suture procedure. This is particularly suitable for patients with a broad boxy or even bifid nasal tip with firm strong alar cartilages. The skin may be thin with little intervening subcutaneous tissue. This technique aims at the *preservation* and *reorientation* of the nasal tip structures, conserving the structural anatomy of the alar cartilages (Tardy, Patt and Walter, 1993).

Surgical steps include both intercartilaginous and marginal incisions with elevation of the overlying skin to allow full delivery of the lower laterals. The intercartilaginous incisions may be continuous with the transfixion incision at the caudal end of the septum. The external or open approach as described below may be used but it is not essential to do so. The upper margin of the lower laterals may be reduced as necessary, but the minimum amount of cartilage is removed, as this technique relies primarily on the repositioning of existing cartilage. Interdomal soft tissue is removed.

A 4–0 clear PDS suture is now placed from medial to lateral through first the left dome, passing back from lateral to medial. The needle and suture end are then passed through the interdomal area and the procedure repeated on the opposite side. A knot can now be gently tied which will lie buried deep in the interdomal area. The orientation of the lower laterals can now be assessed before locking the knot. If the new position appears unsatisfactory, the suture can be removed and the procedure repeated until a satisfactory shape is achieved.

With nasal tips that require less marked narrowing, it is not necessary to suture both alar domes together. A suture to each individual dome near the apex, between the lateral and medial crura, is used in these cases for tip narrowing. The marginal incisions are carefully resutured with 4–0 plain catgut.

The saddle nose

The cartilaginous septum and maxillary bony crest form the main supports of the lower two-thirds of the nasal dorsum. If there is insufficient cartilage to give

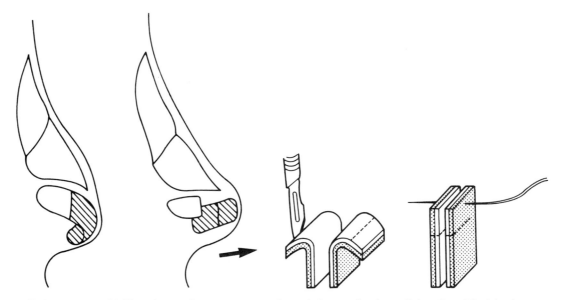

Figure 17.15 Diagram of Goldman's tip technique – suturing the medial crura plus the medial portion of the lateral crura back-to-back to increase tip projection

support, either due to absence or fibrosis of the carti-laginous part of the septum, nasal saddling to various degrees will result. Nasal saddling is, therefore, com-monly seen after septal haematomas, following septal surgery or injury and, if the haematoma becomes infected, nasal collapse is almost inevitable. Patients should of course be warned prior to drainage of a septal abscess or haematoma that some degree of nasal saddling may occur. Immediate grafting is advo-cated by some (Huizing, 1986) but, in most instances grafting of the dorsum is deferred until the degree of saddling is evident. Loss of septal support for the nasal dorsum, although resulting mainly from trauma, may follow many of the chronic inflamma-tory conditions which involve cartilage such as sar-coidosis, tuberculosis, polychrondritis and syphilis. Malignant granuloma may also damage septal carti-lage and lead to nasal dorsum collapse; some degree of saddling may also be a familial or racial characteristic.

When considering management of a nasal saddle, one's first thought tends to be of a suitable graft material. It should be remembered, however, that many small saddles are accentuated by a nasal hump and simple removal of the hump suffices to solve the saddle defect resulting in a smaller nose which may be a bonus, particularly in the female patient (Figure 17.16). In some instances, it may be possible to remove a dorsal hump and use this to graft the saddle. With more severe saddling, however, an im-plant is required to restore an acceptable nasal con-tour. The problem is to select from the great number of alternatives the most acceptable and reliable long-term graft. When the saddle is due to loss of cartilagi-nous support, a 'soft' cartilaginous graft is preferable to the harder implants such as bone and synthetics. When the saddle defect involves the entire dorsum, that is both bone and cartilage, one of the harder implants is probably to be preferred.

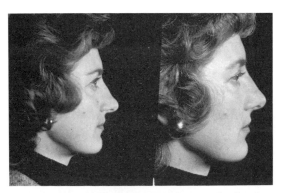

Figure 17.16 Pre- and postoperative photographs showing how a small saddle is accentuated by a hump and may be corrected by removal of the hump with no augmentation

Iliac crest bone grafts are still widely used and advocated in many standard texts, although their long-term survival is doubtful. When the saddling involves the bony skeleton of the nose, iliac crest grafts have a place but they are usually unsatisfactory for the cartilaginous saddle, producing a rather rigid and wide unnatural appearance. The donor site gives some considerable pain initially and produces a scar.

Autografts are probably the most useful graft mater-ial for the majority of nasal saddle defects. For the small saddles, sufficient cartilage may be obtained from the nasal septum. Usually, however, the cause of the saddle defect makes the likelihood of sufficient residual septal cartilage being available improbable. The bone of the septum from the vomer and ethmoid is thin and less satisfactory to fashion than the cartilage. Rib cartilage may be needed for the large saddle defects, but the harvesting risks of pneumo-thorax, postoperative pain and scar are among other disadvantages. Rib cartilages may twist, whatever manoeuvres are taken to avoid this troublesome long-term possibility.

Aural conchal cartilage is the most useful graft for the majority of saddle defects and can be obtained with minimal deformity, if necessary, from both ears. The shape of the conchal cartilage lends itself well to restoring good contour to saddle deformity. Although this cartilage gives many good results, it is a viable graft and change in shape and bulk may occur, so, as with all implants, it is not totally reliable. It is arguable whether this graft should be used for sad-dling related to chronic inflammatory diseases such as sarcoid, relapsing polychondritis or with malignant granuloma. It is not always possible to be certain that the disease is quiescent and the implanted graft may become involved in the inflammatory process and cause a complex deformity with the cartilage involved in the chronic inflammatory process.

Irradiated preserved cartilage is also advocated and impressive reports are available (McGlynn and Sharpe, 1981). Synthetic implants have a place in the management of nasal saddling, although there are those who oppose their use with almost religious fervor. It is curious that, for chin augmentation, synthetic implants are almost universally used with little in the way of criticism. The thick overlying soft tissue present over the chin implant, however, makes extrusion unlikely and conceals minor displacement. Synthetic implants underlying the nasal dorsal skin are close to the nasal cavity and to the exterior. Even with minimal infection, therefore, extrusion of the graft either externally or through a sinus inside the nose is possible. The firm synthetic implants may also move and their asymmetry of outline is obvious and aesthetically unacceptable. It is not true, how-ever, to say that most synthetic nasal implants ex-trude. Long-term follow up of cases shows that this is not evident if certain precautions are taken (Mackay and Bull, 1983). An implant inserted through a midline vertical columella incision into a pocket underlying the dorsum of the nose with few or no other rhinoplasty steps undertaken concurrently will almost certainly remain *in situ*. Telangiectasia of the skin may occur and displacement from the midline position gives rise to asymmetry. The synthetic meshes, such as Supramid, also act as a satisfactory filling material in the nose and good results have been demonstrated (Beekhuis, 1975). These materials, however, cannot easily be fashioned or shaped. If infection does occur, the extrusion of solid implants results in a return to the status quo and surgical removal is also simple. With the mesh implants, however, complete removal may be difficult or impossible. The same problem of surgical removal arises with an infected bone or cartilage graft.

Firm synthetic implants are useful in saddling involving the nasal bones and cartilage and are particularly applicable in some cases where a saddle appearance is an unwanted racial characteristic. With thin or scarred skin, synthetic implants are better avoided and any skin blanching overlying the implant at the time of insertion is to be avoided for the skin may later break down at this site.

There is probably no single ideal implant for all saddle deformities, but conchal cartilage grafts suffice and are possibly the most suitable graft at present to select for the moderate cartilaginous saddles. However, there is insufficient ear cartilage for gross saddle defects and, in this situation, a synthetic, rib or iliac crest graft is required.

The deviated nose

Correcting a deviated nose is one of the more difficult procedures in rhinoplasty. This is in part due to the fact that two-thirds of the nose is made up of cartilage which, unlike bone, does not 'stay put' but tends to spring back to its former position. In many cases, extensive septal surgery will be required which can considerably complicate any rhinoplasty procedure; lastly any inequality or asymmetry of the bony side walls may not be corrected by the usual medial and lateral osteotomies. Regrettably, although the procedures required to correct a deviation may be complex, this is seldom fully appreciated by the patient, whose attitude can often be summarized by the statement: 'I don't want the shape changed, just straighten it!' As with all rhinoplasty surgery, it is well worth spending more time explaining the limitations than the expectations of any proposed surgery and this is particularly true of the deviated nose, when it should be carefully explained that no guarantee can be given that the nose will be perfectly straight but that certainly one hopes to achieve an improvement.

As long ago as 1845, Dieffenbach advocated division of the upper lateral nasal cartilages from the

septum, the nose being held in its new position with bandages. In 1889, Trendelenberg was performing sophisticated procedures to correct the deviated nose by undertaking endonasal lateral osteotomies, percutaneous superior osteotomies and dividing the septum from the nasal crest using a fine osteotome. Joseph described a technique in 1907 whereby bilateral lateral osteotomies were undertaken in addition to removing a triangular wedge of bone from the 'long side'. A similar 'wedge-technique' together with an asymmetrical hump reduction was described by Foman in 1936 and later modified in 1960 (Foman, 1936, 1960). Cottle's description in 1960 of a high lateral osteotomy on the broad side and low osteotomy on the short side, together with a septoplasty and 'push down', although apparently effective, was criticized on the basis that it could lead to a 'step deformity'.

The techniques required to correct a deviated nose may be considered under four headings:

1 Correction of the septum and upper lateral cartilages
2 Dealing with deviation and asymmetry of the nasal bones
3 The nasal tip
4 Augmentation, i.e. filling a depression to give an appearance of straightening the nose.

The last of these would not be suitable on its own if there is any functional element, but is a useful supplementary technique used in conjunction with the former three and may occasionally be all that is required to correct a purely aesthetic deformity.

The nasal septum and upper lateral cartilages

The septum is dealt with more fully in Chapter 11. When the septum, although deviated, is itself reasonably straight, i.e. it may bend at one particular point only or it is straight within the nose but both nose and septum deviate to one side of the face, then the so-called 'septoplasty technique' can be usefully employed. A mucoperichondrial flap is elevated from both sides of the nasal septum or completely on one side with superior and inferior tunnels on the other. If mucoperichondrium is left attached to one side, it may reduce the chance of resorption of cartilage at a later date although, in practice, this seems rarely to occur. Leaving the flaps attached one side but not on the other, however, may lead to unequal scarring and later contracture which it is felt by some could lead to further deviation of the nose and septum at a later date. The septum is then separated from each upper lateral nasal cartilage above, divided at the 'bend' posteriorly, repositioned onto the maxillary crest below, or the crest itself repositioned following an osteotomy if it is not in the midline and, finally, the septum repocketed anteriorly into a slot incised behind the columella.

Skin overlying the upper lateral nasal cartilages and nasal bones is elevated in the normal way via an intercartilaginous incision and, following detachment of the upper laterals from the septum, any inequality can be corrected by lowering the 'long' side and possibly even augmenting the 'short' side with a cartilage graft.

Septoplasty techniques are less satisfactory for dealing with deviations which are maximal at the valve area, where there is generalized 'ballooning' of the septum towards one side or where there is gross buckling and distortion of the nasal septum. In these cases, it may be necessary to undertake a submucosal resection of as large a portion of septal cartilage as possible which can then be repositioned and replaced as a free graft, or it may need to be completely replaced with an autograft from the ear or a homograft of banked septal cartilage. In these cases, there is a serious risk of supratip depression and saddling developing at a later date and, when possible, it is better not to separate the upper lateral cartilage attachment to the septum. This will, however, make it impossible to correct any inequality of the upper laterals and more difficult to correct any deviation of the middle third of the nose. Very occasionally, it may be necessary to stage the procedure in these circumstances.

The septum may, in some instances, be dislocated to one side of the columella anteriorly, but the remaining septum may be in a satisfactory position. Providing there is adequate support for the columella, which can readily be checked by pressing a finger in the columella, then any displaced cartilage must be surplus to requirement and may be excised together with its covering mucous membranes, provided this is excised parallel with the septum to ensure that no useful cartilage is removed. If the cartilage is excised at a right-angle to the septum, too much caudal border may be removed leading to unsightly columella retraction.

Deviation of the upper third – nasal bones

Correction of the bony upper third should not in theory present too much of a problem, as it should be possible to refracture, manipulate and immobilize the nasal bones into any desired position. In practice, however, residual deviation in this area is not uncommon and this may, in many cases, be due to the fact that medial, lateral and superior osteotomies will not correct the deformity.

Trauma to one side of the nose will often result in a curved deformity and, if one considers the nasal

bones individually, each can be considered as 'canoe-shaped' or 'banana-shaped' – medial, lateral and superior osteotomies will simply result in two fragments, each still with the same curved shape (Figure 17.17).

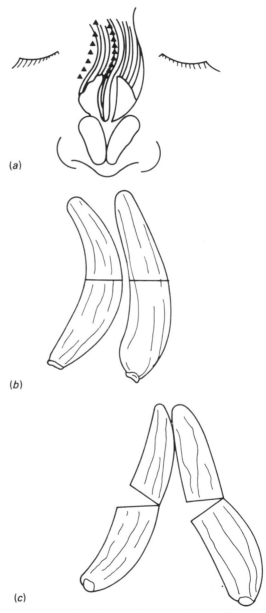

Figure 17.17 (*a*) With gross deviation of the nasal bones the standard medial and lateral osteotomies lead to 'banana-shaped' fragments; (*b*) transverse intermediate osteotomies are required; (*c*) the nasal bones can now be realigned

Tardy and Denneny (1984) described the use of vertical intermediate osteotomies using a 2 or 3 mm osteotome endonasally. While this certainly results in greater mobilization of the fragments, it may still not be ideal because a transverse or horizontal intermediate osteotomy is more logical. This is difficult to perform endonasally, but can easily be performed using a percutaneous technique.

The nose is prepared in the normal way; a small stab incision is then made in the midpoint of the desired osteotomy. Through this single incision, the osteotome is then moved up and down along the proposed line scoring the periosteum, and then tapped through in three or four positions to complete the osteotomy. The same technique can be used for the lateral and superior osteotomies. A medial osteotomy is undertaken in the normal manner. Following this, the nasal bones are infractured or outfractured into the desired position. It is important to note that skin and mucoperiosteum must not be widely elevated as these are required to splint the relatively small fragments of nasal bones. Intermediate osteotomies, whether longitudinal or transverse, must be completed before any other osteotomies. There may be further comminution of the nasal bones, but this need not be a disadvantage and, indeed, was the basis of a technique described by Kazanjian and Converse (1972) who advocated covering the nose with cottonwool, protecting the eye with wadding and refracturing the nose with a strong blow from a mallet.

Nasal tip

The cartilage-splitting technique described above can at times be used to correct a tip deformity by an asymmetrical reduction, either removing more cartilage from one side than the other or reducing the tip only on the side to which the nose deviates. Occasionally, a tip can be reduced and the cartilage removed used to augment the other side.

Where the tip not only deviates to one side but also requires projection, the technique described by Goldman (1965) may be useful. A rim incision is performed and the overlying skin elevated. Skin and cartilage are then incised at a point some 2 mm lateral to the dome; the two sides are then sutured back-to-back in such a way that they can not only project the tip but also twist it back to the midline (Figure 17.18).

Augmentation

In addition to augmentation of the tip, as described above, it may at times also be useful to consider augmentation on the concave side of the nose over the upper lateral cartilage and nasal bones (Figure 17.19). It is always wise to consider the need for this carefully at the *preoperative* planning stage as, following infiltration and elevation of the skin together with a certain amount of inevitable oedema of the tissues during surgery, the need for augmentation after undertaking various other manoeuvres can be difficult to visualize. One can frequently be disappointed with long-term results in a case where a graft was considered preoperatively, but deemed to be unnecessary at the time of surgery.

Autografts are preferrable to homografts and it is usually not difficult to find a suitable piece of cartilage. It is often necessary to remove cartilage from the nasal septum while correcting a deviated nose, and this makes ideal graft material. Where this is not available, however, conchal cartilage from the ear is equally suitable.

Whenever possible, these grafts should be positioned into a pocket which has been fashioned to the exact size of the graft to prevent the latter being displaced. While this is highly desirable, it is not always practical: e.g. if it has been necessary to elevate the skin over the dorsum to remove a hump, it is then impossible to fashion any pocket in the supratip region. In these circumstances, it is possible to secure the graft with 4–0 plain catgut sutured through the skin and secured with Steri-strip.

Deviation associated with gross deformity of the nose

Where there is gross deviation, particularly if this is associated with severe septal deformity, as with the cleft-lip nose, an external rhinoplasty approach should be considered. This allows excellent exposure of the septum, together with direct visualization of the nasal anatomy. It is, however, simply an approach and does not in itself offer an advantage other than improved exposure and access. The principles outlined above will still need to be followed in order to correct the deformity.

Alar collapse

Alar collapse is the phenomenon whereby the alae nasi collapse inwards on inspiration in a valve-like manner, causing nasal obstruction. It is most common in elderly patients with a drooping tip, loss of elasticity of the cartilage and atrophy of the dilator muscles. It may occur after rhinoplasty, if too much lower lateral nasal cartilage has been excised. Loss of vestibular skin may result in gross scarring and contracture in the valve area.

Conductance is proportional to the fourth power of the diameter of a vessel and a very small change in the width of the nostril will markedly affect the flow. As air passes inwards through the nose the nostrils are drawn inwards due to Bernoiulli's

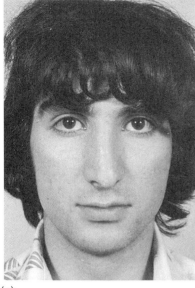

(a)

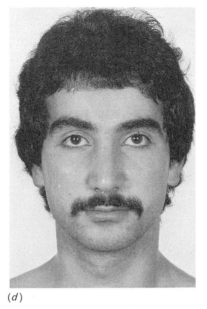

(d)

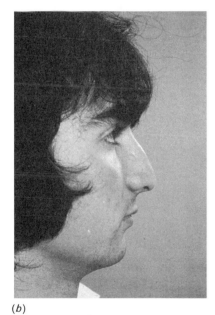

(b)

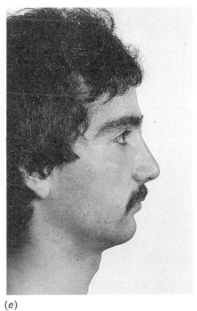

(e)

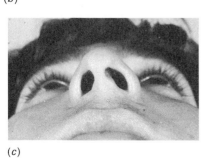

(c)

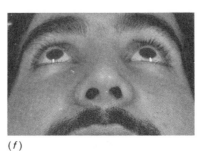

(f)

Figure 17.18 (a, b, c) Pre- and (d, e, f) postoperative views to demonstrate deviation of tip corrected by the Goldman technique – suturing medial crura and the medial portion of the lateral crura back-to-back

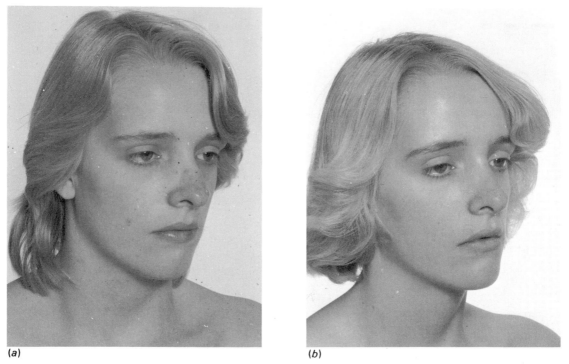

(a) **(b)**

Figure 17.19 (*a*) Pre- and (*b*) postoperative views to demonstrate augmentation of the nose with a cartilage autograft to fill a depression over the upper lateral nasal cartilage

principle; as this occurs, the resistance will increase tending to cause further indrawing until the nostrils eventually close off completely. In the normal subject, this will occur if inspiration through the nose is sufficiently forceful and a diagnosis of alar collapse should be reserved for those patients unable to achieve inspiration at physiological flow rates.

While a relatively small decrease in the diameter of the airway may greatly increase resistance, the converse is also true and a relatively minor alteration of the nasal septum in the valve area or narrowing of the columella may be sufficient to prevent the initiation of this phenomenon. One can test the relative significance of a wide columella (Figure 17.20) by gently squeezing it between the two limbs of a Thudicum speculum. If this improves the situation, it is a simple matter to excise an ellipse of skin to include the herniating portion of the medial crus of the lower lateral cartilage. The skin is then gently undermined and closed with sutures.

In addition to narrowing caused by the medial crus, the lateral crus may at times herniate inwards, causing obstruction (Figure 17.21); this cannot be corrected by simple excision, however, but needs to be dissected free and repositioned into a new pocket

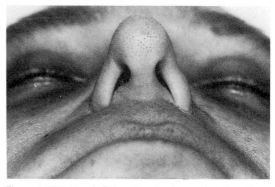

Figure 17.20 Nasal obstruction due to a wide columella

slightly more lateral and superior to its former position.

Apart from these supplementary techniques, the methods used to correct this problem fall into three groups:

1 Prostheses
2 Modification of existing cartilage
3 Grafting additional material.

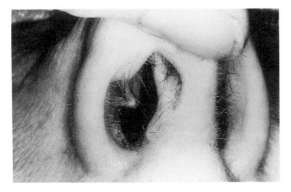

Figure 17.21 Nasal obstruction due to inward herniation of the lateral crus of the lower lateral cartilage

Prosthetic devices

Many prostheses have been tried over the years from quills and reeds to the silver wire alae nasi dilator used by Clement Francis at The Metropolitan Ear, Nose and Throat Hospital (Figure 17.22). Not one of them has, however, found lasting favour. More recently, Davenport, Brain and Hunt (1981) have reported greater success using acrylic materials. A mould is made with silicone putty which is then cast in clear acrylic resin through which a hole is drilled to provide an airway.

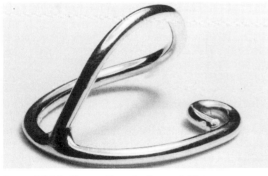

Figure 17.22 Clement Francis alae nasi dilator

Modification of existing cartilage

In some cases, alar collapse is due to slit-like narrowness between the septum and the upper lateral nasal cartilages. Walter (1976b) has described a technique whereby the valve can be enlarged by dividing the upper laterals from the septum and covering the defect with a flap from the upper border of the lower lateral cartilage.

The skin is elevated over the upper lateral nasal cartilages which are then divided, together with the underlying mucosa, from the septum on both sides.

A flap of cartilage and vestibular skin is then fashioned, based on the dome and retaining a 2–3 mm strip of cartilage along the lower border undisturbed. This flap is then rotated upwards to fill the defect between the septum and lower lateral cartilages (Figure 17.23).

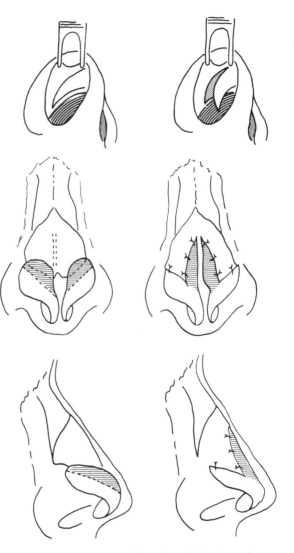

Figure 17.23 A medial based flap of vestibular skin and lower lateral cartilage is elevated and rotated upwards to fill the defect formed by dividing the upper lateral cartilage from the septum to widen the valve area (after C. Walter)

Rettinger and Masing (1981) noted that the medial crus and lateral crus of the lower lateral cartilages lie in the same plane, in many patients with alar collapse, and this is particularly true in the elderly patient with a drooping tip. They also observed the tension lines in a plastic model under polarized light.

By rotating the two limbs of the model in opposite directions, they noticed that these tension lines were distributed over a larger surface increasing the stability of the system. These principles were applied to the problem and the lateral border of the lower lateral cartilage was rotated upwards into a more cephalic position.

A rim incision is performed and the lateral crus dissected free of both overlaying skin and underlying vestibular skin until the whole of the lateral crus remains attached only at the dome. A pocket is developed above the upper lateral and sesamoid cartilages and the lateral crus rotated upwards by means of a traction suture. The cartilage can then be maintained in its new position either with a mattress suture tied over Teflon foil or with fibrin glue (Figure 17.24).

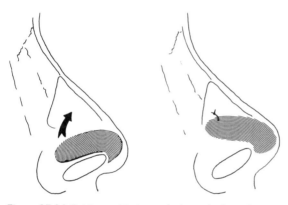

Figure 17.24 Rettinger–Masing technique; the lateral crus of the lower lateral cartilage is rotated upwards and sutured into position

Rettinger and Masing reported an initial success rate of 18 out of 19 patients with a minimum follow-up period of 6 months and pre- and postoperative rhinomanometry confirmed this improvement in the four patients on whom this was performed.

Cartilage grafts

In some cases, there is insufficient cartilage to reposition; this is particularly true following excessive excision of cartilage during rhinoplasty. In other cases, although present, the cartilage appears to have atrophied and lost all its elasticity such that repositioning is unlikely to be beneficial. In these cases, it is necessary to graft new cartilage either from the septum or from the conchal cartilage of the ear, which is probably better as the latter is suitably curved and elastic. Where support alone is needed, a cartilage graft will suffice; if vestibular lining is needed in addition to support, a composite graft will be required.

An ellipse of cartilage is taken from the concha of the ear and inserted into a pocket prepared at the site where support is lacking. A small incision is made in the vestibular skin and a pocket fashioned with curved pointed scissors – the size of which should exactly match that of the graft to prevent the graft wandering into the wrong position. The pocket is then closed with a few fine sutures.

Composite cartilage graft

Alar collapse with stenosis may follow rhinoplasty, although it should not occur if the principles outlined here are followed; in particular, vestibular skin should not be excised. In addition to surgery, other trauma and in particular burns, sometimes following cautery for epistaxis, may result in this deformity.

Aural conchal composite grafts offer the most effective method to correct this difficult problem. Although composite grafts were described many years ago (Konig, 1902), it is due to Claus Walter's more recent innovative work that the wider application of these grafts has been developed (Walter, 1976a).

For the more minimal stenosis involving the apex of the vestibule alone, two separate elliptical composite grafts may be used. The vestibular skin is incised and undermined, on either side, but no skin is removed; the composite graft is then sutured into the defect. When stenosis is associated with saddling, a large composite graft can be used, with a small strip of skin removed from the midline of the graft where it 'bridges' the septum. This can provide cartilage to fill the saddle, cartilage to prevent alar collapse and skin to replace the stenosed vestibule as a simple procedure. The external rhinoplasty approach may facilitate the securing of these grafts.

External rhinoplasty

The standard rhinoplasty techniques, evolved from Joseph's and Roes original operations, involve no external incisions on the nose or face. The technique is, however, to some extent blind and certainly placing intranasal sutures or accurate securing of grafts is not always easy via these standard incisions.

Rethi (1956) demonstrated that an excellent exposure and access to all nasal structures could be achieved with elevation of the nasal skin via a transverse columella incision linking the cartilage rims. The transverse incision across the columella is, however, invariably ugly and conspicuous and almost impossible to revise effectively. In 1974, Goodman of Toronto demonstrated that an inverted 'V'-shaped incision resulted in an almost imperceptible scar. Vertical columellar incisions are barely perceptible whereas transverse incisions are very obvious.

This small change in the incision led to a resurgence of interest in the external or 'open' rhinoplasty operation. In certain gross deformities, marked deviation, revision surgery and in particular the management of cleft lip nasal deformities, the external rhinoplasty has become an accepted alternative to the traditional endonasal approach (Anderson and Ries, 1986; Johnson and Toriumi, 1990; Zijlker and Hade, 1993). It has the advantage of demonstrating the anatomy clearly so that correction can be better controlled and sutures accurately placed. For the insertion of composite or intranasal grafts and possibly access for repair of a septal perforation, this approach should be considered (Figure 17.25). It also forms an excellent access for excision, with minimal scarring, for lesions and swellings under the nasal dorsum which may hitherto have been approached by a direct incision through nasal skin.

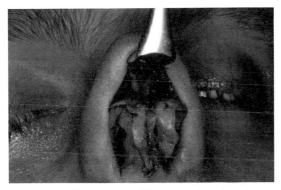

Figure 17.25 The exposure of the nose achieved by the external rhinoplasty approach

Marginal incisions are connected across the columella by way of a 'w', 'v' or step-shaped incision (Figure 17.26). The skin is then elevated over the

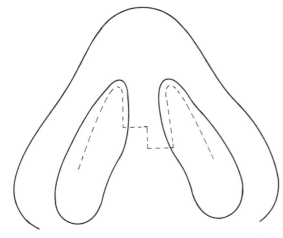

Figure 17.26 Diagram of a 'step' incision which joins the two marginal incisions across the columella

lower lateral and upper lateral cartilages and gently retracted with a retractor such as a Cottle alar retractor in such a way that the whole of the underlying nasal skeleton can be clearly visualized.

The alar cartilages may now be sculptured and refashioned under direct vision. If there is any evidence of asymmetry such as is seen in the cleft lip nose, cartilage may be taken from one side and used to augment the other. Sutures may be used to reorientate the cartilages such as the interdomal suture described above. Cartilage harvested more posteriorly from the septum can be placed under direct vision between the medial crura of the lower laterals as a columella strut to reinforce this area before augmenting the tip.

If there is insufficient cartilage available from the septum, a graft may be harvested from auricular conchal cartilage. The 'shield' graft was introduced by Sheen (1975) and has continued to be enthusiastically advocated by others, particularly via the external approach which it is claimed allows for better placement and easier fixation (Johnson and Quatella, 1987; Arden and Crumley, 1993).

Once harvested the cartilage is sculptured to shape according to the needs of the case, but in general terms it will resemble a heart or shield with the two upper corners measuring some 6–8 mm apart, which will form the two tip defining points. It narrows to the base where it measures 3–4 mm and is approximately 10–12 mm in length with the thickness varying from 1 to 3 mm (Zijlker and Hade, 1993). A shield graft does not increase tip support and when this is needed, a columella strut between the medial crura may be necessary in addition to this graft which acts more as a 'filler'. The graft can be temporarily held in place with fine hypodermic needles which are passed through the graft into the underlying tissues after it has been placed into the correct position. It is then sutured in place using 6–0 prolene sutures (Figure 17.27).

Dressings, splints and plasters

Prior to the application of any dressings, one should ensure that any cartilage-splitting incisions have been sutured and that mucoperichondrial flaps are replaced and secured. It is not usually necessary to suture the intercartilaginous incisions.

Splints

Silastic splints may be required to immobilize the nasal septum and help to maintain this in the midline. These should be thick enough to provide rigid support, of sufficient length to support the entire length of the septum, but should not be too wide as they may otherwise cause pain due to pressure between

matic instrument for the lateral osteotomy and its use predisposes to this deformity: an osteotome is to be preferred.

If asymmetrical excision of the alar cartilage is carried out and the rim of the cartilage remaining is too narrow, particularly near the dome, 'bossing' or asymmetry of the nasal tip becomes obvious. If the medial and lateral crura are divided when the overlying nasal tip skin is thin, irregularities or highlights will show. Asymmetrical division of the cartilages, or division on one side only, is particularly likely to predispose to this unsatisfactory appearance. Morcellizing techniques of the tip cartilages are also at risk of producing tip irregularities with thin overlying skin.

Intranasal complications of rhinoplasty also occur. The standard rhinoplasty technique correctly carried out does not prejudice the nasal airway. Over 500 patients assessed postoperatively at The Royal National Throat, Nose and Ear Hospital had no complaint of nasal obstruction following rhinoplasty. Nonetheless, vestibular stenosis following revision rhinoplasty or excessive incisions inside the nasal vestibule, particularly if coupled with excision of vestibular skin, will lead to stenosis and narrowing of the airway which may be very severe.

Failure to excise the caudal portion of the upper lateral cartilage may result in a projection of this cartilage into the vestibule with an area of vestibulitis.

Synechiae should not occur but trauma to the lateral nasal wall skin and mucosa, if coupled with damage to the septal mucosa, may predispose to this and careful use of instruments is a relevant factor. Excessive lowering of the upper lateral cartilage along its dorsal margin also predisposes to webbing of the nasal valve with nasal obstruction.

Rhinoplasty and septoplasty, however, are operations which, if correctly applied, give excellent results achieving both an improvement in nasal airway and an acceptable and natural improvement in the external nasal shape.

References

ANDERSON, J. R. and RIES, W. R. (1986) *Rhinoplasty: Emphasizing the External Approach*. New York: Thieme Inc.

ARDEN, R. L. and CRUMLEY, R. L. (1993) Cartilage grafts in open rhinoplasty. *Facial Plastic Surgery*, 9, 285–294

BEEKHUIS, S. G. J. (1975) Surgical correction of saddle nose deformity. *Transactions of the American Academy of Ophthalmology and Otolaryngology*, 80, 596–607

COTTLE, M. H. (1960) *Corrective Surgery. Nasal Septum and Pyramid*. Chicago: American Rhinologic Society. pp. 53–60, 72–73

DAVENPORT, J. C., BRAIN, D. J. and HUNT, A. T. (1981) Treatment of alar collapse with nasal prostheses. *Journal of Prosthetic Dentistry*, 45, 435–437

DIEFFENBACH, J. F. (1845) *Operative Chirurgie Bd* 1s.367

FOMAN, S. (1936) The treatment of old unreduced nasal fractures. *Annals of Surgery*, 107–117

FOMAN, S. (1960) *Otolaryngology*, vol. 3. Baltimore, MD: Harper and Row. pp. 74–75

GOLDMAN, I. B. (1965) Rhinoplastic sequelae causing nasal obstruction. *Archives of Otolaryngology*, 83, 151

GOODMAN, W. S. (1974) External approach to rhinoplasty. *Laryngoscope*, 84, 2195–2201

HUIZING, E. H. (1986) The management of septal abscesses. *Monographs in Facial Plastic Surgery*, 3, 243–252

JOHNSON, C. M. and QUATELLA, V. C. (1987) Nasal tip grafting via the open approach. *Facial Plastic Surgery*, 4, 301–316

JOHNSON, C. M. and TORIUMI D. M. (1990) *Open Structure Rhinoplasty*. Philadelphia: WB Saunders Company

JOSEPH, J. (1907) Die korrektur der Schiefnase. *Deutsche Medizinische Wochenschrift*, 49, 2035–2040

KAZANJIAN, V. H. and CONVERSE, J. M. (1972) *The Surgical Treatment of Facial Injuries*. Baltimore, MD: Williams and Wilkins

KONIG, F. (1902) Zur Deckung Von Defecten der Nasenflugel. *Klinische Wochenschrift*, 7, 137–138

MCGLYNN, M. J. and SHARPE, D. T. (1981) Cialit preserved homograft cartilage in nasal augmentation: a long-term review. *British Journal of Plastic Surgery*, 34, 53–57

MACKAY, I. S. and BULL, T. R. (1983) The fate of Silastic in saddle deformity of the nose. *Journal of Laryngology and Otology*, 97, 43–47

RETHI, A. (1956) Operationen wegen entstellender Sattelnose. *Chirurg*, 27, 356–360

RETTINGER, G. and MASING, H. (1981) Rotation of the alar cartilage in collapsed alae. *Rhinology*, 19, 81–86

SHEEN, J. H. (1975) Achieving more nasal tip projection by the use of a small autogenous vomer or septal graft. *Plastic and Reconstructive Surgery*, 56, 35–40

SHEEN, J. H. (1978) *Aesthetic Rhinoplasty*. New York: C. V. Mosby Co.

TARDY, M. E. and DENNENY, J. C. (1984) Micro-osteotomies in rhinoplasty. *Facial Plastic Surgery*, 1, 137–145

TARDY, M. E., PATT, B. S. and WALTER, M. A. (1993) Transdomal suture refinement of the nasal tip: long-term outcomes. *Facial Plastic Surgery*, 9, 275–284

TRENDELENBERG, F. (1989) *Verhandlungen der deutsch Gesellschaft fur chirurgie Bd*, 19, 82

WALTER, C. (1967a) Survey of the use of composite grafts in the head and neck. *Otolaryngologic Clinics of North America*, 5, 571–602

WALTER, C. (1976b) Plastische und Wiederherstellend Chirurgie Zum Thema: Nasenflugelkollaps. *Laryngologie, Rhinologie, Otologie und Ihre Grenzgebiete*, 55, 447–449

ZIJLKER, T. D. and HADE, V. (1993) Cartilage grafts for the nasal tip. *Clinical Otolaryngology*, 18, 446–458

18

Epistaxis

J. C. Watkinson

History

Epistaxis is mentioned in medical literature dating back to early times. Hippocrates (fifth century BC) was probably the first to appreciate that pressure on the alae nasi was an effective method of controlling nose bleeds, although in some cases he resorted to nasal packing and the application of cold fomentations to the shaved head. He regarded the complaint as being primarily of young persons, and was the first to describe vicarious menstruation.

Ali Ibn Rabban Al-Tabiri (AD 850) devoted a chapter of his massive work *The Paradise of Wisdom* to epistaxis. In it he wrote: 'The complaint of nose bleeding is due to swelling of a vein and its rupture, or perhaps a reduction in the force which confines the blood within'. He implied that some of the medications inserted into the nose owed their efficacy as much to their temperature as to their pharmacological properties. Morgagni (1769) recognized 'the extremely turgid blood vessels about that part where the alae nasi are formed with the bone, about a finger's breadth more or less from the bottom of the nostril'. He was reported to have stopped nose bleeds by introducing his finger and 'pressing that part whereupon the blood ceased to flow, so that it was not even discharged by the posterior nostril into the fauces'. Morgagni drew his inspiration from his former teacher Valsalva and for this reason Little's area is referred to as '*Locus Valsalvae*' in Italian circles. Morgagni's records also contain the suggestion, previously entertained by Valsalva, that nasal haemorrhage might be arterial in origin for it was his practice to 'syringe the nose with cold water and to apply the spirit of wine, especially to contract the mouths of swollen arteries'.

Mahomed (1880–81) who pioneered the development of the sphygmomanometer stated that 'the frequency with which severe epistaxis occurs in old people with high arterial pressure is striking and for them very fortunate for if their noses did not bleed their brains would'. In 1879, Little published his case reports in the *Hospital Gazette* (Rainey, 1952) in which he identified the site of bleeding as being at the caudal end of the septum, and a year later Kiesselbach made similar observations. However, even after the introduction of modern histological methods, investigations into the mechanism of epistaxis were few and relatively uninformative, so that until recently very little was known about the pathology of nasal blood vessels.

The first attempts at arterial ligation were in 1868 (Bartlett and McKittrick, 1917) when Pilz of Breslau tied the common carotid artery, and it was much later that external carotid ligations were performed for the control of nose bleeds. Seiffert (1928) introduced ligation of the internal maxillary artery via a transantral approach and Goodyear (1937) was the first to tie the anterior ethmoidal artery.

Recent advances in endoscopic and microvascular surgery, laser technology and interventional radiology mean the otolaryngologist now has an extensive treatment armamentarium to offer the patient with epistaxis.

This chapter outlines current thinking on the aetiology and treatment of epistaxis.

Vascular anatomy of the nose

Textbook descriptions of the vascular anatomy of the human nose are largely based on Zuckerkandl's original and comprehensive studies of the subject (1892) and this has been supplemented by the further work of others (Burnham, 1935). A detailed up-to-date account of the vascular supply of the nose is available in the literature (Lund, 1996). The nose is vascularized by the internal and external carotid arteries via their respective branches, there being a confluence of the two systems, particularly at the caudal end of the septum where a number of arteries anastomose with each other (Little's area, 1879; Kiesselbach's plexus, 1880; Stell, 1977).

This classical description of dual blood supply is often stated to be based on Zuckerkandl's work. This is not true. He did not recognize the significance of the supply from the two independent systems but stated that the nasal cavity is supplied by an anterior nasal artery, the sphenopalatine artery and both ethmoidal arteries but that the sphenopalatine artery was the most important and that the other two only supplied collaterals (Stell, 1977).

With the exception of Little's area, the middle turbinate has for a long time been regarded by clinicians as the dividing line between the internal and external carotid distributions, with a corresponding imaginary line of demarcation at the same level on the nasal septum (Weddell *et al.*, 1946). This landmark has served as a guide in deciding which of the two areas is responsible for the epistaxis, and has allegedly helped the surgeon to decide which artery to ligate in severe cases of epistaxis.

The dividing line between the two carotid distributions may not, however, coincide exactly with the level of the middle turbinate. The work of Zuckerkandl (1892) and Burnham (1935) indicates that the blood supply to the middle turbinate is derived exclusively from the external carotid artery and that anastomosis between the two carotid distributions occurs above and anterior to its attachment to the lateral nasal wall, and not within it. They also described an artery inferior to the superior turbinate and meatus, with a corresponding vessel on the septum, both of which originate from the nasopalatine branch of the sphenopalatine artery.

Shaheen (1967) confirmed the presence of a branch from the nasopalatine artery supplying the superior meatus, turbinate and corresponding septum by X-raying the excised nasal fossae of cadavers which had been previously injected with barium–gelatin mixtures (Figure 18.1). It would therefore seem that the area designated as receiving blood from the internal carotid artery is smaller than previously supposed. Certainly the gross disproportion between the diameters of the anterior ethmoidal and sphenopalatine arteries at their points of entry into the nose would corroborate this view. The surgeon who lacerates the anterior ethmoidal artery in an external ethmoidectomy rarely has difficulties with haemorrhage; similarly those who deliberately ligate this vessel for epistaxis are always impressed by its small size. By contrast the terminal segment of the internal maxillary artery is a much larger vessel (Shaheen, 1967) (Figure 18.2). The calibre of the posterior ethmoidal artery is also small, so that its contribution to the nasal blood supply is unlikely to be significant even if it varies reciprocally in size with the anterior ethmoidal vessel as suggested by Batson (1935).

It is noteworthy that the anterior ethmoidal artery was found to be absent unilaterally in 14% of cadaver dissections, and bilaterally in 2.5% of cases, the canal being either imperforate or filled with fibrous tissue or nerves (Shaheen, 1967).

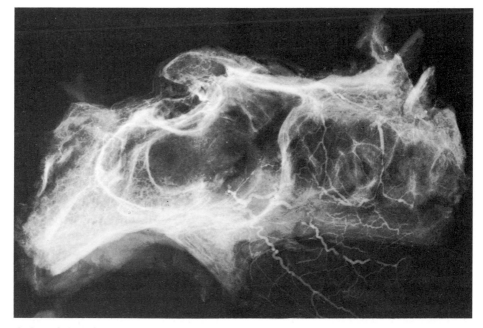

Figure 18.1 The branch from the nasopalatine artery which supplies the superior turbinate and equivalent area of the nasal septum, anastomosing with the arcades formed by the ethmoidal vessels

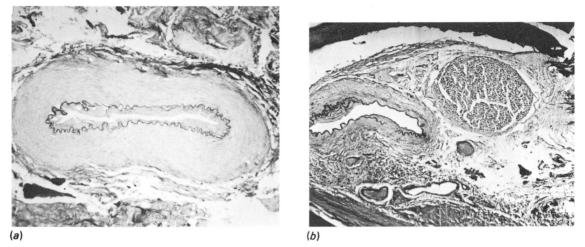

(a) **(b)**

Figure 18.2 (*a, b*) The maxillary artery and anterior ethmoidal neurovascular bundle at their points of entry in the nose (× 80)

This supports the contention that these vessels contribute very little to the blood supply of the nose, even if a somewhat larger posterior ethmoidal artery is found doubling for the missing anterior vessel and running a similar course to it, as sometimes happens. In this connection, the surgeon who sets out to ligate the ethmoidal vessels should be aware that, when the anterior vessel is missing, the posterior ethmoidal artery may arise directly from the circle of Willis and may, therefore, not be encountered in the orbit at all. This arrangement conforms much more to the state of affairs in early embryonic life when the posterior ethmoidal artery is the dominant vessel of the nose, dwarfing not only the anterior ethmoidal artery but the nasopalatine vessel as well (Shaheen, 1967) (Figure 18.3).

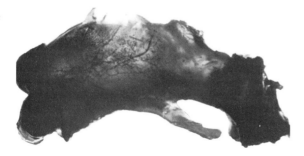

Figure 18.3 The nasal septum of a 3-month-old fetus which has been injected with a silicose elastomer, showing the dominance of the ethmoidal vessels and in particular the posterior ethmoidal artery

Burnham (1935) in his description of the anatomy of the lateral nasal wall claimed that the arteries to the inferior and middle turbinates and their respective branches lay partly embedded in the bone of these structures. In the case of the inferior turbinate, he found the bony canals containing the branches of the inferior turbinate artery extended along the central three-fifths of the bone. The middle turbinate artery and its branches were protected by a bony covering in the posterior half of the concha. Thus a considerable segment of both of these arteries and their branches is unlikely to give rise to epistaxis even if rupture occurs. By the time the arteries have emerged from their bony channels to lie beneath the mucous membrane, they will have diminished considerably in size.

Recent studies on the blood supply to this region (Padgham and Vaughan-Jones, 1991) have confirmed much of Burnham's work (1935). The supply to the middle and inferior turbinates is from the main descending branch of the sphenopalatine artery which is given off in the sphenopalatine foramen (which was also found to be under cover of the middle turbinate rather than behind it). While under cover of the posterior part of the attachment of the middle turbinate, a substantial branch is given off medially to enter the middle turbinate and supply it with anterior and posterior branches running close to the bone. The descending main arterial trunk then passes down to enter the inferior turbinate on the superior aspect of its lateral attachment between 1.0 and 1.5 cm from its posterior tip. Here the artery enters a bony canal, branches into two (upper and lower) which then run forward for much of the turbinate's length. As previously stated by Burnham (1935), frequent large branches are given off to pierce the bone but, despite this, the main artery in the bony canal increases in size as it passes anteriorly suggesting a significant additional anterior arterial anastomosis.

Ogura and Senturia (1949) found in a series of patients with epistaxis that the bleeding point arose on the lateral wall in 28 out of 88 cases, and more recently other authors have similarly implicated the lateral wall as a common site for bleeding (Padgham, 1990). Shaheen (1967), on the other hand, was unable to find any cases of bleeding from the lateral wall of the nose in 117 cases, and his anatomical dissections and serial sections of the nose confirmed the findings of Burnham (1935) (Figure 18.4).

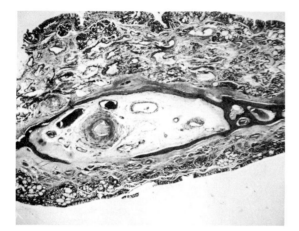

Figure 18.4 The middle turbinate artery in transverse section, encased in its shell of bone (× 25)

The vast majority of patients who suffer from arterial epistaxis bleed from the nasal septum, and chiefly from the area where anastomosis of the nasopalatine, greater palatine, anterior ethmoidal, and coronary arteries takes place (Shaheen, 1967) (Figure 18.5). This plexus was originally described by James Little in 1879 (McKenzie, 1914) and it is important to note that bleeding from it is arterial in origin, and not venous as some reports suggest. The venous bleeding, which is common in young persons, arises from the vein which lies immediately behind the columella at the anterior edge of Little's area. It runs vertically downwards and crosses the floor of the nose obliquely before joining the venous plexus on the lateral wall of the nose.

Other recognized sources of bleeding include haemorrhagic nodules (Padgham and Parham, 1993), the septal turbinate and the naso-nasopharyngeal (Woodruff's) plexus (Woodruff, 1949). Haemorrhagic nodules consist of an aneurysmal dilatation of an unusually sited muscular artery with evidence of hypertensive changes in the wall and thrombus and haemorrhage in the adjacent connective tissue. They may occur in any nasal location and once identified as the source of epistaxis can be dealt with by local excision or cautery.

The septal turbinate represents an area (often visible on CT) of engorged vascular nasal mucosa on the septum. It may be unilateral or bilateral and can be a source of profound epistaxis. Its location may explain why a submucous resection cures some cases of septal epistaxis.

Woodruff's plexus is a collection of rather large blood vessels found in many people in the lateral wall of the inferior meatus posteriorly. These vessels appear to originate from the posterior pharyngeal wall and are venous in origin. They are a well recognized cause of epistaxis which responds to treatment by tamponade.

Vascular physiology of the nose

The vascular physiology of the nose is well documented in the literature (Drake-Lee, 1996).

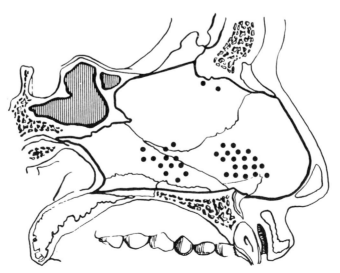

Figure 18.5 Scattergram of bleeding points showing the large number of arterial ruptures which occur in Little's area

The dynamics of the nasal circulation depend to a large extent on the presence of arterioarterial anastomoses between the various arteries which contribute to the vascular supply of the nose. The branches of the anterior and posterior ethmoidal arteries join in a series of arcades in the upper one-third of the nose and the branches of the sphenopalatine artery anastomose with those of the ethmoidal arteries above the level of the middle turbinate. Opposing heads of pressure meet in the anastomoses with a sharp interface between the two, which can be displaced by dropping the pressure in one or other of the opposing systems. Shaheen (1967) demonstrated, by means of dye injections into the carotid vessels of live humans, that the dispersion of dye in the nasal mucous membrane could be affected by dropping the pressure in the system not being injected. For instance, dye injected into the internal carotid artery failed to appear in the nose, confirming the poor circulation of the ethmoidal vessels, but when the external carotid was occluded at the time of injection the entire upper half of the nose was suffused with dye from above downwards (Figure 18.6). The rapidity with which such dye displacement takes place, confirms the importance of the arterioarterial anastomoses within the nose.

The importance of possible anastomoses across the midline also must not be overlooked, either at the nasopharyngeal end or between the two anterior ethmoidal arteries at the crista galli. These observations could well explain the many documented reports of failed ligation in which surgeons assumed, probably incorrectly, that they had tied the wrong vessel simply because bleeding had not stopped after ligation.

The arteriovenous anastomoses which are present at the anterior end of the inferior turbinate and septum at a microscopical level are probably of little importance in the aetiology and persistence of epistaxis, but their precise role remains unclear.

Epidemiology

Epistaxis is extremely common and affects all age groups. Its prevalence in random samples of the population was found in one study to be between 10 and 12% (Shaheen, 1967). Anterior epistaxis is more common in the child or young adult, whereas posterior nasal bleeding is more often seen in the older adult with hypertension or arteriosclerosis. Accordingly, the age distribution in that study showed an increase in frequency between the ages of 15 and 25 years, and later from 45 to 65 years (Figure 18.7) with no evidence of sex predilection (Shaheen, 1967). The incidence of epistaxis is higher during the colder winter months when upper respiratory tract infections are more frequent and fluctuations in both temperature and humidity are most dramatic (Nunez, McClymont and Evans, 1990). It is also more common in hot dry climates with low humidity.

Patients who suffer from rhinosinusitis of whatever cause are more prone to epistaxis because the nasal mucosa is more inflamed and friable. In addition, changes from a cold outside environment to a warm dry one (i.e. housing, car, office, etc.) result in variations of the normal nasal cycle of alternating congestion and decongestion. This in turn leads to sinonasal congestion and infection, engorgement of the nasal mucosa and ultimately epistaxis. The causes of epistaxis are listed in Table 18.1.

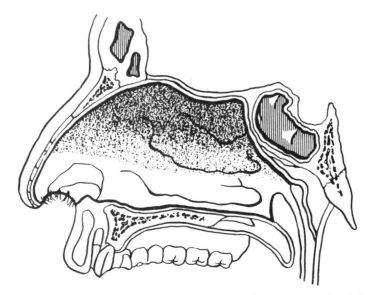

Figure 18.6 Diffusion of dye from above downwards when the internal carotid artery is injected with dye while the external carotid artery is occluded

Table 18.1 Causes of epistaxis

Local

Congenital
  Unilateral choanal atresia
  Meningocoele
  Encephalocoele
  Glioma

Acquired
  Infective
    Acute
      viral
      bacterial
      fungal
    Chronic
      specific
        tuberculosis
        syphilis
        leprosy
        rhinoscleroma
      non-specific   (ozaena)
  Inflammatory
    Rhinosinusitis (allergic/vasomotor),
    nasal polyposis
  Trauma
    Iatrogenic
    Facial trauma
    Foreign body
    Surgery
  Idiopathic
    Little's area
    Superior part of nose
    Middle meatus
    Woodruff's plexus
  Neoplastic
    Benign
      Transitional cell papilloma, angiofibroma, others
    Malignant
      Squamous cell carcinoma, adenocarcinoma, adenoid
      cystic carcinoma, olfactory neuroblastoma,
      melanoma, lymphoma
  Drug-induced
    Rhinitis medicamentosa (topical decongestants/
    cocaine)
  Inhalants
    Tobacco, cannabis, heroin, chrome, mercury,
    phosphorus, wood dust

General

1 *Bleeding disorders*
A Coagulopathies
   (i) inherited   coagulation factor deficiencies, i.e. factor
                    VII (haemophilia A, B) and factor IX
                    deficiency
   (ii) acquired   anticoagulants, liver disease, vitamin K
                    deficiency, disseminated intravascular
                    coagulation (DIC), acquired inhibitor

B Platelet disorders
   (i) Thrombocytopenia   congenital
                            acquired   marrow failure, i.e.
                                        aplasia, drugs,
                                        infiltration
                                        increased
                                        consumption, i.e.
                                        immune, DIC,
                                        hypersplenism.
                                        massive blood loss
   (ii) Platelet dysfunction   congenital
                                 Von Willebrand's disease,
                                 Bernard Soulier syndrome,
                                 Glanzmann's
                                 thrombasthenia
                               acquired
                                 myeloproliferative disease/
                                 leukaemia,
                                 uraemia,
                                 dysparaproteinaemias
                               Drugs: aspirin, NSAIDs
                               Acquired storage pool
                               disease, i.e. bypass

C Blood vessel disorders
   congenital   osteogenesis imperfecta, hereditary
                haemorrhagic telangiectasia
   acquired   amyloid, vasculitis, vitamin C deficiency

D Hyperfibrinolysis
   congenital α_2 antiplasmin deficiency
   acquired   malignancy, DIC, fibrinolytic therapy, i.e.
                streptokinase

2 *Drugs* (see 1B)
   Aspirin
   Anticoagulants
   Chloramphenicol
   Methotrexate
   Immunosuppression
   Alcohol
   Dypyrimadole

3 *Neoplasms* (see 1B)

4 *Idiopathic*
   Inflammatory disorders
   Sarcoidosis
   Wegener's
   Lethal midline granuloma

5 *Others*
   Liver failure
   Hypothyroidism
   HIV

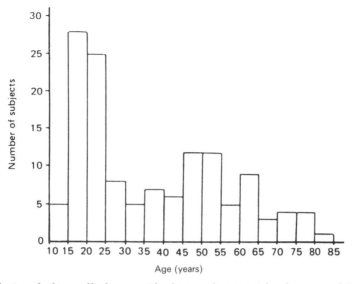

Figure 18.7 Age distribution of subjects of both sexes with a history of epistaxis taken from a population survey

In only a small number of cases can epistaxis be attributed to a well-defined primary cause, such as a blood dyscrasia, a blood vessel abnormality, or local nasal pathology. In the majority of cases bleeding arises from an artery or a vein without any obvious abnormality to account for it; hence the terms 'spontaneous' or 'idiopathic epistaxis' which have been coined to cover this, the xcommonest category of epistaxis.

Certain contributory factors may be implicated in the onset of bleeding in cases of so-called 'spontaneous epistaxis', such as nose blowing, sneezing, coughing, straining, pregnancy and, as stated previously, coryza and sinusitis. They all share one thing in common, namely a sudden rise in vascular pressure.

Venous epistaxis from the retrocolumellar vein tends to occur in subjects under the age of 35 years, whereas arterial epistaxis occurs in the older age groups. The duration of bleeding, as might be expected, is short-lived in venous epistaxis, and quite prolonged in bleeding of arterial origin (Shaheen, 1967) (Table 18.2). Furthermore, there is an inverse relationship between the frequency and duration of epistaxis, the more severe arterial haemorrhages recurring rarely more than once or twice. No correlation can be established between the prevalence of epistaxis in random samples of the population and their blood pressure status (Figure 18.8), although there is some correlation between the severity of epistaxis and the degree of vessel wall disease as judged by retinoscopy (Shaheen, 1967). There is also a correlation between mild or moderate (Padgham. 1990). The finding of a high proportion of subjects with high blood pressures in hospital practice signi-

fies, not that hypertension causes epistaxis, but rather that patients with higher blood pressures have more severe or persistent bleeding and are therefore eligible for admission to hospital.

Table 18.2 The striking difference in duration between venous and arterial epistaxis

	10 minutes or under	Over 10 minutes and under 2 hours	Over 2 hours
Subjects over 35 years	10	18	44
Subjects under 35 years	28	13	4

The pathology of nasal arteries

Examination of the medium and smaller nasal arteries of persons dying in middle and old age has shown that these are subject to a progressive replacement of the muscle tissue in the tunica media by collagen (Shaheen, 1967). This change varies from interstitial fibrosis (Figure 18.9) to almost complete replacement of the muscle by scar tissue (Figure 18.10). It seems that persons giving a history of epistaxis exhibit the more severe changes, but this is not to say that these changes are necessarily responsible for vessel rupture. They could, however, account for the lengthy duration of arterial haemorrhages, presumably because of a failure of the vessel to contract down in the absence of sufficient muscle in the tunica media.

It is also apparent that larger vessels of the calibre of the maxillary artery are prone to calcification (Mönckeberg's sclerosis). The resulting lack of elasticity could well contribute to the pathogenesis of small vessel rupture by the creation of a local systolic hypertension.

The precise mechanism of bleeding is thought to be a dissecting aneurysm of the nasopalatine artery or one of its branches, but the factors initiating this process have, so far, not been identified (Figure 18.11).

It is also a mystery why bleeding should occur from the retrocolumellar vein in young subjects. Careful inspection of the site shortly after a bleed sometimes reveals a tiny area of local ballooning overlying the vein, and this could possibly signify an area of vessel wall weakening, perhaps as a result of localized ischaemia and/or trauma.

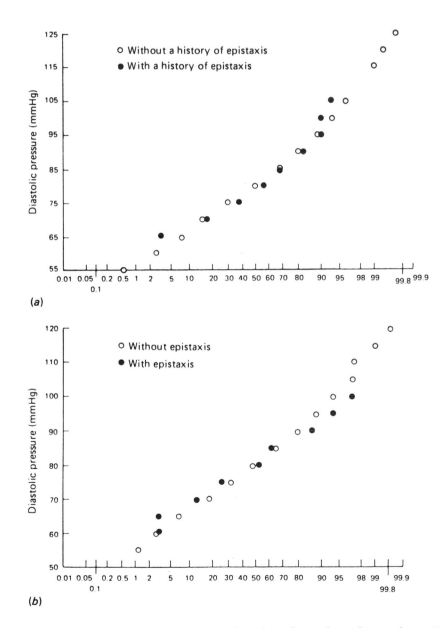

Figure 18.8 (*a, b*) Cumulative distribution of diastolic pressures for males with or without a history of epistaxis taken from two population surveys

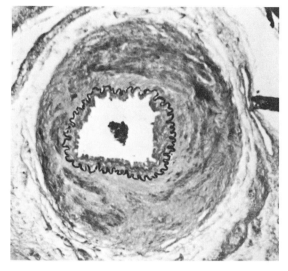

Figure 18.9 Interstitial fibrosis of the tunica media of a nasal artery seen in transverse section (× 110)

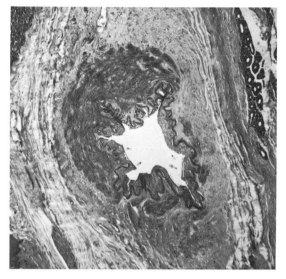

Figure 18.10 Severe segmental loss of muscular tissue with replacement by collagen in the tunica media of a nasal artery seen in transverse section (× 90)

Clinical management of spontaneous epistaxis

The young person with recurrent bleeding

After taking a careful history to establish that the bleeding may not be secondary to systemic disease (and, therefore, warrant further investigation), the nose is carefully examined for signs of recent bleeding and for local abnormalities. Examination should be

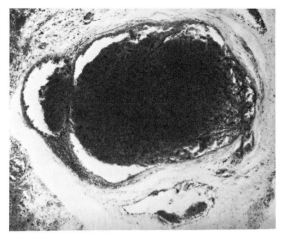

Figure 18.11 Transverse section of the nasopalatine artery to show a dissecting aneurysm (× 120)

as extensive as possible including flexible and rigid endoscopy. In the absence of any obvious local disease, attention is turned to the septum which will often reveal an engorged vein at the anterior end of Little's area just behind the columella. If bleeding has been quite recent, a microaneurysm may be seen in the musosa overlying the vein. Prominent vessels may also be seen within Little's area itself. Subsequent treatment is controversial. Conventionally, topical anaesthesia with 5% cocaine followed by cauterization with a silver nitrate stick and a 7-day course of Naseptin cream has been recommended although recent evidence (Ruddy *et al.*, 1991) suggests that Naseptin given alone for 4 weeks is as effective.

Whichever method is adopted, what is equally important is advising the patient regarding 'nose picking', only blowing one nostril at a time and the use of Vaseline applied to the nasal vestibule and Little's area twice a day indefinitely. Vaseline is supposed to decrease recurrent nose bleeds by keeping the vessels moist thereby preventing them becoming dry and friable. However, what is probably more important is once a child has picked his nose and tasted the Vaseline, he is unlikely to do so again.

The above techniques will usually suffice to control all but the most difficult cases of epistaxis. However, some cases are particularly obstinate and may require more than one application of a caustic agent. In these cases it may be more effective to use trichloro-acetic acid. Great care must be taken to ensure that none of the acid comes into contact with the nasal vestibule, as this will leave a particularly painful burn. There are some patients who bleed in spite of seemingly adequate attempts at cauterization, and the best policy is to coagulate the offending vessel with diathermy under general anaesthesia. Galvano-cautery under local anaesthesia is not to be recommended in children, and even adults may find the experience unpleasant, with the sight of the heated filament, the sensation of heat within the nose, and the smell of charred mucosa.

The adult person with recurrent bleeding

The initial approach to the adult with recurrent epistaxis is similar to that in the child regarding the history and examination. However, it is important in the history to ask about alcohol, current medication and blood pressure problems (Mittelman *et al.*, 1986; Jackson and Jackson, 1988; Watson and Shenoi, 1990) (see Table 18.1). Habitual bleeders should be screened for a bleeding disorder (Beran, Stigendal and Petruson, 1987).

Epistaxis in older persons does not recur with the same frequency as it does in younger people. Some patients only have the one major bleed, and when examined afterwards there may be very little to see. In such cases, there is nothing to be gained by cauterizing Little's area, unless it is certain that bleeding previously originated from this part of the septum.

Assessment of the cardiovascular system is important, however, and the patient should be referred to a physician if any abnormality such as hypertension is discovered. This is not so much to prevent further epistaxis, as to protect the individual from the harmful effects of the raised blood pressure.

Treatment is initially with nasal cautery under local anaesthetic using silver nitrate followed by a week's course of Naseptin. Similar advice is given as to a child regarding nose picking, etc. Treatment by Naseptin alone is not usually effective. A recent study compared electro- and chemical cautery in the treatment of anterior epistaxis and showed both to be equally effective so that chemical cautery is usually the initial mode of treatment used (Toner and Walby, 1990). Resistant cases can be treated by electro-cautery under local anaesthesia but most surgeons favour electrocautery or diathermy under general anaesthesia. Alternative treatments include submucosal resection, transection of varicose vessels (Beran and Petruson, 1986), and diathermy and excision of haemorrhagic nodules. The submucosal resection/septoplasty operation probably works for a number of reasons. These include transection of varicose vessels, interruption of blood supply to haemorrhagic nodules, the septal turbinate, Little's area and the removal of any septal spurs.

Management of acute epistaxis in the young

The management of epistaxis at any age is well summarized by the age-old dictum: resuscitate the patient, establish the site of bleeding, stop the bleeding, treat the cause.

In the young, resuscitation is uncommon in all but the complex cases so that pinching the nostrils is the time-honoured method of stopping venous bleeding from the caudal end of the septum. Once bleeding has ceased, the nose can be cocainized and the offending vessel (venous or arterial) is cauterized. Sometimes the vessel may bleed during this process of applying the caustic agent so that perseverance is required until bleeding finally stops. Advice then follows as for the young person with recurrent bleeding.

Very occasionally, the bleeding persists despite simple measures and this often occurs in children with associated haematological problems. The nose should then be packed and depending on the age of the child, this can be with Vaseline gauze, a BIPP (bismuth iodoform paraffin paste) pack, nasal balloons or calcium sodium alginate (Kaltostat). The latter is particularly useful in the very young since it can be inserted without local anaesthetic, it is relatively atraumatic and is absorbed locally. Similarly, nasal balloons are useful in children due to their ease of insertion (Guarisco and Graham, 1989). Sustained bleeding despite adequate packing should be treated on its merits. Very occasionally postnasal packs, diathermy under general anaesthetic and arterial ligation may be necessary. Specialist advice may also be required regarding haematological replacement therapy (i.e. factor VIII) and subsequent treatment (i.e. desmopressin (DDAVP)) (Brown, 1986).

Management of acute epistaxis in the elderly

Resuscitation becomes a paramount consideration in the elderly patient with epistaxis (Figure 18.12). Observations of pulse, blood pressure, and general condition are made in order to gauge the extent of any blood loss. Subsequent estimation of the packed-cell volume in conjunction with the haemoglobin will guide the clinician as to the need for replacing any blood loss, although early transfusion should be approached with caution (Birzgalis and Saeed, 1991). If a blood dyscrasia is suspected, concurrent investigations of bleeding and clotting times along with a platelet count should be requested.

The nose is examined, preferably with the patient sitting upright in a chair. Proper precautions to avoid HIV contamination should be taken in high risk individuals (see later). A plastic cover is draped around the patient's neck and a bowl placed in the hands. Inspection of the nose may show a spurting blood vessel on the nasal septum, but usually the site of bleeding is smothered in blood. Cocainizing

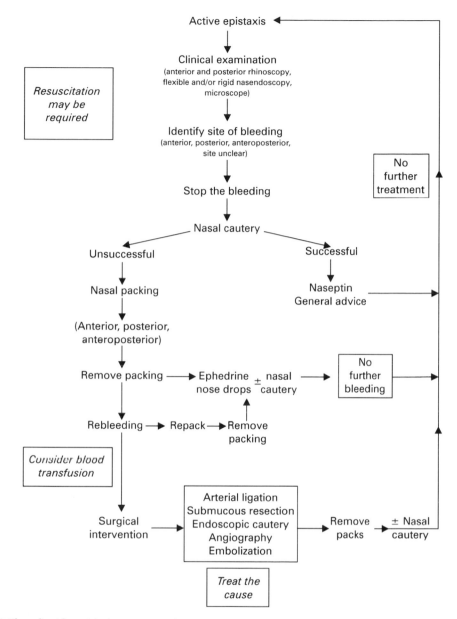

Figure 18.12 Flow chart for epistaxis management

the nose with a 5% spray serves two purposes, namely to allow the introduction of a catheter so that the blood can be sucked away, and to stop bleeding by vasoconstriction. This gives the examiner the opportunity of locating the site of bleeding, but if this has stopped, suspect areas can be gently rubbed with orange sticks loaded with cotton wool in an attempt to cause further bleeding. Formal examination should be completed with the use of flexible nasopharyngoscopy, rigid endoscopes or the

microscope (Borgstein, 1987; Bingham and Dingle, 1991; Nicolaides, Gray and Pfleiderer, 1991).

Any bleeding points are cauterized if accessible but, quite frequently, they are situated far back on the septum or behind a spur so that cauterization is technically impossible. Access posteriorly is greatly improved using the flexible nasopharyngoscope (Premachandra, 1991).

If the bleeding cannot be stopped or recurs, then the nose should be packed.

Patients with epistaxis that require such action should be admitted to hospital. When the bleeding is thought to be anterior (and sometimes it is difficult to be sure), then packing of *both* sides of the nose should be performed. There is currently considerable controversy regarding the choice of nasal packing but Vaseline gauze or ribbon gauze impregnated with the antiseptic BIPP appear to be cheaper and as effective as anything else available at present. Vaseline gauze packs should not be left for longer than 48 hours without antibiotic cover. The advantage of BIPP packing is it can be left undisturbed (without antibiotic cover) for several days without fear of the patient developing complications.

When the bleeding is deemed to be posterior (or both anterior and posterior) then it is advisable to use a balloon catheter, such as a Foley, as an additional postnasal pack. This is inserted along the floor of the nasal cavity on the side of bleeding until the catheter tip is just visible below the soft palate. The balloon is inflated with 15 ml of sterile water or air and then withdrawn to impact at the posterior choana. Deflation can be delayed or prevented by the use of umbilical clamps placed on the catheter at the anterior nares. Dental rolls or similar material should be placed between the clamps and skin to prevent ulceration and scarring. Both nasal cavities are then packed anteriorly as described above. Very occasionally, when the bleeding is severe, bilateral and posterior, Foley catheters can be inserted bilaterally. Although this sounds easy in theory it may be more difficult in practice and usually one Foley catheter will suffice in the first instance.

The old-fashioned method of controlling epistaxis by sitting the patient up with a cork between his teeth (Trotter's method) and allowing him to bleed until he becomes hypotensive is to be condemned. Death from coronary thrombosis secondary to hypotension is a well-recognized complication of epistaxis and regularly appears in the Registrar General's mortality statistics. It must be emphasized that old patients with cardiovascular disease cannot tolerate severe and prolonged blood loss.

Some clinicians prefer to insert an inflatable balloon or packing other than ribbon gauze into the nose. This is because the latter is abrasive to the nasal mucosa and can cause damage during both its insertion and removal. There are many intranasal catheters (along with alternative packing) currently on the market and they are listed in Table 18.3 and shown in Figure 18.13.

Several clinical studies have associated nasal packing in the treatment of epistaxis with a number of complications that range in severity from being an uncomfortable and inconvenient nuisance to causing life-threatening hypoxia (Elwany, Kamel and Mekhamer, 1986). Current dissatisfaction with conventional nasal packing led to the development of pneumatic nasal balloons and it was hoped that these

Table 18.3 List of commonly used products currently available for nasal packing

	Cost*
Vaseline gauze	£1.51
BIPP	£6.50 for 1.25 × 100 cm
Postnasal pack	£1.00
Foley catheter	£0.73
Simpson balloon	£10.00
Brighton balloon	£12.93
Bivona balloon (triple lumen)	£22.75
Kaltostat	2 g cavity dressing (£2.77)
Merocel nasal tampon	4.5 cm (£2.37) 8 cm (£3.00)

*All costs are approximate in 1994

would be associated with increased efficacy and fewer complications. Although there are several balloon catheters on the market, their exact mode of action is unclear. They are supposed to act by neatly occupying the nasal cavity or snugly fitting into the anterior and posterior nasal choanae and many manufacturers actually depict this in their drawings. Given the complexity of nasal anatomy, it is highly unlikely that they work in such a way and indeed recent studies have confirmed this.

McGarry and Aitken (1991) showed that balloons do not conform to the contours of the nasal cavity but expand along pathways of least resistance and prolapse into the nasopharynx. These findings may explain complications such as headache and eustachian tube obstruction. It is unlikely that nasal tamponade is their true mode of action and they probably act by a combination of factors rather than a specific design feature relating to pressure effects.

Despite the claimed advantages of nasal balloons (ease of insertion, less pain, less sedation required, less hypoxia), there seems very little reason to recommend their use over conventional packing with BIPP or Vaseline gauze in the routine case. Balloons are not without their complications, necrosis of nasal mucosa and septum, alar necrosis and respiratory obstruction have all been described, and all balloons are significantly more expensive than conventional treatment. However, they may have their uses in isolated cases as can the less traumatic packing such as Kaltostat (McGlashan *et al.*, 1992) and Merocel. Although there are many balloon catheters on the market (see Figure 18.13), those with a triple lumen are probably the most useful since they combine anterior and posterior compression with a central channel to allow for both breathing and suction.

Postnasal packing may be helpful in those cases where anterior packing alone has failed to control the bleeding. It is particularly indicated in the control

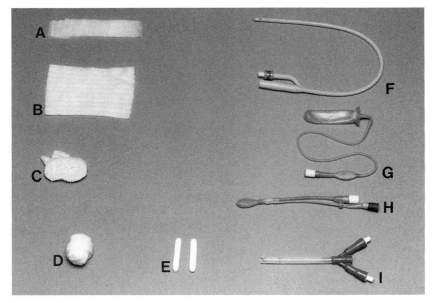

Figure 18.13 Various nasal packs, balloons and catheters currently available to pack the nose: A: Vaseline gauze; B: Kaltostat; C: BIPP pack; D: Postnasal pack; E: Merocel nasal tampons; F: Foley catheter; G: Simpson balloon; H: Brighton balloon; I: Bivona epistaxis catheter (triple lumen)

of haemorrhage following adenoidectomy. It is normally undertaken under general anaesthesia but can be accomplished under local anaesthesia in the cooperative patient. A small catheter is passed through each nostril from anteriorly backwards into the oropharynx. These are then drawn out through the mouth, and tied to two tapes which are secured to the pack. The catheters and attached tapes are then pulled forward through the nose, and tied across a bolster or dental roll which protects the columella. A piece of thread, previously attached to the lower edge of the pack is brought out through the mouth and secured to the cheek with adhesive tape. The anterior nasal cavities can then be packed with BIPP. The patient should be covered with a suitable broad-spectrum antibiotic and, after the bleeding has been controlled for a few days, the anterior packing removed. After cutting the tapes knotted across the columella, the pack can be removed through the open mouth, by pulling downwards on the lower central thread.

After 2–3 days the packing (in whatever form) can be removed and in most instances the bleeding will have stopped completely so that nasal cautery (if required) along with ephedrine nose drops and subsequent general advice is all that is required. If recurrent bleeding occurs, however, the pack will have to be reinserted and antimicrobial therapy commenced. Rebleeding is more common in those patients on aspirin, alcohol and those with elevated blood pressure (Jackson and Jackson, 1988). Patients in this

category, together with those suffering from prolonged epistaxis and who are elderly and/or generally unfit, should always be admitted to hospital. They should be nursed sitting up, given ice to suck and/or an ice pack and they *may* be sedated to allay their anxiety and lower their blood pressure. Sedatives should not, however, be used overzealously since heavy sedation not only increases the risks of confusion but may also allow blood to drip unnoticed into the pharynx, larynx and tracheobronchial tree with the possibility of subsequent bronchopneumonia and its inevitable consequences.

The choice of sedative is a matter of individual preference, but opiates such as Omnopon (morphine) are popular, although they can sometimes cause vomiting. Diazepam either orally or by injection is also effective. When elevated blood pressure is a significant problem, sublingual nifedipine may be helpful. If bleeding persists in spite of adequate anterior and posterior nasal packing, then serious consideration must be given to the need for surgical intervention.

Risk of infection and epistaxis

Patients with epistaxis represent a potential hazard with regard to the spread of hepatitis, HIV and AIDS. The most effective way of controlling the spread of HIV is by means of universal blood and body fluid precautions (HMSO, 1990). Spontaneous epistaxis represents a significant infective risk due to the spraying of large amounts of blood.

Gloves, an apron and eye protection (Euroguard Visor) should all be worn by the health care worker. Disposable suckers and tubing, bibs, aprons and vomit bowls should be used for the patient. It is ideal for an area to be set aside for treatment of patients which is as uncluttered and bare of instruments as possible. A tray of instruments which can be opened, used and cleared away is desirable to prevent contamination of other instruments by dirty gloves. It is preferable for both a nurse and a doctor to be present to give adequate support to the patient and to ensure safety of the treatment area.

Where gloves are worn they should be latex rubber since these have been shown to be more durable than plastic. Euroguard Face Visors are available which cover the eyes, nose and mouth. Smaller spectacles may be better for tracheal suction as only small amounts of blood are likely to be involved and care should be taken not to damage further the patient's image.

In those patients who are HIV positive or who have AIDS, if universal precautions are followed there is no need for any additional precautions to be taken or for patients to be isolated except in cases of uncontrollable blood loss in a confused patient, when a communicable opportunistic infection such as open pulmonary or laryngeal tuberculosis is present or when the patient's immune status requires protective isolation.

Surgical intervention

The patient who continues to bleed every time the pack is removed or when bleeding persists with the pack *in situ* will generally have to be transfused. If, over a period of 4–5 days, bleeding has not stopped or sooner in case of profuse haemorrhage, surgical intervention should be considered. In the absence of definite knowledge about the whereabouts of the bleeding point, it is reasonable to interrupt the external carotid system, since this supplies as much as 90% of the nasal mucosa. Bleeding from the ethmoidal region is in fact very uncommon and is rarely of a severity to merit arterial ligation, in spite of the occasional report describing severe ethmoidal bleeding.

Arterial ligation

Conventionally this has been the method of choice to treat surgically persistent epistaxis. The arteries which can be ligated are the external carotid artery, the internal maxillary artery and the anterior and posterior ethmoidal arteries. Although interruption of the internal maxillary artery has become fashion-able, it is by no means certain that this is necessarily more effective than ligation of the external carotid artery and it is a matter of personal preference which operation is performed.

The drop in local blood pressure which occurs following maxillary artery ligation is greater than that observed following external carotid ligation and this is thought to be due to the fact that the former artery is nearer the source of bleeding. From this, dividing the maxillary artery should, in theory, be more effective, but the drop in pressure almost certainly encourages the displacement of blood from other areas of the nose via arterial anastomoses with the possibility of persistent bleeding.

Pearson, Mackenzie and Goodman (1969) also pointed out that continued haemorrhage after maxillary artery ligation could result from retrograde blood flow by way of arterioarterial anastomoses between branches of the maxillary artery in the pterygopalatine fossa. Such distortions of flow would by-pass the interrupted segment of the maxillary artery thereby contributing to the persistence of haemorrhage. The descending branch of the sphenopalatine artery was particularly singled out as being a possible source of retrograde bleeding into the final portion of the maxillary artery, the theory being that not only should the main trunk be ligated as close to the nose as possible, but that as many branches as possible should be interrupted.

Failure to stop the bleeding is often due to ligation of the non-dominant maxillary artery, failure to identify the maxillary artery in the pterygomaxillary space, blood flow through partially closed clips, bleeding from posterior ethmoidal arteries and revascularization of the nasal blood supply (Metson and Lane, 1988; Premachandra and Sergeant, 1993).

By contrast, ligation of the external carotid artery does not produce quite the same blood pressure reduction distally and is, therefore, less effective in controlling bleeding, although blood flow from the ethmoidal to the nasopalatine areas may, in fact, be less. There is no doubt that external carotid ligation is easier and quicker to perform than maxillary artery ligation so it is often the operation of choice in the elderly and debilitated. If bleeding persists after ligation of the maxillary artery, it is logical to proceed to interruption of the anterior ethmoidal artery with the prospect of arresting the bleeding permanently. The addition of ethmoidal artery ligation to external carotid ligation for persistent haemorrhage is less likely to be as effective, since the cause of the persistent bleeding in this case is probably inadequate drop of pressure in the distal external carotid, rather than displacement of blood from one area of the nose to another. In cases of hypertension, it would be reasonable to ligate the maxillary and anterior ethmoidal arteries empirically at the same sitting. When anterior ethmoidal ligation is performed for protracted, severe and/or recurrent bleeding, it is probably advantageous to carry out posterior ethmoidal ligation at the same time (Strutz and Schumacher, 1990).

Ligation of the internal maxillary artery

This operation is usually performed under general anaesthesia. A sublabial incision is made and then as large an opening as possible is made in the anterior antral wall without compromising the infraorbital nerve. The thin posterior bony wall of the antrum is penetrated with a gouge and removed piecemeal with punch forceps to reveal the underlying periosteum on the posterior wall of the maxilla. This is incised horizontally from side to side and the fat of the ptergyopalatine fossa teased out with long straight artery forceps until the tortuous maxillary artery is seen. The artery is divided between clips as close to the sphenopalatine foramen as possible and clips are placed on any large adjacent branches. The creation of an antrostomy is optional (Shaheen, 1987).

Ligation of the external carotid artery

This is performed through a curved incision which follows one of the skin folds in the neck centred over the bifurcation of the common carotid artery at the upper border of the thyroid cartilage. The deep cervical fascia is divided along its attachment to the sternomastoid muscle so that the carotid sheath can be exposed lying between it and the infrahyoid muscles. The carotid sheath is opened, the carotid bulb identified and the carotid bifurcation can be seen at the upper border of the thyroid cartilage. The hypoglossal nerve should be identified and preserved where it crosses lateral to both arteries having turned round the sternomastoid branch of the postauricular artery. Once the bifurcation has been found, the external carotid artery is identified by one of its branches. The level of the greater cornu of the thyroid bone serves as a useful landmark for the facial and lingual arteries. The external carotid is then ligated in continuity with a 3/0 silk or linen thread to include the ascending pharyngeal artery. The wound is closed in layers with a small vacuum drain (Wright, 1986).

Ligation of the anterior ethmoidal artery

This is performed through an external ethmoidectomy incision. After ligating branches of the angular vein, the incision is continued down to the periosteum which is then incised in the line of the incision. The periosteum is elevated posteriorly, first off the lacrimal fossa, then the lamina papyracea of the ethmoid. The medial orbital periosteum is retracted laterally together with the lacrimal sac and held out of the way by a self-retaining retractor (Talbot or

Kwango). The artery is identified as a funnelling of orbital periosteum into the ethmoid labyrinth at the junction of the medial and superior walls of the orbit about half-way back from the orbital margin. It is coagulated and divided, and the incision closed without drainage. The posterior ethmoidal artery is located 1 cm behind the anterior ethmoidal artery and is dealt with in a similar fashion.

Other methods of treatment

Although other methods of surgical treatment are currently available to treat epistaxis, at present none has been widely evaluated or is generally available so management strategies vary from one centre to another. At present, it seems reasonable to suggest that all patients should be investigated thoroughly (to include fibreoptic, flexible and rigid nasopharyngoscopy) in an attempt to identify and treat conventionally any bleeding site(s). If this fails, then the nose should be packed. Refractory or recurrent bleeding should then be treated either by arterial ligation or other methods of appropriate surgical intervention.

Angiography and embolization

The increasing availability of angiography and subsequent embolization means that this technique is becoming generally recognized as the investigation and treatment of choice for epistaxis due to congenital arteriovenous malformations, aberrant arterial vessels (Figure 18.14), rebleeding after arterial ligation, nasal tumours, facial trauma and intractable cases, particularly those involving posterior epistaxis (Breda *et al.,* 1989; Heeneman, Parnes and Vinuela, 1987; Solomons and Blumgart, 1988; Siniluoto *et al.,* 1993).

Embolization following localization cannot be used for anterior epistaxis since the blood supply to the anterior septum is from the anterior and posterior ethmoidal arteries in most cases (branches of the internal carotid system). There are many advantages to arterial embolization. These include direct visualization of the bleeding site close to the source and the vessel can be occluded close to the site of bleeding which can decrease the effects of collateral blood flow. In addition, the technique is repeatable. In experienced hands the success rate is reported to be 90% or more. Complications occur in less than 0.1%. Possible problems include cerebrovascular accidents and facial nerve paralysis (De Vries *et al.,* 1986). Embolization is contraindicated in the presence of angiographic evidence of significant anastomoses with the internal carotid system, severe atheromatous disease and allergy to contrast material.

Angiography may be performed directly via the

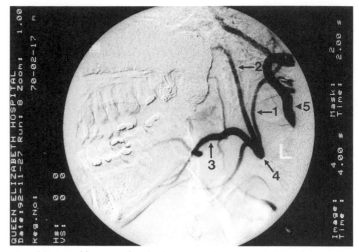

Figure 18.14 Angiogram in a 23-year-old man with refractory secondary epistaxis following functional endoscopic sinus surgery, inferior turbinate reduction and bilateral antral washout. He had undergone a septoplasty 1 year earlier. His epistaxis had persisted despite two attempts at nasal packing under general anaesthetic, left external carotid artery and anterior ethmoidal artery ligation and then right external carotid and left maxillary artery ligation. Four vessel angiography showed ligated right and left external carotid arteries, a substantial left occipitovertebral anastomosis which filled the external carotid artery above the level of ligation. The retrograde flow from this anastomosis indirectly supplied a prominent patent left maxillary artery via the left external carotid artery distal to the site of ligation. 1. Occipital artery; 2. maxillary artery; 3. facial artery; 4. external carotid artery at the site of ligation; 5. vertebral artery. His epistaxis stopped following subsequent surgery ligating the abnormal anastomotic occipital artery and religation higher up of the left external carotid artery. The left maxillary artery was embolized with Spongistan and then ligated and both sphenopalatine foramina were diathermized. (Reproduced with kind permission of Mr A. P. Johnson and the Editor of the *Journal of Laryngology and Otology*)

percutaneous route or indirectly using digital substraction techniques. Materials such as polyvinyl alcohol, Gelfoam particles of different sizes and coiled springs can all be used for embolization. Once the site of bleeding has been identified using direct angiography, embolization may be considered depending on the site of bleeding, presence of anastomoses, atheroma or contrast allergy.

Submucous resection

A submucous resection has long been advocated to treat epistaxis (Shaheen, 1987). This is because there is some evidence to suggest that submucous resection of the septum may be helpful when bleeding originates behind a prominent septal spur, to improve access for inspection, cautery and packing and to interrupt the blood supply to Little's area, haemorrhagic nodules and the septal turbinate. A recent prospective study suggested patients who did not respond to 48 hours of nasal packing were treated more successfully and more economically by submucous resection of the nasal septum than by delayed arterial ligation (Cumberworth, Narula and Bradley, 1991).

Endoscopic cautery and ligation

The advent of endoscopic nasal surgery using rigid endoscopes has facilitated greater diagnostic accuracy regarding bleeding nasal sites and can facilitate both endoscopic cautery, unipolar diathermy or the laser as well as endoscopic ligation of the sphenopalatine artery (Sulsenti, Yanez and Kadiri, 1987; Wurman *et al.*, 1988). The carbon dioxide, argon, potassium titanyl phosphate (KTP), neodymium yttrium-aluminium-garnet (Nd–YAG) and KTP–YAG lasers have all been used (Kluger *et al.*, 1987; Haye and Austad, 1991).

Further evaluation of these techniques in the acute setting is awaited but early results are encouraging and suggest they may have a role in the management of refractory and recurrent epistaxis.

Unusual causes of epistaxis

Many of the unusual causes of epistaxis are listed in Table 18.1. Some of the more familiar ones will be discussed further.

Osler's diseases – haemorrhagic familial telangiectasia

This is a familial autosomal dominant complaint in which sufferers develop prominent telangiectatic formations recognized as red spots on the lips and the mucous membranes of the mouth (especially the tongue) as well as on the face and in the nose.

The defects within the nose are liable to cause severe epistaxis and bleeding is rarely from one site alone. These nasal telangiectases consist of dilated venules located just beneath the basement membrane. They are lined with endothelium without elastic tissue and appear spiderlike, punctate or nodular. The condition may be complicated by the presence of bleeding lesions in the gut, lungs and genitourinary tract.

Recognized treatment modalities have included oestrogens, radiotherapy, diathermy cautery, laser cautery, cryosurgery, microembolization, septal dermoplasty and radical surgery (to include amputation) with reconstruction. Harrison (1957) showed that high doses of oestrogen will lessen the frequency and severity of nose bleeds, probably by inducing a squamous metaplasia of the nasal mucous membrane. However, this treatment is unsuitable in male patients and is not without potential side effects.

Mild cases of epistaxis should be treated using conventional techniques regarding packing and repeated transfusions. Packing should be carried out as atraumatically as possible and Kaltostat can be particularly useful. Laser (argon, KTP or YAG) or diathermy cautery can be used in mild resistant cases. Several treatments may be necessary. Refractory cases can be treated by either oestrogens (in women) or progesterones such as Provera (medroprogesterone acetate) in men and women. Side effects of progesterones are not as severe as oestrogens but can include fluid retention and pruritus. Dosage is usually between 10 and 30 mg but can be increased to 100 mg daily.

More severe cases may require septal dermaplasty where the whole mucous membrane (if appropriate) on one side of the nose can be removed including vestibular skin since this is often the site of troublesome bleeding. Repair is usually with split skin grafted onto the perichondrium or occasionally free flap transfer may be necessary (Bridger and Baldwin, 1990). Using skin may lead to postoperative crusting which can occasionally be troublesome so that buccal mucosa is an acceptable alternative. Septal dermaplasty should be carried out on one side of the nose at a time to avoid septal necrosis.

An alternative to septal dermaplasty for intractable epistaxis is Young's procedure (Young, 1967; Brooker and Cinnamond, 1991). This is bilateral nasal closure which stops bleeding by preventing repeated nasal trauma. Early results are encouraging, not only for patients with Osler's disease but for those with severe epistaxis from other causes such as chronic atrophic rhinitis and large septal perforations. Complete closures can be reopened eventually with a good outcome and in some cases partial openings remain as a satisfactory result (Shah *et al.*, 1974). Some workers have now suggested that Young's procedure should be the treatment of choice for severe refractory epistaxis in Osler's disease (V. Lund, personal communication).

Radiotherapy is also successful for a time in controlling nose bleeds but is rarely used nowadays.

Haemorrhage in this condition may sometimes be severe and may require repeat transfusions to keep up with the blood loss. In some patients the disease runs a relatively mild course, whereas in others it may become increasingly debilitating, with the development of chronic anaemia and hypertension.

Bleeding diatheses

Epistaxis may be a manifestation of a clotting defect, increased fragility of capillaries, or a deficiency in platelets. The possible causes of these and other conditions are outlined in Table 18.1. A history of prolonged bleeding after trauma or dental extraction is suggestive as is bruising or bleeding into joints. When suspected, the patient should have a full clinical examination and a careful search made for signs of purpura, bruising and swollen joints; a Hess's test and platelet count are carried out and the bleeding and clotting times are measured. If required, specific tests for coagulation factor deficiencies can be performed to rule out Christmas disease and haemophilia. In elderly patients Waldenstrom's macroglobulinaemia should be excluded. Early referral to a haematologist is recommended.

Treatment depends to a large extent on the individual case of the blood dyscrasia, but in the short term, blood transfusion is often necessary. Particular caution should be exercised in packing the nose of patients with bleeding diatheses as clumsy handling will result in trauma to the mucous membranes, leading to further haemorrhage so that in these situations nasal packing can do more harm than good. This is particularly true in children where Kaltostat may be extremely useful.

Nasopharyngeal angiofibroma

This condition arises in male adolescents and is thought to be a vascular malformation. It is characterized by severe epistaxis resulting in anaemia, local sepsis and general debility. The diagnosis is confirmed by anatomical imaging (MRI if possible) followed by arteriography. The correct treatment is surgical removal either using an external incision or, preferably, the midfacial degloving technique (Howard, 1992). Embolization may be helpful prior to treatment and in the recurrent case.

Acknowledgement

I would like to acknowledge freely the help and assistance Mr Omar Shaheen has given me in the preparation of this chapter and for his kind permission to reproduce Figures 18.1–18.11 and Table 18.2.

References

BARTLETT, W. and MCKITTRICK, O. F. (1917) A study of secondary haemorrhage treated by ligation of the common carotid cartery. *Annals of Surgery*, **65**, 715–719

BATSON, O. V. (1935) Anatomical anomalies of importance to otolaryngologists. *Annals of Otology, Rhinology and Laryngology*, **44**, 939–947

BERAN, M. and PETRUSON, B. (1986) Transection of varicose vessels in the nasal mucosa of patients with recurrent epistaxis. A 2-year follow-up. *Clinical Otolaryngology*, **11**, 369–372

BERAN, M., STIGENDAL, L. and PETRUSON, B. (1987) Haemostatic disorders in habitual nose-bleeders. *Journal of Laryngology and Otology*, **101**, 1020–1028

BINGHAM, B. and DINGLE, A. F. (1991) Endoscopic management of severe epistaxis. *Journal of Otolaryngology*, **20**, 442–443

BIRZGALIS, A. R. and SAEED, S. (1991) The effect of early blood transfusion on severe epistaxis. *Clinical Otolaryngology*, **16**, 501–503

BORGSTEIN, J. A. (1987) Epistaxis and the flexible nasopharyngoscope. *Clinical Otolaryngology*, **12**, 49–51

BREDA, S. D., CHOI, I. S., PERSKY, M. S. and WEISS, M. (1989) Embolisation in the treatment of epistaxis after failure of internal maxillary artery ligation. *Laryngoscope*, **99**, 809–813

BRIDGER, G. P. and BALDWIN, M. (1990) Microvascular free flap in hereditary hemorrhagic telangiectasia. *Archives of Otolaryngology – Head and Neck Surgery*, **116**, 85–87

BROOKER, D. S. and CINNAMOND, M. J. (1991) Young's procedure in the treatment of epistaxis. *Journal of Laryngology and Otology*, **105**, 847–848

BROWN, O. E. (1986) The use of desmopressin in children with coagulation disorders. *International Journal of Paediatric Otorhinolaryngology*, **11**, 301–305

BURNHAM, H. H. (1935) Anatomical investigations of blood vessels of lateral nasal wall and their relation to turbinates and sinuses. *Journal of Laryngology and Otology*, **50**, 569–593

CUMBERWORTH, V. L., NARULA, A. A. and BRADLEY, P. J. (1991) Prospective study of two management strategies for epistaxis. *Journal of the Royal College of Surgeons of Edinburgh*, **36**, 259–260

DE VRIES, N., VERSLUIS, R. J. J., VALK, J. and SNOW, G. B. (1986) Facial nerve paralysis following embolization for severe epistaxis. *Journal of Laryngology and Otology*, **100**, 207–210

DRAKE-LEE, A. B. (1996) The physiology of the nose and paranasal sinuses. In: *Scott-Brown's Otolaryngology*, 6th ed, vol. 1, edited by M. Gleeson. Oxford: Butterworth-Heinemann. Ch. 6

ELWANY, S., KAMEL, T. and MEKHAMER, A. (1986) Pneumatic nasal catheters: advantages and drawbacks. *Journal of Laryngology and Otology*, **100**, 641–647

GOODYEAR, H. M. (1937) Nasal haemorrhage: ligation of anterior ethmoidal artery. *Laryngoscope*, **47**, 97–99

GUARISCO, J. L. and GRAHAM, H. D. (1989) Epistaxis in children: causes, diagnosis, and treatment. *Ear, Nose and Throat Journal*, **68**, 522–538

HARRISON, D. F. N. (1957) Familial haemorrhagic telangiectases: a survey of a series treated by oestrogen therapy. *Journal of Laryngology and Otology*, **71**, 577–596

HAYE, R. and AUSTAD, J. (1991) Hereditary hemorrhagic teleangiectasia – argon laser. *Rhinology*, **29**, 5–9

HEENEMAN, H., PARNES, L. S. and VINUELA, F. (1987) Percutaneous embolization for control of nasal blood circulation. *Laryngoscope*, **97**, 1312–1315

HIPPOCRATES. Translation by JONES, W. H. S. (1923–1931) *Aphorisms V*, 33, 4, 167. *Airs, Waters and Places IV*, 1, 79. London: Wellcome Historical Museum

HMSO (1990) *Guidance for Clinical Health Workers: Protection Against Infection with HIV and Hepatitis viruses*. Recommendations of the expert advisory Group on AIDS. London: HMSO

HOWARD, D. J. (1992) Mid-facial degloving technique (sublabial approach) for nasal and paranasal sinus resection. In: *Rob and Smith's Operative Surgery*, 4th edn. Head and Neck (Part 2), edited by I.A. McGregor and D.J. Howard. Oxford: Butterworth-Heinemann. pp. 571–575

IBN RABBAN AL-TABIRI, A. (AD 850) *Paradise of Wisdome*, book 4, maquala 3, chapter 9

JACKSON, K. R. and JACKSON, R. T. (1988) Factors associated with active, refractory epistaxis. *Archives of Otolaryngology – Head and Neck Surgery*, **114**, 862–865

KLUGER, P. B., SHAPSHAY, S. M., BOHIGIAN, R. K. and HYBELS, R. L. (1987) Neodymium-YAG laser intranasal photocoagulation in heriditary hemorrhagic telangiectasia: an update report. *Laryngoscope*, **97**, 1397–1401

LUND, V. J. (1996) Anatomy of the nose and paranasal sinuses. In: *Scott-Brown's Otolaryngology*, 6th edn, vol. 1, edited by M. Gleeson, Oxford: Butterworth-Heinemann. Ch. 5

MCGARRY, G. W. and AITKEN, D. (1991) Intranasal balloon catheters: how do they work? *Clinical Otolaryngology*, **16**, 388–392

MCGLASHAN, J. A., WALSH, R., DAUOD, A., VOWLES, A. and GLEESON, M. J. (1992) A comparative study of calcium sodium alginate (Kaltostat) and bismuth tribromophenate (xeroform) packing in the management of epistaxis. *Journal of Laryngology and Otology*, **106**, 1067–1071

MCKENZIE, D. (1914) Little's area of a locus Kiesselbachi. *Journal of Laryngology and Otology*, **29**, 21

MAHOMED, F. A. (1880–81) Chronic Bright's disease without albuminuria. *Guy's Hospital Reports*, **25**, 295–416

METSON, R. and LANE, R. (1988) Internal maxillary artery ligation for epistaxis: an analysis of failures. *Laryngoscope*, **98**, 760–764

MITTELMAN, M., LEWINSKI, U., OGARTEN, U. and DJALDETTI, M. (1986) Dipyridamole-induced epistaxis. *Annals of Otology, Rhinology and Laryngology*, **95**, 302–303

MORGAGNI, J. B. (1769) *The Seats and Causes of Diseases Investigated by Anatomy* (1761). Translated by Alexander, B. Letter XIV. Articles 24, 23, 25. London: Wellcome Historical Museum. Book 1, pp. 336–340

NICOLAIDES, A., GRAY, R. and PFLEIDERER, A. (1991) A new approach to the management of acute epistaxis. *Clinical Otolaryngology*, **16**, 59–61

NUNEZ, D. A., MCCLYMONT, L. G. and EVANS, R. A. (1990) Epistaxis: a study of the relationship with weather. *Clinical Otolaryngology*, **15**, 49–51

OGURA, J. H. and SENTURIA, B. H. (1949) Epistaxis. *Laryngoscope*, **59**, 743–763

PADGHAM, N. (1990) Epistaxis: anatomical and clinical correlates. *Journal of Laryngology and Otology*, **104**, 308–311

PADGHAM, N. P. and PARHAM, D. M. (1993) Haemorrhagic nasal nodules. *Clinical Otolaryngology*, **18**, 118–120

PADGHAM, N. and VAUGHAN-JONES, R. (1991) Cadaver studies of the anatomy of arterial supply to the inferior turbinates. *Journal of the Royal Society of Medicine*, **84**, 728–730

PEARSON, B. W., MACKENZIE, R. G. and GOODMAN, W. S. (1969) The anatomical basis of transantral ligation of the maxillary artery in severe epistaxis. *Laryngoscope*, **79**, 969–984

PREMACHANDRA, D. J. (1991) Management of posterior epistaxis with the use of the fibreoptic nasolaryngoscope. *Journal of Laryngology and Otology*, **105**, 17–19

PREMACHANDRA, D. J. and SERGEANT, R. J. (1993) Dominant maxillary artery as a cause of failure in maxillary artery ligation for posterior epistaxis. *Clinical Otolaryngology*, **18**, 42–47

RAINEY, J. J. (1952) James Lawrence Little, forgotten pioneer. *Archives of Otolaryngology*, **55**, 451–452

RUDDY, J., PROOPS, D. W., PEARMAN, K. and RUDDY, H. (1991) Management of epistaxis in children. *International Journal of Paediatric Otorhinolaryngology*, **21**, 139–142

SEIFFERT, A. (1928) Unterbindung der arteria maxillaris interna. *Zeitschrift für Hals-Nasen und Ohrenheilkunde*, **22**, 323–325

SHAH, J. T., KARNIK, P. P., CHITALE, A. R. and NADKARNI, M. S. (1974) Partial or total closure of the nostrils in atrophic rhinitis. *Archives of Otolaryngology*, **100**, 196–198

SHAHEEN, O. H. (1967) Epistaxis in the Middle-Aged and Elderly. *Thesis*. London: University of London

SHAHEEN, O. H. (1987) Epistaxis. In: *Scott Brown's Otolaryngology*, 5th edn, vol. 4, edited by I. S. MacKay and T. R. Bull. London: Butterworths. pp. 272–282

SINILUOTO, T. M. J., LEINONEN, A. S. S., KARTTUNEN, A. I., KARJALAINEN, H. K. and JOKINEN, K. E. (1993) Embolization for the treatment of posterior epistaxis. *Archives of Otolaryngology – Head and Neck Surgery*, **119**, 837–838

SOLOMONS, N. B. and BLUMGART, R. (1988) Severe late-onset epistaxis following le Fort 1 osteotomy: angiographic localization and embolization. *Journal of Laryngology and Otology*, **102**, 260–263

STELL, P. M. (1977) Epistaxis. A review. *Clinical Otolaryngology*, **2**, 263–273

STRUTZ, J. and SCHUMACHER, M. (1990) Uncontrollable epistaxis. *Archives of Otolaryngology – Head and Neck Surgery*, **116**, 697–699

SULSENTI, G., YANEZ, C. and KADIRI, M. (1987) Recurrent epistaxis: microscopic endonasal clipping of the sphenopalatine artery. *Rhinology*, **25**, 141–142

TONER, J. G. and WALBY, A. P. (1990) Comparison of electro and chemical cautery in the treatment of anterior epistaxis. *Journal of Laryngology and Otology*, **104**, 617–618

WATSON, M. G. and SHENOI, P. M. (1990) Drug-induced epistaxis? *Journal of the Royal Society of Medicine*, **83**, 162–164

WEDDELL, G., MACBETH, R. G., SHARP, H. S. and CALVERT, C. A. (1946) The surgical treatment of severe epistaxis in relation to the ethmoidal arteries. *British Journal of Surgery*, **33**, 387–392

WOODRUFF, G. H. (1949) Cardiovascular epistaxis and the naso-nasopharyngeal plexus. *Laryngoscope*, **59**, 1238–1247

WRIGHT, D. (1986) Ligature of the external carotid artery. In: *Rob and Smith's Operative Surgery*, 4th edn, edited by J.C. Ballantyne and D.F.N. Harrison. London: Butterworths pp. 397–399

WURMAN, L. H., SACK, J. G., PAULSON, T. O. and FLANNERY, J. V. (1988) 'How I Do It' – selective endoscopic electrocautery for posterior epistaxis. *Laryngoscope*, **98**, 1348–1349

YOUNG, A. (1967) Closure of the nostrils in atrophic rhinitis. *Journal of Laryngology and Otology*, **81**, 515–524

ZUCKERKANDL, E. (1892) *Normale und Pathologische Anatomie der Nasenhöhle*. Leipzig: W. Braumuller

19

Snoring and sleep apnoea

Charles B. Croft and Michael B. Pringle

As long ago as 1836 Charles Dickens observed the association between obesity and daytime sleepiness in his description of Joe the servant boy in the *Pickwick Papers*. In 1889 William Hill described this association and added to it the symptoms of snoring and restless sleep (Hill, 1889). Osler recorded the syndrome in his text book of medicine in 1906 but it was not until 1956 that Burwell coined the phrase the 'Pickwickian syndrome' describing obesity, hypersomnolence, alveolar hypoventilation and cor pulmonale. The 1950s saw a great increase in sleep research and by 1960 sleep stages had been described with recognition of rapid eye movement (REM) sleep, non-REM sleep and characteristic EEG patterns. In 1965 Gastaut related the findings in the Pickwickian syndrome to sleep and demonstrated that apnoeic episodes occurred which were related to episodic upper airway obstruction (Gaustat, Tassinari and Duran, 1965). The sleep apnoea syndrome was described by Guilleminault, Eldridge and Dement in 1973 and it was this group in Stamford who established one of the first sleep clinics for the investigation of patients with sleep complaints. Since that time there has been a burgeoning interest in sleep-related disorders. This is well illustrated by the fact that between 1975 and 1992 there have been 3222 papers on the subject of 'sleep apnoea' and that in the USA there is now a dedicated board-certified sleep disorder specialist known as a clinical polysomnographer. Chest physicians, cardiologists, neurologists, anaesthetists, maxillofacial surgeons and otolaryngologists can all be involved in the investigation and treatment of patients with sleep apnoea, but unfortunately at the present time communication between these specialties is sometimes limited.

Definitions

Snoring: a noise generated from the upper airway due to partial upper airway obstruction.

An apnoea is the cessation of airflow at the nostrils and mouth for at least 10 seconds.

The apnoea index [AI] is the number of apnoeas per hour of sleep.

An hypopnoea is a reduction in tidal volume. There is disagreement as to the exact definition of an hypopnoea. Gould *et al.* (1988) suggest it is a 50% reduction in thoracoabdominal movement lasting for 10 seconds in the presence of continued air flow. However, some authors describe it as a decrease in airflow associated with oxygen desaturation (Block *et al.*, 1979; Guilleminault *et al.*, 1984).

The sleep apnoea syndrome (SAS): 30 or more apnoeic episodes during a 7-hour period of sleep or an apnoea index equal to or greater than 5. This is an arbitrary definition and, with increasing experience of the condition, others have suggested that an apnoea index of 10 (Lavie, Ben-Yousef and Rubin, 1984; Shore and Millman, 1984; Fletcher *et al.*, 1985) or an 'apnoea + hypopnoea' index of 15 (Gould *et al.*, 1988) should be present before diagnosing the sleep apnoea syndrome.

The American Sleep Association grade sleep apnoea as follows:

- Mild = 5–20 apnoeas per hour
- Moderate = 20–40 apnoeas per hour
- Severe = > 40 apnoeas per hour.

There are two very distinct types of sleep apnoea: central sleep apnoea and obstructive sleep apnoea. Some apnoeic episodes will exhibit elements of both types and are thus known as mixed apnoeas.

Obstructive sleep apnoea: the cessation of airflow in the presence of continued respiratory effort.

Central sleep apnoea: no flow of air at the nose or mouth associated with a cessation of all respiratory effort. These patients may or may not snore. It is not abnormal to see short-lived central apnoeas in drowsy patients who are going to sleep or in REM sleep. Central apnoeas may be seen in patients with heart failure, frontal lobe damage or brain-stem lesions. Often no apparent cause for the central apnoea can be found and it is thought to be related to an instability of the respiratory control mechanisms.

Mixed apnoea: this usually begins as a central type of apnoea with no airflow or respiratory effort followed by increasingly forceful respiratory efforts again with no airflow until the airway clears.

Obstructive apnoea is far more common than central apnoea though any individual may demonstrate one or more of the above forms of apnoea during a night's sleep.

High upper airways resistance syndrome: this group of patients have episodes of marked partial upper airway obstruction but do not actually completely obstruct the airway. They are able to maintain their oxygen saturation but need so much respiratory effort to overcome the partial obstruction that they induce frequent microarousals. They will not be picked up on simple pulse oximetry screening or limited polysomnography yet they may have considerable cardiovascular strain from the excessive and prolonged respiratory effort and are likely to suffer marked daytime sleepiness (Stoohs and Guilleminault, 1990).

Nocturnal hypoventilation and hypoxia: some patients with a normal respiratory rhythm and no apnoeic episodes hypoventilate at night and in those with a pre-existing hypoxia from pulmonary or cardiac disorders this can lead to significant arterial desaturation. Chronic obstructive airway disease, pulmonary fibrosis, cystic fibrosis and respiratory muscle weakness due to myasthenia gravis, polio or Guillain-Barré syndrome should all be excluded.

Prevalence

In a study of almost 6000 Italians, Lugaresi found that 24% of men and 14% of women were 'habitual snorers'. With respect to age only 10% of men under 30 snored compared with 60% of men over 60. More than half of the patients who weighed 15% over ideal body weight developed 'habitual snoring' (Lugaresi *et al.*, 1980). A recent American survey looking at a random sample of 602 adults aged 30–60 years found that overall 24% of men and 9% of women had an apnoea–hypopnoea score of greater than 5. With respect to the middle-aged workforce the figures were 4% of men and 2% of women (Young *et al.*, 1993). Others have found similar prevalence figures for mild obstructive sleep apnoea (Cirignotta *et al.*, 1989; Stradling and Crosby, 1991). The prevalence of moderate to severe obstructive sleep apnoea is about 2% of men (Lavie, 1983) and the prevalence of severe obstructive sleep apnoea is about 0.3% of men in the 35–65 age group (Gislason, 1988a; Stradling and Crosby, 1991). In the UK this

would mean about 36 000 people with severe obstructive sleep apnoea.

At present because of the lack of normative data the dividing line between 'normal' and what should be considered obstructive sleep apnoea remains unclear.

Aetiology and pathophysiology

It is not fully understood why people snore or develop upper airway obstruction. Male sex, increasing age and obesity are all well recognized associations. Both conditions are exacerbated by alcohol and sedative medication.

The pathophysiology of snoring and obstructive sleep apnoea is determined by a number of interrelated factors (Figure 19.1). The onset of inspiration triggers a reflex increase in the EMG activity of the pharyngeal dilator muscles (e.g. genioglossus, geniohyoid, palatoglossus, medial pterygoids) (Mathur *et al.*, 1992). These muscles are activated rhythmically during daytime respiration (Sauerland and Mitchell, 1975) and hold the airway open preventing collapse. In common with other skeletal muscles they become hypotonic during sleep, especially REM sleep. However, in patients with obstructive sleep apnoea EMG activity is further decreased during an obstructive episode and can sometimes completely disappear (Sauerland and Harper, 1976; Guilleminault *et al.*, 1978). Any excessive reduction in upper airway muscle tone or any incoordination between reflex EMG activity in these muscles and onset of inspiration results in an increased susceptibility of the upper airway to collapse.

Upper airway resistance is determined by the diameter of the airway which in turn is dependent on the patient's craniofacial morphology and any anatomical defects or space-occupying lesions. Anything narrowing the airway will increase the resistance. In order to pull air through the narrowing greater respiratory effort will be needed resulting in the generation of a higher negative intraluminal pressure which, in turn, encourages collapse. Increased compliance of the pharyngeal tissues results in collapse at a lower negative pressure.

As the airway narrows so the rate of airflow through it increases and, on the basis of the Venturi principle, there is a further drop in the intraluminal pressure again encouraging collapse.

Any space-occupying lesion from the nasal vestibule to the glottis can predispose to obstructive sleep apnoea (Table 19.1). Despite this long list of causes most adult patients with obstructive sleep apnoea have no evident predisposing abnormality (Rivlin *et al.*, 1984). It is probably the case that most patients with snoring and obstructive sleep apnoea, while not having obvious skull base and facial skeletal anomalies, have more subtle anatomical variations which

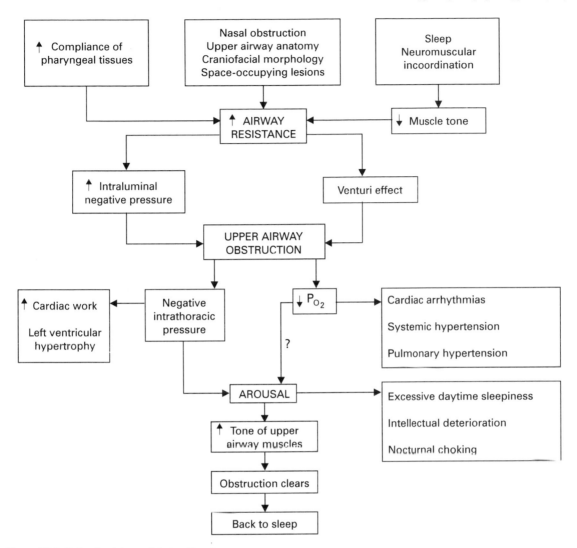

Figure 19.1 Pathophysiology of obstructive sleep apnoea

means that they fall at one end of the normal distribution of pharyngeal dimensions. Studies of patients with obstructive sleep apnoea using CT scanning would seem to confirm this theory (Crumley, Stein and Gamsu, 1987; Bohlman, Haponik and Smith, 1983).

The clinical features and complications (see Table 19.2) associated with the obstructive sleep apnoea syndrome essentially result from the two main effects of the obstructive episode. These effects are:

1 Oxygen desaturation
2 The generation of high negative intrathoracic pressures.

Hypoxia

During an apnoeic episode no air flows into the lungs, thus if the episode is long enough the patient will become hypoxic and hypercapnic. The degree of hypoxia will be determined by the duration of the apnoeic event, lung volume (which is reduced in obesity) and any coexistent neuromuscular or cardiopulmonary disorders.

Hypoxia is associated with a rise in sympathetic output (Hedner *et al.*, 1988) and catecholamine production (Fletcher *et al.*, 1987) and the resulting peripheral vasoconstriction causes transient pulmonary and systemic hypertension. However, the relationship

Table 19.1 Causes of obstructive sleep apnoea

Nose
Nasal polyps
Deviated nasal septum
Rhinitis
Nasal packing

Pharynx
Nasopharyngeal tumour
Enlarged adenoids
Enlarged palatal tonsils
Enlarged lingual tonsils
Retropharyngeal mass
Large tongue
   myxoedema
   acromegaly
Micrognathia/retrognathia
Obesity

Larynx
Tumours
Oedema
Shy-Drager syndrome

between night-time hypoxia and established systemic hypertension is controversial (Shiner *et al.*, 1990). Long-standing pulmonary hypertension was thought to develop only in patients with coexisting chronic obstructive airways disease (Krieger *et al.*, 1989) but, recently, it has been found in patients without respiratory problems (Laks, Krieger and Podszus, 1992).

Hypoxia can cause a variety of cardiac arrhythmias which range from bradycardias to ventricular ectopics. During an obstructive episode the effort of trying

Table 19.2 Clinical features of obstructive sleep apnoea syndrome

Common
Snoring
Excessive daytime sleepiness
Obstructive episodes

Less common
Morning headaches
Personality change
Intellectual deterioration
   poor memory
   difficulty in concentrating
Abnormal body movements
Frequent waking
Nocturnal choking
Nocturnal enuresis
Impotence
Systemic hypertension
Pulmonary hypertension
Right heart failure
Cardiovascular mortality

to inspire against a closed glottis results in increased vagal activity with subsequent bradycardia. The presence of hypoxia significantly worsens this bradycardia (Zwillich *et al.*, 1982; Shepard, Garrison and Grither, 1985).

Polycythaemia associated with prolonged hypoxia is thought to develop only in patients with coexistent daytime oxygen desaturations (Stradling and Lane, 1983).

Negative intrathoracic pressure

Arousals

The efforts of the respiratory system to overcome upper airway obstruction result in the generation of high negative intrathoracic pressures. The main symptomatic consequence of these high negative pressures is that they stimulate arousals and the termination of an obstructive episode is thought to depend heavily on arousal (Phillipson and Sullivan, 1978; Remmers *et al.*, 1978). Despite a number of human and animal studies the place of hypoxia or hypercapnia as mechanisms for arousal remains unclear. It was thought that arousal was caused by hypoxia stimulating carotid body receptors or hypercapnia stimulating CNS receptors. However, it is now recognized that obstructive episodes can result in arousal without there being any associated hypoxia or hypercapnia. Recent studies suggest that the main factor producing arousal is the high level of negative intrathoracic pressure generated by increased respiratory effort associated with airway obstruction (Vincken *et al.*, 1987; Gleeson, Zwillich and White, 1990; Gleeson and Zwillich, 1992). Hypoxia and hypercapnia will contribute to this by stimulating increased ventilatory effort. When the degree of inspiratory effort reaches a certain threshold in a given subject, arousal occurs, resulting in a return of tone to the upper airway muscles and the obstruction clears. The patient is often unaware of these arousals which can occur many hundreds of times throughout the night. The effect of repeated arousals is a very disturbed sleep pattern which is reflected in the symptom of excessive daytime sleepiness, one of the commonest symptoms of obstructive sleep apnoea.

Excessive daytime sleepiness also occurs in patients with higher upper airways resistance syndrome and in some patients who snore loudly without any obstructive episodes. Presumably these patients are generating sufficiently high negative intrathoracic pressures from their partial obstruction to stimulate arousals frequently enough during the night to disturb sleep.

The threshold for arousal is elevated during REM sleep such that obstructive episodes are more prolonged and severe during this sleep stage.

Cardiovascular consequences

The generation of high negative intrathoracic pressures has cardiovascular consequences. The heart has to work hard to pump against these subatmospheric pleural pressures as well as against an increased pulmonary and systemic arterial resistance. The dilating force on the heart will tend to aspirate venous blood into the right heart but, at the same time, increase the preload of the left heart and there is evidence that the heart enlarges during an obstructive episode (Lugaresi, Cirignotta and Coccanga, 1984). However, cardiac output falls during an obstructive episode, mainly as a result of the bradycardia (Guilleminault *et al.*, 1986). When the obstruction clears and the negative pressure is released the heart will continue to pump against a high peripheral resistance until this also returns to normal. Whether these events have any permanent effect on cardiovascular function is unknown but, clearly, for this excessive workload to continue throughout the night is extremely abnormal. In some patients left ventricular wall thickening has been observed (Hedner, Ejnell and Caidahl, 1990). The increase in cardiac work may be reflected in ischaemic changes sometimes seen on ECG recordings during obstructive episodes.

There is a high prevalence of hypertension among patients with obstructive sleep apnoea reaching above 40% in some studies (Guilleminault, Tilkian and Dement, 1976). Similarly the prevalence of sleep apnoea among hypertensive patients ranges between 26% and 47% (Kales *et al.*, 1984; Lavie, Ben-Yousef and Rubin, 1984; Fletcher *et al.*, 1985; Williams *et al.*, 1985) which is much higher than the prevalence of sleep apnoea in the general population. However, it is still unknown whether this relationship between obstructive sleep apnoea and hypertension is causative or due to associated factors such as age, obesity (Jeong and Dimsdale, 1989; Hoffstein, Chan and Slutsky, 1991; Levinson and Milliman, 1991) or antihypertensive medication (Warley, Mitchell and Stradling, 1988). The most serious consequence of untreated obstructive sleep apnoea is increased cardiovascular morbidity and mortality. This is the reason why it is so important to exclude or establish the diagnosis. A long-term study by He *et al.* (1988) found that untreated patients with obstructive sleep apnoea with an apnoea index of > 20 had an 8-year cumulative probability of survival of 63% compared with a probability of survival of 96% in those with an apnoea index of < 20. None of the patients treated with nasal continuous positive airway pressure or tracheostomy died and interestingly uvulopalatopharyngoplasty did not seem to improve survival. Partinen, Jamieson and Guilleminault (1988) found that in a group of patients with obstructive sleep apnoea followed for 5 years all the deaths occurred in the group treated conservatively with weight loss as compared with the group treated with tracheostomy in which there were no deaths. Another report suggested an increased incidence of cerebrovascular accidents, angina and myocardial infarct in snorers (Koskenzuo, Partinen and Sarnas, 1985). This was an unselected group that presumably included some patients with obstructive sleep apnoea. The long-term effects of mild obstructive sleep apnoea are unknown.

Social consequences

As well as daytime sleepiness the combination of disturbed sleep and chronic hypoxia is also responsible for other psychological and intellectual changes that patients with obstructive sleep apnoea may exhibit. These include personality change, poor memory and difficulty in concentrating. These complications combined with the loud snoring can result in serious social consequences. Examples include marital stress sometimes leading to divorce, interference with the performance of the patient's job possibly leading to loss of employment and an unwillingness to stay in hotels often limiting business and leisure pursuits. Far more serious is the increased incidence of accidents, especially road traffic accidents because of daytime sleepiness and poor concentration (Haroldson *et al.*, 1990; George *et al.*, 1987; Findley *et al.*, 1989).

Clinical features and differential diagnosis

Snoring is the cardinal symptom of the obstructive sleep apnoea syndrome and essentially all patients with this syndrome snore. Of course, by no means do all patients who snore have obstructive sleep apnoea syndrome. By far the commonest associated symptom is excessive daytime sleepiness. Other symptoms that may be present are listed in Table 19.2.

Snoring and obstructive episodes

The classic snoring noise is due to partial upper airway obstruction causing turbulent airflow with resultant vibration of the soft palate and uvula, the faucial pillars, the lateral pharyngeal walls and sometimes the tongue base. Where the narrowing is primarily at the tongue base level or is associated with a high upper airways resistance syndrome the noise has a different, less vibrant quality. In the obstructive sleep apnoea syndrome the bed partner will describe periods of very loud snoring interspersed with periods of silence during apnoeic episodes. These apnoeic episodes usually last 20–60 seconds but can last up to a couple of minutes, though most partners will not usually wait this long and will rouse the patient. During an episode there is no flow of air at the nose or mouth yet the patient can be seen to be making marked respiratory efforts associated with tracheal tug, paradoxical abdominal and chest movements and suprasternal recession. Respiratory efforts become more strenuous as time passes until the silence is broken by a loud snorting, grunting noise followed by some deep breaths as the patient clears the airway. The snoring then resumes before the next apnoeic episode begins.

Although the minimum criteria for diagnosis of obstructive sleep apnoea is > 5 apnoeic episodes per hour some patients will experience many hundreds of episodes throughout the night and those that are symptomatic will usually have an apnoea index of > 20.

Excessive daytime sleepiness

The presumed cause of excessive daytime sleepiness, also known as hypersomnolence, is discussed above. The symptom can vary from a feeling of being generally tired to actually falling asleep during important activities. In the mild form patients will complain of falling asleep during activities such as watching television or trying to read a novel. More seriously they may fall asleep during important events such as meetings and even during face-to-face conversations and most seriously while driving or operating machinery. The authors have treated a lecturer who fell asleep while giving a lecture and a teacher who fell asleep in front of the class. Patients are often not good at assessing their degree of daytime sleepiness and talking to the partner may give a more accurate indication of the degree of the problem.

The Epworth sleepiness scale (ESS) (Table 19.3) is a self-administered questionnaire which provides a measurement of the patient's general level of daytime sleepiness. ESS scores increase with the severity of OSA and are more closely related to the apnoea index than the degree of hypoxaemia (Johns, 1990). Normal patients score between 2 and 10 whereas total ESS scores greater than 16 are found only in patients with moderate or severe OSA, narcolepsy or idiopathic hypersomnia (Johns, 1991). However, a small minority of patients with moderate or severe OSA score in the normal range so a low score alone cannot exclude OSA. As with many assessments related to OSA the results should not be interpreted in isolation.

Other conditions should be considered in patients who fall asleep during the day (Table 19.4.) A rare condition causing daytime sleepiness is narcolepsy in which there are episodes of sudden onset of sleep usually lasting about 15 minutes. This disease usually starts between the ages of 10–20 years and affects both sexes equally. It can be associated with cataplexy, sleep paralysis and hallucinations at the onset of sleep (hypnogogic) or when waking up. Snoring is not usually a feature and the diagnosis is confirmed using EEG which shows REM stage at the onset of sleep.

Table 19.3 The Epworth sleepiness scale (Johns, 1991)

Name: _____

Today's date: _____Your age (years): _____

Your sex (male = M; female = F): _____

How likely are you to doze off or fall asleep in the following situations, in contrast to just feeling tired? This refers to your usual way of life in recent times. Even if you have not done some of these things recently try to work out how they would have affected you. Use the following scale to choose the *most appropriate number* for each situation:

0 = would *never* doze
1 = *slight* chance of dozing
2 = *moderate* chance of dozing
3 = *high* chance of dozing

Situation	Chance of dozing
Sitting and reading	_____
Watching TV	_____
Sitting, inactive in a public place (e.g. a theatre or a meeting)	_____
As a passenger in a car for an hour without a break	_____
Lying down to rest in the afternoon when circumstances permit	_____
Sitting and talking to someone	_____
Sitting quietly after a lunch without alcohol	_____
In a car, while stopped for a few minutes in the traffic	_____

Thank you for your cooperation

Table 19.4 Differential diagnosis of excessive daytime sleepiness

Sleep apnoea syndrome
Narcolepsy
Nocturnal myoclonus (periodic movements of sleep)
Depression
Drugs
Sleep deprivation
Idiopathic hypersomnolence
Hypoglycaemia
Severe anaemia
Hypothyroidism
Cerebral tumours

Morning headaches

These are often quoted as a common symptom but in our experience this is not the case.

Intellectual deterioration and personality change

As with excessive daytime sleepiness a more accurate picture will be obtained from the partner as opposed to the patient.

Abnormal body movements

These can vary from isolated movements of an arm or leg and restlessness of the body to thrashing of the limbs which can be so disruptive that the partner is driven to seek refuge in another room.

Nocturnal enuresis and impotence

These are also often quoted yet rarely volunteered symptoms.

Chronic obstructive airways disease, congestive cardiac failure and pulmonary fibrosis can all mimic sleep apnoea and in some cases may coexist in patients with sleep apnoea. A good history and examination should alert one to these other conditions.

Obesity

Most patients with symptomatic obstructive sleep apnoea are obese, one review suggesting up to 70% (Guilleminault, Tilkian and Dement, 1976). Though the widespread use of sleep laboratories has detected many patients with obstructive sleep apnoea who are not significantly overweight it seems true that the more obese the person the more likely it is that he will have obstructive sleep apnoea.

Obesity is defined as a body weight at least 20% above the ideal (White, 1982), and morbid obesity as being 45 kg above ideal or twice ideal body weight (Kral and Hymsfields, 1987). The ideal body weight is usually defined using life insurance company tables where the ideal weight is that which is associated with the lowest mortality for an individual of specific height and sex. Two ways of calculating desirable body weight without the need for charts are shown in Table 19.5. The body mass index (BMI) correlates with body fat and adjusts body weight for individual differences in stature.

An increase of one standard deviation in any measure of body habitus is related to a threefold increase in the risk of having an apnoea index of 5 or greater (Young *et al.*, 1993).

Sugerman (1986) and Victor *et al.* (1984) both described patients reaching a critical weight, unique to each individual, at which obstructive sleep apnoea developed or worsened. Below this weight improvement in symptoms occurred. Obesity is thought to encourage obstructive sleep apnoea by a number of mechanisms. Excess weight on the abdomen and chest wall decreases lung compliance and lung volume and increases the work of breathing, and fatty infiltration in the diaphragm and intercostal muscles decreases the strength of the respiratory effort. Also obesity is associated with a depression of the genioglossus muscle reflex (Remmers *et al.*, 1978) and a decrease in the hypercapnic and hypoxic ventilatory responsiveness (Harman and Block, 1986). This last feature is seen in the Pickwickian syndrome which is a combination of morbid obesity, excessive daytime sleepiness, right heart failure and alveolar hypoventilation resulting in hypercapnia and hypoxia. Essentially this group of patients suffers with obstructive sleep apnoea. The suggestion that obesity is related to fat deposition in the soft palate and pharyngeal walls has not been confirmed on CT scans (Kuna and Remmers, 1985). Obesity clearly has an important role in sleep disordered breathing.

Management philosophy

A patient with a unilateral sensorineural hearing loss may have an acoustic neuroma, a potentially life-threatening condition which should be excluded. In the same way a patient presenting with snoring may have obstructive sleep apnoea syndrome another possibly life-threatening condition either directly because of its long-term cardiovascular effects or indirectly because of excessive daytime sleepiness leading to road traffic accidents or other injuries. Presented with a snoring patient one should consider the possibility of obstructive sleep apnoea which cannot be reliably excluded on the basis of history (Crocker, Olson and Saunders, 1990; Viner, Szalai and Hoffstein, 1991), examination (Viner, Szalai and

Table 19.5 Two methods for calculating desirable body weight

Body mass index (BMI)	*American Diabetes Association method*

$$\frac{\text{weight in kilograms}}{\text{height in metres}^2} = \frac{kg}{m^2}$$ for men BMI should be < 27.8 for women BMI should be < 27.3	Desirable body weight for:
	
	 • A man of 5 ft tall = 106 lb
	       + 6 lb for every extra inch
	       (i.e. a man 5′ 10″ ideal wt = 166 lb)
	
	 • A woman of 5ft tall = 100 lb
	       + 5 lb for every extra inch
	       (i.e. a woman 5′ 5″ ideal wt = 125 lb)
	
	 in both cases ± 10% dependent on body frame

Hoffstein, 1991) or observation during sleep (Haponik *et al.*, 1984) alone. The extent of any investigations will obviously be influenced by resources and locally available facilities. However, to perform surgery, such as uvulopalatopharyngoplasty, on a snoring patient without any attempt to exclude obstructive sleep apnoea will deprive some patients of an important warning sign (i.e. snoring) that they have a potentially life-threatening condition. A condition that may well not be cured by surgery but for which there are successful alternative treatments if the condition is identified.

A multidisciplinary problem requires a multidisciplinary approach and ideally the otolaryngologist managing these patients needs to forge close links with a local physician, neurologist or anaesthetist who has an interest in the medical aspects of sleep apnoea and with a maxillofacial surgeon who has an interest in the oral surgical aspects. A management plan is suggested in Figure 19.2.

Diagnosis
History

In order to obtain an accurate history it is extremely important for the bed partner to be present. The symptoms they describe can make the diagnosis.

The details that need to be obtained in the history are listed in Table 19.6.

Is the snoring positional, i.e. does this only occur when the patient is supine or in any position. It is important to enquire about nasal obstruction which may be persistent because of septal deviation or nasal polyps, or fluctuating due to rhinitis which is often worse at night because of bedroom allergens. It is essential to determine alcohol intake. It is well recognized that alcohol can induce snoring in non-snorers (Tasson, Block and Boysen, 1981), cause snorers to obstruct (Mitler, Dawson and Henriksen, 1988) and exacerbate established obstructive sleep apnoea (Issa and Sullivan, 1982). Any sedative drugs such as

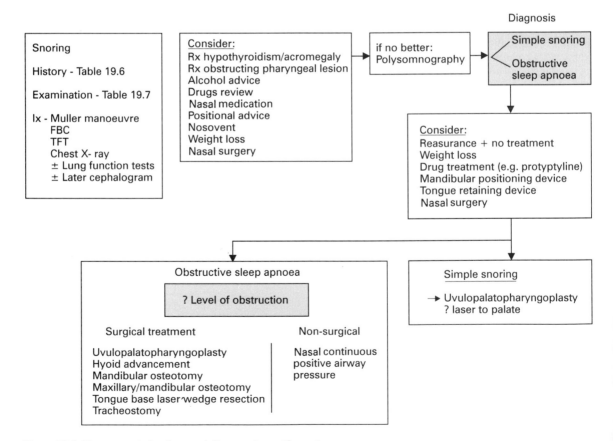

Figure 19.2 Management plan for an adult presenting with snoring

Table 19.6 Important points in the history

Partner must be present
Snoring
Positional
Obstructive episodes
Arousals/nocturnal choking
Excessive daytime sleepiness
Intellectual deterioration/personality change
Abnormal motor movements
Morning headaches
Nocturnal enuresis/impotence
Nasal obstruction
Drugs
Alcohol intake
Cardiovascular symptoms
Respiratory symptoms
Thyroid symptoms
Social history

barbiturates, hypnotics, anticonvulsants, narcotics or antihistamines may have similar effects. Sleep apnoea may be a presenting feature of hypothyroidism so symptoms suggestive of this disorder should be excluded. Any coexistent cardiovascular or respiratory disorder needs to be recorded. Finally one should bear in mind the possibility that snoring is being used as an excuse by the spouse to leave the marital bed such that when the patient is investigated minimal or no snoring is found. This possibility has been recognized for many years (Dengrove, 1939).

Examination (Table 19.7)

The patient's general appearance will indicate the extent of any obesity and may suggest conditions such as acromegaly or myxoedema. Height, weight, neck circumference and blood pressure need to be

Table 19.7 Important aspects of the examination

General appearance
Weight
Height
Blood pressure
Craniofacial morphology
Nasal airway
Tongue size
Soft palate/uvula/tonsils
Nasopharynx – adenoids/polyps/cyst/tumour
Hypopharynx – lingual tonsils/vallecula, epiglottic or supra-glottic cysts/tumour
Larynx – vocal cord mobility

recorded. Craniofacial morphology is assessed looking for retrognathia or micrognathia. Nasal examination will allow assessment of the nasal airway and reveal any causes of nasal obstruction. Oral cavity examination allows assessment of the size of the tongue, soft palate, uvula and tonsils. Patients with obstructive sleep apnoea often have a classic picture of an enlarged, swollen oedematous uvula and soft palate (Plate 4/19/I). One must be very cautious about seeing this as an invitation to perform a uvulopalatopharyngoplasty as this appearance can represent part of a multisegmental upper airway problem for which alternative treatment may be preferable, so a full assessment is required before any surgery. The nasopharynx is examined to exclude adenoidal tissue, polyps, cysts or tumours. The oropharynx often appears congested and there may be redundant mucosa and prominent lateral pharyngeal bands. The hypopharynx and larynx must be examined to look for any lesions that may be narrowing the airway such as enlarged lingual tonsils, cysts or tumours. A normal glottis with mobile vocal cords must be confirmed. In most patients no obvious obstructive lesion is found and, in a few patients with obstructive sleep apnoea the oropharyngeal inlet appears completely normal and widely patent.

Investigations

The reasons for investigations in this condition are threefold:

1 To assess the patient's general condition
2 To differentiate between simple snoring and sleep apnoea and determine the presence, type and severity of any apnoeas or hypopnoeas
3 To assess the site of obstruction.

1 To assess the patient's general condition

- FBC: to look for polycythaemia/anaemia/mean corpusular volume (MCV) (?alcohol)
- Thyroid function tests: if hypothyroidism is suspected
- Chest X-ray: to detect cardiomegaly or pulmonary disorders
- ECG: if there is any suggestion of associated cardiac disease
- Blood gases: if there is any suspicion of daytime hypoventilation and hypoxaemia then arterial P_{O_2} and P_{CO_2} need to be determined.
- Lung function tests: performed if there is suspicion of a coexisting pulmonary disorder. The finding of a 'saw-tooth' pattern on a flow volume loop is thought to be very suggestive that the patient has obstructive sleep apnoea (Sanders *et al.*, 1981).

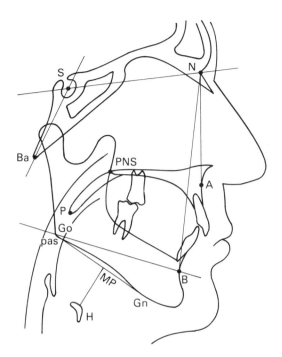

Figure 19.4 Measurements made on a lateral cephalogram. S: sella; N: nasion; PNS: posterior nasal spine; SNA: angle of lines from sella to nasion to point A; P: tip of soft palate; Go: gonion; pas: posterior airway space; SNB: angle of lines from sella to nasion to point B; MP: mandibular plane; H: hyoid; Gn: gnathion. (From Partinen *et al.*, 1988, *Chest*, **93**, 1199–1205, by kind permission of the publishers)

1985; Ryan, Dickson and Lower, 1990) with others finding no correlation between the above parameters and surgical success (Gislason *et al.*, 1988b; Croft and Golding-Wood, 1990). Cephalometry allows assessment of any maxillomandibular hypoplasia and is obviously essential if considering maxillofacial surgery.

CT scan

Measurements of the pharynx in awake patients have shown that those with obstructive sleep apnoea tend to have a narrower cross-sectional area and that this narrowing can occur at various levels (Haponik, Smith and Bohlman, 1983; Suratt, Dee and Atkinson, 1983). Performing CT of the upper airway in patients undergoing uvulopalatopharyngoplasty Shepard and Thawley (1989) found that patients with a minimum cross-sectional area of < 1 cm located 20 mm below the hard palate (i.e. at the lower velopharynx) had a high chance of obtaining a good result with uvulo-palatopharyngoplasty. Others however have found that no particular airway measurements could accurately differentiate responders and non-responders (Gislason *et al.*, 1988b).

Sleeping patients

Fibreoptic nasendoscopy

Borowiecki *et al.* (1978) and Rojewski *et al.* (1982) used simultaneous videoendoscopy and polysomnography as research tools to try to determine what happens in the upper airway during an obstructive event. Patients with moderate to severe obstructive sleep apnoea had a nasendoscope inserted into the upper airway and then supported on a frame above the bed while they fell asleep. Video recordings of the upper airway were made throughout the night. Different patients exhibited different levels of obstruction. However, because of the restricted movement of the suspended scope and the relatively limited view, this technique was not used routinely. Croft and Pringle (1991) have devised an outpatient technique known as 'sleep nasendoscopy' which involves inducing sleep with a small dose of sedative then examining the upper airway during obstructive episodes. Experience with this procedure has allowed the formulation of a grading system based on site of obstruction (Pringle and Croft, 1993). Patients who obstruct primarily at the velopharyngeal level can be identified and offered uvulopalatopharyngoplasty whereas those who have multisegmental collapse or tongue base collapse can be offered alternative treatment. The investigation is best reserved for those in whom obstructive sleep apnoea has already been diagnosed on overnight sleep study as these patients often require much smaller doses of sedative to induce sleep.

Somnofluoroscopy

In this technique sleeping patients with obstructive sleep apnoea are monitored with polysomnography and during obstructive episodes their upper airway is visualized using an image intensifier. The results are recorded on videotape and later analysed. Use of this technique has allowed classification of patients into groups on the basis of site of obstruction (Figure 19.5) and allowed the successful selection of which patients with obstructive sleep apnoea would respond to uvulopalatopharyngoplasty (Katsantonis and Walsh, 1986; Hegstrom *et al.*, 1988). A fat or short neck may hinder adequate visualization.

Cine CT

The Imatron C-100 rapid sequence scanner allows 8 cm of upper airway to be scanned in 240 ms and this can be repeated at 0.7 s intervals. One can obtain a record of the upper airway changes throughout an obstructive episode. Cine CT performed on eight sleeping patients with obstructive sleep apnoea (Stein *et al.*, 1987) demonstrated that they fell into two groups – those with soft palate level obstruction alone, and those with multisegmental obstruction. At the present time cost, availability and X-ray exposure

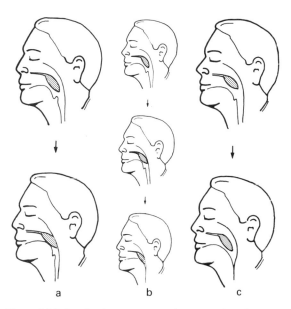

Figure 19.5 Levels of upper airway obstruction based on somnofluoroscopy. (a) Type-1 airway obstruction. Obstruction occurs at level of soft palate only during somnofluoroscopy. (b) Type-2 airway obstruction. Obstruction occurs initially at level of soft palate followed by closure of more distal airway. (c) Type-3 airway obstruction. Obstruction initially occurs distal to soft palate. Airway at soft palate level may close or remain open. (From Hegstrom *et al.*, 1988, *American Journal of Radiology*, **150**, 67–69, by kind permission of the publishers)

mean that this investigation will remain a research tool.

Pharyngeal manometry

Using a series of three catheters to measure upper airway pressure Chaban, Cole and Hoffstein (1988) identified two groups of patients: one group in whom the lower limit of obstruction was at the soft palate and the other in whom the lower limit was at the tongue base.

Hudgel and Hendricks (1988) using slightly different manometry techniques found that, during sleep, normal non-snoring, non-obese men develop increased upper airway resistance at either the palate level or the hypopharyngeal level. Patients with obstructive sleep apnoea had a similar pattern of palatal or hypopharyngeal narrowing except that it was quantitatively greater (Hudgel, 1986).

All the methods described above for determining site of obstruction reach the same conclusion. There are two main groups of patients with obstructive sleep apnoea, those in whom the obstruction is primarily at the velopharyngeal level and those in whom it is either multisegmental or at the tongue base. The

former group have the potential of benefiting from uvulopalatopharyngoplasty and thus possibly being saved from a lifetime of nasal continuous positive airway pressure. This highlights the importance of assessing the site of obstruction in patients with obstructive sleep apnoea when considering surgery and explains why uvulopalatopharyngoplasty, which is aimed at the velopharynx, performed on unselected patients with obstructive sleep apnoea has only about a 50% success rate in reducing the apnoea/hypopnoea index.

The advent of miniaturized solid state pressure transducers for improved manometry, acoustic analysis of snoring noise and MRI scanning for the production of detailed sagittal images of the upper airway are all possible future developments.

The search continues for a simple, safe, cheap, objective and reliable method for determining the level of obstruction.

Treatment

Treatment choice depends on a number of factors:
1 Is it simple snoring or obstructive sleep apnoea?
2 What does the patient want?
3 The severity of the obstructive sleep apnoea and the presence of complications, i.e. apnoea index/ degree of oxygen desaturation/apnoea associated cardiac arrhythmias/associated cardiopulmonary pathology
4 The level of obstruction.

No treatment

With increased patient awareness of the possible consequences of snoring some patients will seek advice for reassurance that their health is not at risk. If there is no daytime sleepiness and investigations exclude the presence of obstructive sleep apnoea or cardiac arrhythmias and the patient is not concerned by the snoring noise then he can be reassured and no further treatment will be necessary. As yet there is no evidence for encouraging 'prophylactic' surgical treatment of snoring.

Medical management (Table 19.10)

The first step in medical management is to diagnose and treat any systemic disorders such as *hypothyroidism* or *acromegaly*. It is well recognized that *alcohol* can induce or exacerbate sleep apnoea and avoidance of alcohol may achieve significant improvement in apnoea severity. As little as 85 ml (3 oz) of 80 proof alcohol can significantly increase the severity of mild sleep apnoea (Scrima, Broudy and Nay, 1982).

Table 19.10 Medical treatment

Exclude hypothyroidism/acromegaly
Alcohol advice
Drug review
Weight loss
Nasal medication
Nosovent
Drug treatment (e.g. protriptyline)
Positional advice
Mandibular positioning device
Tongue retaining device
Nasal continuous positive airway pressure

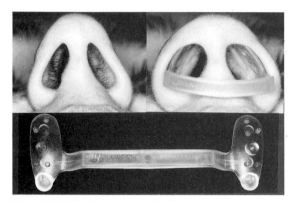

Figure 19.6 The Nozovent nasal splint

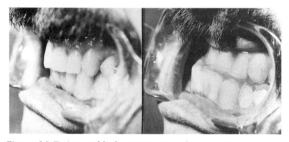

Figure 19.7 A mandibular positioning device. (*a*) Normal occlusion; (*b*) device *in situ*. (Courtesy of Air Commodore T. Negus)

Sedative medication should be avoided, especially in high risk patients. The effects of obesity have been discussed above and *weight loss* should be encouraged in those patients with obstructive sleep apnoea who are obese. However, the effects of weight loss on the severity of obstructive sleep apnoea are variable. In mild to moderately obese patients loss of 10 kg often yields improvements in apnoea severity and daytime sleepiness (Smith, Gold and Meyers, 1985), however

others have found no consistent benefit with weight loss (Guilleminault, Eldridge and Tilkian, 1977; Harman, Wynne and Block, 1982). In reality many patients find sufficient weight loss extremely difficult and to achieve effective weight loss that is then maintained patients need advice about long-term changes in attitude, perception, diet and activity. In some patients with morbid obesity and life-threatening obstructive sleep apnoea, referral for surgical procedures to achieve weight loss may be appropriate (Sugerman *et al.*, 1981). *Nasal obstruction* due to rhinitis may improve sufficiently with the use of intranasal steroid sprays to have a beneficial effect on symptoms (McNicholas, Tarlo and Cole, 1982). The *Nozovent*, a silastic splint (Figure 19.6) that dilates the nasal valve and reduces nasal resistance, is reported to reduce snoring noise in some patients (Petruson, 1990). Many *drugs* have been tried in the treatment of sleep apnoea syndromes including acetazolamide, theophylline, doxapram, buspirone, medroxyprogesterone, nicotine and protriptyline (Erman, 1991). The last of these is the most widely used. Protriptyline is a non-sedating tricyclic antidepressant which also has the effect of suppressing REM-stage sleep. Apnoeic episodes tend to be more severe during this stage of sleep and the theory is that less REM sleep will mean less of the severe apnoeas. Other theories about its action include a primary respiratory stimulant property (Series and Cormier, 1990) and a capacity to increase muscle tone (Borona, St John and Bledsoe, 1985). However, its anticholinergic side effects limit patient compliance. Side effects and the lack of evidence of reduction in either morbidity or mortality essentially means that drugs play no part in the treatment of sleep apnoea syndromes (Douglas, 1993).

Some patients find that snoring or sleep apnoea occur or are worse when they are supine. In these individuals *positional therapy* is worth trying. This can range from behavioural therapy using electronic devices to detect position (Cartwright, 1985) to simply stitching a tennis ball into a pocket on the back of the night shirt. Two types of custom-made orthodontic device are being investigated, the 'tongue-retaining device' and the 'mandibular positioning device'. The latter is like an upper and lower gum shield fixed together so that the mandible is protruded and held forward (Figure 19.7) Protruding the mandible pulls the tongue forward and widens the posterior airway space. There have been some encouraging results (Bonham *et al.*, 1988; Ichioka *et al.*, 1991), but long-term effects on the temporomandibular joint remain uncertain. The tongue-retaining device holds the tongue forward by suction generated by squeezing the air out of a plastic bulb inserting the tongue then releasing the bulb. The bulb is attached to a gum shield and is worn throughout the night (Figure 19.8) (Cartwright, 1985).

Nasal continuous positive airway pressure (nasal

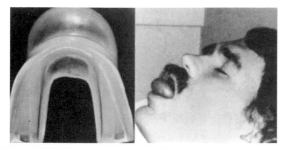

Figure 19.8 The tongue retaining device

CPAP) was first described by Sullivan *et al.* in 1981. This is the 'gold standard' treatment for obstructive sleep apnoea and challenges tracheostomy in effectiveness. It will prevent apnoeas in 99% of patients who can tolerate it (Chambers, Birkenmeier and Walsh, 1986; Sullivan and Grunstein, 1989; Douglas, 1993). If the patient fails to report a subjective improvement with nasal CPAP, the original diagnosis should be questioned. The patient wears a tightly fitting mask over the nose (Figure 19.9). The mask is connected by a tube to a small pump that sits at the bedside. The pump blows air into the upper airway at pressures of between 7 and 15 cm H_2O. This is thought to act as a pneumatic splint and hold the walls of the upper airway apart thus preventing collapse and obstruction. Continuous positive airway pressure will obviously not work in the presence of severe nasal obstruction. The first night of CPAP should be performed under controlled conditions in the sleep laboratory. This is because the first night of unobstructed sleep can produce intense and prolonged REM sleep and such low arousal levels that potentially dangerous hypoxaemia can occur (Krieger *et al.*, 1983; Labyah and Aldrich, 1989). It also allows the correct air pressure to be determined because too low a pressure will not only result in failure but may worsen hypoxaemia. The main problem with CPAP is one of patient compliance. A number of studies have found compliance rates of between 50 and 90%. The commonest problem is nasal mucosal irritation. Other problems include noise from the machine, mask discomfort, air leak causing sore eyes, abdominal bloating and feelings of claustrophobia. The use of customized masks to improve comfort, smaller quieter machines and active follow up and counselling, all improve compliance. Recently the introduction of nasal BiPAP (bi-level positive airways pressure) in which the pressure is reduced during expiration is claimed to improve comfort and compliance. Nasal CPAP also prevents snoring so may be useful for patients who do not want surgery but sleep away from home frequently and find their snoring an embarrassment.

Surgical management

Anaesthetic considerations

Patients with obstructive sleep apnoea can present anaesthetic problems. They can be sensitive to sedatives and narcotics and these drugs should be avoided in the premedication. They often have short thick necks making intubation difficult and, during induction, the upper airway can start to collapse and obstruct. Mask ventilation may then be inadequate requiring prompt intubation. A nasopharyngeal tube can be used to maintain airway patency during induction. In some patients with associated chronic obstructive airway disease high oxygen concentration and ventilation may blow off carbon dioxide which can reduce or abolish spontaneous ventilation by depressing ventilatory drive. Paralysing agents can exacerbate this and should be avoided. Postoperatively, because of the possibility of a depressed ventilatory drive and the swelling often associated with surgery, the patient can continue to obstruct risking the development of severe hypoxia. Extubating the patient when he is fully awake, leaving a nasopharyngeal airway in place, constant P_{O_2} monitoring and the avoidance of narcotic analgesia will help prevent these problems.

Nasal surgery

There is good evidence that nasal obstruction can contribute to obstructive sleep apnoea syndrome. Induced nasal obstruction in normal people results in disturbed sleep both subjectively and objectively (Olsen, Kern and Westbrook, 1981; Zwillich *et al.*, 1981; Lavie *et al.*, 1983). It can cause a marked increase in the number of obstructive apnoeas, hypopnoeas and arousals. Some individuals were found to be affected significantly more than others indicating that it takes more than nasal obstruction alone to induce obstructive sleep apnoea. In patients with predisposing factors such as neuromuscular incoordination or upper airway narrowing, additional nasal

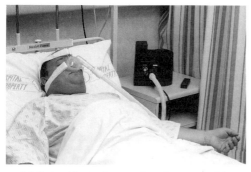

Figure 19.9 A patient using nasal continuous positive airway pressure

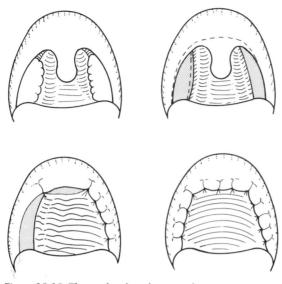

Figure 19.10 The uvulopalatopharyngoplasty operation

obstruction may be the initiating factor. Acoustic rhinometry on a group of snorers and patients with obstructive sleep apnoea found inferior turbinate hypertrophy in 97% (Lenders, Schaefer and Pirsig, 1991). The cross-sectional area was smaller in the region of the head of the inferior turbinate than in the region of the isthmus nasi, the usual site of the minimum cross-sectional area of the nasal cavity. Interestingly only one-third of those with moderate or marked nasal obstruction on acoustic rhinomanometry were aware of it. However, there was no correlation between severity of nasal obstruction and apnoea index again suggesting that the onset and degree of obstructive sleep apnoea is dependent on other predisposing factors being present. Nasal obstruction probably acts as a high upstream resistance necessitating the generation of high negative intrathoracic pressures to pull air through the narrowing. As the nose becomes more obstructed the patient will start to breathe through the mouth. Opening the mouth causes the tongue to move posteriorly thus narrowing the posterior airway space and further contributing to the conditions necessary for collapse.

The effects of nasal surgery on snoring and obstructive sleep apnoea are variable (Lavie *et al.*, 1982; Caldarelli, Cartwright and Lillie, 1985; Ellis *et al.*, 1992). This may be because nasal obstruction is an extremely common condition and so will be purely coincidental in some patients with snoring and obstructive sleep apnoea. Alternatively, it is possible that in some patients the nasal obstruction is the initiating factor but, after a prolonged period of high intraluminal negative pressures, the upper airway becomes 'stretched' and excessively compliant so that even if the nasal obstruction is corrected the snoring or obstructive sleep apnoea will continue. Despite this we feel that any nasal obstruction that does not respond to medical treatment should be corrected surgically. It would seem reasonable to assume that failure to do so, thus leaving an area of high upstream resistance in the system, would risk the long-term effectiveness of pharyngeal surgery such as uvulopalatopharyngoplasty.

Uvulopalatopharyngoplasty

Removal of the uvula and rim of soft palate to treat snoring was developed by Dr Ikematsu (1964) a Japanese surgeon but was modified and popularized in America by Fujita *et al.* (1981). The uvulopalatopharyngoplasty (UPPP) operation essentially involves removing the tonsils, trimming the faucial pillars if required, removing the uvula and a variable amount of soft palate, then suturing the posterior to the anterior faucial pillar and the posterior soft palate mucosa to the anterior soft palate mucosa (Figure 19.10). This results in the removal of excessive and 'space-occupying' tissue with a corresponding increase in the cross-sectional area of the velopharynx. The resistance to flow through a tube is inversely proportional to the fourth power of the radius so even a small increase in the size of this area will significantly reduce the resistance. This along with some stiffening from subsequent scarring of the remaining tissues is thought to prevent the vibration that is responsible for snoring noise and the collapse that is responsible for obstruction.

The indications for UPPP are:

1 Socially disruptive 'simple' (non-apnoeic) snoring
2 Obstructive sleep apnoea where the obstruction is primarily at the velopharyngeal or upper oropharyngeal level.

The problems of selecting such patients are discussed above. UPPP is quoted as having 85–90% success rates in curing snoring (Fairbanks, 1984; Macaluso *et al.*, 1989; Pelausa *et al.* 1989; Sharp *et al.*, 1990), but its ability significantly to reduce apnoea index in unselected patients with obstructive sleep apnoea varies from as low as 23% (de Berry-Borowiecki, Kukwa and Blanks, 1985) up to 77% (Dickson and Blokmanis, 1987), the average being around 50–60% (Fujita *et al.*, 1985; Katsantonis *et al.*, 1985; Gislason *et al.*, 1988b; Macaluso *et al.*, 1989). Its effectiveness in improving excessive daytime sleepiness has been demonstrated by Haroldson *et al.* (1991) who have found improved simulated long-term driving performance in patients treated with UPPP. It is a generally safe operation (Pelausa and Tarshis, 1989) though not withought some morbidity (Croft and Golding-Wood, 1990). The operation has a reputation for being extremely painful. This is not always the case and early postoperative

Colour plates

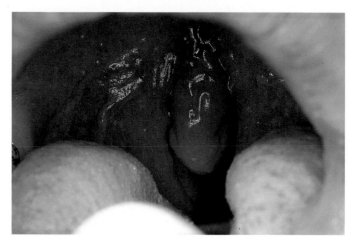

Plate 4/19/I Congested oropharynx in a patient with obstructive sleep apnoea

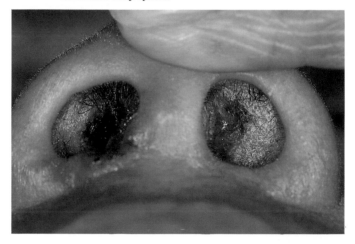

Plate 4/20/I Tuberculosis. Lesion affecting vestibular skin

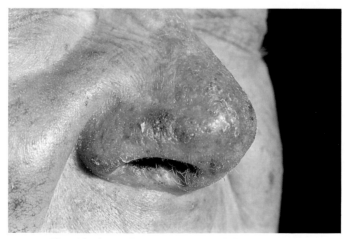

Plate 4/20/II Leishmaniasis. Lesions of skin of external nose

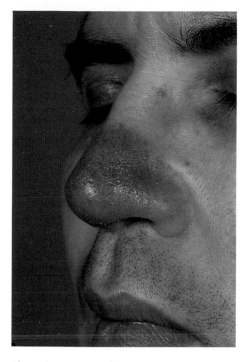

Plate 4/20/III Sarcoidosis. Typical appearances of nasal lupus pernio

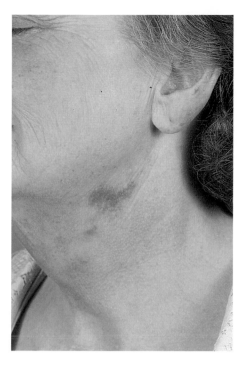

Plate 4/20/V Sarcoidosis. Typical appearances of lesions on cervical skin

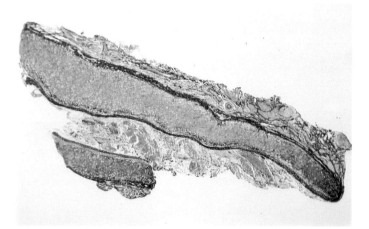

Plate 4/20/IV Sarcoidosis. Coronal section through nasal septal cartilage showing erosion by granulomatous lesions

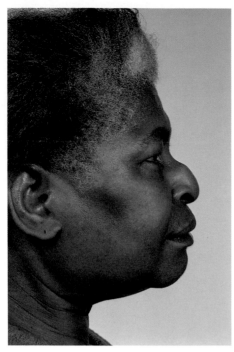

(a)

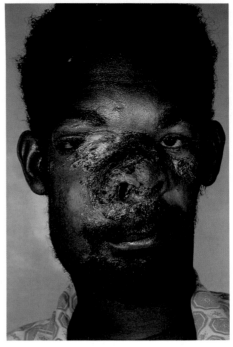

(c)

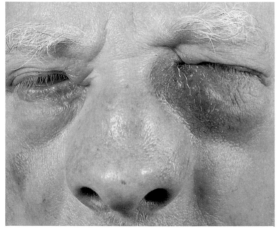

(b)

Plate 4/20/VI Lymphoma. The range of clinical manifestations of lymphoma are illustrated in the following cases: (*a*) B-cell lymphoma presenting as a mass on the bridge of the nose; (*b*) B-cell lymphoma presenting in the antrum, with involvement of the nasolacrimal region; (*c*) T-cell lymphoma affecting the midface, with ulceration; (*d*) T-cell lymphoma of the midface, with significant central destruction

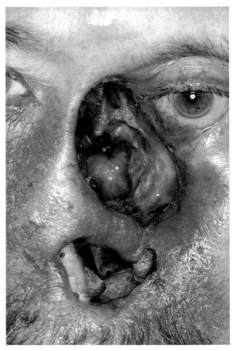

(d)

pain can be helped by infiltration of the wound with Marcain at the end of the procedure. Complications include nasal regurgitation of food or fluid, a dry throat, disturbance of taste and hypernasal speech. Nasal regurgitation is uncommon and rarely a long-term problem. Probably the most serious complication is velopharyngeal stenosis and it is for this reason that UPPP and adenoidectomy must never be performed simultaneously. Patients with obstructive sleep apnoea must be very carefully monitored in the postoperative period. The place of UPPP in the treatment of obstructive sleep apnoea is still not fully defined and though UPPP may eliminate snoring in these patients it has been shown not to improve long-term mortality (He *et al.*, 1988). This reinforces the importance of patient selection and late postoperative reassessment when using UPPP to treat patients with moderate obstructive sleep apnoea. Any figures produced with regard to the long-term efficacy of UPPP must be viewed in the light of the quality of preoperative assessment and patient selection.

Palatal procedures

A recently developed procedure for the treatment of patients with simple snoring involves an attempt to stiffen the soft palate by removing a longitudinal strip of mucosa from its oral surface using an Nd-YAG laser (Ellis, Williams and Shneerson, 1993). The procedure is not recommended in the treatment of obstructive sleep apnoea.

Kamami describes a method of treating snoring using the CO_2 laser (Kamami, 1990). He progressively enlarges the oropharyngeal airspace by successive 'vaporizations' of the uvula, soft palate, posterior tonsillar pillars and any redundant posterior pharyngeal mucosa. The 'vaporizations' are performed on successive occasions under local anaesthetic in the out patient clinic, the number of sessions being determined by the patient's response. Again this technique is recommended for snorers without OSA.

A full thickness excision of a horizontal strip from the central part of the soft palate with three-layer closure has also been reported (Crestinu, 1991).

Maxillofacial techniques

Robert Riley and Nelson Powell have written extensively on the use of maxillofacial surgery in the treatment of obstructive sleep apnoea. In a review of UPPP failures they concluded that the base of the tongue was the cause of continued obstruction (Riley *et al.*, 1985) and the procedures they employ attempt to widen the hypopharynx by advancing the tongue base (Powell and Riley, 1991). The simplest procedure is an *infrahyoid myotomy with suspension of the hyoid* 15 mm anterosuperiorly by a strip of fascia lata wrapped around the hyoid body and fixed to the inferior border of the mandible. Advancing the hyoid more than 15 mm is likely to cause dysphagia. *Mandibular osteotomy and genioglossus advancement* (Figure 19.11a) is usually combined with the above procedure, and with a UPPP if there is evidence of coexistent soft palate obstruction. A segment of mandible that includes the geniotubercle, which is the site of attachment of the genioglossus and the geniohyoid muscles, is freed and advanced forward so the lingual cortex locks on the labial cortex. It is then fixed with titanium screws and wires. Advancement of 8–18 mm is possible (Riley, Powell and Guilleminault, 1987, 1989). *Bimaxillary and mandibular advancement* (Figure 19.11b) is reserved for patients with severe obstructive sleep apnoea who have failed other forms of medical or surgical treatment, including the above procedures. The patients were often morbidly

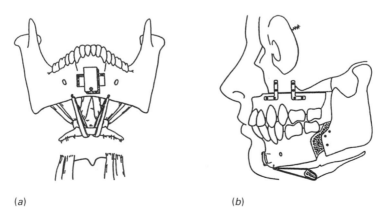

(a)   (b)

Figure 19.11 Maxillofacial techniques for treatment of tongue base obstruction. (*a*) Inferior sagittal osteotomy with infrahyoid myotomy and suspension with fascia lata. (*b*) Mandibular, maxillary and hyoid advancement. (From Riley and Powell, 1990, *Journal of Oral and Maxillofacial Surgery*, **48**, 20–26, by kind permission of the publishers)

obese with BMIs of > 33. In this surgery the standard maxillofacial technique of a LeFort 1 osteotomy with advancement and a sagittal split ramus osteotomy with advancement is modified by maximizing the distances that the segments are moved and filling the defects with calvarial bone grafts. The overall average advancement of the genial tubercle is 21 mm. The authors claim a response rate for this surgery of over 90% (Riley and Powell, 1990).

Midline laser glossectomy

This procedure, devised to tackle the problem of hypopharyngeal collapse, is an alternative to the maxillofacial procedures described above. After a covering tracheostomy, a CO_2 laser is used via an operating microscope and a rectangular area of the tongue base excised down to the valecculla. Further tongue base, hypertrophic lingual tonsils or redundant aryepiglottic folds are also excised using the laser (Fujita, 1991).

Tracheostomy

Tracheostomy cures 100% of patients with obstructive sleep apnoea. It is indicated in severe apnoea where conservative therapy has failed and there are associated complications such as cor pulmonale, disabling daytime sleepiness, and chronic alveolar hypoventilation. In the case of serious cardiac arrhythmias it can be a life-saving procedure. The relief of symptoms is dramatic and many patients are delighted despite the problems often encountered. Many of those requiring tracheostomy have short thick necks making the technique difficult and often resulting in problems with postoperative healing and long-term care. The trachea is often deep in the neck such that a standard tube is easily displaced. Also the excessive amounts of neck fat can be associated with granulation formation around the stoma. To overcome these problems it is advisable to remove excessive fatty tissue at the tracheostomy site and to create skin flaps that tunnel down and can be sutured to the edges of the tracheal defect (Maisel and Goding, 1991). Complications include haemorrhage, granulation tissue formation, stenosis, recurrent chest infections and psychological problems (Conway *et al.*, 1981). Postoperatively patients will need extensive support and education about tracheostomy care. They can wear a speaking valve during the day and leave the tube open at night. A tracheostomy will allow many patients to return to a near normal lifestyle.

References

BLOCK, A. J., BOYSON, P. G., WYNNE, J. W. and HUNT, L. A. (1979) Sleep apnoea, hypopnoea and oxygen desaturation in normal subjects. A strong male preponderance. *New England Journal of Medicine*, **300**, 513–517

BOHLMAN, M. E., HAPONIK, E. F. and SMITH, P. L. (1983) CT demonstration of pharyngeal narrowing in adult obstructive sleep apnoea. *American Journal of Radiology*, **140**, 543–548

BONHAM, P. E., CURRIER, G. F., ORR, W. C., OTHMAN, J. and NANDA, R. S. (1988) The effect of a modified functional appliance on obstructive sleep apnoea. *American Journal of Orthodontics and Dentofacial Orthopedics*, **94**, 384–392

BORONA, M., ST JOHN, W. and BLEDSOE, T. (1985) Differential elevation by protriptyline and depression by diazepam of upper airway respiratory motor activity. *American Review of Respiratory Diseases*, **232**, 41–45

BOROWIECKI, B., POLLACK, C. P., WEITZMAN, E. D., RAKOFF, S. and IMPERATO, J. (1978) Fibro-optic study of pharyngeal airway during sleep in patients with hypersomnia obstructive sleep apnoea syndrome. *Laryngoscope*, **88**, 1310–1313

BURWELL, C., ROBIN, E. D., WHALEY, R. D. and BICKLEMAN, A. (1956) Extreme obesity associated with alveolar hypoventilation: A Pickwickian syndrome. *American Journal of Medicine*, **21**, 811–818

CALDARELLI, D. D., CARTWRIGHT, R. D. and LILLIE, J. K. (1985) Obstructive sleep apnoea: variations in surgical management. *Laryngoscope*, **95**, 1070–1073

CARTWRIGHT, R. (1985) Predicting response to the tongue retaining device for sleep apnoea syndrome. *Archives of Otolaryngology*, **111**, 385–388

CHABAN, R., COLE, P. and HOFFSTEIN, V. (1988) Site of upper airway obstruction in patients with idiopathic obstructive sleep apnoea. *Laryngoscope*, **98**, 641–647

CHAMBERS, G. W., BIRKENMEIER, N. and WALSH, J. K. (1986) Nasal continuous positive airways pressure (CPAP) and home compliance. *Sleep Research*, **16**, 112

CIRIGNOTTA, F., D'ALESSANDRO, R., PARTINEN, M., ZUCCONI, M., CRISTINA, E. and CACCIATORE, F. M. (1989) Prevalence of every night snoring and obstructive sleep apnoea among 30–69 year old men in Bologna, Italy. *Acta Psychiatrica Scandinavica*, **79**, 366–372

CONWAY, W. A., VICTOR, L. D., MAGILLIGAN, D. J., FUJITA, S., ZORICK, F. J. and ROTH, T. (1981) Adverse effects of tracheostomy for sleep apnoea. *Journal of the American Medical Association*, **246**, 347–350

COOPER, B. G., VEALE, D., GRIFFITHS, C. J. and GIBSON, G. J. (1991) Value of nocturnal oxygen saturation as a screening test for sleep apnoea. *Thorax*, **46**, 586–588

CRESTINU, J. M. (1991) Intrapalatine resection in the treatment of sleep apnoea and snoring. In: *Sleep Apnoea and Rhonchopathy 3rd World Congress on Sleep Apnoea and Rhonchopathy*, edited by K. Togawa *et al.* Basel: Karger. pp. 41–44

CROCKER, B. D., OLSON, L. G. and SAUNDERS, N. A. (1990) Estimation of the probability of disturbed breathing during sleep before a sleep study. *American Review of Respiratory Diseases*, **142**, 14–18

CROFT, C. B. and GOLDING-WOOD, D. G. (1990) Uses and complications of uvulopalatopharyngoplasty. *Journal of Laryngology and Otology*, **104**, 871–875

CROFT, C. B. and PRINGLE, M. B., (1991) Sleep nasendoscopy: a technique of assessment in snoring and obstructive sleep apnoea. *Clinical Otolaryngology*, **16**, 504–509

CRUMLEY, R., STEIN, M. and GAMSU, G. (1987) Determination of obstructive site in obstructive sleep apnoea. *Laryngoscope*, **97**, 301–308

DE BERRY-BOROWIECKI, B., KUKWA, A. A. and BLANKS, R. H. I. (1985) Indications for palatopharyngoplasty. *Archives of Otolaryngology*, **111**, 659–663

DENGROVE, E. (1939) Snoring (letter). *British Medical Journal*, **1**, 808

DICKSON, R. I. and BLOKMANIS, A. (1987) Treatment of obstructive sleep apnoea by uvulopalatopharyngoplasty. *Laryngoscope*, **97**, 1054–1059

DOUGLAS, N. J. (1993) The sleep apnoea/hypopnoea syndrome and snoring. *British Medical Journal*, **306**, 1057–1060

DOUGLAS, N. J., THOMAS, S. and JAN, M. A. (1992) Clinical value of polysomnography. *Lancet*, i, 347–350

ELLIS, P. D., WILLIAMS, J. E. and SHNEERSON, J. M. (1993) Surgical relief of snoring due to palatal flutter: a preliminary report. *Annals of the Royal College of Surgeons of England*, **75**, 286–290

ELLIS, P. D. M., HARRIES, M. L., FFOWCS WILLIAMS, J. E. and SHNEERSON, J. M. (1992) The relief of snoring by nasal surgery. *Clinical Otolaryngology*, **17**, 525–527

ERMAN, M. K. (1991) Conservative treatment modalities for obstructive sleep apnoea *Operative Techniques in Otolaryngology – Head and Neck Surgery*, **2**, 120–126

FAIRBANKS, D. N. F. (1984) Snoring: surgical versus non-surgical management. *Laryngoscope*, **94**, 1188–1192

FINDLEY, L. J., FABRIZIO, M., THOMMI, G. and SURRAT, P. M. (1989) Severity of sleep apnoea and automobile accidents. *New England Journal of Medicine*, **320**, 868–869

FLETCHER, E. C., DE BEHNKE, R. D., LOVOI, M. S. and GORIN, A. B. (1985) Undiagnosed sleep apnoea in patients with essential hypertension. *Annals of Internal Medicine*, **103**, 190–195

FLETCHER, E. C., MILLER, J., SCHAAF, J. W. and FLETCHER, J. G., (1987) Urinary catecholamines before and after tracheostomy in patients with obstructive sleep apnoea and hypertension. *Sleep*, **10**, 35–44

FUJITA, S., CONWAY, W., ZORICH, F. and ROTH, T. (1981) Surgical correction of anatomic abnormalities in obstructive sleep apnoea syndrome: uvulopalatopharyngoplasty. *Otolaryngology – Head and Neck Surgery*, **89**, 923–934

FUJITA, S. (1991) Midline laser glossectomy with linguoplasty: a treatment of obstructive sleep apnoea syndrome. *Operative Techniques in Otolaryngology – Head and Neck Surgery*, **2**, 127–131

FUJITA, S., CONWAY, W., ZORICH, F., SICKLESTEEL, J. M., ROEHRS, T. A., WITTIG, R. M. *et al.* (1985) Evaluation of the effectiveness of uvulopalatopharyngoplasty. *Laryngoscope*, **95**, 70–74

GASTAUT, H., TASSINARI, C. A. and DURAN, B. (1965) Polygraphic study of episodic diurnal and nocturnal manifestations of the Pickwickian syndrome. *Review of Neurology*, **112**, 568–579

GEORGE, C. F., MILLARM, T. W. and KRYGER, M. H. (1988) Identification and quantification of apnoeas by computer based analysis of oxygen. *American Review of Respiratory Diseases*, **137**, 1238–1240

GEORGE, C. F. NICKERSON, P. W., HANLEY, P. J., MILLAR, T. W. and KRYGER, M. H. (1987) Sleep apnoea patients have more automobile accidents. *Lancet*, ii, 447

GISLASON, T., ALMQVIST, M., ARIKSSON, G., TAUB, A. and BOMAN, G. (1988a) Prevalence of sleep apnoea among Swedish men. An epidemiological study. *Journal of Clinical Epidemiology*, **41**, 571–576

GISLASON, T., LINDHOLM, C. E., ALMQVIST, M., BIRRING, E., BOMAN, G., ERIKSSON, G. *et al.* (1988b) Uvulopalatopharyngoplasty in the sleep apnoea syndromes. *Archives of Otolaryngology and Head and Neck Surgery*, **114**, 45–51

GLEESON, K. and ZWILLICH, C. W. (1992) Adenosine stimulation, ventilation and arousal from sleep. *American Review of Respiratory Diseases*, **145**, 453–457

GLEESON, K., ZWILLICH, C. W. and WHITE, D. P. (1990) The influence of increasing ventilatory effort on arousal from sleep. *American Review of Respiratory Diseases*, **142**, 295–300

GOULD, G. A., WHYTE, K. F., AIRLIE, M. A. A., RHIND, G. B., CATERALL, J. R., SHAPIRO, C. M. *et al.* (1987) Criteria for diagnosing abnormal breathing during sleep (abstract). *Thorax*, **42**, 722

GOULD, G. A., WHYTE, K. F., RHIND, G. B., AIRLIE, M. A. A., CATTERALL, J. R., SHAPIRO, C. M. *et al.* (1988) The sleep hypopnoea syndrome. *American Review of Respiratory Diseases*, **137**, 895–898

GUILLEMINAULT, C., ELDRIGE, F. L. and DEMENT, W. C. (1973) Insomnia with sleep apnoea: a new syndrome. *Science*, **181**, 856–858

GUILLEMINAULT, C., ELDRIGE, F. L. and TILKIAN, A. (1977) Sleep apnoea due to upper airway obstruction. *Archives of Internal Medicine*, **137**, 296–300

GUILLEMINAULT, C., TILKIAN, A. and DEMENT, W. C. (1976) The sleep apnoea syndromes. *Annual Review of Medicine*, **27**, 465–484

GUILLEMINAULT, C., HILL, M. W., SIMMONS, B. and DEMENT, W. (1978) Obstructive sleep apnoea: electromyographic and fibreoptic studies. *Experimental Neurology*, **62**, 48–67

GUILLEMINAULT, C., CONNOLLY, S., WINKLE, R., MELVIN, K. and TILKIAN, A. (1984) Cyclical variation of the heart rate in sleep apnoea syndrome. *Lancet*, i, 126–131

GUILLEMINAULT, C., MOTTA, J., MIHM, F. and MELVIN, K. (1986) Obstructive sleep apnoea and the cardiac index. *Chest*, **89**, 331–334

HAPONIK, E. F., SMITH, P. L., MYERS, D. A. and BLEEKER, E. R., (1984) Evaluation of sleep disordered breathing: is polysomnography necessary? *American Journal of Medicine*, **77**, 671–677

HAPONIK, E. F., SMITH, P. L. and BOHLMAN, M. E. (1983) Computerised tomography in obstructive sleep apnoea syndrome. *American Review of Respiratory Diseases*, **127**, 221–226

HARMAN, E. and BLOCK, A. (1986) Why does weight loss improve the respiratory insufficiency of obesity? *Chest*, **90**, 153

HARMAN, E., WYNNE, J. W. and BLOCK, A. (1982) The effect of weight loss on sleep disordered breathing and oxygen desaturation in morbidly obese men. *Chest*, **82**, 291

HAROLDSON, P., CARENFELT, C., LAURELL, H. and TORNROSS, J. (1990) Driving vigilance simulator test. *Acta Otolaryngologica*, **110**, 136–140

HAROLDSON, P., CARENFELT, C., PERSSON, H. E., SACHS, C. and TORNROSS, J. (1991) Simulated long term driving performance before and after uvulopalatopharyngoplasty. *Oto-Rhino-Laryngology*, **53**, 106–110

HE, J., KRYGER, M. H., ZORICK, F. J., CONWAY, W. and ROTH, T. (1988) Mortality and sleep apnoea in obstructive sleep apnoea. *Chest*, **94**, 9–14

HEDNER, J. A., EJNELL, H. and CAIDAHL, K. (1990) Left ventricular hypertrophy independent of hypertension in patients with obstructive sleep apnoea. *Journal of Hypertension*, **8**, 941–946

HEDNER, J. A., EJNELL, H., SELLGREN, J., HEDNER, T. and WALLIN, G. (1988) Is high and fluctuating muscle nerve sympathetic activity in the sleep apnoea syndrome of pathogenic importance for the development of hypertension. *Journal of Hypertension*, **6**, 529–531

HEGSTROM, T., EMMONS, L. L., HODDES, E., KENNEDY, T., CHRISTOPHER, K., COLLINS, T. *et al.* (1988) Obstructive sleep apnoea syndrome: preoperative radiologic evaluation. *American Journal of Radiology*, **150**, 67–69

HILL, W. (1889) On some cases of backwardness and stupidity in children. *British Medical Journal*, **2**, 711–712

HOFFSTEIN, V., CHAN, C. K. and SLUTSKY, A. S. (1991) Sleep apnoea and systemic hypertension: a causal association. *American Journal of Medicine*, **91**, 190–196

HUDGEL, D. W. (1986) Variable site of airway narrowing among obstructive sleep apnoea patients. *Journal of Applied Physiology*, **61**, 1403–1409

HUDGEL, D. W. and HENDRICKS, C. (1988) Palate and hypopharynx – sites of inspiratory narrowing of the upper airway during sleep. *American Review of Respiratory Diseases*, **138**, 1542–1547

ICHIOKA, M., YOSHIZAWA, M., CHIDA, M., MIYAZATO, I., TANIAI, S., MARUMO, F. *et al.* (1991) A dental device for the treatment of obstructive sleep apnoea: a preliminary study. *Otolaryngology – Head and Neck Surgery*, **104**, 555–558

IKEMATSU, T. (1964) Study of snoring, 4th report: therapy. *Journal of Japanese Otorhinolaryngology*, **64**, 434–435

ISSA, F. G. and SULLIVAN, C. E., (1982) Alcohol, snoring and sleep apnoea. *Journal of Neurology, Neurosurgery and Psychiatry*, **45**, 353–359

JEONG, D. and DIMSDALE, J. E. (1989) Sleep apnoea and essential hypertension: a critical review of the epidemiological evidence for co-morbidity. *Clinical and Experimental Hypertension – Theory and Practice*, **11**, 1301–1323

JOHNS, M. W. (1990) Daytime sleepiness, snoring and obstructive sleep apnoea. The Epworth sleepiness scale. *Chest*, **103**, 30–36

JOHNS, M. W. (1991) A new method for measuring daytime sleepiness: The Epworth sleepiness scale. *Sleep*, **14**, 540–545

KALES, A., BIXLER, E. O., CADIEUX, R. J., SCHNECK, D. W., SHAWL, L. C. and LOCKE, T. W. (1984) Sleep apnoea in a hypertensive population. *Lancet*, **ii**, 1005–1008

KAMAMI, Y. V. (1990) Laser CO2 for snoring. Preliminary results. *Acta oto-Rhino-Laryngologica Belgica*, **44**, 451–456

KATSANTONIS, G. P., WALSH, J. K., SCHWEITZER, P, K. and FRIEDMAN, W. H. (1985) Further evaluation of uvulopalatopharyngoplasty in the treatment of obstructive sleep apnoea syndrome. *Otolaryngology, Head and Neck Surgery*, **93**, 244–250

KATSANTONIS, G. P. and WALSH, J. K. (1986) Somnofluoroscopy: its role in the selection of candidates for uvulopalatopharyngoplasty. *Otolaryngology, Head and Neck Surgery*, **94**, 56–60

KOSKENZUO, M., PARTINEN, M. and SARNAS, S. (1985) Snoring as a risk factor for hypertension and angina pectoris. *Lancet*, **i**, 893–896

KRAL, J. G. and HYMSFIELDS, S. (1987) Morbid obesity: definitions, epidemiology and methodological problems. *Gastroenterology Clinics of North America*, **16**, 197–206

KRIEGER, J., SFORZA, E. and APPRILL, M., LAMPERT, E., WETZENBLUME, E. and RATOMAHARO, J. (1989) Pulmonary hypertension, hypoxaemia and hypercapnia in obstructive sleep apnoea patients. *Chest*, **96**, 729–737

KRIEGER, J., WEITZENBLUME, E., MONASSIER, J., STOECKEL, C. and KURTZ, D. (1983) Dangerous hypoxaemia during continuous positive airway pressure treatment of obstructive sleep apnoea *Lancet*, 1429–1430

KRIPKE, D., MASON, W., BLOOMQUIST, J., COBARRUBIAS, M., ENGLER, R. and ANCOLI-ISRAELS, S. (1988) Relationship of Respitrace apnoea-hypopnoea counts and 4% desaturations. *Sleep Research*, **17**, 208

KUNA, S. T. and REMMERS, J. E. (1985) Neural and anatomic factors related to upper airway occlusion during sleep. *Medical Clinics of North America*, **69**, 1221–1242

LABYAH, S. E. and ALDRICH, M. S. (1989) Phasic REM activity and cardiac arrhythmias during initial CPAP treatment of sleep apnoea. *Sleep Research*, **18**, 254

LAKS, L., KRIEGER, J. and PODSZUS, T. (1992) Pulmonary hypertension in obstructive sleep apnoea: retrospective multicentre analysis. *American Review of Respiratory Diseases*, **145**, A865

LAVIE, P. (1983) Incidence of sleep apnoea in a presumably healthy working population. *Sleep*, **6**, 312–318

LAVIE, P., BEN-YOUSEF, R. and RUBIN, A. E. (1984) Prevelance of sleep apnoea syndrome amongst patients with essential hypertension. *American Heart Journal*, **108**, 373–376

LAVIE, P., ZOMER, J., ELIASCHARI, I., JOACHIM, Z., HALPERNE, E., RUBIN, A. E. *et al.* (1982) Excessive daytime sleepiness and insomnia. Association with deviated nasal septum and nocturnal breathing disorders. *Archives of Otolaryngology*, **108**, 373–377

LAVIE, P., FISCHEL, N., ZOMER, J. and ELIASCHAR, I. (1983) The effects of partial and complete mechanical occlusion of the nasal passages on sleep structure and breathing in sleep. *Acta Otolaryngologica*, **95**, 161–166

LENDERS, H., SCHAEFER, J. and PIRSIG, W. (1991) Turbinate hypertrophy in habitual snorers and patients with obstructive sleep apnoea: findings of acoustic rhinometry. *Laryngoscope*, **101**, 614–618

LEVINSON, P. D. and MILLMAN, R. P. (1991) Causes and consequences of blood pressure alterations in obstructive sleep apnoea. *Archives of Internal Medicine*, **151**, 455–462

LUGARESI, E., CIRIGNOTTA, F. and COCCANGA, G. (1984) Clinical significance of snoring. In: *Sleep and Breathing*, edited by N. A. Saunders and C. E. Sullivan. New York: Dekker. pp. 283–98

LUGARESI, E., CIRIGNOTTA, F., COCCANGA, G. and PIANNA, C. (1980) Some epidemiological data on snoring and cardiocirculatory disturbances. *Sleep*, **3**, 221–224

MACALUSO, R. A., REAMS, C., GIBSON, W. S., VRABEC, D. P. and MATRAGRANO, A. (1989) Uvulopalatopharyngoplasty: postoperative management and evaluation of results. *Annals of Otology, Rhinology and Laryngology*, **98**, 502–507

MCNICHOLAS, W. T., TARLO, S. and COLE, P. (1982) Obstructive sleep apnoea during sleep in patients with seasonal allergic rhinitis. *American Review of Respiratory Diseases*, **126**, 625–628

MAISEL, R. H. and GODING, G. S. (1991) Tracheostomy for obstructive sleep apnoea: indications, techniques and selection of tubes. *Operative Techniques in Otolaryngology Head and Neck Surgery*, **2**, 107–111

MATHUR, R., JAN, M. A., MASTROPASQUA, B. and DOUGLAS, N. J. (1992) Upper airway dilator muscle reflex to negative pressure stimuli (abstract). *British Sleep Society Meeting*, 14–16 September, University of Leicester, p. 29

MITLER, M., DAWSON, A. and HENRIKSEN, S. (1988) Bedtime ethanol increases resistance of upper airways and produces sleep in asymptomatic snorers. *Alcohol Clinical and Experimental Research*, **12**, 801–805

OLSEN, K. D., KERN, E. B. and WESTBROOK, P. R. (1981) Sleep

and breathing disturbance secondary to nasal obstruction. *Otolaryngology Head and Neck Surgery*, **89**, 804–810

OSLER, W. (1906) *The Principles and Practice of Medicine*. New York: Appleton. p. 431

PARTINEN, M., GUILLEMINAULT, C., QUERA-SALVA, M. A. and JAMIESON, A. (1988) Obstructive sleep apnoea and cephalometric roentgenograms. The role of anatomic upper airway abnormalities in the definition of abnormal breathing during sleep. *Chest*, **93**, 1199–1205

PARTINEN, M., JAMIESON, A. and GUILLEMINAULT, C. (1988) Long term outcome for obstructive sleep apnoea syndrome patients. *Chest*, **94**, 1200–1204

PELAUSA, E. O. and TARSHIS, L. M. (1989) Surgery for snoring. *Laryngoscope*, **99**, 1006–1010

PETRUSON, B. (1990) Snoring can be reduced when the nasal airflow is increased by the nasal dilator Nozovent. *Archives of Otolaryngology Head and Neck Surgery*, **116**, 462–464

PHILLIPSON, E. A. and SULLIVAN, C. E. (1978) Arousal: the forgotten response to respiratory stimuli. *American Review of Respiratory Diseases*, **118**, 807–809

POWELL, N. and RILEY, R. (1991) Maxillofacial techniques for hypopharyngeal obstruction in obstructive sleep apnoea. *Operative Techniques in Otolaryngology – Head and Neck Surgery*, **2**, 112–119

PRINGLE, M. B. and CROFT, C. B. (1991) A comparison of sleep nasendoscopy and the Muller manoeuvre. *Clinical Otolaryngology*, **16**, 559–562

PRINGLE, M. B. and CROFT, C. B. (1993) A grading system for obstructive sleep apnoea based on sleep nasendoscopy. *Clinical Otolaryngology*, **18**, 480–484

REMMERS, J. E., DEGROOT, W. J., SAUERLAND, E. K. and ANCH, A. M. (1978) Pathogenesis of upper airway occlusion during sleep. *Journal of Applied Physiology*, **44**, 931–938

RILEY, R. and POWELL, N. (1990) Maxillofacial surgery and obstructive sleep apnoea. *Otolaryngology Clinics of North America*, **23**, 809–826

RILEY, R., POWELL, N. and GUILLEMINAULT, C. (1987) Current surgical concepts for treating obstructive sleep apnoea syndrome. *Journal of Oral and Maxillofacial Surgery*, **45**, 149–157

RILEY, R., POWELL, N. and GUILLEMINAULT, C. (1989) Maxillofacial surgery and obstructive sleep apnoea: a review of 80 patients. *Otolaryngology Head and Neck Surgery*, **101**, 353–361

RILEY, R., GUILLEMINAULT, C., POWELL, N. and SYMMONS, F. B. (1985) Palatopharyngoplasty failure, cephalometric roentgenograms and obstructive sleep apnoea. *Otolaryngology Head and Neck Surgery*, **93**, 240–244

RIVLIN, J., HOFFSTEIN, V., KALBFLEISH, J., MCNICHOLAS, W., ZAMEL, N. and BRYAN, A. C. (1984) Upper airway morphology in patients with idiopathic obstructive sleep apnoea. *American Review of Respiratory Diseases*, **129**, 355–360

ROJEWSKI, T. E., SCHULLER, D. E., CLARK, R. W., SCHMIDT, H. S. and POTTS, R. E. (1982) Synchronous video recording of the pharyngeal airway and polysomnograph in patients with obstructive sleep apnoea. *Laryngoscope*, **92**, 246–250

RYAN, C. F., DICKSON, R. I., and LOWER, A. A. (1990) Upper airway measurements predict response to uvulopalatopharyngoplasty in obstructive sleep apnoea. *Laryngoscope*, **100**, 248–253

SANDERS, M. H., MARTIN, R. J., PENNOCK, B. E. and ROGERS, R. M. (1981) The detection of sleep apnoea in the awake patient. The 'saw tooth sign'. *Journal of the American Medical Association*, **245**, 2414–2418

SAUERLAND, E. K., and HARPER, R. M. (1976) The human tongue during sleep, electromyographic activity of the genioglossus muscle. *Experimental Neurology*, **51**, 160–170

SAUERLAND, E. K. and MITCHELL, S. P. (1975) Electromyographic activity of intrinsic and extrinsic muscles of the human tongue. *Texas Report on Biological Medicine*, **33**, 445–455

SCRIMA, L., BROUDY, M. and NAY, K. (1982) Increased severity of obstructive sleep apnoea after bedtime alcohol ingestion: diagnostic potential and proposed mechanism of action. *Sleep*, **5**, 318–328

SERIES, F. and CORMIER, Y. (1990) Effects of protriptyline on diurnal and nocturnal oxygenation in patients with chronic obstructive pulmonary disease. *Annals of Internal Medicine*, **113**, 507–511

SHARP, J. T., JALALUDIN, M., MURRAY, J. A. M. and MARAN, A. G. D. (1990) The uvulopalatopharyngoplasty operation: the Edinburgh experience. *Journal of the Royal Society of Medicine*, **83**, 569–570

SHEPARD, J. W., GARRISON, M. W. and GRITHER, D. A. (1985) Relationship of ventricular ectopy to nocturnal oxygen saturation in patients with obstructive sleep apnoea. *Chest*, **88**, 335–340

SHEPARD, J. W. and THAWLEY, S. E. (1989) Evaluation of the upper airway in patients undergoing uvulopalatopharyngoplasty for obstructive sleep apnoea. *American Review of Respiratory Diseases*, **140**, 711–716

SHER, A. E., THORPY, M. J., SHPRINTZEN, R. J., SPIELMAN, A. J., BURACK, B. and MCGREGOR, P. A. (1985) Predictive value of Muller manoeuvre in selection of patients for uvulopalatopharyngoplasty. *Laryngoscope*, **95**, 1483–1487

SHINER, R. J., CARROLL, N., SAWICKA, E. H., SIMMOND, A. K. and BRAITHWAITE, M. A. (1990) Role of nocturnal hypoxaemia in the genesis of systemic hypertension. *Cardiology*, **77**, 25–29

SHORE, E. T. and MILLMAN, R. P. (1984) Abnormalities in the flow volume loop in obstructive sleep apnoea sitting and standing. *Thorax*, **39**, 775–779

SMITH, P., GOLD, A. and MEYERS, D. (1985) Weight loss in mildly to moderately obese patients with obstructive sleep apnoea. *Annals of Internal Medicine*, **103**, 580–585

STEIN, M. G., GAMSU, G., DE GEER, G., GOLDEN, J. A., CRUMLEY, R. L. and WEBB, W. R. (1987) Cine CT in obstructive sleep apnoea. *American Journal of Radiology*, **148**, 1069–1074

STOOHS, R. and GUILLEMINAULT, C. (1990) Obstructive sleep apnoea syndrome or abnormal upper airway resistance during sleep. *Journal of Clinical Neurophysiology*, **7**, 83–92

STRADLING, J. R. and CROSBY, J. H. (1991) Predictors and prevalence of obstructive sleep apnoea and snoring in 1001 middle aged men. *Thorax*, **46**, 85–90

STRADLING, J. R. and LANE, D. J. (1983) Nocturnal hypoxaemia in chronic obstructive pulmonary disease. *Clinical Science*, **64**, 213

SUGERMAN, H. J. (1986) Pulmonary function in morbid obesity. *Gastroenterology Clinics of North America*, **90**, 225–237

SUGERMAN, H. J., FAIRMAN, R. P., LINDEMAN, A. R., MATHERS, J. A. and GREENFIELD, L. J. (1981) Gastroplasty for respiratory insufficiency of morbid obesity. *Annals of Surgery*, **193**, 677–683

SULLIVAN, C. E. and GRUNSTEIN, R. G. (1989) Continuous positive airway pressure in sleep disordered breathing. In: *Principles and Practice of Sleep Medicine*, edited by M. H. Kryger, T. Roth and W. C. Dement. Philadelphia: W. B. Saunders. p. 559

SULLIVAN, C. E., ISSA, F. G., BERTHON-JONES, M. and EVES, L. (1981) Reversal of obstructive sleep apnoea by continuous positive airway pressure applied through the nares. *Lancet*, i, 862–865

SURATT, P. M., DEE, P. and ATKINSON, R. L. (1983) Fluoroscopic and computed tomography features of the pharyngeal airway in obstructive sleep apnoea. *American Review of Respiratory Diseases*, **127**, 487–492

TASSON, V., BLOCK, A. and BOYSEN, P. (1981) Alcohol increases sleep apnoea and oxygen desaturation in asymptomatic men. *American Journal of Medicine*, **71**, 240–245

VICTOR, M. D. W., SARMIENTO, C. C., YANTA, M. M. and HALVERSON, J. D. (1984) Obscurtive sleep apnoea in the morbidly obese. *Annals of Surgery*, **119**, 970–972

VINCKEN, W., GUILLEMINAULT, C., SILVESTRI, L., COSIO, M. and GRASSINO, A. (1987) Inspiratory muscle activity as a trigger causing the airways to open in obstructive sleep apnoea. *American Review of Respiratory Diseases*, **135**, 372–377

VINER, S., SZALAI, J. P. and HOFFSTEIN, V. (1991) Are history and physical examination a good screening test for sleep apnoea? *Annals of Internal Medicine*, **115**, 356–359

WARLEY, A. R. H., MITCHELL, A. H. and STRADLING, J. R. (1988) Prevelance of nocturnal hypoxaemia in men with and without hypertension. *Queensland Journal of Medicine*, **68**, 637–644

WHITE, J. H. (1982) An overview of obesity. Its significance to nursing – definition, prevelance, etiological concerns and treatment strategies. *Nursing Clinics of North America*, **17**, 191–199

WILLIAMS, A. J., HOUSTON, D., FINBERG, S., LAM, C., KINNEY, J. L. and SANTIAGO, S. (1985) Sleep apnoea syndrome and essential hypertension. *American Journal of Cardiology*, **55**, 1019–1022

YOUNG, T., PALTA, M., DEMPSEY, J., SKATRUD, J., WEBER, S. and BADR, S. (1993) The occurrence of sleep disordered breathing among middle aged adults. *New England Journal of Medicine*, **328**, 1230–1235

ZWILLICH, C., DEVLIN, T., WHITE, D., DOUGLAS, N. J., WEIL, J. and MARTIN, R. I. (1982) Bradycardia during sleep apnoea. *Journal of Clinical Investigation*, **69**, 1286–1292

ZWILLICH, C., PICKETT, C., HANSON, F. N. and WEIL, J. V. (1981) Disturbed sleep and prolonged apnoea during nasal obstruction in normal men. *American Review of Respiratory Diseases*, **124**, 158–160

20

Non-healing granulomas

David Howard

Granulomatous lesions of the nose and sinuses still give rise to some of the greatest confusion and diagnostic difficulty encountered in otorhinolaryngology and its allied specialties. Indeed, their tremendous diversity causes difficulties even for the most experienced pathologist. However, this situation continues to improve with the advances in histopathology techniques and the clearer understanding of the natural history of these pathologies.

Historically the principal components of a granulomatous lesion are considered to be macrophages, epithelioid cells and multinucleated giant cells. However, many of the granulomatous lesions encountered in the nose and sinuses do not have the features of a typical granuloma. Necrosis and vasculitis are also variable features and previous therapies may have altered the situation so that a conclusive 'diagnostic' biopsy is frequently not obtained by the clinician. It therefore remains important that the clinician obtains a detailed clinical history, undertakes a thorough physical examination, and requests the appropriate radiological, haematological, microbiological and histological evaluations. Only then will it be possible effectively to separate the granulomas of the nose and sinuses into those caused by specific infective agents and those which are non-specific and in many instances of unknown aetiology (Table 20.1).

Infection

As a result of the increasing numbers of people travelling internationally throughout the world and settling in other countries it is essential for all otorhinolaryngologists to be aware of the possibility of encountering unusual infective lesions of the nose and paranasal sinuses, although they may not be common entities in the local community where the

Table 20.1 Nasal granulomas

Specific
  Tuberculosis
  Leprosy
  Syphilis
  Yaws
  Scleroma
  Actinomycosis
  Aspergillosis
  Mucormycosis
  Rhinosporidiosis
  Leishmaniasis
  AIDS

Non-specific
  Sarcoidosis
  Wegener's granulomatosis
  Sinonasal lymphoma

clinician is practising. While many of these infective diseases have decreased in frequency in the developed countries they still remain important diseases in large areas of the world.

Tuberculosis

Tuberculosis involving the nasal mucosa remains rare and is almost always associated with primary pulmonary tuberculosis. Macroscopically the lesions in the nose usually take the form of ulcers, although polyps may also occur, and the lesions are most commonly found on the anterior part of the septum, inferior turbinate and anterior choanae. Microscopically the characteristic features of tuberculosis are usually present with epithelioid granulomas, Langhan's giant cells and extensive caseation. Acid-alcohol-fast bacilli are present in the granulomas and their presence is necessary in order to confirm the diagnosis. Other mycobacteria such as *Mycobacterium balnei* and *Mycobacterium leprae* can cause granulomatous lesions in the nose and sinuses. Lupus vulgaris is the name given to tuberculous lesions of the skin of the nose and may cause epitheliomatous reaction of the squamous epithelium giving rise to a misdiagnosis of squamous cell carcinoma (see Plate 4/20/I) (Michaels, 1987).

Leprosy

Leprosy remains an important tropical disease with a worldwide distribution. Almost 1200 cases of leprosy were notified between 1951 and 1985 in England and Wales and all these patients had contracted the disease in other countries (Younus, 1986). The nose is frequently involved in leprosy, and is often the site of first manifestation, although the disease is best known for its effects on skin and peripheral nerves. It is caused by the bacillus *Mycobacterium leprae* which is less acid-fast resistant than *Mycobacterium tuberculosis* but not alcohol fast. When infected the nose may be an important site of discharge of the bacilli. There is a wide spectrum of the disease, ranging between the so-called lepromatous form in which large quantities of mycobacteria are present and tuberculoid leprosy where few organisms are detected.

The precise form of leprosy in any given individual seems to depend on the state of the patient's immune response. Macroscopically the most common changes are a nodular thickening of the mucous membrane and perforation of the cartilaginous septum. In tuberculoid leprosy it is important not to misinterpret the lesion as sarcoidosis or scleroma as the leprae bacilli are much fewer and can be difficult to demonstrate. Dapsone 44, diamenodythenal sulphone (DDS) remains the most widely used drug. It may require administration for many years, particularly in lepromatous leprosy.

Syphilis

The treatment of venereal disease with antibiotics has resulted in a significant diminution of syphilitic lesions. However, one of the inevitable consequences of this improved treatment has been the less frequent consideration of syphilis in the differential diagnosis. Syphilis may be transmitted venereally or congenitally and, in the latter, the nose is always involved. Congenital syphilis does not usually present until several weeks after birth with acute inflammation and persistent catarrh; subsequently by the age of 3–4 years the characteristic saddle nose deformity develops. In acquired nasal syphilis primary chancre of the nasal cavity is rare; when it does occur it involves the anterior part of the septum or skin of the vestibule. Secondary lesions are essentially the same as those which occur on mucous membranes elsewhere and they appear as white, 'mucous patches' and usually present in association with oral and cutaneous lesions.

Tertiary lesions may appear at any time following the secondary stage and their manifestations may be delayed for 20 years or more. Destructive extension of these lesions often leads to ultimate collapse of the bridge of the nose producing the characteristic 'saddle' deformity. Nasal obstruction and blood-stained discharge are common forms of presentation. The anterior nares may be involved by indolent, brawny ulcerating granulations which can be confused with lupus vulgaris, squamous carcinoma, basal cell carcinoma or T-cell lymphoma. The sites most commonly affected in tertiary syphilis are the septum, inferior turbinates and floor of the nose. The localized gummatous form usually produces ulceration and a posterior septal perforation but diffuse syphilitic infiltration may cause swelling and extensive necrosis of nasal and facial tissues. The collapse of the bridge of the nose is not the outcome of destruction of the septum but is due to involvement of the nasal bones which have gradually collapsed because of contraction of scar tissue.

Tertiary lesions are of particular interest as they may present problems of differential diagnosis. Microscopically there are areas of necrosis alternating with granulation tissue which ranges from a non-specific appearance to epithelioid manifestations including multinucleated giant cells mimicking a tuberculoid granuloma. These lesions require the standard serological tests for syphilis and careful culture to exclude mycobacterial infection. In the non-gummatous, diffuse form of tertiary syphilis there are diminished numbers of glands which are hypoactive. Their diminished secretory activity can be ascertained by staining with alkaline phosphatase and periodic-acid-Schiff (PAS) alcian blue staining, this is useful when serological tests are inconclusive.

Yaws

Yaws is an extragenital, treponemal infection occurring in tropical countries and usually beginning in childhood. It is characterized by papillomatous and ulcerated skin nodules and subsequent involvement of lymph nodes and bone. Later there may be gummatous destruction within the nose and paranasal sinuses which has a similar clinical and histological pattern to that of acquired syphilis. In many cases there may be a positive Wassermann reaction but the differential diagnosis relies strongly on the case history. The majority of patients with syphilis and yaws are still treated with penicillin.

Scleroma

This condition was first reported in the nasal cavity by Hebra (1870). Mikulicz (1887) presented a detailed account of the histological picture and the large vacuolated cells which bear his name. However, the condition has a tendency to involve other parts of the upper respiratory tract, most notably the larynx and trachea, and the disease should correctly be called scleroma rather than rhinoscleroma. Von Frisch (1882) observed organisms within the Mikulicz cells and identified *Klebsiella pneumoniae*, subspecies rhinoscleromatis. This latter finding provoked much speculation and argument as to the aetiology of this lesion – and indeed the debate continues. Scleroma is a chronic condition which, in the early part of this century, was most commonly seen in eastern and central Europe. However the disease is rare in these areas nowadays and is most commonly encountered in Central and South America, parts of the Middle East and Far East.

The disease occurs most commonly in the third decade of life and there are essentially three stages. The initial catarrhal rhinitic stage gives symptoms similar to a common cold but often the granulomatous changes in the mucosa are already occurring and the disease may have similar features to atrophic rhinitis. During the second stage, nodular granulomatous masses appear within the nasal cavity and the disease may extend into the sinuses, nasopharynx, larynx, trachea, nasolacrimal system and even intracranially. The nasal tip and ala may be involved producing severe disfigurement, the so-called Hebra nose. The third stage is characterized by fibrosis and cicatricial scarring with consequent distortion. The cellular component, particularly the Mikulicz cells, become less evident leading to difficulty in histological diagnosis.

Mikulicz cells are the characteristic morphological feature and probably derive from a macrophage. Ultrastructural studies show these cells to contain distended vesicular structures and a variable amount of granular material. The bacilli are usually difficult to demonstrate in ordinary haemotoxylin and eosin (H & E) staining and are better demonstrated by silver impregnation stains such as Warthin–Starry or a Giemsa stain. *Klebsiella rhinoscleromatis* is a Gram-negative encapsulated diplococcus, 2–3 μm long. Other types of klebsiella have been identified in patients and proposed as causative organisms. Indeed, a number of other infectious diseases can be mistaken for scleroma illustrating further the initial point made in this chapter of the difficulty of diagnosis between granulomatous conditions. A lepra cell may simulate the Mikulicz cell and mycotic infection, such as rhinosporidiosis, and protozoal infection, such as leishmaniasis, may also be confused with scleroma. The granulomatous second stage may be interpreted as tuberculosis, syphilis, malignancy or Wegener's granulomatosis. Bacterial confirmation is therefore essential in the diagnosis of scleroma and an important aid to diagnosis is the immunohistochemical detection of klebsiella capsular antigen III.

Kouwenaar (1956) pointed out that the clinical picture in scleroma varies according to the geographical location. The Hebra nose is common in Indonesia but rare elsewhere while laryngeal involvement is more common in Europe and America. In the granulomatous phase, masses of inflammatory tissue may cause pressure erosion of bone and extension into the orbit and cranial cavity has been reported. Scleroma responds in a variable manner to streptomycin treatment, although the organism is normally sensitive. The essential problem is access of the antibiotic to the organism and the combination of irradiation to destroy the organisms and streptomycin to improve the mucosal defence mechanisms was found to be the best method of treatment by Toppozada and Gaafar (1986).

Actinomycosis

Actinomycosis in man is usually caused by *Actinomyces israelii*, and over 50% of the cases occur in the head and neck region but reports involving the nose and sinuses are rare. The organisms are now considered to be bacteria – by tradition their description often remains in the section of books dealing with mycoses. The disease most commonly involves the cervicofacial tissues.

The usual site of the rare infection in the nose and sinuses is the maxillary antrum. Irrigation may reveal foul pus containing the causal organism. Granular lesions may be seen in the nose and under certain circumstances the diagnosis of actinomycosis can be made on tissue sections. The appearance of so-called sulphur granules surrounded by a purulent exudate is the hallmark of actinomycosis. The morphological diagnosis of actinomycosis is confirmed if Gram-positive filaments can be identified in the sulphur granules. Infection of the maxillary sinus may also be caused by an anaerobic species of actinomyces, sometimes identified as *Actinomyces bovis* which has long been established as the cause of the granulomatous lesion of the tongue and jaw in cattle. Erosion of bone may occur even at an early stage (Lewis and Manning, 1949), brawny swelling of the cheek with the appearance of fistulae through the skin has been documented.

Nocardiosis

This condition is very rare within the nose and sinuses and is caused by aerobic varieties of actinomyces. Friedmann and Osborn (1982) described a case causing granular lesions on the middle and inferior turbinates which contained many multinucleated giant cells of the Langhan's type and sometimes forming tuberculoid type lesions; culture, however, produced aerobic actinomyces. Penicillin remains the drug of choice.

Fungal disease

Of the many potentially pathogenic fungi, aspergillus is the one principally affecting the nose and sinuses. Others are rare but occur in certain regions of the world. There is an increasing incidence of mycotic infections in immunosuppressed patients and under these circumstances a high tendency for dissemination to other organs. Awareness of the possibility of fungal infection is essential as initial symptoms are often non-specific and the diagnosis may require the use of special stains. With experience the histopathologist can make a correct diagnosis and often place the fungus in its correct genus, this does not however replace mycological studies and this has to be borne in mind and requires adequate specimens to be taken from these patients. A number of these fungal conditions can produce prominent inflammatory changes within the nose including granulomas.

Michaels (1987) clearly divides mycotic infections of the nose and paranasal sinuses into four clinical groups:

1 A fungus ball of aspergilli in the maxillary antrum accompanied by low grade inflammation (aspergillosis)
2 A slowly progressive process with fibrosis involving the nasal and paranasal sinus mucosa spreading externally into the subcutaneous tissues of the nose, orbit and nasopharynx. This lesion is caused by a zygomycete, *Conidiobolus coronatus*
3 A fulminating disease, often occurring in diabetics, but not exclusively, which spreads rapidly from the nose to the base of the skull and brain and caused by a zygomycete, *Rhizopus oryzae*. This fungal infection is commonly known as mucormycosis or rhinocerebral zygomycosis
4 In the fourth group chronic granulomatous lesions of the nasal and paranasal sinus cavities occur and are caused by *Rhinosporidium seeberi* (rhinosporidiosis). Candidosis may rarely also become chronic and cause a candida granuloma.

Protozoal infection

Leishmaniasis

Leishmaniasis is an endemic, infectious disease caused by a protozoan. It is widely distributed in tropical and subtropical countries, but is particularly a problem in Central and South America. It is seen in three forms. A visceral form caused by *Leishmania donovani*, a cutaneous form caused by *Leishmania tropica*, and the mucocutaneous form caused by *Leishmania braziliensis*.

The most common primary sites in patients with mucocutaneous leishmaniasis are the forearm, leg, trunk and nose. The nasal manifestations are probably the result of implantation by contaminated fingers. The nasal lesions may be ulcerative or nodular involving the anterior nares and spreading backwards into the nasal fossa and downwards into the upper lip (see Plate 4/20/II). They may also involve the nasopharynx and cause marked destruction. After inoculation the parasites multiply within histiocytes which later rupture with release of leishmania into the tissue. Biopsy specimens may contain the organisms intracellularly or free in the tissue. In later stages the morphological picture may be strikingly tuberculoid with numerous inflammatory cells but few organisms. Any tuberculoid lesions in the nose and sinuses in a patient coming from endemic areas should be examined for *Leishmania*. The mucosal infection becomes a chronic condition unless treatment is applied. In the early stages the lesions do respond to antimony compounds but if left the nose may become deformed and there may be massive destruction of midfacial tissues and death from bronchopneumonia.

Viruses

AIDS

The otolaryngological manifestations of HIV infection can occur at any stage of the disease but a granular rhinitis may be seen in the nasal cavity similar to sarcoid and often associated with sinusitis. There is usually other, more obvious evidence of HIV elsewhere. The infecting organisms are the common pathogens. In the fully developed AIDS syndrome, Karposi's sarcoma can occur on any part of the skin or mucous membrane but is rarely found in the nose (Maran and Lund, 1990).

Granulamatous conditions
Sarcoidosis

In his original description of sarcoidosis, Boeck (1899), noted that four of his nine patients had nasal sarcoidosis that preceded the skin lesions. Sarcoidosis is a systemic condition of unknown aetiology, it may affect any part of the body but most frequently lymph nodes, skin, lungs, eyes, liver, spleen and small bones of the hands and feet. It is found throughout the world although there is higher incidence in the south east USA and Scandinavia and it is more common in coloured races.

Sarcoid lesions may affect the nose in three different ways. The skin of the nose may be affected by sarcoid lesions; deep granulomatous plaques may occupy the full thickness of the dermis to produce bulbous red or violet skin lesions (Figure 20.1 and see Plates 4/20/III, 4/20/IV and 4/20/V). The nasal bones may be affected by sarcoid lesions in a similar manner to those of the hands and feet. The nasal bridge becomes swollen and plain X-rays may show translucent deposits. Separate from, or in addition to the above two changes, the most common form of nasal sarcoid includes involvement of the nasal mucosa usually on the nasal septum or inferior turbinates. The lesions may be relatively inconspicuous in their early stages comprising of yellow or greyish slightly raised nodules. The patient complains of obstruction, mucopurulent and sometimes blood-stained discharge and crusting. Saddling of the nose, synechiae and stenosis may occur. Investigations include ESR, serum calcium, and serum angiotensin converting enzyme measurements. A chest X-ray is mandatory and sinus X-rays frequently show mucosal thickening. A Kviem test, which consists of an intradermal injection of filtered extract of spleen from a case of sarcoid, followed 6 weeks later by skin biopsy, shows positive histology in 90% of cases but is a test which remains open to criticism on the grounds of non-specificity.

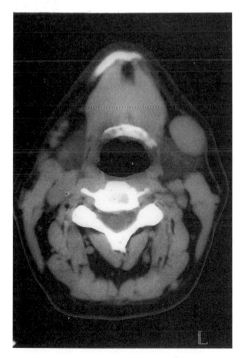

Figure 20.1 Sarcoidosis. Axial CT scan of neck showing cervical lymphadenopathy in submandibular region, confirmed by fine needle aspirate

The nasal granulomas normally tend to be smaller than those found in Wegener's granulomatosis and histologically are characterized by the presence of epithelioid cell tubercles without caseation, which are converted into hyaline fibrous tissue. In fact the granulomas may have some central necrosis but no caseous necrosis as in tuberculosis. Implicit in the diagnosis is the exclusion of any other aetiological basis for the granuloma. The aetiology of sarcoidosis remains unknown and treatment of nasal symptoms is best achieved using alkaline douches and betamethasone drops. Some patients will also require oral corticosteroids to control other symptoms of their sarcoidosis and at times the nasal lesions will seem to improve with this.

Wegener's granulomatosis

As is frequently the case in medicine Frederick Wegener was not the first person to describe the syndrome which now bears his name. Heinz Klinger (1931) reported post-mortem studies on two patients who died of disseminated vasculitis and he proposed that this was an atypical form of polyarteritis nodosa. Wegener (1936, 1939) reported further cases and gave a detailed account of the natural history of this condition under the name of rhinogenic granulomatosis. The patients died between 4 and 7 months after diagnosis of irreversible renal disease – a situation which fortunately we rarely see nowadays. The disease was later clearly defined as a condition characterized by granulomas within the nasal cavity and the respiratory tract, a generalized vasculitis and a focal form of glomerulonephritis (Fahey, Leonard and Churg, 1954). It was also realized that this was a generalized condition that could involve any organ. The issue of more localized forms of Wegener's granulomatosis remains under debate but localized Wegener's granulomatosis in the lungs was first described by Carrington and Liebow (1966). Although presentation in a single system remains a clinical entity many of these patients go on to develop generalized Wegener's granulomatosis. Nowadays patients remain well for long periods in the absence of glomerulonephritis.

The aetiology of Wegener's granulomatosis remains unknown. Its inflammatory nature and its resemblance to polyarteritis nodosa indicate that it represents some form of hypersensitivity reaction with an immune response to an unknown stimulus. It has been postulated that this may be related to inhaled bacteria, explaining the frequency with which the respiratory tract is involved. The deposition of the immune complexes is thought to be responsible for vasculitis in other conditions but they have only been demonstrated in a small proportion of patients with Wegener's granulomatosis. McDonald and De-Remee (1983) studied biopsies subjected to immunofluorescence microscopy, but rarely found deposits of immunoglobulin or complement. From an aetiological and diagnostic point of view the most important finding of recent years was that reported by der

Woude, Rosmussen and Witt (1985). These workers found antibodies reacting with the cytoplasm of ethanol-fixed granulocytes and monocytes in 25 patients with Wegener's granulomatosis. Lockwood, Baker and Jones (1987) have since shown that patients with polyarteritis also have circulating autoantibodies to neutrophil cytoplasmic antigens (ANCA). These autoantibodies may be fundamental to the development of systemic vasculitis. Although the pathogenicity of ANCA has not been completely proven they are far more readily detected in patients with Wegener's granulomatosis, particularly those who are not receiving treatment with either steroids or cytotoxic medications. The ANCA antibodies have been reported to be present in almost every patient with Wegener's granulomatosis but disappear when the disease is treated or regresses. Recent reports confirm that these antibodies are not entirely specific for Wegener's granulomatosis but present in some patients with polyarteritis and Churg-Strauss syndrome. Debate continues with regard to their use in monitoring treatment of the patients.

Clinical features

The age distribution of Wegener's granulomatosis shows a wide spectrum and all large reported series range from adolescence to the eighth decade of life. Most series also report significant numbers of the patients to be under 25 years of age and these young patients usually present with the generalized form. Most reports confirm that this disease predominates within the respiratory tract and kidneys, although any system may be involved and, in active cases, this involvement may be multiple at the onset or they may become rapidly affected. The frequency with which different sites are involved, both at presentation and subsequently, varies with the interests and specialty of the reporting physicians.

As late as the early 1970s Wegener's granulomatosis remained a serious and a lethal disease with patients frequently dying within a 6–8-month period. Even today this classical presentation with vasculitis of the respiratory tract and fulminating glomerulonephritis is recorded. It remains of great importance since rapid progression with a fatal outcome can occur in as little as 48 hours. The duration of symptoms before a diagnosis is made remains highly variable and can be more than a year in some cases. All otorhinolaryngologists should be aware that granulomas of the upper respiratory tract are the most common presenting feature. They may be associated with variable degrees of epistaxis, nasal obstruction and the appearance of bloody crusts in the nose. These may continue with destruction of intranasal structures including the septum and, eventually, nasal collapse. Minor nasal surgery and repeated biopsies during this period may add to the problem. Many patients present with a short history of progressive malaise, pyrexia, weight loss and notably feel very unwell. They may have minimal physical findings under these circumstances which often results in delay in diagnosis. The nose and sinuses are involved in more than 80% of patients. With the widespread availability of the ANCA test it is important that patients in this category have, at the very least, an ESR, ANCA test, chest X-ray and examination of their urine. Failure to consider Wegener's granulomatosis, or at worst to make a misdiagnosis of some other granulomatous nasal condition, may result in delay of treatment allowing considerable progression of the disease. It is important to point out that, while there is intranasal destruction of bone and cartilage in some patients with Wegener's granulomatosis with associated septal perforation and external saddle deformity, there are none of the *gross* destructive changes of midfacial skin seen in T-cell lymphomas and basal cell carcinomas.

Pulmonary symptoms

The majority of patients with active disease experience pulmonary symptoms at some point; cough, haemoptysis or pleuritic pain. The pulmonary lesions often cavitate and can be seen radiologically in most patients. These may be the presenting symptoms and the diagnosis may be aided by flexible bronchoscopy and lung biopsy. Encapsulated lung abscess formation can occur.

Renal symptoms

Between 30 and 90% of patients will develop renal symptoms, although the organs may be spared in more limited forms of the disease. Both casts and red cells appear in the urine and early treatment is vital since damage is irreversible. Microscopic evaluation of a mid-stream specimen of urine remains a simple but important test in the diagnosis and management of Wegener's granulomatosis. Renal biopsy is not essential and it must be remembered that Wegener's granulomatosis is one of a number of diseases which produces segmental or diffuse glomerulonephritis.

Ocular symptoms

The commonest ocular manifestation of Wegener's granulomatosis is orbital involvement but optic neuritis and retinal artery occlusion also occur. Conjunctivitis, dacrocystitis, episcleritis and corneal ulceration have also been described. Approximately 20% of patients may experience proptosis from an orbital mass or extension from surrounding paranasal sinuses. Delayed or inadequate treatment is responsible for failure to control many orbital symptoms and loss of vision has been frequently documented.

Oral symptoms

A wide variety of oral lesions have been described. The commonest is a hyperplastic granular lesion of the gingiva, beginning in the area of the interdental papillae. If a tooth is lost the socket fails to heal. Extensive ulcerative stomatitis has also been reported.

Otological symptoms

Approximately one-third of patients may develop serous otitis media or acute otitis media. There may be deafness, pain and suppuration. Facial nerve paralysis has also been recorded. Both conductive and sensorineural hearing loss occur and while a secretory otitis media may be secondary to inflammatory changes within the nasal cavity, Wegener's granulomatosis of the temporal bone, with necrotizing granulation tissue filling the tympanic cavity, has been documented.

Laryngeal and tracheal symptoms

Laryngeal involvement is unusual but when present the subglottis and upper trachea are most commonly affected. This may present a serious problem with laryngotracheal obstruction. Biopsies frequently show only non-specific changes, and dilatation and resection are unsatisfactory and usually unsuccessful. Localized disease and a positive ANCA test have been well documented (Hoare *et al.*, 1989).

Other symptoms

The generalized vasculitis may produce ulceration of the skin, particularly of the distal arms and legs. Polymyalgia and polyarthritis have been described. Direct nervous system involvement occurs in 10–15% of patients in some series. This latter is caused by granulomatous invasion of neural tissues, intracerebral or meningeal granulomas, as well as neuritic vasculitis. Any cranial nerve may be involved. Multiple case reports describe solitary examples of involvement to most of the organs in the body with Wegener's granulomatosis making it a possible diagnosis in a wide range of obscure and bizarre clinical presentations.

Investigations

As soon as the disease is suspected an ESR, ANCA test, chest X-ray and examination of the urine for blood cells and casts is mandatory. Other investigations such as sinus X-rays, renal biopsies etc. will depend on the sites and extent of involvement. While the ANCA test is not specific for Wegener's granulomatosis, in the untreated patient it is a particularly valuable diagnostic tool for the early diagnosis of

disease. When coupled with a high ESR (over 80 mm/h), positive nasal findings, or chest X-ray changes, it is important to consider immediate treatment with steroids and cytotoxics.

Nasal biopsy

Nasal involvement in Wegener's granulomatosis is by no means specific and the typical clinical appearance with extensive nasal mucosal swelling, ulceration and crusting is not always present. The crusts are usually foul smelling, rather large, green and often bloody. They may completely cover the area of ulceration. It is important to obtain representative biopsy material and ideally the surgeon should take several biopsies from the septum and turbinates. The crusts are microscopically non-specific and should be cultured for microorganisms. The histopathologist must be provided with an adequate, minimally traumatized sample but the absolute diagnosis of Wegener's granulomatosis does not rely on this biopsy material. It is simply a clue which will often help in the differential diagnosis. The main histological features in Wegener's granulomatosis are:

1 Vasculitis is mandatory for the diagnosis and fibrinoid vascular necrosis is a common finding
2 The granulomas are of the epithelial cell type being large, irregular and lined with histiocytes. They may show fibrinoid necrosis but can also be non-necrotic
3 Multinucleated giant cells are often present and eosinophils are numerous.

Treatment

The report of Fahey, Leonard and Churg (1954) suggesting that steroids and a variety of cytotoxic drugs could improve short-term prognosis has subsequently resulted in over 90% of patients with Wegener's granulomatosis obtaining prolonged remission. Renal damage prior to commencing treatment is the major prognostic factor and therapy should be begun as soon as the diagnosis is suspected rather than waiting for histological verification. While debate on the usefulness of the ANCA test to monitor therapy continues, there is no doubt that the ESR has been a most useful method for assessing response to treatment. The majority of patients, at the active stage when first diagnosed, feel generally very unwell and it is interesting to see the rapidity with which this feeling resolves when they begin treatment. Progress is monitored by ESR and ANCA estimations. The latter frequently becomes negative with the disease under control. Although a sign of renal involvement is the presence of red cells, protein and casts in an uncontaminated specimen of urine, it is important to establish renal function early in the disease using creatinine clearance estimations.

Unfortunately, despite many reports of good initial control of Wegener's granulomatosis using a combination of prednisolone and either cyclophosphamide or azathioprine, the majority of long-term studies emphasize the continuing problems that these patients face. Harrison's experience during 27 years at The Royal National Throat, Nose and Ear Hospital (Harrison and Lund, 1993) showed the varied course which this disease can take. Prednisolone 60–80 mg/day with cyclophosphamide 2 mg/kg or azathioprine 200 mg/day should produce a dramatic improvement in acute disease. The ESR may fall slowly and gradual reduction of both drugs has to be based on clinical and laboratory assessment. It is not possible to generalize, but with the exception of the fulminating, progressive cases, initial control is now the norm. In Harrison and Lund's series, azathioprine with prednisolone has produced 100% immediate control in 48 cases and, over a 20 year follow-up in some patients, no patients have had significant complications such as alopecia, leucopenia or iatrogenic haemorrhagic cystitis. In contrast, a major complication of cyclophosphamide is leucopenia, and alopecia may occur even with low dosage. Approximately 40% of patients taking this drug may have some bladder bleeding which is a considerable disadvantage in patient management when the urine is being assessed for the possibility of red cells. In view of the unavoidable side effects of continued steroid and cytotoxic treatment, there is an obvious desire by both the patient and doctor to reduce or stop treatment as soon as possible. However, there is no doubt that this is a cyclical disease and clinical flare up may result in considerable tissue reaction, damage and subsequent fibrosis. These are best avoided. Outstanding examples of this are the fibrosis which, in the orbit can result in painful proptosis, visual defects or blindness, and in the lungs with increasing pulmonary fibrosis with consequent severe dyspnoea. Although both ESR and ANCA tests are of value in monitoring the disease, change can occur suddenly and the patient is often aware of variations in their well-being in the absence of altered haematological tests and, in our experience, some are particularly sensitive to changes in dose. They should therefore be listened to with care and their medications altered appropriately.

In Harrison and Lund's series, there are patients who have, after many years, managed to stop their medications but it has been impossible to predict the likelihood of any individual patient suffering late recurrence, particularly after immunological challenges such as influenza or pregnancy. It requires a delicate balance between the intrinsic risks of a hazardous relapse against the surety of drug toxicity, and for the moment permanent follow up remains essential.

Sinonasal lymphoma (non-healing midline granuloma, midfacial destructive lesion)

The vast majority of the lesions previously reported as non-healing midline granuloma, lethal midline granuloma, midfacial granuloma syndrome, midfacial destructive lesion, Stewart's granuloma, polymorphic reticulosis, midline malignant reticulosis, lymphatoid granulomatosis, necrosis with atypical cellular exudate, etc. were probably, in fact, malignant lymphomas of the sinonasal region. Harrison (1987), Michaels (1987) and Hellquist (1990) all strongly stated that probably all destructive midline granulomatous lesions previously described by this wide variety of terminology are manifestations of malignant lymphoma and should be treated as such. And, in the light of our present knowledge, it is now extremely doubtful whether any subgroup of 'idiopathic', inflammatory, destructive lesion exists. It is important to differentiate between the different types of malignant lymphoma in this region (see Plate 4/20/VI).

1 Generalized lymphoma involving the sinonasal tract
2 Lymphomas of Waldeyer's ring, extending into the nasal cavity and sinuses
3 Peripheral, extranodal sinonasal lymphoma which causes the well-known destruction of midfacial structures.

Generalized lymphoma involving the nasal tract

The nose and sinuses are rarely involved in generalized malignant lymphoma of both non-Hodgkin's and Hodgkin's type, although Waldeyer's ring is often involved. In cases where this happens there is seldom any destruction of facial structures and the diagnosis is already established on a lymph node biopsy. Biopsy specimens from Waldeyer's ring are frequently taken in patients with malignant lymphoma when assessing the clinical stage of the disease.

Malignant lymphomas of Waldeyer's ring

In Waldeyer's ring most of the lymphomas are the large cell histiocytic type, more than 85% being diffuse (Barton *et al.*, 1984; Burk, 1988), but all forms of Hodgkin's lymphomas may occur. Most of these are of the B-cell lineage. When histiocytic lymphomas of Waldeyer's ring involve the nasal and paranasal cavities they are not as destructive as peripheral T-cell lymphomas and frequently only cause nasal obstruction, epistaxis or swelling of the maxillary area.

Peripheral, sinonasal, T-cell lymphoma

It is this tumour which is responsible for the classical destruction of the midface and which previously caused great controversy with clinical and pathological debate. It was first described by McBride (1896), with a subsequent comprehensive account of the clinical and histological features by Stewart (1933). Inconsistencies in terminology and histopathological criteria caused much confusion and, at times, similarities with Wegener's granuloma were suggested. However, the situation is now clear and we now know that nasal T-cell lymphomas are responsible for the slow progressive destruction of the nose and midfacial region by what seems an apparent chronic inflammatory response. There is remarkably little systemic disturbance and in complete contrast to Wegener's granulomatosis no evidence of pulmonary or renal involvement. In the past, death has eventually followed intercurrent infection or disseminated lymphoma. Inadequate diagnosis or inadequate radiotherapy and chemotherapy still make this an unsatisfactory lesion.

The nasal T-cell lymphoma still presents a diagnostic problem because the atypical cell infiltrates are often dispersed in necrotic areas. Good quality biopsy material from tissue beneath the crust is essential. The formalin-fixed biopsies are insufficient and it is advisable to arrange for fresh tissue and for the pathologist to be forewarned. Peripheral T-cell lymphomas possess an extremely heterogeneous histological appearance. In good quality biopsy material there should be an abundance of atypical lymphocytes which show positive immunohistochemical reactivity to T-cell markers. With the fresh tissue a substantial panel of monoclonal antibodies against T-cell differentiation antigen should be applied as approximately 80% of the peripheral T-cell lymphomas will show aberrant phenotypes. Histologically the infiltrates are polymorphic and atypical cells tend to be arranged in a necrotizing angioinfiltrative growth pattern. Infiltrates consist of neoplastic atypical T lymphocytes mixed with plasma cells, small lymphocytes, histiocytes, eosinophils and also some immunoblasts (Hellquist, 1990). Granulomas and giant cells are not present in T-cell lymphomas; thrombosis and necrosis are, however, common findings. The exact classification of these peripheral T-cell lymphomas remains under evaluation – as too does their treatment.

These lesions, previously described as 'midline granulomas' were initially treated with low doses of radiotherapy. This occasionally produced a dramatic response but no long-term cures. Nowadays we recommend that all patients must be treated with radical dose radiotherapy of 5500 cGy or more with wide field coverage including, nose, sinuses and palate. Recurrence or the development of disseminated lymphoma worsens the prognosis and it is possible that a regimen of chemotherapy may be advocated with further experience in those lesions classified as high grade.

Eosinophilic granuloma

Debate continues as to whether eosinophilic granuloma is a localized manifestation of histiocytosis X or represents an entity in its own right. The aetiology is unknown but the basic process for all three conditions in histiocytosis X, i.e. Hand–Schüller–Christian disease, Letterer–Siwe disease, and eosinophilic granuloma, is a hyperplasia of Langhans cell type histiocytes. The eosinophilic granuloma lesions predominantly occur in bone with the skull being involved in almost one-half of patients. While all areas can be affected the temporal, frontal and parietal bones are the common sites.

A wide age range from infancy to over 80 years has been recorded but the majority of patients are young children (Appling, Jenkins and Patton, 1983). The usual presentation is a painful swelling of the involved bone, often present for many months. This is commonly associated with cervical lymphadenopathy. Mandibular lesions produce toothache, gum ulceration and loose teeth. Radiological evaluation shows punched out bony lesions and in the jaws the radiolucent areas surrounding the teeth produce a most dramatic appearance. Macroscopically the lesions are soft and yellow or red-brown in colour and biopsy material is best obtained by curettage. Microscopically there are numerous histiocytic cells and eosinophils with associated fibrosis. The greater the number of eosinophils the more likely a reasonable prognosis.

Treatment depends on whether or not the eosinophilic granulomatous lesion is localized, and often solitary. This is termed 'type 2' disease in recent publications and approximately 25% of cases present in this manner (Cinberg, 1978). With unifocal disease the combination of curettage/excision and radiotherapy is usually curative provided that no new lesions develop within approximately one year. However, a proportion of the patients will develop a generalized disease with hepatosplenomegaly, lymphadenopathy, skin lesions and further osseous lesions, so-called 'type 1'. The course of this disease can be rapid with a poor prognosis. Survival with multifocal disease is improved in the older age group, patients with no visceral involvement, and patients with a high number of eosinophils in the lesions. Chemotherapy has understandably been advocated for this type 1 disease in addition to surgery and radiotherapy. At present the most effective chemotherapy regimen appears to be etoposide and steroids.

These may need to be given for periods of 12 months or more depending on the response (Benz-Lemoine, 1989). Recently alpha interferon and bone marrow transplantation have also been used successfully.

Giant cell reparative granuloma

These lesions commonly occur in children and young adults but are benign osseous lesions despite the presence of mitoses which may cause the inexperienced pathologist difficulties. The giant cells do not contain multiple nuclei as in a true giant cell tumour. In contrast a giant cell tumour is rare in children and young adults and the giant cells contain large numbers of nuclei and are surrounded by spindle-celled elongated nuclei. Giant cell tumours are benign but must be completely excised to prevent recurrence. Giant cell lesions mimicking reparatory granuloma are also found in association with hyperparathyroidism and appropriate biochemical tests are required to exclude this diagnosis.

Cholesterol granuloma

Cholesterol granulomas are most commonly found in the mastoid air cells and paranasal sinuses, the frontal sinus being the commonest latter site. They are a granulomatous reaction to cholesterol crystals which have been precipitated in the tissue following haemorrhage. The appearances are typical with granulation tissue containing foreign-body-type giant cells surrounding clefts created by the cholesterol crystal. Cholesteatoma may coexist with cholesterol granuloma in the ear and this occasionally gives rise to confusion. Adequate surgical removal is curative for cholesterol granuloma and the majority are found by chance at surgical exploration.

Allergic granulomatosis

This syndrome was first described by Churg and Strauss in 1951 and frequently carries their name. They described asthma associated with pulmonary infiltrates seen on chest X-ray which on biopsy show necrotizing giant cell vasculitis, interstitial granulomas and eosinophilic pneumonia-like areas. Subsequently it was realized that these patients often have nasal involvement (in approximately two-thirds of the cases), exhibiting rhinitis, polyp formation and occasionally septal perforation (Olsen *et al.*, 1980). Nasal biopsies show necrotizing granulomas surrounded by an abundance of eosinophils, giant cells and plasma cells but usually without vasculitis. Presence of the profound eosinophilia and a strong clinical history of asthma helps to separate this rare syndrome from other granulomatous disorders of the nose, such as Wegener's granulomatosis. Treatment consists of systemic and local corticosteroids and, occasionally, nasal polyps may require removal.

Plasma cell granuloma

It is appropriate to finish this chapter with this confusing and inaccurate term. There are no granulomas in this lesion, which may occur in the mucosa of the sinuses. In severe chronic sinusitis with gross inflammation, the mucosa may become heavily infiltrated by plasma cells which appear to form lymphoid follicles, not normally present in the mucosa of the sinuses. This may present a trap for the unwary pathologist and an incorrect diagnosis of lymphoma may be made under these circumstances. However, with the advent of modern immunohistochemical stains, as was indeed stated in the very first paragraph of this chapter, a polyclonal plasma cell population can be easily demonstrated indicating the true nature of the inflammatory lesion.

References

APPLING, D., JENKINS, H. A. and PATTON, G. A. (1983) Eosinophilic granuloma in the temporal bone and skull. *Otolaryngology, Head and Neck Surgery*, **91**, 358–365

BARTON, J. H., OSBORNE, B. M., BUTLER, J. J., MEOZ, R. T., KONG, J., FULLER, L. M. (1984) Non-Hodgkins lymphoma of the tonsil. A clinopathological study of 65 cases. *Cancer*, **53**, 86–95

BENZ-LEMOINE, E. (1989) Prognostic factors in histiocytosis X. *Annals de Pediatrie (Paris)*, **36**, 499–503

BOECK, C. (1899) Multiple benign sarcoid of the skin. *Journal of Cutaneous and Genito-Urinary Diseases*, **17**, 543–550

BURK, J. S. (1988) Lymphomas. In: *Pathology of the Head and Neck*, edited by D. R. Gnepp. Edinburgh: Churchill Livingstone. pp. 335–358

CARRINGTON, C. B. and LIEBOW, A. A. (1966) Limited forms of angiitis and granulomatosis of Wegener's type. *American Journal of Medicine*, **41**, 497–527

CHURG, J. and STRAUSS, I. (1951) Allergic granulomatosis, allergic angiitis and periarteritis nodosa. *American Journal of Pathology*, **27**, 277–301

CINBERG, J. Z. (1978) Eosinophilic granuloma in the head and neck: a five year review with report of an instructive case. *Laryngoscope*, **88**, 1281–1289

DER WOUDE, F. J., ROSMUSSEN, N. and WITT, A. (1985) Auto antibodies against neutrophils and monocytes: tool for diagnosis and marker of disease activity in Wegener's granulomatosis. *Lancet*, i 424–429

FAHEY, J., LEONARD, E. and CHURG, J. (1954) Wegener's granulomatosis. *American Journal of Medicine*, **17**, 168–170

FRIEDMANN, I. F. and OSBORN, D. A. (1982) Other mycotic and parasitic infections: In: *Pathology of Granulomas and Neoplasms of the Nose and Paranasal Sinuses*. Edinburgh: Churchill Livingstone. pp. 70–83

HARRISON, D. F. N. (1987) Midline destructive granuloma: fact or fiction. *Laryngoscope*, **97**, 1049–1053

HARRISON, D. F. N. and LUND, V. J. (1993) Wegener's granulomatosis. In: *Tumours of the Upper Jaw.* Edinburgh: Churchill Livingstone. pp. 283–293

HEBRA, F. (1870) Über ein eigenthümliches neugebilde an der naserhinosklerom. *Wiener medizinische Wochenschrift,* 20, 1–5

HELLQUIST, H. B. (1990) Granulomatous lesions of the nose and sinuses. In: *Pathology of the Nose and Paranasal Sinuses.* London: Butterworths. pp. 60–81

HOARE, T. J., JAYNE, D., EVANS, P. R. and HOWARD, D. J. (1989) Wegener's granulomatosis, subglottic stenosis and antineutrophil cytoplasm antibodies. *Journal of Laryngology and Otology,* 103, 1187–1191

KLINGER, H. (1931) Grenzformen der periarteritis nodosa. *Frankfurt Journal of Pathology,* 42, 450–458

KOUWENAAR, W. (1956) Rhinoscleroma: a review of the present situation. *Documenta de medecina Geographica et Tropica,* 8, 13–22

LEWIS, R. B. and MANNING, E. L. (1949) Actinomycosis involving ethmoid and maxillary sinuses. *Archives of Otorhinolaryngology,* 49, 423–430

LOCKWOOD, C. M., BAKER, D. and JONES, J. (1987) Association of alkaline phosphatase with an autoantigen recognized by circulating anti-neutrophil antibodies in systemic vasculitis. *Lancet,* i, 716–719

MCBRIDE, P. (1896) A case of rapid destruction of the nose and face. *Journal of Laryngology and Otology,* 12, 64–66

MCDONALD, T. J. and DEREMEE, R. A. (1983) Wegener's granulomatosis. *Laryngoscope,* 93, 220–231

MARAN, A. D. G. and LUND V. J. (1990) *Clinical Rhinology.* Stuttgart: Thieme Medical Publishers. p. 60

MICHAELS, L. (1987) Miscellaneous conditions. In: *Ear, Nose and Throat Histopathology.* Berlin: Springer Verlag. pp. 227–236

MIKULICZ, J. (1887) Uber das rhinosklerom (Hebra). *Archives für Klinische Chirurgie,* 20, 485–534

OLSEN, K. D., NEEL, H. B. (lll), DEREMEE, R. A. and WEILLARD, L. H. (1980) Nasal manifestations of allergic granulomatosis and angiitis (Churg-Strauss syndrome). *Otolaryngology, Head and Neck Surgery,* 88, 85–89

STEWART, J. P. (1933) Progressive lethal granulomatous ulceration of the nose. *Journal of Laryngology and Otology,* 48, 657–701

TOPPOZADA, H. H. and GAAFAR, H. A. (1986) The effect of streptomycin and irradiation on rhinoscleroma. (Electron micrsocopy study.) *Journal of Laryngology and Otology,* 100, 809–815

VON FRISCH., A. (1882) Zur Aetiologie des Rhinoscleroms. *Wiener Medizinische Wochenschrift,* 32, 969–972

WEGENER, F. (1936) Uber generaliserlez septische geffasserkrankugen. *Verhandlungen der Deutschen gesselschaft für Pathologie,* 42, 202–210

WEGENER, F. (1939) Uber eine eigenartige rhinogene granulomatese mit besonderer beteilgung des arterier systems und der mieren. *Beitrage zur Pathologie,* 102, 36–68

YOUNUS, M. (1986) Leprosy in ENT. *Journal of Laryngology and Otology,* 100, 1437–1442

21

Facial pain and headache

N. S. Jones

The patient with facial pain presents a diagnostic challenge. Difficulties arise because of the frequency of referred pain and the overlap in symptoms between different conditions. It is essential to take a structured history in order not only to reach the correct diagnosis but to avoid misguided treatments, especially surgical, which only complicate the picture. The range of disorders which present to general practitioners, oto-rhinolaryngologists, neurologists, ophthalmologists, and oral-maxillofacial surgeons varies considerably and it may appear that each specialty is presented with a completely different subgroup of patients. However, diseases are not limited by the specialty on the sign of the outpatient clinic, and it is therefore essential to keep an open mind.

Painful stimuli affecting facial structures are mostly transmitted via afferents in the trigeminal nerve to the spinal tract in the brain stem. Pain afferents from the VIIth, IXth and Xth cranial nerves also relay in the spinal tract. The majority of these fibres are unmyelinated and therefore produce a poorly localized dull ache, rather than the sharp, well-defined pain produced by the myelinated fibres which supply the skin of the face. Referred pain, on the other hand, represents incorrect central interpretation, probably due to stimulation of the same group of cells in the central posterior nucleus of the thalamus, although a more peripheral interaction cannot be excluded.

Facial pain has a special emotional significance. This means that while pathology is often present, symptom interpretation by the patient forms part of the diagnosis: e.g. a young woman who is assaulted and has her nose fractured may have it reduced, but subsequent nasal symptoms, whether directly related to this incident or not, may be coloured by her traumatic experience. She may feel that the damage which she has sustained cannot be repaired in physical terms alone and the underlying anxiety which she has about her condition or her unresolved feeling relating to the incident may influence the expression of her symptoms.

The history from the patient is often the only source of information on the nature of the pain, and the patient's description and affect are vital clues in interpreting what is going on. Melzack and Wall (1965) postulated a mechanism by which emotional factors can lower the pain threshold, by decreasing activity in the normal central inhibitory efferents and thereby opening the synaptic gate to transmit pain impulses.

For a few patients, facial pain may be the channel by which they express emotional distress, anxiety, or the psychological harm caused by disease, trauma or surgery. It may be the means by which they demand attention or obtain secondary gain. However, there is no distinct division between somatic and psychogenic pain and few patients suffer exclusively from one or the other. The presence of a marked psychological overlay does not mean that there is no underlying organic problem, but it should make one wary about initiating surgery.

If there is a big discrepancy between the patient's affect and the description of the pain, one may find that the organic component of the illness may be of relatively minor importance. Pain which remains constant for many months or years, or which extends either across the midline or across defined dermatomes, is less likely to have a physical basis. However, pain associated with clear exacerbating or relieving factors, whose onset was clearcut and whose site does not vary during the consultation, usually has an organic cause.

Should the diagnosis remain obscure, re-taking the history at the next consultation may be helpful, or a symptom chart kept by the patient may be of use. On the other hand, manifest uncertainty on the part of the doctor may induce anxiety, and although it may be tempting to keep the patient under review, this runs the risk of medicalizing a minor symptom and generating dependence. If a patient's ability to function is severely impaired by chronic pain he or she should be referred to a pain clinic which may be able to offer a variety of approaches to the problem.

The essence of the problem is how to diagnose the cause relatively quickly, efficiently and methodically. A careful history is central in establishing a correct diagnosis.

Twelve questions form the basis of a mental algorithm which helps to reduce the differential diagnoses.

1 Where is the pain and does it radiate anywhere?
Asking the patient to point with one finger to the site of the pain is helpful, not only because it localizes the pain, but also because the gesture made often relays information about its nature, and the facial expression indicates its emotional significance to the patient. The commonest diagnoses to be missed are temporomandibular joint dysfunction presenting as deep aural pain or tension headache as a frontal headache.

2 Is it deep or superficial?
Pain from the skin tends to be sharp and well-defined, while deep pain is dull and poorly localized.

3 Is the pain continuous or intermittent?
The periodicity of symptoms may be a pointer to the diagnosis, e.g. being woken in the early hours by severe facial pain which lasts up to 2 hours suggests cluster headache. On the other hand, pain which is unrelenting over a long period and is unaffected by analgesics often has a large non-organic component.

4 How did the pain begin?
A nagging ache under the nasal bridge initiated by an upper respiratory infection implies a rhinological cause. An aura followed by nausea preceding unilateral facial pain or headache are typical of migraine.

5 How often does the pain occur?
Recurrent bouts of aching of the ear and upper neck with sharp twinges is a pattern characteristic of temporomandibular joint dysfunction, while monthly premenstrual headaches are typical of migraine.

6 What is the pattern of the attacks and are they progressing?
The relentless progression of a headache, in particular if associated with nausea or effortless vomiting is worrying, and an intracranial lesion should be sought. The response to the question whether the symptoms are worsening or improving broadly indicates whether conservative management is appropriate or more intervention is called for.

7 How long is each episode?
Frontoethmoidal sinusitis can cause symptoms of variable duration, while the sharp multiple attacks of facial pain in chronic paroxysmal hemicrania last no more than 15 minutes and the stabbing pain of trigeminal neuralgia is momentary.

8 What precipitates the pain?
Chewing commonly exacerbates temporomandibular joint dysfunction and trigeminal neuralgia is always initiated by a specific trigger point. An enquiry about precipitating factors in migraine is often productive and can help in treatment as well as diagnosis.

9 What relieves the pain?
Tension headaches do not respond to analgesics, whereas patients presenting with migraine often report that taking aspirin and going to sleep in a quiet, dark room has enabled them to limit their misery.

10 Are there any associated symptoms?
A specific enquiry as to whether the nausea and the pain are synchronous is worthwhile as it is characteristic, although not diagnostic, of migraine. Inexplicably, patients with migraine often fail to volunteer this symptom.

11 What effect does it have on daily life and sleep?
Should the patient describe a severe unrelenting pain but have an apparently normal life and pattern of sleep, atypical facial pain should be considered in the differential diagnosis. Facial pain causing early morning waking which is severe enough to make the patient, often a man, want to bang his head against a wall is typical of cluster headache.

12 What treatment has been tried and with what effect?
Tension headache and atypical facial pain fail to respond to analgesics; this in isolation does not clinch the diagnosis but is a useful pointer. Chronic paroxysmal hemicrania specifically responds to indomethacin, and trigeminal neuralgia to carbamazepine.

The whole subject has been complicated by an array of eponymous syndromes which have been described in an attempt to correlate clinical and neurophysiological findings. As many of these are rare or doubtful entities, the following descriptions are an attempt to rationalize them into main groups of syndromes, placing them in the context of the commonest forms of facial pain. It is helpful to classify facial pain into the following categories, despite the use of both anatomical and pathological criteria: rhinological, dental, vascular, neuralgic, central, ophthalmic and miscellaneous.

Rhinological pain

Patients not infrequently complain of 'sinus', believing that they have had sinusitis: the latter term, often used loosely by patients and doctors, should be treated with scepticism. Chronic sinusitis is often painless, causing postnasal catarrh or nasal obstruction except during acute episodes. Symptoms of a dull ache around the medial canthus of the eye, the lower part of the forehead, or under the nasal bridge are often related to sinus disease. The symptom of 'blockage' under the nasal bones may present in the absence of airflow obstruction and this symptom may be due to mucosal disease in the ethmoid sinuses with obstruction of the ostiomeatal complex and subsequent under-aeration of the sinuses. Such symptoms are often exacerbated by upper respiratory tract infections, although the primary pathology is just as likely to be allergic as infective. Acute sinusitis often causes pain which is exacerbated by bending down. It is common for the maxillary teeth to ache and while the maxilla may be slightly tender to palpation, marked swelling of the cheek is rare and suggests dental infection. Symptoms of pain high on the calvarium or over the temples is less readily recognized as being due to sinus disease but can arise from the sphenoid or posterior ethmoidal cells and needs consideration in the differential diagnosis. Frontal pain can be caused by obstruction of the frontonasal recess, and in particular by disease in the very anterior ethmoidal air cells called the agger nasi cells.

Acute episodes are usually initiated by infection, but the mucosal swelling of allergic rhinitis can contribute to sinus obstruction, pressure symptoms and mucus retention. A history of asthma, eczema or hay-fever in a first-degree relative increases the likelihood of an allergic element in mucosal disease. Itchy eyes, or an improvement in symptoms with topical steroids or antihistamines also support an allergic element. Although a seasonal history of an exacerbation of symptoms with high pollen counts, pets or house dust indicates atopy; allergic rhinitis can produce perennial symptoms, often attributable to house dust mite, dust or feathers. Anatomical variations can contribute to obstruction and inadequate ventilation and drainage of the sinuses, e.g. a deviated septum, paradoxical middle turbinate, or a concha bullosa. Maxillary dental infections can initiate and perpetuate maxillary sinusitis: therefore premolar and molar teeth need inspection.

Radiology has a very limited role in the diagnosis of rhinosinusitis. Radiographs showing a 'thickened lining', may be due to allergic nasal mucosa or sinus infection, but is *not* diagnostic of the latter. Plain radiographs have both poor specificity (true negatives / false positives + true negatives) and poor sensitivity (true positives / true positives + false negatives) (Davidson, Brahme and Gallagher, 1989). Rigid endoscopy provides more accurate information regarding the extent of sinus disease.

Until recently attention has centred on the maxillary sinus; however, there is a resurgence of the idea that disease at the ostiomeatal complex is responsible for sinus-related symptoms and disease (Stammberger and Wolf, 1988). Although its place awaits clarification, functional endoscopic sinus surgery is based on the concept of helping normal mucociliary flow patterns through the natural ostia by opening the ostiomeatal area and removing diseased air cells along with any structural abnormalities which impede aeration and drainage of the sinuses. However, it should be remembered that approximately 30–40% of asymptomatic people have changes in one or more of their sinuses on CT scan (Lloyd, 1990). While a decision about the extent of planned surgery may be influenced by CT findings, the decision whether or not to operate should primarily be based on a detailed history and outpatient endoscopic examination and it should only be considered *where a full course of medical treatment has failed*. An inferior meatal antrostomy often helps facial pain but it does little for catarrh and nasal obstruction as it does not address ethmoidal disease and the floor of the maxillary sinus lies below the nasal floor thus forming a sump for infected mucus. In theory, a middle meatal antrostomy is physiologically more sound, as mucociliary flow is directed towards it, but prospective trials are needed to verify the clinical benefit.

Occasionally, following a nasal fracture, pain or paraesthesiae can persist over the nasal bridge. The cause of this is unclear, it may be due to a neuroma in the scar tissue, but again it seems to be influenced by the degree of distress the patient continues to feel about the insult he has received. Not infrequently patients who are dissatisfied with the appearance of their nose are reluctant to present this as their primary problem. They may provide an array of other symptoms, only to appear greatly relieved when asked if they think adjustment of any apparent external structural abnormality would help.

Carcinoma of the maxilla is rare. Patients unfortunately often present late when the disease has spread beyond the confines of the sinus. Unilateral bloody purulent nasal discharge is the most frequent presentation. Less common symptoms are infraorbital paraesthesiae, loose teeth or ill-fitting dentures, proptosis, deformity of the cheek, nasal obstruction or epistaxis. Pain is a late feature.

Nasopharyngeal carcinoma is also rare, but presents most commonly in young adults from the Far East. It often presents with cervical lymphadenopathy and middle ear effusions; however, its spread can involve the Vth and VIth cranial nerves, causing facial pain or a lateral rectus palsy. It can also spread posteriorly to involve the IXth–XIIth cranial nerves.

The tumour may cause:

Trotter's triad

Unilateral middle ear effusion, elevation and immobility of the ipsilateral soft palate, and pain in the ear, jaw or tongue.

If a nasopharyngeal tumour extends intracranially, it may cause:

Godtfredsen's syndrome

Ophthalmoplegia, pain in the distribution of the trigeminal nerve and tongue paralysis.

Pterygopalatine fossa syndrome

This is caused by malignant infiltration in this area producing maxillary dental pain, infraorbital and palatal anaesthesia, pterygoid muscle paralysis and blindness.

Foix's syndrome

In this syndrome there is also ophthalmoplegia and trigeminal pain but without any tongue signs. It can be caused by an aneurysm abutting, a tumour invading or a thrombosis of the cavernous sinus.

Tolosa Hunt syndrome (recurrent painful ophthalmoplegia) (Tolosa, 1954; Hunt *et al.*, 1961; Scott Brown *et al.*, 1990)

This occurs equally in both sexes at any age. It presents with gnawing unilateral orbital pain with relapsing and remitting paralysis of the IIIrd, IVth and VIth cranial nerves. Occasionally there is paraesthesia of the forehead. It is caused by a lesion in the region of the cavernous sinus or the superior orbital fissure. It should be differentiated from ophthalmoplegic migraine, painful diabetic oculomotor palsy and malignancy. Although this condition often responds to steroids, this is not diagnostic.

Dental pain

Afferent fibres from the dental pulp, being small and unmyelinated, produce poorly localized pain, which often radiates to surrounding structures, but rarely crosses the midline. However, dentino-enamel defects produce a sharp and usually well localized excruciating pain which is often followed by a dull ache. These symptoms may arise from a cervical erosion or a lost or cracked filling, and may be induced by a temperature change, osmotic or mechanical stimuli.

Once the periodontium is involved, the pain becomes more localized. The periodontium may be affected either by the formation of a periapical abscess involving the periodontium at the apex of the tooth or by infection in a pocket around the tooth where there has been long-standing gingival and periodontal inflammation. The tooth throbs and is tender to percussion. Infection of a periodontal pocket will usu-ally result in swelling and erythema of the gingivae and the tooth may show increased mobility if there has been erosion of surrounding bone with periodontal disease. With periodontal disease the tooth is rarely hypersensitive to hot or cold stimuli.

Acute pulpitis causes a dull ache with exacerbations of excruciating pain and often radiates or is referred to the adjacent ipsilateral jaw. Chronic pulpitis causes a dull ache which is difficult to define and may be worse when lying flat. Usually, clinical examination reveals a carious tooth or leaking restoration, and toothache is either initiated or exacerbated by hot and cold stimuli. Extirpation of the pulp with or without the tooth is the surest way to relieve the patient's suffering.

The transition from an acute to a necrotizing and then to a dead pulp may produce a variety of symptoms and signs with periapical rarefaction or radiolucency taking at least 10 days to occur. The orthopantomogram is a poor second to good periapical X-rays in defining the site of periapical infection. Premolar periapical inflammation can cause pain in the infraorbital or temporal regions while the molar teeth can refer pain to the temporal and preauricular regions.

Pericoronitis around wisdom teeth may alter the bite inducing temporomandibular joint dysfunction, and mislead the clinician as to the primary site of the trouble. Extraction of the opposing wisdom tooth relieves the symptoms, although the overlying gingival flap can be cauterized and along with antibiotics and vigorous mouthwashes leads to symptomatic relief. Unerupted wisdom teeth rarely produce symptoms unless there is a connection with the mouth from a pocket which can become infected. Very occasionally an unerupted impacted tooth can erode an adjacent root and produce pain.

The unpleasant pain caused by a dry socket is progressive and starts 48 hours after an extraction, taking approximately 10 days to settle. The socket is lined with dead bone which looks yellow. None of the topical remedies in current use seems to be consistently effective. Packing the socket with Whitehead's varnish is as effective as anything.

Phantom tooth pain

This is said to follow a dental extraction where there has been incomplete osseous repair. Necrotic bone and neural elements have been found in some patients with this syndrome, while in others there is thought to be a strong psychological element. If the pain is due to a neuroma it can be temporarily blocked with local anaesthesia (Finneson, 1969). It is unusual for buried teeth or odontomes to cause pain, except where there is erosion of dentine in adjacent teeth, or an intraoral connection with infection.

Temporomandibular joint dysfunction (Schwartz 1956)

This is most commonly unilateral (90%) and usually occurs in young adults with a history of bruxism, clenching, trauma, recent dental work, anxiety, enthusiastic kissing, or cradling the telephone between the jaw and the shoulder. Another contributing factor is poor occlusion, as occurs in crossbite, or in a partially edentulous patient without an appropriate denture, or in someone with a completely edentulous mouth whose dentures are very worn or have been made with an inadequate vertical height resulting in overclosure. Pain is caused by pterygoid spasm and is described as a deep dull ache which may masquerade as toothache or earache. There is often a superimposed sharper component which may radiate down the neck, or over the side of the face or temple (Figure 21.1). It is often necessary to ask whether chewing exacerbates the symptoms as this information is rarely volunteered. Spasm may be initiated by a reflex mechanism to avoid an undesirable pattern of malocclusion. Anxiety lowers the threshold for this mechanism, and it often occurs in people under stress. Clicking of the temporomandibular joint is an unreliable sign, whereas pain on palpation of the insertion of the lateral pterygoid is a better indicator. This can be demonstrated with the gloved little finger where the lateral pterygoid muscle can be palpated at the most posterior end of the upper buccal sulcus. Trismus and deviation of the jaw from the midline on opening, as well as evidence of malocclusion or a high shiny spot on a filling, should be sought. Radiographs are normally of little help in making the diagnosis, but where there is a suspicion of an arthropathy they may show degenerative changes in rheumatoid arthritis or gout. Most patients respond when aggravating factors are corrected and if advice to rest the joint is followed, e.g. stifle yawns, avoid prolonged chewing. It is often helpful to reassure patients that they do not have 'arthritis' of the joint – a common anxiety. Occlusal devices such as bite raising appliances often help where simple measures have failed. Condylotomy is a last resort where other measures such as suboccipital transcutaneous nerve stimulation have failed. Costen's syndrome (Costen, 1934), a dull pain in the area of the joint, with tinnitus and an intermittent or continuous impairment of hearing, is not a distinct entity.

Myofascial pain

This causes a widespread, poorly defined aching in the neck, jaw or ear. It is five times more common in women and worse when the patient is tired or stressed. Tender points may be found in the sternomastoid or trapezius muscles and initiating factors include malocclusion or poor deltopectoral posture. This syndrome overlaps to a large degree with temporomandibular joint dysfunction. Reassurance, local heat treatment, ultrasound and massage help. Injection of long-acting local anaesthetics into tender muscle points may induce prolonged periods of relief (Travell and Rinzler, 1952).

Vascular pain

Migraine

Migraine presents in a variety of ways, affecting 8–10% of adults. It is a term which is often wrongly used by patients; the diagnosis needs confirmation by precise questioning. Migraine classically presents with prodromal symptoms including nausea, paraesthesia and visual disturbances such as fortification, scintillating scotoma, blurred vision and flickering fields. A prodromal state is not essential in order to make the diagnosis (Blau, 1982). There is often a family history of migraine. It is said to be due to a primary vasoconstriction of cerebral vessels followed by vasodilatation. It can be induced by stress, diet, premenstrual state and barometric changes, and it is worth asking about these and other trigger factors, although these are often volunteered. Hemifacial pain may occur in the frontal, temporal or parietal regions and starts on the same side in 90% of attacks. Symptomatic relief is often best obtained by soluble aspirin, paracetamol or codeine, taken as early as possible, with rectal or buccal prochlorperazine if nausea is a problem. Ergotamine helps in patients who fail to respond to analgesics but it can make the nausea worse and it should not be given for prophylaxis. Having searched for and excluded precipitating factors, pizotifen often gives good prophylaxis, but it invariably causes some weight gain.

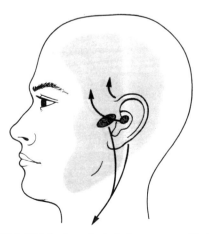

Figure 21.1 Distribution of pain in temporomandibular joint dysfunction

Cluster headache (periodic migrainous neuralgia)

Typical presentation consists of a severe unilateral stabbing or burning pain which may be frontal, temporal, ocular, over the cheek, or even in the maxillary teeth (Figure 21.2). Pain is therefore facial and 'headache' is a misnomer. Nausea is absent but frequently there is rhinorrhoea, conjunctival injection and lacrimation with unilateral nasal obstruction. It is most common in men between the ages of 20 and 50 years. The patient is awakened in the early hours, often walking around the bedroom in distress, with the pain lasting between 30 minutes and 2 hours. Up to three bouts can occur in 24 hours and these may be precipitated by alcohol intake. Myosis or facial flushing may be seen. It has been suggested that the mechanism by which this occurs involves the perivascular neural plexus of the ciliary and sphenopalatine ganglion (Wyke, 1968). One eponym is Horton's syndrome (Horton, 1941). Ergotamine suppositories and methysergide are used for prophylaxis for short periods when there are bouts of attacks. Alcohol should be avoided during a cluster period (Blau, 1982).

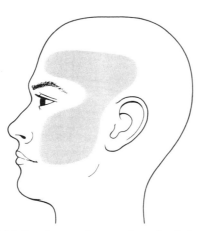

Figure 21.2 Distribution of pain in cluster headache

Chronic paroxysmal hemicrania

This syndrome causes multiple attacks of excruciating pain by day or night in the frontal, temporal or ocular regions (Sjaastad, 1976). It is more common in women and each episode lasts 5–10 minutes with up to 12 episodes occurring in 24 hours. There is nasal obstruction and ptosis. This condition responds to indomethacin.

Temporal arteritis

Temporal arteritis occurs in the over-fifties, the majority being women with malaise, anorexia and a deep boring temporal pain. A low grade fever may be present and classically the temporal artery is tender and feels thickened. (The temporal artery is also tender in migraine, periodic migrainous neuralgia and the underlying temporalis muscle may be in painful spasm in temporomandibular joint dysfunction.) If left untreated, 40% develop a visual loss due to involvement of the ophthalmic artery. Histological examination of a 1-cm length of artery shows intimal hyperplasia and fragmentation of the internal elastic lamina. An elevated ESR is an essential index of the activity of the disease. Steroids should be started where there is strong clinical suspicion, but a biopsy should be obtained within 72 hours of starting treatment for confirmation of the diagnosis. An initial dose of 60 mg/day of prednisolone is required. Pain in the jaw muscles on chewing has been described in this condition, due to claudication.

Carotidynia

Carotidynia presents with a unilateral ache involving the upper neck, face and ear and often occurs with a throbbing headache. It is worse if the common carotid is compressed at or below the bifurcation. Two subgroups are found. The first are younger and middle-aged patients who have neck pain and a tender carotid: their ESR is normal and aspirin provides some relief. The second are elderly patients with recurring attacks of throbbing pain in the area fed by the external carotid artery. Their pain lasts several minutes to hours and responds to ergotamine. It should be noted that the carotid may be tender in migraine. Stellate ganglion block is said to offer relief.

Causalgia (reflex sympathetic dystrophy)

This follows trauma or surgery resulting in an incomplete peripheral lesion. It often produces a constant, diffuse pain, with a burning quality and there may be autonomic changes in the skin (Gross, 1974). It causes much suffering and may be initiated by a variety of stimuli. Some areas of skin may be hyperalgesic. It is thought to be secondary to autonomic afferents which are influenced by central excitation. Sympathetic blockade relieves this condition.

Sphenopalatine neuralgia or Sluder's neuralgia
(Sluder, 1927)

This is thought to be of vascular origin. It is characterized by pain in the forehead, between the eyebrows and over the nasal bones. It is often paroxysmal, with up to three episodes per day. There may be rhinorrhoea, lacrimation, injected conjunctivae, swollen nasal mucous membrane, facial flushing and photophobia. Pain resembles that of sinusitis but no nasal pathology can be found and decongestants do not work. It is postulated that a lesion in the spheno-palatine ganglion is responsible and similar symptoms have been ascribed to a lesion of the vidian nerve. It seems likely that this is not a distinct entity but a group of symptoms. Diagnostically touching the middle turbinate is said to induce the pain and it can be eradicated by cocainization of this region. Submucous resection or cryotherapy are said to be helpful. The author has not seen or heard of a patient with this diagnostic picture who has been helped by this manoeuvre.

Raeder's paratrigeminal syndrome

Presentation is as an intense sharp pain or ache in the area of the ophthalmic division of the trigeminal cranial nerve. There is associated myosis, ptosis and facial hypoaesthesia in the same area. The corneal reflex is reduced, but there is no reduced sweating as in Horner's syndrome. A lesion near the base of the middle cranial fossa at the medial border of the Gasserian ganglion is responsible. It may be due to a carotid aneurysm, metastasis or local invasion by a neoplasm.

Neuralgias

Trigeminal neuralgia

Trigeminal neuralgia (tic douloureux) has an incidence of five per 100 000 per year and is more common in women over 40 years of age with a peak incidence between 50 and 60 years. Patients complain of paroxysms of agonizing lancinating pain induced by a specific trigger point. Repetitive bursts can be triggered usually with a refractory period of more than 30 seconds. In more than one-third of sufferers the pain occurs in both the maxillary and mandibular divisions, while in one-fifth it is confined to the mandibular region and in 3% to the ophthalmic division. A sufferer can always localize the trigger zone but is reluctant to demonstrate it.

Typical trigger sites are the lips and the nasolabial folds but pain may be triggered by touching the gingivae. Some patients report that firm pressure over the trigger point helps and delays a further bout. A flush may be seen over the area in question but there are no sensory disturbances in primary trigeminal neuralgia. Remissions are common but it is not unusual for the attacks to increase in frequency and severity. Carbamazepine is the first line medical treatment, while the addition of phenytoin or antidepressants can help.

Histology shows proliferative and disorganized changes in the myelin sheath of the nerve involved. Janetta (1976) found that a large percentage had vascular compression of the trigeminal nerve; however, this has been noted in many normal cadavers. Beware the dental pain which can mimic trigeminal neuralgia, particularly a fractured tooth, or exposed cervical dentine.

Secondary trigeminal neuralgia is attributable to a discernible pathological cause. In patients under 40 years old, it is most commonly due to multiple sclerosis (Rushton and Olafson, 1965) while over this age a tumour, aneurysm, meningioma and even tabes dorsalis can cause the pain.

Glossopharyngeal neuralgia

This is very uncommon. A stabbing pain is felt in the tonsillar region and ipsilateral ear (rarely in the base of the tongue and angle of the jaw). It is precipitated by swallowing or talking, and bouts last for weeks or months with a tendency to recur (Walker, 1966). Initially, treatment is with carbamazepine; however, avulsion of the nerve via a temporal, tonsillar bed, or posterior fossa approach may be the only way of obtaining a cure. Tympanic plexus neuralgia has been described producing severe paroxysms of earache which is relieved by tympanic plexus neurectomy.

Greater auricular neuralgia

Greater auricular neuralgia not uncommonly follows parotidectomy and is caused by a neuroma on the sectioned nerve. Injection with steroids and a long-acting local anaesthetic may provide long-term relief. Various methods, including burying the sectioned nerve in muscle at the time of surgery have failed to prevent the problem.

Post-herpetic neuralgia

One eighth of patients suffering from herpes zoster infection are left with post-herpetic neuralgia (Rogers and Tindall, 1971); however two-thirds of these recover in the first year. It is defined as pain which persists for more than one month after the eruption and early use of acyclovir may prevent it. It is more common in the elderly, and if it persists for more than a year is unlikely to resolve. It causes a persistent intense burning or lancinating pain, and where there is a sensory loss there is more likely to be associated dysaesthesia. Patients often become depressed and irritable. Histology shows demyelination, together with a disproportionate loss of large nerve fibres and this may allow increased transmission in nocioceptive fibres through the dorsal horn, thus causing pain. Herpes zoster appears to have some effect at the suprathalamic level, as tractotomy at a more peripheral level is of little help. Various medical treatments may be of some benefit including carbamazepine, sodium valproate, anxiolytics, tricyclic antidepressants, transcutaneous nerve stimulation and acupuncture, and again the pain clinic may help.

Mental nerve neuralgia

This can mimic trigeminal neuralgia by producing sharp pain in the lower lip and chin when the lower premolar area is touched in the edentulous patient. It is due to exposure and irritation of the mental nerve branch of the inferior alveolar nerve in a long-standing edentulous patient whose alveolar bone has atrophied. Direct pressure from either a denture or finger can initiate this unpleasant sharp pain. Either bone grafting or re-routing the nerve can help.

Central pain

Stretching of the arterial tree which supplies the proximal portions of the cranial nerves and the dura within 1 cm of any venous sinus induces a headache, but can cause facial pain. The supratentorial vessels and dura refer pain to the ophthalmic division of the trigeminal nerve. Infratentorial structures refer pain to the distribution of the glossopharyngeal and vagus nerves along with the upper three cervical nerve dermatomes.

Space-occupying lesions such as meningiomas, angiomas and intracerebral metastases can induce facial pain by irritation of the trigeminal nerve along its intracerebral course. Syringobulbia, syphilis and multiple sclerosis are rarer causes of central lesions which may cause facial pain. Raised intracranial pressure produces a bursting headache which is worse on coughing or straining and is associated with effortless vomiting. The fundi show papilloedema. Lesions in the posterior cranial fossa produce occipital and upper neck pain, while supratentorial lesions with raised intracranial pressure produce pain at the vertex or over the frontal and temporal region.

Cerebrovascular accidents can cause such pain, but these symptoms may only present when the other more distressing signs and symptoms of a stroke are resolving.

Ophthalmic pain

Uncorrected optical refractive errors can cause headaches, but their importance is exaggerated. Visual acuity is tested, ideally with a Snellen chart, and if there is a refractive problem this can be overcome by testing vision through a pinhole. Disease involving the optic nerve results in reduced acuity and colour vision. Pain on ocular movement is suggestive of optic neuritis or scleritis. It is vital to recognize acute glaucoma which may cause severe orbital pain and headache. The patient may see haloes around lights, and circumcorneal injection can occur as well as systemic upset, especially vomiting. This condition requires urgent treatment as vision is rapidly lost.

Pain is a feature of periorbital cellulitis which may present with lid swelling and erythema if it is preseptal and with chemosis, proptosis and reduced mobility if it arises posterior to the septum. Orbital pain can also be caused by uveitis, keratitis and dry eye syndrome.

Orbital haemorrhage can cause sudden pain, proptosis, nausea and vomiting, along with ecchymosis, reduced mobility and oedema of the optic disc. It may be secondary to an orbital varix, blood dyscrasias, hypertension or trauma.

The term *inflammatory orbital pseudotumour* should not be used for disorders whose aetiology is known (polyarteritis nodosa and vasculitis). This condition probably has an immunological basis and it can produce pain, proptosis, reduced mobility, lid swelling and injection of the eye. Some individuals have recurring bouts and are pain free or have pain with upper respiratory tract infections and may then present to the otorhinolaryngologist as the frontal and ethmoidal sinuses can mistakenly be held responsible. The majority of other causes of proptosis are painless, such as hyperthyroidism and tumours of the orbit or of adjacent structures.

Iatrogenic pain

The surgeon who is faced by a relentless plea from a patient to intervene in some way should resist when no good objective evidence of organic disease can be found or when symptoms do not correspond with signs. It may seem expeditious to agree to surgery, especially when the alternative is to try to explain that you have been unable to find a clear cause for the pain. However, surgery will not only be to no avail but will complicate the clinical picture. Scar tissue from any surgery can result in neuroma formation, but in patients who have a large psychological element to their illness this new pain may not only replace their previous symptoms but become more entrenched than the original one.

Making a 'new' diagnosis where others have failed may fill the surgeon with pride but it is worth substantiating it with investigations or a trial of an appropriate medical treatment wherever possible, before embarking on surgery.

Miscellaneous facial pain

Tension headache

This is typically described as a feeling of tightness, pressure or constriction which varies in intensity, frequency and duration, and may be at the vertex or forehead, eyes or temple, and often has a suboccipital component. It often lasts many hours, is only partly relieved by analgesics and is associated with anxiety, depression or agitated depression. The headaches can last for several days. A sympathetic explanation of the relationship of stress to physical symptoms is sometimes helpful. Low doses of amitriptyline help a proportion of these patients.

Atypical facial pain

This is not a dustbin term and it has many distinguishing features which make it a diagnosis in its own right, not one to resort to in despair. It should only be made reluctantly when organic causes have been excluded. It is often complicated by the effects of surgical procedures performed in an attempt to alleviate symptoms which have been misdiagnosed. The description of symptoms often does not correlate with the patient's affect; there can be unusual associated factors, exaggerated responses to the pain and there are often psychological factors or an excess of unpleasant life events. While psychological factors are always important in any patient's interpretation of facial pain, in this condition they play an overwhelming role. Pain is typically deep and ill-defined, changes location, is unexplainable on an anatomical basis, occurring almost daily and is sometimes fluctuating, sometimes continuous, without any precipitating factors and is not relieved by analgesics. Often more specific questioning about the symptoms results in increasingly vague answers. The pain does not wake the patient up and while the patient reports that she cannot sleep she will often look well rested. It is more common in women over the age of 40 and typically lasts many months. A proportion have symptoms of depressive illness or anxiety neurosis or have problems adjusting to the difficulties which life presents. Some patients appear to be so used to their pain that it is very much part of them and the loss of it would mean that they would have to reappraise their life dramatically.

Confrontation is counterproductive, while sympathetic discussion, close liaison with the general practitioner, and possibly psychiatric help may be beneficial. Tricyclic antidepressants are often of help, in particular when there are symptoms of endogenous depression such as loss of appetite and interest in life, self-neglect, early morning waking and fatigue.

The description of hysterical pain is often ill-defined with unusual neurological symptoms such as weakness and paraesthesia. No physical lesion can be found and the distribution of the neurological loss does not conform with the known anatomy. The pain occurs throughout the day, although fluctuating in severity. It enables the patient to obtain some personal benefit, often by avoiding an unwanted task.

Hypochondriasis

There is often an array of coexisting symptoms elsewhere in the body and the patient frequently expresses an exaggerated concern about the functioning of his or her body. These patients need prompt reassurance.

Eagle's syndrome (Eagle, 1937)

Pain may be felt in the lateral wall of the pharynx, the mandible, the floor of the mouth or the side of the neck. A nagging discomfort lasting seconds to minutes is precipitated on opening the mouth or head turning. An elongated styloid process with a calcified stylohyoid ligament may be palpated laterally or via the tonsillar fossa and can be seen on an oblique radiograph. Relief may be obtained by fracturing the styloid process and surgical removal is advocated by some, but this is not without its own complications (Moffat, Ramsden and Shaw, 1977).

Von Frey's syndrome

Gustatory sweating occurs in 25–95% of patients following superficial parotidectomy. Occasionally paroxysms of burning pain in the temple occur at the same time. No satisfactory treatment has been found except that the sweating can be controlled by topical 20% aluminium chloride hexahydrate in absolute alcohol (Shaheen, 1984).

Glossodynia

This is characterized by a burning sensation in the tongue and there is often disordered taste or the sensation of a dry mouth. The oral cavity should be inspected for any sign of ulceration or erythroplakia and the cause of these investigated and treated. Local irritation, lichen planus, diabetes mellitus, candida, serum iron deficiency, vitamin B_{12} deficiency, irritant mouthwashes, a drug reaction, denture component sensitivity and galvanism should be excluded (Wray and Scully, 1986). In a proportion of patients no cause can be found and this group is over-represented by women over 50 years old, often with a cancer phobia, a history of an emotional disturbance, or a precipitating major life event.

In conclusion, a thorough history will often reveal the diagnosis without resort to expensive investigations. The adage *primum non nocere* is pertinent, in that hasty or incorrect treatments may obscure the diagnosis or be harmful in themselves.

Acknowledgement

To Dr J. N. Blau for his advice in the preparation of this chapter.

References

BLAU, J. N. (1982) A plain man's guide to the management of migraine. *British Medical Journal*, **284**, 1095–1097
COSTEN, J. B. (1934) Syndrome of ear and sinus symptoms dependent upon disturbed function of the temporoman-

dibular joint. *Annals of Otology, Rhinology and Laryngology,* **43,** 1–15

DAVIDSON, T. M., BRAHME, F. J. and GALLAGHER, M. E. (1989) Radiographic evaluation for nasal dysfunction: computed tomography versus plain films. *Head and Neck,* **11,** 405–409

EAGLE, W. W. (1937) Elongated styloid process. *Archives of Otolaryngology,* **25,** 584–587

FINNESON, B. E. (1969) *Diagnosis and Management of Pain Syndromes,* 2nd edn. Philadelphia: W. B. Saunders. pp. 308–309

GROSS, D. (1974) Pain in the autonomic nervous system. In: *Advances in Neurology,* vol 4, *International Symposium on Pain,* edited by J. J. Bonica. New York: Raven Press. pp. 93–103

HORTON, B. T. (1941) Histamine cephalgia: erythromalalgia of the head. *Journal of the American Medical Association,* **116,** 377–383

HUNT, W. E., MEAGHER, J. N., LEFEVER, H. E. and ZEMAN, W. (1961) Painful ophthalmoplegia: its relation to indolent inflammation of the cavernous sinus. *Neurology,* **11,** 56–62

JANETTA, P. J. (1976) Microsurgical approach to the trigeminal nerve for tic douloureux. *Progress in Neurological Surgery,* **7,** 180–200

LLOYD, G. A. S. (1990) CT of the paranasal sinuses: a study of a control series in relation to endoscopic sinus surgery. *Journal of Laryngology and Otology,* **104,** 447–481

MELZACK, R. and WALL, P. D. (1965) Pain mechanisms: a new theory. *Science,* **150,** 971–978

MOFFAT, D. A., RAMSDEN, R. T. and SHAW, H. J. (1977) The styloid process syndrome. Aetiological factors and surgical management. *Journal of Laryngology and Otology,* **91,** 279–294

ROGERS, R. S., and TINDALL, J. P. (1971) Geriatric herpes zoster. *Journal of the American Geriatric Society,* **19,** 495

RUSHTON, J. G. and OLAFSON, R. (1965) Trigeminal neuralgia associated with disseminated sclerosis, report of 35 cases. *Archives of Neurology,* **13,** 383

SCHWARTZ, L. L. (1956) A temporomandibular joint pain dysfunction syndrome. *Journal of Chronic Diseases,* **3,** 284–293

SCOTT BROWN, J., MOSTER, M., KENNING, J. A. and RONIS, M. L. (1990) The Tolosa-Hunt syndrome: a case report. *Otolaryngology – Head and Neck Surgery,* **102,** 402–404

SHAHEEN, O. H. (1984) *Problems in Head and Neck Surgery.* London: Baillière Tindall. pp. 46–47

SJAASTAD, O. (1976) A new clinical headache entity 'chronic paroxysmal hemicrania'. *Acta Neurologica Scandinavica,* **54,** 140–159

SLUDER, G. (1927) *Nasal Neurology, Headches and Eye Disorders.* London: Kimpton

STAMMBERGER, H. and WOLF, G. (1988) Headaches and sinus disease: the endoscopic approach. *Annals of Otology, Rhinology and Laryngology,* **97** (suppl. 134), 3–23

TOLOSA, E. (1954) Peripatetic lesions of the carotid siphon with the clinical features of a carotid infraclinoid aneurysm. *Journal of Neurosurgery and Psychiatry,* **17,** 300–302

TRAVELL, J. and RINZLER, S. H. (1952) The myofascial genesis of pain. *Postgraduate Medicine,* **11,** 425–434

WALKER, A. E. (1966) Neuralgias of the glossopharyngeal, vagus and intermediate nerves. In: *Pain,* edited by R. S. Knighton and P. R. Dumke. Boston: Little, Brown and Co. pp. 421–429

WRAY, D. and SCULLY, C. (1986) The sore mouth. *Medicine International,* **28,** 1134–1137

WYKE, B. (1968) The neurology of facial pain. *British Journal of Hospital Medicine,* **1,** 46–65

22

Aspects of dental surgery for otorhinolaryngology

Philip McLoughlin and Colin Hopper

Disorders of dental development

Abnormalities in the number of teeth

Failure of development of a complete complement of teeth (hypodontia) is relatively common and often hereditary. Most often only one or two teeth are involved and these are most frequently the third molars, second premolars or maxillary lateral incisors. Total failure of development of the dentition (anodontia) is extremely rare. If the permanent dentition is affected, as may occur due to radiotherapy in childhood, then the deciduous teeth can be retained for many years. Hypodontia may be associated with systemic defects. In ectodermal dysplasia the teeth are deficient in number and of simple conical form. These patients also have fine sparse hair, absent sweat glands and defective finger nails. Hypodontia is also a feature in Down's syndrome and in patients with palatal clefts. Additional teeth (hyperdontia) are relatively common. They vary from being simple conical supernumerary teeth to those termed supplemental teeth which are indistinguishable from teeth of the normal series. Supernumerary teeth may delay eruption of an underlying normal tooth and are usually therefore removed. Supplemental teeth often erupt in abnormal positions and are extracted to prevent caries or periodontal disease. Gardner's syndrome and cleidocranial dysplasia are associated with hyperdontia.

Disorders of eruption

Eruption of the deciduous teeth usually starts at about 6 months and is complete by 3 years of age. Delay in eruption of a tooth is most commonly caused by local obstruction such as a supernumerary tooth. In the case of the permanent dentition early loss of a deciduous predecessor may leave inadequate space for correct eruption and alignment. Delayed eruption is associated with cleidocranial dysplasia and the now uncommon rickets. In hereditary gingival fibromatosis the teeth appear not to erupt because they are buried in excessive fibrous gingival tissue. Teeth remaining unerupted may undergo gradual resorption or their follicle may undergo cystic change (see below).

Defects of tooth structure

Defects of tooth structure may be of interest as indications of past disease or as indicators of a multisystem disorder.

Amelogenesis imperfecta is a genetically determined disorder of enamel formation which leads to severe hypoplastic and hypocalcified dental enamel. Appearances vary from vertical ridging on the teeth to a soft chalky appearance. Without extensive preventive and restorative treatment early tooth loss is inevitable.

Dentinogenesis imperfecta, also known as hereditary opalescent dentine, is transmitted as an autosomal dominant disorder. The affected teeth are brown and transluscent and have little or no resistance to wear. Again, unless protected by artificial crowns the teeth soon wear down to gum level. Dentinogenesis imperfecta has a close genetic association with osteogenesis imperfecta.

Notching of the upper incisor teeth (Hutchinson's incisors) and dome-shaped first molar teeth (Moon's molars) are seen in congenital syphilis due to the direct action of *Treponema pallidum* on the dental follicle. In later childhood illness, disturbances of metabolism and drug therapy may result in dental defects. The childhood fevers commonly result in small areas of enamel hypoplasia. The antibiotic, tetracycline, is taken up by calcifying tissues and causes a greyish-brown discoloration when given to children in whom the permanent teeth are calcifying. The permanent anterior teeth calcify from approximately the fourth month to the sixth year of childhood and tetracycline should be avoided if possible during this time.

The sequelae of dental infection

The head and neck is the most common site of acute pain and this very commonly is as a result of the sequelae of dental infection. The mouth is populated by a variety of organisms including streptococci, staphylococci, anaerobes and spirochaetes. However, it is predominantly the effects of the ability of *Streptococcus mutans* to metabolize sugars into acids that cause dental decay.

The initial barrier of dental enamel is variously resistant to acid attack depending upon its content of fluoride ion. This can be incorporated intrinsically during tooth development if fluoride is ingested with the diet or extrinsically from toothpaste or topically applied fluorides after the teeth have erupted. However, with a persistently low pH all enamel will eventually succumb and with progressive tooth loss through dental decay there is exposure of the dentinal tubules. At this stage the patient may experience pain which is particularly noticeable with hot, cold and sweet foods. Later in this process as the dental pulp becomes involved the patient may experience a severe throbbing pain often poorly localized, radiating to other teeth or the ear on the affected side. This usually subsides after a few days as the whole of the dental pulp tissue undergoes necrosis. Following this phase the patient may develop a periapical abscess which will tend to present with localized pain at the site of the tooth with swelling over the root of the tooth possibly involving soft tissues, or as a sinus discharging onto the gum. In severe cases there may be systemic upset with pyrexia and malaise.

Left untreated the infection will spread, the exact path and nature of this will be dictated by muscle insertions that will act as a barrier to infection and create natural soft tissue planes in which it may progress. The most serious example of this is Ludwig's angina which occurs when both submandibular and sublingual spaces are affected, with the result that the tongue is displaced to the roof of the mouth and the airway becomes compromised. This is predominantly a cellulitis and in the early stages there is often little pus. Treatment, in a conventional fashion, by making large incisions into the neck will often therefore make the situation worse. The patient is best treated by adequate doses of intravenous antibiotic and the administration of steroids which will reduce the amount of tissue oedema. That is not to say that the primary cause of the problem should not be addressed and any offending tooth or collection of pus must be dealt with by extraction of teeth and adequate surgical drainage. The organisms responsible for this condition fall into a number of different groups and it is quite possible that this condition represents an inappropriate response to infection rather than being caused by any specific organism. Antibiotics to cover this spectrum should be administered in full therapeutic dose by the intravenous route. A combination of penicillin and metronidazole would be found effective as an initial therapy in most situations.

Infection may also drain through the path of least resistance and manifest as a buccal space infection or may drain onto the skin of the face as a discharging sinus. Spread of purulent exudate in a plane deep to the masseter muscle gives rise to the trismus and pyrexia in the absence of external swelling that is characteristic of a submasseteric abscess. Fluctuant swellings in the floor of the mouth should be treated with particular vigilance. The loose connective tissue of this part of the oral cavity provides a conduit for pus to extend into the sublingual and submandibular spaces but also posteriorly into the connective tissue plane covering the superior pharyngeal constrictor muscles with the formation of a lateral pharyngeal abscess. Periapical infection from maxillary teeth spreads readily into the lax soft tissues of the cheek even involving the periorbital soft tissues giving rise to periorbital oedema or abscess formation (Figure 22.1).

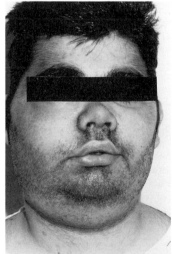

Figure 22.1 Facial and periorbital cellulitis of dental origin

It is important in all instances of cervicofacial infection to examine the mouth to see if there is a dental cause for any facial swellings. It is not uncommon for patients to present late having had previous inappropriate surgery for presumed epidermoid cysts when in fact the cause is simply a sequel to dental infection.

Cysts of the jaws

Radicular cyst

When infection becomes chronic the periapical epithelium can undergo a cystic change giving rise to the radicular cyst, so named due to its intimate association with the tooth root. Cysts which develop in this fashion secrete a variety of interleukins which cause bone resorption. This allows the cyst gradually to expand and it may reach sufficient size to predispose the patient to pathological fracture. Residual cysts may develop even in the absence of a tooth, if it has been extracted at an early stage of cyst formation. Radicular cysts can be treated quite simply by removal of the tooth and the associated cyst or can in fact be treated by performing conventional root canal therapy to the offending tooth in appropriate cases. Local periapical surgery as an adjunct to endodontic treatment may be considered for large cysts especially if there is doubt about the pathology.

It is important in all these cases to be familiar with the radiological features of dental cysts. They should be circumscribed with a clear regular margin and no resorption of the tooth root itself. Any features of irregularity of bone resorption or resorption of adjacent tooth roots should alert one to the possibility that this is something other than straightforward dental pathology and should raise the question of a neoplastic condition (see below).

Radicular cysts also may develop as lateral periodontal cysts. They are relatively uncommon and are formed at the side of the tooth either as a result of inflammation in a gingival pocket or in association with a lateral branch of a root canal. The tooth in question is commonly vital.

Follicular cyst

Cysts may also form around the crowns of developing teeth in the dental follicle. These are the so-called follicular or dentigerous cysts (Figure 22.2). These cysts are relatively common, comprising about 15% of all cysts of the jaw and arise from the remains of the enamel organ after enamel formation is complete. The cyst is attached around the neck of the tooth near the amelocemental junction. The developed tooth can be displaced although if there is sufficient space in the dental arches and the tooth and cyst are favourably placed then the cyst can be removed and the tooth will erupt into a functional position.

Odontogenic keratocyst

These cysts are relatively uncommon (approximately 5% of odontogenic cysts) and arise from the remnants of the dental lamina. They tend to have a characteristic appearance radiographically of a multiloculated radiolucent lesion (Figure 22.3). Histopathologically the

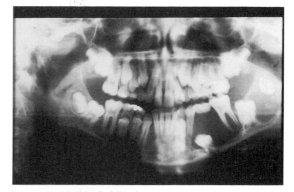

Figure 22.2 Multiple follicular cysts. The patient is a child in the mixed dentition phase and the cysts are associated with unerupted teeth

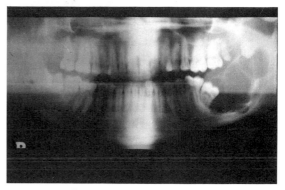

Figure 22.3 Odontogenic keratocyst. A multilocular radiolucency at the left angle of the mandible in a 25-year-old man

lining is thin, being only about eight cells thick. Small daughter or satellite cysts bud from this lining which is also thought to have an inherent growth potential of its own. Because of this it is difficult to remove intact and high recurrence rates following enucleation of these cysts have been reported. The rate of recurrence can be reduced by treating the cyst lining with Carnoy's solution which makes its removal easier. Multiple odontogenic keratocysts occur in the basal cell naevus or Gorlin–Goltz syndrome (Gorlin, 1987). This is an autosomal dominant condition features of which include odontogenic keratocysts and multiple basal cell carcinomas of the skin. Bifid ribs are a particularly characteristic curiosity as is the calcification of the falx cerebri noted on skull X-ray. Many families showing such characteristics are described in the literature.

Calcifying odontogenic cyst

This rare cyst frequently presents with painless swelling, though a large number have been asymptomatic and discovered during routine radiological examination. It occurs as an intraosseous radiolucent area. The outline is quite regular but there is usually an area of irregular radiopacity over the radiolucency. The lesion is treated by surgical enucleation.

Non-odontogenic cysts

These are uncommon cysts though the most common in this group is the nasopalatine cyst. This usually presents as a swelling in the midline posterior to the upper central incisors. Radiographs usually show a pear-shaped radiolucency and the cyst is thought to arise from the epithelium of the nasopalatine ducts in the incisive canal. An arbitrary figure of 5 mm is given to the normal nasopalatine duct. Any canal radiographically larger than this is potentially cystic. Early surgery however is not advised as the natural history of nasopalatine cysts is often to remain small, many of them being just incidental findings. Regular radiographic review is a reasonable policy.

Solitary bone cysts are rare and do not have any epithelial lining. This type of cyst is of unknown aetiology and treatment comprises merely opening the cyst surgically so that there is sufficient intrabony haemorrhage which then resolves. The aneurysmal bone cyst should really be considered as a giant cell lesion. It occurs principally in the mandible and is probably a vascular malformation which, at surgery, has been likened to a blood-filled sponge. Histologically it shows extreme cellularity with numerous giant cells. Thorough curettage is normally the

only treatment required although occasionally these lesions recur, particularly in children.

Neoplastic change

There would appear to be a few well authenticated reports of carcinomas arising in odontogenic cysts. Fortunately, however, this is an extremely rare occurrence.

Soft tissue cysts

The most common of these is a mucous extravasation cyst of a minor salivary gland. These commonly arise in the lower lip or the floor of the mouth (the ranula). The cysts appear as soft bluish swellings. Treatment is by excision in continuity with the offending gland. In the floor of the mouth this generally means removal of the sublingual gland to prevent recurrence. Opening the neck for a plunging ranula is completely unjustified and only results in recurrence of the cyst unless the sublingual gland is removed at the same time.

Sublingual dermoid cyst

These develop between the hyoid bone and the base of tongue. They sometimes present as a midline ranula though the dermoid cyst does not have the characteristic thin bluish appearance as it has developed deeper in the tissues. Treatment is by simple surgical excision.

The principal features of cysts of the jaws are summarized in Table 22.1.

Table 22.1 Summary of the features of common dental cysts

Cyst	Peak age (years)	Sex	Incidence (% of total)	Radiology	Histopathology	Treatment
Radicular	20–40	M:F 1.7:1	55–65	Round or ovoid associated with tooth root	Squamous lining 6–20 cells thick. Cholesterol crystals in cyst fluid	Enucleation with extraction or apicectomy of infected tooth
Follicular	10–35	M:F 1.6:1	13	Unilocular associated with crown of unerupted tooth	Thin, flat cuboidal lining. Cholesterol crystals	Enucleation with the involved tooth
Keratocyst	10–30	M:F 1.6:1	8–11	Scalloped margins so may appear multilocular	Very thin keratinized squamous lining. Squames in cyst fluid	Enucleation and bone curettage or Carnoy's solution
Nasopalatine	30–60	M:F 3:1	12	> 7 mm round or heart-shaped between upper central incisors	Squamous or respiratory epithelial lining	Enucleation if cyst enlarging or diagnosis uncertain

Periodontal disease

Periodontal disease (diseases of the gum) is the most common of all diseases. It is defined as a pathological process affecting the periodontal tissues. It is an inflammatory process manifest by inflammation of the gingival tissues and, in the later stages, characterized by destruction of the periodontal membrane with loss of alveolar bone support with subsequent loosening and even loss of teeth. These conditions are generally slowly progressive though less commonly can present with acute gingivitis or acute periodontitis.

Acute ulceromembranous gingivitis (Vincent's gingivitis) is a specific condition characterized by ulceration of the interdental papillae which then spreads along the gingival margin with rapid destruction of the periodontal tissues. The causative organisms have been assumed to be *Borrelia vincentii* and *Fusobacterium fusiforme*. However these are not the only causative factors and a number of host factors are important. The condition was characteristically common during wartime (trench mouth in the First World War). Smoking, anxiety and concurrent respiratory tract infections have at various times been suggested as aetiological factors. The clinical presentation is of pain and bleeding from the gums, which makes eating difficult, associated with a very unpleasant halitosis. In the Western world the condition is now relatively uncommon and most patients have neglected mouths. Examination of the gingivae usually reveals a characteristic punched-out ulcer on the tips of the interdental papillae. The ulcerated area is usually covered with a yellow-grey slough and bleeding is noted with minimal trauma. This condition responds very quickly to metronidazole and if treatment is started early enough it prevents extensive tissue destruction. Acute bacterial gingivitis needs to be differentiated from other acute infections such as primary herpetic gingivostomatitis. This is an acute viral infection with herpes hominis type 1 which affects children and adolescents. It is associated with a degree of systemic upset and intraoral examination often reveals dome-shaped vesicles which give way to small ulcers. The tongue is usually coated and there is often associated cervical lymphadenopathy. Treatment is essentially supportive with adequate hydration and analgesia but there may be a role for antimicrobials to prevent secondary infection (Main, 1989). The same combination of organisms that produce bacterial acute ulcerative gingivitis can be manifest as the much more serious cancrum oris found in Africa and South America. It has almost totally disappeared from Europe since the last World War. Initially starting as an acute ulcerative gingivitis the disease spreads to destroy large areas of the face. It affects children with a peak age of 2–5 years though sometimes it is a little older. The condition carries a significant mortality rate although this has improved with the use of antibiotics. Major facial disfigurement is however inevitable once the condition is established.

Much more common than acute gingivitis is chronic gingivitis which is almost universally present thoughout the population. The cause is bacterial plaque, especially Gram-negative bacteria. These produce a variety of endotoxic proteolytic enzymes and cytotoxic substances which cause the inflammation. In chronic periodontitis the situation is a little less clear. In addition to the mechanisms outlined above there is almost certainly an immunological response which would play a part in the genesis of this condition. Long-standing periodontal inflammation results in destruction of the ligamentous attachment of the tooth to the alveolar bone and eventually the alveolus itself leading to obvious tooth mobility and ultimately loss.

Treatment of periodontal disease is essentially the elimination of plaque by regular oral hygiene measures though as periodontal disease tends to be a relatively painless condition this simple expedient is often ignored by the majority of patients.

Systemic factors and periodontal disease

Almost any systemic disorder of any magnitude will be reflected by changes in the periodontal health, e.g. a variety of blood disorders from anaemia (which causes atrophic changes) through to acute leukaemia (which cause swelling and ulceration). Nutritional deficiencies, particularly vitamin C, which although uncommon in the Western world, are a well-recognized cause of haemorrhagic gingivitis. A variety of drugs commonly cause changes in the gingival mucosa, most notably phenytoin, cyclosporin and the calcium channel blockers, nifedipine and diltiazem, which produce a fibroepithelial hyperplasia of the gingival mucosa (Figure 22.4).

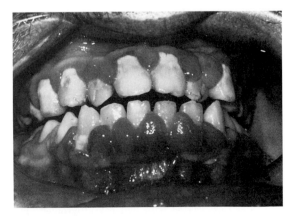

Figure 22.4 Phenytoin induced gingival hyperplasia. Improvement in oral hygiene led to almost complete resolution in this case

Epulides

The term epulis literally means 'upon the gum'. There are three main varieties of epulis.

Fibrous epulis

Irritation of the gum, for instance by calculus, could lead to the formation of a fibrous epulis (Figure 22.5). Similarly, irritation of alveolar or palatal mucosa by a denture may result in the development of a denture granuloma. These lesions are similar in origin and are both merely fibrous nodules. They may be excised at their base.

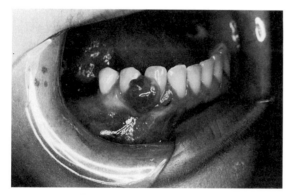

Figure 22.5 A fibrous epulis. Excision resulted in complete cure

Pyogenic granuloma (pregnancy epulis)

This epulis is characterized by its red and haemorrhagic nature. A pregnancy epulis is simply a localized gingival proliferation within an established pregnancy gingivitis.

Giant cell epulis

This is a less common epulis which histologically shows osteoclasts in proliferating granulation tissue. The lesion usually occurs in the anterior permanent dentition and may cause superficial bone resorption. Treatment is excision of the nodule with its base. Most often the giant cell epulis arises as a result of chronic periosteal irritation, however, such lesions have been associated with hyperparathyroidism and it is good practice to check serum bone chemistry when a giant cell epulis has been confirmed histologically.

Tumours of the dental tissues

Ameloblastomas

Ameloblastomas are uncommon slow growing locally invasive neoplasms derived from odontogenic epithelium. They usually present with an expanding lesion of the mandible which is painless. The teeth may become displaced because of root resorption. Radiographically the appearance is of a multilocular cyst (Figure 22.6), though occasionally they may present as a unilocular radiolucency. These tumours account for about 1% of all oral tumours and, despite their locally aggressive behaviour, malignant varieties are very rare (Hjorting-Hansen, 1991). A number of histological subtypes have been described and these are follicular or plexiform. There is also a cystic variety which may be indistinguishable radiographically from any of the other types of unicystic radiolucency. Histologically these tumours consist of islands of odontogenic epithelium in a hypocellular connective tissue stroma. In the follicular variety there are islands of cells which resemble the reticulum of a developing tooth. Squamous metaplasia with keratinization is sometimes found and can give rise to difficulties of diagnosis as there is a superficial resemblance to a squamous cell carcinoma.

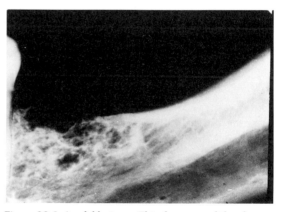

Figure 22.6 Ameloblastoma. This shows a multilocular destructive lesion with early cyst formation. Local resection was the treatment

These are bone dependent tumours that cause resorption of bones and teeth by the production of interleukin IV, among other factors. It is frequently possible to resect the tumour leaving mandibular continuity and wherever possible the bone should be skimmed following tumour removal to prevent recurrence. If the lesion is very extensive then an extraperiosteal resection is recommended with immediate reconstruction.

Adenomatoid odontogenic tumour

This tumour typically presents in the second and third decades, is more common in women than men and most usually affects the anterior maxilla. The tumour presents as a gradually enlarging intrabony swelling, pain is an occasional feature. Radiographically the lesion appears as a unilocular radiolucency. Distinction should be made from a dentigerous cyst as the tumour is sometimes associated with an unerupted tooth. In contrast with the ameloblastoma, the adenomatoid odontogenic tumour shows no tendency to local invasion and does not generally recur following surgical enucleation.

Calcifying epithelial odontogenic tumour (Pindborg tumour)

This is a rare tumour and although occurring in all age groups most commonly manifests in the fifth decade. It has an equal sex incidence and is found most often in the mandibular premolar region. The radiographic appearance is that of a radiolucent tumour with occasional scattered opacities. About half of these lesions are associated with an unerupted tooth. The calcifying epithelial odontogenic tumour progresses to local invasion if left untreated and marginal resection is normally performed.

Odontogenic myxoma

Myxoma of the mandible and maxilla is most usually seen in young adults, most often in women and in the posterior mandible. Lesions in the maxilla may be extensive involving the maxillary antrum and zygomatic process. The lesion usually presents as a painless bony expansion although it may present simply as displacement of teeth. Radiographic examination shows a unilocular or multilocular 'soap bubble' radiolucency, often with a scalloped margin (Figure 22.7). The lesion may resorb the roots of adjacent teeth.

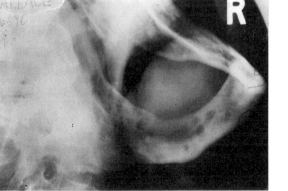

Figure 22.7 This multilocular lesion proved to be an odontogenic myxoma. The patient was edentulous and older than is usual for this lesion

It is interesting now to note the differential diagnosis of multilocular radiolucencies in the jaws. There are four principal lesions that will give this appearance. The odontogenic keratocyst, the ameloblastoma, the odontogenic myxoma and the central giant cell granuloma. Rarely will the diagnosis be a calcifying odontogenic cyst. The distinction is made first by needle aspiration, distinguishing initially between a solid or cystic mass although cystic ameloblastomas certainly occur. Fluid aspirated in the case of an odontogenic keratocyst will contain keratin squames and a low protein content (< 40 g/dl). The distinction between the solid tumours is then made by biopsy under local anaesthesia.

Odontomes

Odontomes are hamartomatous malformations of dental hard tissues. They are classified as compound odontomes containing multiple rudimentary teeth in a fibrous connective tissue and complex odontomes which are merely an irregular mass of all the dental tissues. Both types of odontome typically present in childhood and adolescence, tend to be more common in women and will be seen most usually in the mandibular premolar or molar regions. Odontomes may remain embedded in the jaws and be noticed incidentally on a radiograph. They may erupt through the gum, usually with ulceration of the surrounding mucosa or they may obstruct eruption of other teeth. Odontomes are usually removed if symptomatic.

Intraoral bony swellings

Most intraoral bony swellings are benign. The most common malignant bone tumour in the jaws is a secondary deposit and the bronchus, breast and prostate are the most common primary sites. Primary osteosarcoma of the jaws is very rare indeed.

Bony overgrowths

Localized overgrowths of bone (exostoses) are commonly seen in the mouth. Two specific variants, the torus palatinus and torus mandibularis, develop in characteristic sites.

The torus palatinus occurs in the posterior midline of the hard palate. It is symmetrical and occasionally is grooved in its midline. Patients rarely present before middle age. These lesions are only surgically removed if they interfere with the fitting of a denture.

The torus mandibularis is usually a bilateral exostosis on the lingual aspect of the mandible in the region of the premolar teeth. They are managed similarly to their palatine counterparts.

Osteomas

These are very slow growing tumours of compact lamellar bone or cancellous trabeculated bone. They should be excised if symptomatic or are making the fitting of dentures difficult. Multiple osteomas of the jaws occur in Gardner's syndrome along with multiple unerupted and supernumerary teeth (Carl and Sullivan, 1989). As intestinal polyposis is also a feature of this autosomal dominant trait colonoscopy should take precedence over any dental considerations.

Cemental tumours

Cemental tumours and dysplasias are uncommon causes of intraoral bony swellings. Four main types are described.

Cementoblastoma

A benign neoplasm sometimes producing gross bony swelling and pain. Radiographically a rounded radiopaque mass is seen with a thin radiolucent margin attached to the roots of a tooth. Cementoblastomas do not recur if completely excised and the tooth extracted.

Cementifying fibroma

This lesion is usually seen in the third and fourth decades and more often in women. It is akin to the ossifying fibroma of bone and as such appears as a circumscribed area of radiolucency containing specks of calcification. It usually forms around the roots of mandibular molars and premolars. In the presence of active calcificiation regular follow up is all that is needed as these tumours often completely ossify.

Periapical cemental dysplasia

This is most frequently seen in Negro women. It may affect several sites, usually in the mandibular incisor region. Initially the lesions are radiolucent but gradually calcify starting centrally until the lesion is a mass of sclerotic bone. It is not a progressive lesion and surgery is only usually performed as the lesion is mistaken for chronic periapical odontogenic infection.

Gigantiform cementoma

This is a similar disorder to periapical cemental dysplasia but is rather more florid. The masses of bone are somewhat larger and can affect any part of the oral cavity. Surgical reduction of the lesions is indicated if the mass becomes infected or interferes with denture wearing.

Fibrous dysplasia

Both monostotic and polyostotic fibrous dysplasia cause bony expansion in the jaws. Radiographically a fine orange peel texture of bone is seen with a very thin cortex of expanded bone. The disease, as in other anatomical sites, is self-limiting and the reduction of lesions should, if possible, be delayed until the disease is inactive, although this may not always be possible.

Paget's disease

Paget's disease, although more commonly affecting the skull, may on occasion affect the jaws, usually the maxilla. The usual presentation is of symmetrical expansion of the alveolar process in which the teeth become fused due to hypercementosis. Attempts to extract such teeth may lead to a large portion of alveolus being fractured followed by either severe bleeding from vascular pagetoid tissue or infection of the ischaemic underlying bone. The development of osteosarcoma is a rare but recognized complication of Paget's disease but occurs with extremely low frequency in the jaws.

Central giant cell granuloma

Central giant cell granuloma is a hyperplastic condition and probably represents a developmental disorder in which collections of giant cells may be found. The lesion is most common in females in the first and second decades. The mandible anterior to the first molar teeth is the most commonly affected site. A painless swelling is usually all that it is found although growth may sometimes occur at a rapid rate. Radiography reveals a well circumscribed cystic area which is often loculated or gives a soap bubble appearance. The roots of teeth are often displaced and uncommonly resorbed. Serum bone chemistry is found to be normal. Curettage of giant cell granulomas is adequate. Recurrence is unusual, even following incomplete removal and even then only limited surgery or calcitonin therapy is required.

Central haemangiomas of the jaws

These are rare and mostly occur in the mandible, principally in women. They cause a progressive painless swelling which may become pulsatile as the alveolus becomes thin with resorption. Radiographically the haemangioma is usually round or pseudo-loculated. Histologically haemangiomas of the jaws are usually of the cavernous type, although intrabony arteriovenous malformations can occasionally be found. The treatment of these lesions usually involves a combined approach utilizing radiological embolization and local surgery.

Problems following the extraction of teeth

As the most common dental operation is tooth extraction it follows logically that most complications seen in dental and oral surgical practice are related to this procedure. General complications such as socket infection or dry socket (alveolar osteitis) will occur irrespective of which tooth is removed. Other complications will be more specific and related directly to the local anatomy of that part of the mouth.

Post-extraction haemorrhage

This most usually represents primary haemorrhage at the time of extraction although an equivalent to surgical reactionary haemorrhage does occur. In dental local anaesthetic practice it is customary to use fairly high local concentrations of vasoconstrictor, e.g. adrenalin in concentrations of 1:80 000 and as this vasoconstrictor loses its effect after the surgery, capillaries may reopen and further haemorrhage may ensue. However, both types of bleeding are managed similarly.

Local pressure will usually arrest most post-extraction haemorrhage. The patient simply bites on a gauze pack placed over the socket for at least 10 minutes. The patient is told to rest and sit in an upright position which often involves raising of the dental chair. If these initial measures fail to stop the bleeding, oxidized regenerated cellulose (Surgicel) or fibrin foam (Oxycel) when placed in the socket are useful adjuncts to haemostasis. Apposition of the socket mucosal margins using a tightly placed mattress suture will tense the mucoperiosteum effectively strangling its blood vessels and arresting an otherwise persistent haemorrhage. Should all these measures fail a systemic coagulopathy should be suspected.

Dry socket (alveolar osteitis)

This is a common complication of dental extraction affecting some 4% of sockets in total and over 10% of sockets where a wisdom tooth has been removed. Some patients seem to be particularly prone to this complication. Smoking and poor oral hygiene have been cited as relevant risk factors. The condition typically presents 2–5 days after tooth removal with an increasingly painful tooth socket which, on inspection, is denuded of protective blood clot. Alveolar bone often is visible hence the term dry socket. The aetiology of the condition is uncertain although it probably represents merely a localized inflammation rather than infection. However, left untreated the condition may progress to a full blown osteomyelitis, particularly in the immunocompromised. The drug, metronidazole, given as 400 mg eight-hourly for 3 days by mouth, has been shown to be effective, both in the prophylaxis of dry socket in those predisposed, as well as reducing the socket healing time in those already affected. Alveolar osteitis is an extremely painful condition and local measures aimed at reducing discomfort should be encouraged. Various topical pastes have been developed, none of which has been shown to be of any greater benefit than simple irrigation of the socket with warm saline. Large areas of denuded bone may be covered with ribbon gauze soaked in Whitehead's varnish.

Oroantral communication (fistula)

An oroantral communication most often occurs following removal of a posterior maxillary tooth. Anatomically the second molar is most closely related to the maxillary antrum although most oroantral communications occur after removal of the first molar, simply because this tooth is more often extracted. Particular caution should be exercised where a single standing posterior maxillary molar tooth is to be removed. Suspicions should be aroused if the patient develops an epistaxis following extraction and on occasion prolapsing antral mucosa or even polypoid tissue may be seen in the socket. If the patient performs the Valsalva manoeuvre a gust of air will blow through the communication. In the absence of any infection the treatment of choice is primary closure of the defect. This can be accomplished by a variety of means although three currently stand pre-eminent:

1 Buccal advancement flap: a wide-based flap is raised based on the buccal sulcus. A transverse releasing incision of the flap periosteum will allow advancement of the flap over the socket to be sutured without tension to the palatal mucosa. If necessary a small amount of the socket rim is removed to facilitate this manoeuvre.
2 Palatal flap: this has the advantage that it does not interfere with the depth of the buccal sulcus. It involves raising a finger-shaped flap of palatal mucosa based on the anterior palatine artery. This is transposed over the oroantral communication and sutured to the buccal mucoperiosteum. It leaves a small area of exposed bone in the palate which is left to granulate.
3 Buccal fat pad flap: this is a relatively new technique in which the buccal fat pad is mobilized through a gingival flap, again based on the buccal sulcus (Samman, Cheung and Tideman, 1993). The fat pad is brought into the mouth and sutured across the open socket. Within a few weeks the mucosa has seeded on to the flap and gives an excellent healed result.

Disorders of the temporomandibular joint
Temporomandibular joint pain (facial arthromyalgia)

Facial arthromyalgia is a symptom complex of pre-auricular and facial pain associated with difficulty in mouth opening and clicking or locking of the jaw joint. Occasional cases have a traumatic aetiology but the majority are associated in some way with psychological stress. The condition may be due to a true internal derangement of the joint with rupture of meniscal ligaments and anterior displacement of the fibrocartilaginous disc. Such a condition may progress to and merge imperceptibly with an osteoarthrosis. Initial management of facial arthromyalgia is with low dose tricyclic antidepressants. These have been shown to be very effective in symptomatic relief, regardless of the aetiology of the condition. A biochemical basis for their action would appear to exist in that the tricyclic antidepressants inhibit production of cytokines responsible for pain in the temporomandibular joint. Symptom control is usually achieved within 3 months. When this is not successful and symptoms referable to the joint still persist temporomandibular joint arthroscopy with intrajoint lysis and lavage is effective for most minor internal derangements. Open joint surgery is reserved for the most severe and resistant cases.

Osteoarthrosis

Temporomandibular joint osteoarthrosis is a common condition, although symptomatic in approximately 30% of those so affected. Collectively patients with osteoarthrosis are older than the group presenting with facial arthromyalgia, although 10% of patients with degenerative joint disease are under 25 years of age. The essential features are of pain in the jaw, crepitus and radiographic features of articular surface erosions and osteophytes. Treatment is with conservative measures in the first instance followed similarly by arthroscopic surgery with the most severe cases proceeding to open joint surgery and even joint replacement. As this is a degenerative rather than an inflammatory condition there is no place here for intra-articular corticosteroid injections.

Rheumatoid arthritis

Although the temporomandibular joint may be involved in arthritis associated with any of the connective tissue disorders it is most commonly seen associated with rheumatoid arthritis because of the predominance of this condition. One-half to two-thirds of patients with rheumatoid arthritis will have temporomandibular joint involvement, although only a few of these will complain of symptoms. Pain is the usual feature, often associated with crepitus. Management is conservative in the first instance with non-steroidal anti-inflammatory agents and in severe cases intra-articular steroids may be of benefit. Open arthroplasty may be required for cases not responding to these measures or where ankylosis has ensued. The use of intracapsular steroids in the management of temporomandibular joint disease is nowadays restricted to the immunologically mediated arthritides which, in common practice, is rheumatoid arthritis and the arthritis associated with psoriasis.

Dislocation of the temporomandibular joint

Dislocation of the temporomandibular joint occurs when the condyle is displaced anterior to the articular eminence. Usually this is self-reducing, i.e. a subluxation. This is often seen recurrently in hypermobility disorders such as the Ehlers–Danlos syndrome. Occasionally the jaw becomes locked in the dislocated position with the mouth fixed open and the mandible protruded. Reduction is by gripping the angle of the mandible extraorally with the fingers and placing thumbs on the retromolar pad of both sides intraorally. The best position for the operator is in front of a patient who is seated upright. The initial movement is to *open* the jaw, the mandibular angle is then pressed firmly downwards and backwards, taking the condyle back into the glenoid fossa. Occasionally cases may require sedation with an intravenous benzodiazepine before suitable cooperation and muscle relaxation can be achieved. Occasionally surgery may be required to correct cases of recurrent dislocation.

Dry mouth (xerostomia)

The causes of dry mouth are summarized in Table 22.2.

The management of patients with severe xerostomia centres around the control of oral and dental infection and symptomatic measures to alleviate the discomfort of a parchment-like mucosa.

Table 22.2 The common causes of xerostomia

Drugs: tricyclic antidepressants, antihistamines, phenothiazines, lithium

Conditions causing dehydration: diabetes, diarrhoea and vomiting

Psychogenic: anxiety, depression

Salivary gland disease: Sjögren's syndrome, irradiation damage, infections, e.g. mumps, AIDS, sarcoidosis

Control of infection

Oral candidosis is common in severe xerostomia and antifungal agents such as fluconazole or amphotericin lozenges may be prescribed. If the patient is a denture wearer miconazole gel or nystatin ointment may be spread on the denture before it is inserted. As a free flow of saliva is necessary for adequate dental cleansing and plaque control, oral hygiene measures have to take account of this. The use of fluoride mouth rinses and gels is effective in preventing dental caries in dentate patients. Similarly the use of aqueous chlorhexidine mouth washes on a daily basis is essential to control periodontal disease.

Symptomatic treatment

This is based along two main lines of therapy. First, drugs that directly stimulate salivation, or alternatively the use of synthetic saliva substitutes. Cholinergic drugs, such as pilocarpine, used as a mouth rinse are effective in stimulating any remaining salivary tissue. Non-specific cholinergic side effects such as bradycardia and lacrimation tend to limit the use of pilocarpine in some patients. Ametholetrithione is a drug that increases cholinergic receptors in salivary glands and may have some benefit clinically. Salivary substitutes vary from simple sips of water taken as frequently as the patient wishes, to salivary replacements based on methylcellulose, mucin or lemon and glycerine. They are presented as a spray (Glandosane, Saliva Orthana) or in tablet form (Salivix).

References

CARL, W. and SULLIVAN, M. A. (1989) Dental abnormalities and bone lesions associated with familial adenomatous polyposis: report of cases. *Journal of the American Dental Association*, 119, 137–139

GORLIN, R. I. (1987) Naevoid basal cell carcinoma syndrome. *Medicine*, 66, 98–113

HJORTING-HANSEN, E. (1991) Benign tumours of the jaws. *Current Opinion in Dentistry*, 1, 296–304

MAIN, D. M. G. (1989). Acute herpetic stomatitis: referrals to Leeds Dental Hospital 1978–1987. *British Dental Journal*, 166, 14–16

SAMMAN, N., CHEUNG, K. and TIDEMAN, H. (1993) The buccal fat pad in oral reconstruction. *International Journal of Oral Maxillofacial Surgery*, 22, 2–6

23

Trans-sphenoidal hypophysectomy

R. A. Williams

Operations on the pituitary gland are for the removal of pituitary tumours. This form of pituitary surgery is not a complete hypophysectomy, as ideally the normal pituitary tissue is not removed. However, the term 'hypophysectomy' is too widely used and accepted to suggest any redefinition.

Pituitary operations are performed 'from below', which is trans-sphenoidally, or 'from above', which involves a craniotomy. The sphenoid sinus has been approached in a variety of ways, but two have emerged as the most satisfactory. The transethmoid method is used by otolaryngologists; it has the advantage of a wider access and exposure, but the disadvantage of a facial scar. The sublabial trans-septal route is mostly used by neurosurgeons, and there are some centres where otolaryngologists and neurosurgeons operate together.

History

The leading text books of 100 years ago described the pituitary gland as surgically inaccessible. Horsley (1906) was the first to decompress, by the transcranial route, a pituitary tumour which was causing blindness, but did not record this in print for some years. The threat of blindness was then the indication for operation. A number of surgeons tried modifications of the transcranial route, both intradurally and extradurally. Schloffer (1906, 1907) for example made an external incision across the eyebrows and then down to join a lateral rhinotomy. However, these operations seriously damaged nasal function and produced unacceptable scars on the face. In 1909 Cushing started his sublabial trans-septal operation. At about the same time, Hirsch (1911a,b) described an operation through the nose which was later modified to become much the same as the

Cushing operation. Cushing (1932) continued with a large series of 159 trans-septal operations and 88 transfrontal operations. The 5-year recurrence rate was 35% from below and 13% from above. He therefore returned mainly to the transfrontal route in 1928. His overall mortality was only 5.8%. His name stands out as a great pioneer of pituitary surgery.

Chiari performed the first transethmoid trans-sphenoid operation in 1912, and this approach was taken-up later, in the 1950s, by a number of otolaryngologists who were removing the pituitary gland as part of the treatment for carcinoma of the breast and prostate. Angell James (1967a, b), Bateman (1962, 1963), Briant (1964, 1968) and Williams (1978) had large series of operations at that time and it was their experience that reintroduced the transethmoid operations for pituitary tumours. Other approaches from below, such as the transantral operation described by Hamberger et al. (1959, 1960, 1961) and the transpalatal operation by Trible and Morse (1965) have not generally been continued.

Treatment of pituitary tumours

Surgery was initially the only method of dealing with pituitary tumours. Later radiotherapy by external beam with X-rays (Jenkins, Ash and Bloom, 1972) or protons (Kjellberg et al., 1968; Lawrence et al., 1963, 1973) and by implantation of radioactive gold or yttrium (Wright et al., 1970) became effective and safe. Both surgery and radiotherapy were at first non-selective, just destructive. Microdissection to remove the neoplastic portions and leave the normal parts was introduced, and the idea had great promise. However, for reasons discussed later, this is not always so successful. Radiotherapy is not selective and does not completely destroy a tumour leaving the normal gland intact, especially in the case of well differentiated neoplasms, but it does have a useful and effective role to play sometimes. It is possible to shrink certain pituitary tumours medically and this applies particularly to prolactinomas where bromocriptine can be very effective. However, the management of pituitary tumours today still requires the use of surgery, radiotherapy, and medication. It should be for the endocrinologist to decide how best to treat each case, as described by Levy and Lightman (1994).

Surgical indications for removal of pituitary tumours

The indications for the removal of pituitary tumours may be for their local effects. If a pituitary tumour enlarges upwards, it will result in bitemporal hemianopia and restriction of the visual fields leading to total blindness. There will of course be the intracranial pressure effects of headache and papilloedema. When these tumours extend laterally into the cavernous sinus they will affect the cranial nerves III, IV and VI. Large downward extensions may present in the nasopharynx and sometimes cause cerebrospinal fluid leaks and recurrent meningitis. It may be necessary therefore to decompress, if not completely remove, large pituitary tumours for their serious local effects.

Medical indications for the removal of pituitary tumours

Acromegaly and gigantism

If it is possible to remove the tumour completely by trans-sphenoid surgery, this is now the most effective treatment for acromegaly. There are large series reported by Hardy (1973, 1975, 1979; Hardy, Beauregard and Robert, 1978; Hardy and Somma, 1979) and Williams (1974; Williams *et al.*, 1975) indicating nearly 80% cure, that is reduction of growth hormone to normal, by surgery. High energy radiotherapy and especially proton beam therapy are certainly partially effective treatments for tumours causing acromegaly. Medical treatment for acromegaly has met with some success. It is sometimes possible to shrink these tumours and lower the growth hormone to a variable extent but the results of medical treatment are not predictable. Maybe in the future the medical treatment of acromegaly will become as effective as it is with prolactin-secreting tumours.

Cushing's disease and Nelson's syndrome

Cushing's syndrome may be caused by a pituitary tumour, adrenal gland tumour, ectopic ACTH-produc-

ing tumour, and the administration of steroids or certain other drugs. The diagnosis of the cause of Cushing's syndrome is not always straightforward. However, the endocrinologist may ask the surgeon to treat Cushing's syndrome by removing a pituitary tumour. These tumours may be microtumours not apparent on plain X-ray but showing on computerized tomography (CT) and magnetic resonance imaging (MRI) scans, or they may be large invasive tumours. Usually the tumour is small and provides the possibility of a successful microdissection with removal of the tumour and sparing the normal pituitary. Large invasive tumours are very difficult to cure surgically or in any other way. If an adrenalectomy has been performed for Cushing's syndrome primarily due to a small pituitary tumour, then some months or years later the pituitary tumour is liable to grow. The result is high adrenocorticotropic hormone (ACTH) and melanocyte-stimulating hormone (MSH) levels with generalized pigmentation as well as the local problems associated with the development of the pituitary tumour – this is Nelson's syndrome (Nelson *et al.*, 1958; Nelson Menkin and Thorn, 1960). The results of trans-sphenoid surgery for Cushing's disease can be highly satisfactory with a complete cure of a very serious medical condition. These patients may, however, be extremely unwell on first presentation and it may be advisable to block the production of cortisol medically for some weeks or months until the patient is fit for operation.

Prolactinoma

Before the discovery of prolactin, these tumours were included with chromophobe tumours and it was thought that they did not have any hormonal effects. Prolactin-secreting tumours as their name implies actually secrete the hormone directly in large quantities. However, any suprasellar tumour interfering with the control of prolactin can cause hyperprolactinaemia, but the prolactin level in this case is not as high as with a prolactin-secreting tumour. In women, hyperprolactinaemia mainly causes amenorrhoea and infertility, but sometimes galactorrhoea as well. In men, hyperprolactinaemia may cause impotence, gynaecomastia and skin changes. Before medical treatment for prolactinoma became so effective, surgery was widely used, especially in the USA and Canada. This is where microdissection first came into its own and pressure was put on the surgeon by the endocrinologist to remove the tumour to allow a woman to become pregnant, but not to remove all the normal pituitary. The results of microdissection were sometimes most satisfactory but they depended on the size of the adenoma. Hardy (1979) had a cure rate of 90% with non-invasive tumours of less than 10 mm size, dropping to zero for large invasive tumours. A microadenoma with a piece of normal pituitary attached, which was thought to have been completely removed, is shown in Figure 23.1. However, with special staining it was possible to show that in other parts of this pituitary there were abnormal clumps of prolactin-secreting cells which could have grown into another microadenoma. Prolactin-secreting tumours are now generally treated medically and it is only when this medical treatment cannot be tolerated by the patient that surgery is occasionally necessary. Even large tumours causing pressure effects will shrink with medical treatment.

Chromophobe tumours (adenoma and germinoma) in children

These tumours do not have any direct hormone effects but they may raise the prolactin level indirectly by pressure on the prolactin controlling mechanism. A germinoma is a rare pituitary tumour occurring in childhood and pituitary surgery is sometimes necessary to make the diagnosis so that the patient can then be treated with radiotherapy.

Other pituitary tumours

There are other rare pituitary tumours producing a mixture of hormones and these may have to be treated surgically.

Craniopharyngioma and cordoma

These tumours may occasionally require trans-sphenoid surgery.

Contraindications

It is not safe to proceed with trans-sphenoid hypophysectomy in the presence of nasal or sinus infection, and this should be cleared up first. Partial pneumatization or non-pneumatization of the sphenoid is frequently quoted as a contraindication to trans-sphenoid hypophysectomy. This is not the case. Figure 23.2 shows an X-ray of a boy with a germinoma and a partially pneumatized sphenoid, who had an uneventful trans-sphenoid pituitary operation. It is not difficult to pneumatize the sphenoid with a drill. The soft cancellous bone can be removed until the more compact wall of the sphenoid is encountered. Once the shape of the pituitary fossa has been identified the operation can proceed normally. Upward extensions of more than a few millimetres anteriorly or 1 cm posteriorly are not accessible from below, and this is usually a contraindication to a trans-sphenoid operation. The exception is a dumb-bell tumour, needing surgery from below and above. It has been found better to stage these operations, starting trans-sphenoidally.

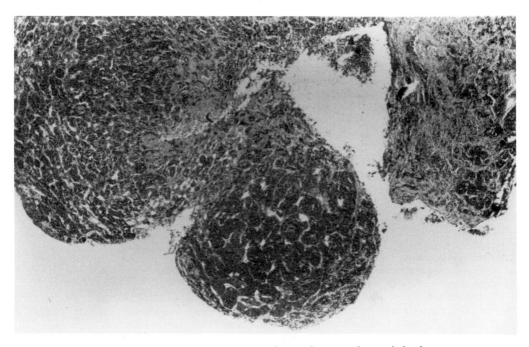

Figure 23.1 A microadenoma apparently completely removed with a good margin of normal gland

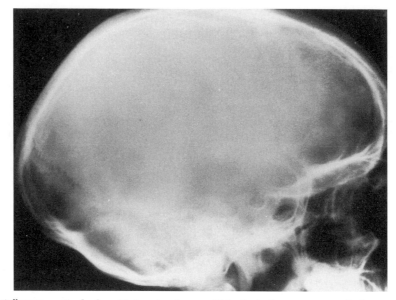

Figure 23.2 A partially pneumatized sphenoid sinus in a boy aged 13 who had a germinoma which required pituitary surgery

Preoperative investigations

Medical investigations include measuring all pituitary hormone levels and often an oral or intravenous glucose tolerance test with measurements of serum growth hormone and insulin levels, as well as blood sugars. These tests are usually arranged by the referring endocrinologist.

Serum electrolytes are required, because in some conditions, such as Cushing's disease, the potassium levels may be dangerously low for general anaesthesia. It is safer to have two units of blood crossmatched. Although blood transfusion is hardly ever required, it may be vital if there is serious bleeding from the cavernous sinus or carotid artery.

Imaging

Routine skull X-rays will show the outline of the pituitary fossa, the pneumatization of the sphenoid, and the size of the frontal sinuses. Sinus X-rays should also be taken to exclude infection. For pituitary tumours it is necessary to show the outline of the upper part of the gland, and the first method for doing this was by an air encephalogram. However, this investigation was not entirely without risk and has now been completely abandond in favour of CT and MRI scans. High quality CT and MRI scans with sagittal reconstructions show the whole pituitary gland very satisfactorily (Figure 23.3). The degree of upward extension is important when deciding whether trans-sphenoid surgery is appropriate (Figures 23.4 and 23.5). MRI scans show some pituitary tumours better than CT scans, especially where there is an empty sella with a rim of tumour or a lateral extension (Figures 23.6 and 23.7). Hardy (1979) has shown that growth-hormone-secreting tumours are more often in the lateral parts of the fossa inferiorly; prolactin-secreting tumours in the lateral part of the gland superiorly; and ACTH-secreting tumours more

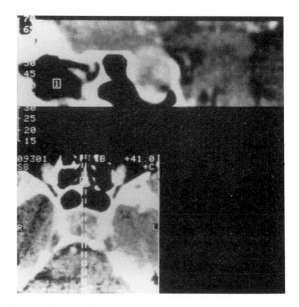

Figure 23.3 A CT scan of a tumour with a small upward extension accessible from below

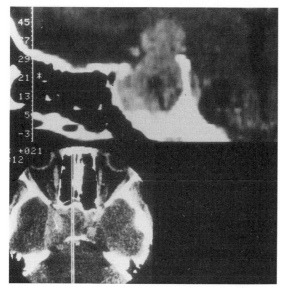

Figure 23.4 A CT scan of a dumb-bell tumour not all accessible from below

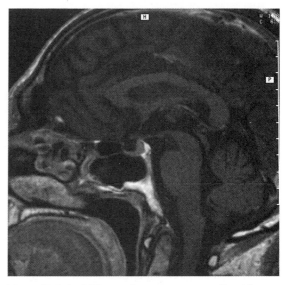

Figure 23.6 An MRI scan showing an empty sella with some tissue posteriorly, which could be tumour or normal gland

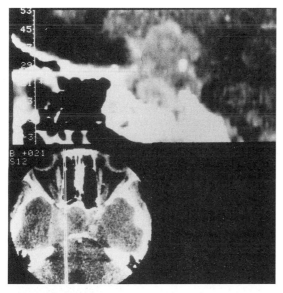

Figure 23.5 A CT scan of a large right-sided upward extension, requiring a craniotomy

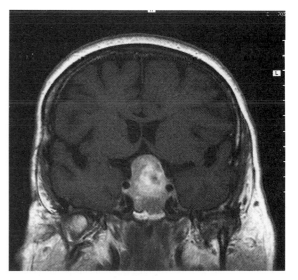

Figure 23.7 An MRI scan showing a large upward and some lateral extensions of the tumour

often central. The author has not found that this can be relied upon. Neurosurgeons prefer to have arteriography of the internal carotid arteries to show their position. There is certainly one occasion where this can be most informative, and that is if a tumour has been treated medically and has apparently regressed.

The carotid arteries can then move towards the midline and the space between them may be only a few millimetres, with the residual tumour below. Although the carotid arteries can be identified positively during surgery it is helpful to know where to expect to find them.

Visual fields

Visual field defects begin to appear when the tumour extends upwards to the optic chiasma; this is an important sign as it usually means the trans-sphenoid operation is not indicated and that surgery is better performed from above. It is good practice to have visual fields routinely recorded and to compare them with any subsequent tests, in case for example there is a recurrence of the tumour.

Drugs

Adequate doses of steroids must be given to cover the operation and the postoperative period. Experience has shown that if trans-sphenoid surgery is covered by prophylactic antibiotics, infection is extremely rare. A pack will normally be left in the nose for about 9 days and to prevent infection the combination of a broad-spectrum antibiotic and an antibiotic which diffuses easily into the cerebrospinal fluid is effective. These antibiotics should be continued until the pack is removed. Desmopressin (DDAVP) should be available for the first few postoperative days to treat diabetes insipidus. Water intoxication is however more dangerous than diabetes insipidus, so this drug should only be given when necessary. Urine osmolarity is used as a guide, but also when the specific gravity of the urine is low and the urinary output exceeds 500 ml/h for 3 consecutive hours, this is a reasonable indication for the injection of desmopressin 2 μg. Also, a total output of more than 5 litres in 24 hours may indicate that the diabetes insipidus should be treated. Some patients may have been told that they may become thirsty and because of this they drink so much that they can simulate a diabetes insipidus.

Anaesthesia

Intubation during anaesthesia may be difficult because of the large tongue in patients with acromegaly, and large laryngoscopes and long endotracheal tubes should be available. Whether the ventilation is spontaneous or controlled is for the anaesthetist to decide, providing that the venous pressure can be kept low. Air embolism does not seem to be a problem because under direct vision it is possible to see if blood is coming from the cavernous sinus or if air is entering it, and the ventilation pressure can be adjusted accordingly. In the author's experience it is not necessary to monitor the neck veins with Doppler probes for air embolism. Hypotension can be most helpful during the dissection of the pituitary. However, in the early stages of the operation it is better to have a normal blood pressure so that all the superficial bleeding can be thoroughly controlled to avoid a subcutaneous haematoma.

The operation

Transethmoid approach

The operating table is tipped about 25° head-up, and the neck slightly flexed to face the surgeon who stands on the right hand side of the patient. It may be necessary to perform a submucous resection of the nasal septum for access to the right side of the nose. An external incision is made, curved round the medial side of the orbit. The incision is deepened towards the nose medially, so that the lacrimal sac is avoided (Figure 23.8).

Superiorly the supratrochlear nerve is also avoided by straightening the upper 1 cm of the incision. The incision is deepened to the bone by dividing the periosteum, which is then separated from the bone and dissected back past the orbital rim until the anterior ethmoidal artery is exposed.

This artery runs through the frontoethmoidal suture and represents the upper limit of the roof of the ethmoids (Figure 23.9). The artery is sealed above and below by unipolar diathermy and is divided. Bipolar diathermy should not be used here as it is not so effective. There is usually no bleeding but there may be a small extravasation of fat. The dissection continues to the posterior ethmoidal artery which is left as a landmark. The lacrimal sac is lifted out of its groove and mobilized to avoid tension, when the retractor is inserted. A Luongo retractor is then placed in position (Figure 23.10). The paper plate of the ethmoid is removed up to the anterior ethmoidal arery and if necessary back as far as the posterior ethmoidal artery (Figure 23.11); the orbital rim is taken away with a drill or gouge. The frontonasal duct must not be

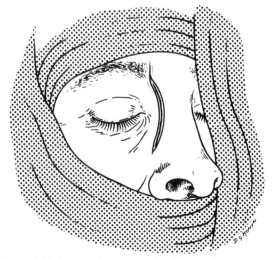

Figure 23.8 Incision for a transethmoid operation

opened widely in acromegalic patients for the soft
tissues may later prolapse and obstruct the duct. This
removal continues downwards as far as the posterior
edge of the lacrimal fossa. A complete external ethmoidectomy is performed. It is convenient to use forceps
either through the external opening or through the
nose lateral to the middle turbinate. It is not necessary

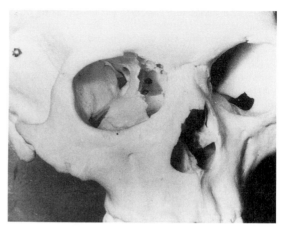

Figure 23.11 Skull with an ethmoidectomy and
sphenoidotomy performed as it would be for a transethmoid
operation

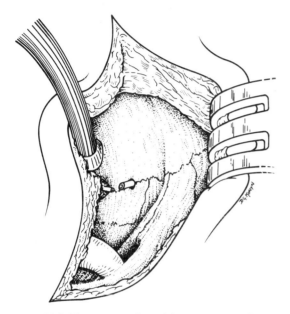

Figure 23.9 The anterior ethmoidal artery is exposed in
the frontoethmoidal suture

to remove the middle turbinate unless a wide access
is required for the larger tumours, when this step is
indicated. The sphenoid sinus is opened through the
posterior ethmoid cell and usually the right sphenoid
is entered first. The position of the intersphenoid
septum can be seen on the submentovertical X-ray of
the skull, and it is nearly always necessary to remove
this septum. The opening into the sphenoid sinus is
widened and the rostrum of the vomer is removed
either with back biting Ostrum's forceps or a drill,
until full exposure of the front of the pituitary fossa is
achieved.

Trans-septal approach (Cushing's)

A gingival incision is made (Figure 23.12). The periosteum is elevated with the mucosa to expose the
mucosa of the pyriform opening and floor of the

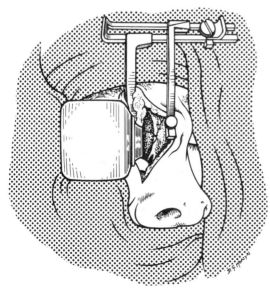

Figure 23.10 A Luongo retractor in position holding the
lacrimal sac aside

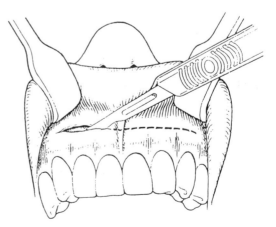

Figure 23.12 The sublabial (Cushing's) incision

nose. The dissection is continued to the front of the
nasal septum (Figure 23.13). Firm retraction is
needed to elevate the upper lip and tip of the nose,
using small right-angled retractors. The mucosa is
separated from the floor of the nose, to both sides
and from the nasal septal cartilage. The bony opening
of the front of the nose is thus exposed, and can then
be enlarged inferolaterally with a bone punch or
drill. This is not always necessary, and may cause
temporary or occasionally permanent denervation of
the incisior teeth. A submucous resection of the nasal
septum is then performed, holding the flaps apart
with a large Killian's speculum. A Hardy bivalve
speculum is inserted. The anterior wall of the sphenoid sinus is opened with a gouge or drill and removed laterally as far as possible (Figure 23.14). The
pituitary fossa is not identified as easily from this
angle as from the ethmoids, especially if the pneumatization is not full. From this point the operation is the
same whichever approach is used, except that with
the transethmoid approach straight instruments can
be used, but with the sublabial approach angled
instruments are better. This is because the microscope
view and all instrumentation are through the same
relatively small opening trans-septally.

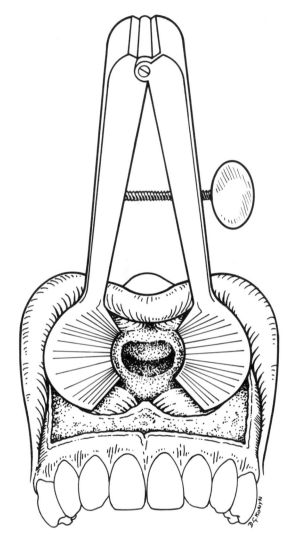

Figure 23.14 A Hardy retractor in position, and the
sphenoid sinus opened

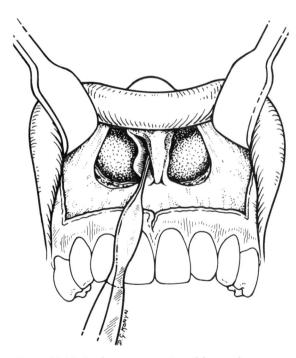

Figure 23.13 A submucous resection of the nasal septum,
as in the Cushing's approach

Opening the pituitary fossa and dissection

A Zeiss operating microscope with a 300 mm objective lens is positioned, viewing through the external

incision where a transethmoid approach has been
used. The bone over the pituitary fossa is drilled
away using a small cutting burr as this does not
damage the dura. A layer of bone is removed extending above to the top of the sphenoid sinus, sideways
until the bone thickens, and the full width of the fossa
is reached, and downwards to the floor. The floor
is not removed, as this is needed to support the muscle
plug at the end of the operation. Large tumours often
erode through the bone and sometimes through the
dura presenting in the sphenoid sinus. At this stage
the front of the pituitary fossa may be seen as a
pulsating sheet of dura. The carotid arteries are
occasionally exposed laterally and can be identified by their thicker appearance. The cavernous and

intercavernous sinuses can usually be seen through the dura and the incision made to avoid them. Bleeding from the cavernous sinuses can be a problem but is lessened by good anaesthetic technique and adequate head-up position. The author has never found it necessary to abandon an operation because of bleeding. The venous sinuses are less obvious with expanding tumours than with small normal-sized pituitary glands. If there is an almost 'empty sella', care must be taken to enter the gland or tumour and not the subarachnoid space. If possible a cruciate incision is made, but if there is insufficient space between the superior and inferior intercavernous sinuses, a transverse incision is adequate (Figure 23.15). A diathermy incision helps to seal the two layers of dura, but some surgeons prefer a knife.

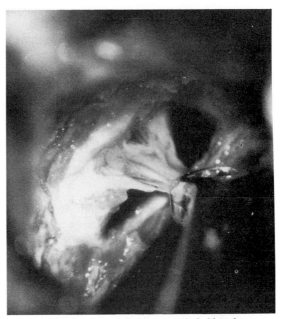

Figure 23.16 Pituitary stalk being gently held in the diaphragm, with a small piece of normal gland. Some tumour is present above, on the patient's right side

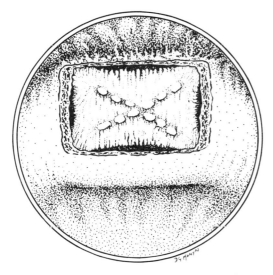

Figure 23.15 The bone of the front of the pituitary fossa is drilled away, exposing the dura. The cavernous and intercavernous sinuses are visible through the dura. Diathermy dots show where the dura will be opened

drilled away under direct vision. Lateral extensions are more difficult and it is often not possible to see completely the lateral extent of a tumour. Dissection therefore has to be blind. For this situation Hardy curettes are useful but great care has to be taken not

When the gland is opened a tumour will extrude whereas a normal-sized gland just presents itself. Angell–James dissectors are especially shaped to separate the floor and sides of the gland and are useful for microdissection. Where a large tumour is present the normal pituitary is not easy to find, and probably enough of it resides in the diaphragm where the stalk emerges. It is best therefore to remove all the tumour that can be found but not to clean the diaphragm too thoroughly, if tumour does not appear to be attached to it (Figure 23.16). Where there is some upward extension, and when the tumour has been decompressed, the diaphragm may well come down into view (Figure 23.17). Downward extensions can be followed easily and removed; they may even extend out into the basisphenoid and occiput, and can be

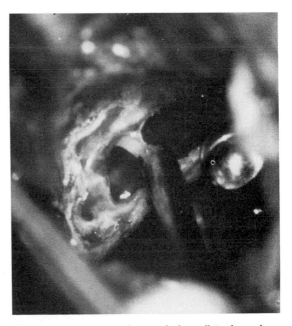

Figure 23.17 An empty fossa with the stalk in the sucker

to curette too firmly out of sight, or serious bleeding can result. For microtumours, microdissection is often possible. This involves removing the tumour and leaving an adequate quantity of normal pituitary gland behind. The tumour can usually be identified as a separate adenoma appearing different from the normal gland. Experience is required to be confident about this identification but the tumour may be whiter and of a softer consistency. A plane of cleavage may appear, but it is advisable to take some adjacent normal pituitary for it has been shown histologically that, if a cleavage plane is followed, some tumour may be left behind. If there is doubt in identifying the tumour from the normal gland small pieces may be sent for frozen section. Cerebrospinal fluid will escape if the diaphragm is breached. This can be sucked away until pressure is lowered so the flow will then stop, and the operation can proceed.

Insertion of a piece of muscle into the fossa stops bleeding and escape of cerebrospinal fluid. It also supports the diaphragm and prevents postoperative headache due to stretching. This muscle should be placed in the fossa lightly rather than packed tightly. A large plug may extrude. The muscle can then be covered with Sterispon to prevent adherence of the pack. A 1.25 cm (half-inch) ribbon gauze pack is inserted into the sphenoid sinus, coming out through the right side of the nose. More packing should be placed in the nose to keep the sphenoid pack in position. The sphenoid pack stays in for 9 days but the nasal packs can be removed sooner especially with a Cushing's approach, depending on the stability of the sphenoid pack. With the transethmoidal operation the pack should fill the ethmoid and not bulge into the orbit. Only the skin requires suturing. Padding and bandaging the eye for 12 hours helps to reduce postoperative swelling, but care must be taken not to apply the bandage too tightly and compress the eye.

Postoperative care

The patient's temperature often rises during the first 12 hours but this does not necessarily indicate infection and it is probably due to some hypothalamic disturbance. From the second to about the eighth postoperative day the temperature is often subnormal for the same reason. After the packs are removed on the ninth day, the treatment is the same as for any other intranasal operation. It is sometimes necessary to remove crusts from the nose, but with saline nose sniffs for 2 or 3 weeks the nose usually becomes clean and healed. Looking into the nose the pulsations of the pituitary may be seen for up to one month postoperatively. Medically, steroids ought to be continued until the normal pituitary function has been tested, usually about 6 weeks after operation. The preoperative tests are repeated to assess the effect of the operation and whether it is necessary to continue with steroids and/or thyroxine. After

surgery for large pituitary tumours about 25% of patients have some pituitary hormone deficit and require replacement therapy.

Complications

Some patients develop a superficial haematoma or black eye but this is outside the orbital periosteum. It may look alarming for a few days but usually settles within 5 days. If the eye becomes completely closed it is important to test the vision and eye movements to exclude excessive intraorbital pressure. Temporary diabetes insipidus occurs in up to one-third of patients. Cerebrospinal fluid leaks are rare but if they occur following removal of the packs the treatment should be conservative, with the continuation of the antibiotics. The leakage usually settles within 3 weeks. Only if the muscle pack has come out completely would it be necessary to take the patient back to the operating theatre and insert another muscle plug. In the author's experience this has only occurred once in over 300 tumours operated on and the reason was that the patient decided to restore himself to his normal health. It was on the fiftieth press-up on the tenth postoperative day that the cerebrospinal fluid started to leak. This was followed by meningitis. No other case of meningitis has been encountered in this series and it is generally a very rare complication. Frontal sinusitis occurs especially in acromegalic patients if the frontonasal duct has been opened too widely. With proper operative technique this should be avoided but if it does occur, an operation some months or years later to reopen the frontonasal duct may be necessary. In experienced hands the mortality of this operation is less than 1%.

Conclusion

Trans-sphenoid pituitary surgery is a most effective way of treating some pituitary tumours which extend downwards into the sphenoid sinus. Neurosurgeons usually approach the sphenoid via the nasal septum, but otolaryngologists use an external ethmoidectomy approach. CT and MRI scans have made it possible to localize microtumours which can often be dissected leaving the normal pituitary intact. The overall management of pituitary tumours should be by an endocrinologist, with a surgeon who can operate trans-sphenoidally, a neurosurgeon and a radiotherapist. The treatment of pituitary tumours should be restricted to centres where these specialists are available.

References

ANGELL–JAMES, J. (1967a) Transethmoidal hypophysectomy. *Archives of Otolaryngology*, **86**, 256–264

ANGELL–JAMES, J. (1967b) The Semon lecture: the hypophysis. *Journal of Laryngology and Otology*, **81**, 1283

BATEMAN, G. H. (1962) Transsphenoidal hypophysectomy. A review of 70 cases treated in the past 2 years. *Transactions of the American Academy of Ophthalmology and Otolaryngology*, **66**, 103

BATEMAN, G. H. (1963) *Proceedings of the Royal Society of Medicine*, **56**, 389

BRIANT, J. D. R. (1964) Transsphenoidal hypophysectomy. *Proceedings of the Canadian Otolaryngology Society*, **18**, 159

BRIANT, J. D. R. (1968) Transethmoidal sphenoidal hypophysectomy. *Laryngoscope*, **78**, 649

CHIARI, O. (1912) Uber eine Modifikation der Schlofferschen Operation von Tumoren der Hypophyse. *Wiener klinische Wochenschrift*, **25**, 5

CUSHING, H. (1909) Partial hypophysectomy for acromegaly: with remarks on the function of the hypophysis. *Annals of Surgery*, **50**, 1002

CUSHING, H. (1932) The basophil adenomas of the pituitary body and their clinical manifestations (pituitary basophilism). *Bulletin of the Johns Hopkins Hospital*, **50**, 137

HAMBERGER, C. A., HAMMER, G., NORLEN, G. and SJOGREN, B. (1959) Hypophysectomy in acromegaly (letter). *Journal of Clinical Endocrinology and Metabolism*, **19**, 1500

HAMBERGER, C. A., HAMMER, G., NORLEN, G. and SJOGREN, B. (1960) Surgical treatment of acromegaly. *Acta Otolaryngologica Supplementum*, **158**, 168

HAMBERGER, C. A., HAMMER, G., NORLEN, G. and STOGREN, B. (1961) Transantrosphenoidal hypophysectomy. *Archives of Otolaryngology*, **74**, 2–8

HARDY, J. (1973) Transsphenoidal surgery of hypersecreting pituitary tumors. *Excerpta Medica International Congress Series*, **303**, 179–194

HARDY, J. (1975) Transsphenoidal microsurgical removal of pituitary microadenoma. *Progress in Neurological Surgery*, **6**, 200

HARDY, J. (1979) Transsphenoidal microsurgical treatment of pituitary tumours. *Recent Advances in the Diagnosis and Treatment of Pituitary Tumours*, edited by J. A. Linfoot. Raven Press: New York. Vol. 28, pp. 375–388

HARDY, J. and SOMMA, M. (1979) Acromegaly: surgical treatment by transsphenoidal microsurgical removal of the pituitary adenoma. In: *Clinical Management of Pituitary Disorders*, edited by G. T. Tindall and W. F. Collins. New York: Raven Press. pp. 209–217

HARDY, J., BEAUREGARD, H. and ROBERT, F. (1978) Prolactin-secreting pituitary adeonomas: transphenoidal microsurgical treatment. In: *Progress in Prolactin Physiology and Pathology*, edited by C. Robin and M. Harter. Amsterdam: North Holland. p. 361

HIRSCH, O. (1911a) Ueber endonasale Operations-methode bei Hypophysis-Tumoren mit Bericht uber 12 operiete falle. *Berlin klinische Wochenschrift*, **48**, 1933

HIRSCH, O. (1911b). Ueber Methoden der operativen Behandlung von Hypophysistumoren auf endonasalem Wege. *Archiv für Laringologie und Rhinologie*, **24** 129

HORSLEY, V. (1906) On the technique of operations on the central nervous system. *British Medical Journal*, **2**, 411

JENKINS, J. S., ASH, S. and BLOOM, H. J. G. (1972) Endocrine function after external pituitary irradiation in patients with secreting and non-secreting pituitary tumours. *Quarterly Journal of Medicine*, **41**, 57

KJELLBERG, R. H., SHINTANI, A., FRANTZ, A. G. and KILMAN, B. (1968) Proton-beam therapy in acromegaly. *New England Journal of Medicine*, **278**, 689

LAWRENCE, J. A., TOBIAS, C. A., BORN, J. L., GOTTSCHALK, A., LINFOOT, J. A. and KLING, R. P. (1963) Alpha particle and proton-beams in therapy. *Journal of the American Medical Association*, **186**, 236

LAWRENCE, J. H., CHONG, C. Y., LYMAN, J. T., TOBIAS, C. A., BORN, J. L., GARCIA, J. F. *et al.* (1973) Treatment of pituitary tumors with heavy particles. In: *Diagnosis and Treatment of Pituitary Tumors*, edited by P. O. Kohler and G. T. Ross. New York: Elsevier, p. 253.

LEVY, A. and LIGHTMAN, S. L. (1994) Diagnosis and management of pituitary tumours. *British Medical Journal*, **308**, 1087–1091

NELSON, D. H., MEAKIN, J. W., DEALY, J. B., MATSON, D. D., EMERSON, K. and THORN, G. W. (1958) ACTH-producing tumour of the pituitary gland. *New England Journal of Medicine*, **259**, 161

NELSON, D. H., MENKIN, J. W. and THORN, G. W. (1960) ACTH-producing pituitary tumors following adrenalectomy for Cushing's syndrome. *Annals of Internal Medicine*, **52**, 560

SCHLOFFER, H. (1906) Zur Frage der Operation en an der Hypophyse. *Beitrage zur klinische Chirurgie*, **50**, 767

SCHLOFFER, H. (1907) Erfolgreiche Operation eines Hypopharynxtumors auf nasalem Weg. *Wiener klinische Wochenschrift*, **20**, 621

TRIBLE, W. M. and MORSE, A. E., (1965) Transpalatal hypophysectomy. *Laryngoscope*, **75**, 1116

WILLIAMS, R. A. (1974) Hypophysectomy for pituitary tumours. *Proceedings of The Royal Society of Medicine*, **67**, 881–892

WILLIAMS, R. A. (1978) Hypophysectomy. *Clinical Otolaryngology*, **3**, 201–212

WILLIAMS, R. A., JACOBS, H. S., KURTZ, A. B., MILLAR, J. G. B., OAKLEY, N. W., SPATHS, G. S. *et al.* (1975) The treatment of acromegaly with special reference to transsphenoidal hypophysectomy. *Quarterly Journal of Medicine*, **44**, 79–98

WRIGHT, A. D., HARTOG, M., PALTER, H., TEVAARWERK, G., DOYLE, F. H. and ARNOT, R. (1970) Use of yttrium-90 implantation in the treatment of acromegaly. *Proceedings of the Royal Society of Medicine*, **63**, 221

24

The orbit

V. J. Lund

The orbit is an area of considerable interest to the otorhinolaryngologist, an interest which has been heightened by the advent of endoscopic sinus surgery. There is potential overlap of pathology arising in the nose, paranasal sinuses and orbit, and surgery may involve the orbit both intentionally and accidentally. However, armed with a clear understanding of the anatomy and careful clinical and radiological assessment, it is an area in which the otorhinolaryngologist should be confident to operate and an area of beneficial cooperation with ophthalmic colleagues.

Applied surgical anatomy (Figure 24.1)
(Wolff, 1976; Doxanas and Anderson, 1984; Kanski, 1989; Roper-Hall, 1989)

The importance of the anatomy of the orbit to the otolaryngological surgeon lies mainly in its relationships with the anterior cranial fossa lying superiorly, the nasal cavity and ethmoidal labyrinth medially, the maxillary sinus and occasionally ethmoidal cells (Haller) inferiorly, and laterally, the infratemporal fossa and middle cranial fossa, rather than its contents. The apex of the orbit leads directly into the middle cranial fossa.

The orbit is a quadrilateral pyramid, with its base facing forwards, laterally and slightly inferiorly. It contains the globe, extraocular muscles, nerves, vessels and some associated structures such as the lacrimal apparatus. The average volume of the adult Caucasian orbit is 30 ml, 70% of which is occupied by retrobulbar and peribulbar structures. As it constitutes a fixed bony cavity, an increase of orbital volume of only 4 ml produces 6 mm of proptosis (Gorman, 1978).

Medial wall

This wall is of most significance to the otorhinolaryngologist. It is composed of:

- The frontal process of the maxilla
- The lacrimal bone
- The lamina papyracea of the ethmoid
- The body of the sphenoid.

Anteromedially lies the fossa for the lacrimal sac, demarcated by anterior and posterior lacrimal crests. Through the frontoethmoid suture, where the medial wall junctions with the roof, foramina for the anterior and posterior ethmoidal vessels and nerves are located. Their position is variable, but a rule of 24–12–6 has been suggested, based respectively on the average distance in millimetres from the anterior lacrimal crest to the anterior ethmoidal foramen, from the anterior to the posterior ethmoidal foramen, and from the posterior ethmoidal foramen to the optic canal (Rontal, Rontal and Guildford, 1979). The ethmoidal foramina are also taken as an indication of the level of the cribriform plate but are only a rough guide as 16% of individuals have no anterior ethmoidal foramen, 30% have multiple foramina and 4.6% have none (Shaheen, 1967). The medial wall is extremely thin in parts and may be naturally dehiscent. It is thus a poor anatomical barrier to the spread of sinonasal pathology.

Inferior wall

The floor is composed of three bones:

- The large orbital plate of the maxilla
- The zygomatic orbital plate anterolaterally
- The orbital process of the palatine bone.

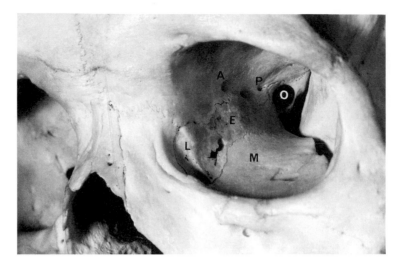

Figure 24.1 Photograph showing orbit. A: anterior ethmoid, P: posterior ethmoid, O: optic canal, L: lacrimal bone, E: ethmoid (lamina papyracea), M: maxilla

The infraorbital foramen is vertically in line with the superior orbital notch, lying half-way along the inferior rim and is continuous with the infraorbital canal. The anterior and occasionally middle superior alveolar nerves are given off from the infraorbital nerve within the canal, which if damaged may lead to denervation of the upper dentition (Wood Jones, 1939; Harrison, 1971). Lateral to the nasolacrimal canal is a pit marking the origin of the inferior oblique muscle which is the only extrinsic muscle to take origin from the front of the orbit and which is encountered in a Patterson's external ethmoidectomy. In 9% the origin of the muscle is intraperiosteal with no bony attachment which facilitates dissection. The floor is generally thin (0.5–1 mm) and the infraorbital canal is the commonest site for blow-out fractures. The distance between the infraorbital foramen and the optic canal varies considerably with an average distance of 46 mm, and an average distance from the posterior wall of the maxilla to the infraorbital foramen of 25 mm. The floor is encountered in orbital decompression, repair of orbital floor fractures and maxillectomy.

Superior wall

The roof is triangular and composed of the orbital plate of the frontal and the lesser wing of the sphenoid. The bone is thin (generally less than 3 mm) except in the sphenoid region. The extent of frontal and ethmoid sinus invasion is variable but may go as far as the zygomatic process or optic foramen which can be surrounded by ethmoidal (Onodi) cells (Figure 24.2). The superior margin has a supraorbital notch or foramen, transmitting the respective vessels and nerves, and in 50% of the population a frontal notch, lying more medially. The trochlea is a connective tissue sling anchoring the tendinous part of the superior oblique muscle to the orbit. The fovea for the trochlea is a small depression lying close to the superomedial orbital margin. In about 10% of individuals, the ligaments attaching the pulley are ossified. The tendon is enclosed in a synovial sheath within the pulley. Incisions should be placed to avoid damage to the supratrochlear and supraorbital nerves, levator palpebrae superioris muscle and trochlea, all structures related to the superior orbital margin. The superior wall is encountered during frontal sinus trephination, external frontoethmoidectomy, orbital decompression, repair of orbital fractures and orbital clearance or exenteration.

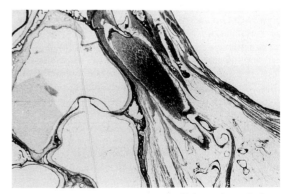

Figure 24.2 Histological section (axial plane) through the optic canal showing the intimate relationship of the posterior ethmoidal cells to optic nerve (haematoxylin and eosin)

Lateral wall

The lateral wall is composed of:

- The greater wing of the sphenoid
- The orbital surface of the zygoma
- The zygomatic process of the frontal bone.

It may be encountered during orbital decompression, infratemporal fossa surgery, exploration of fractures, lateral craniotomy and modified craniofacial resections involving lateral orbitotomy. The superior orbital fissure lies between the greater and lesser wings of the sphenoid. Through it pass cranial nerves III, IV, VI, the ophthalmic branch of V and the ophthalmic vein. The fissure is at least 28 mm from the frontozygomatic suture at the rim and due to this depth and the curvature of the lateral wall, it is rarely at risk in intraorbital procedures. The optic nerve lies 8 mm behind the medial edge of the fissure, so as long as a distance of 25 mm from the frontozygomatic suture is maintained, safe dissection may be carried out on the lateral orbital wall (Rontal, Rontal and Guildford, 1979).

Changes with age

Exploration of the orbit in children is fortunately rare. Growth of the orbit occurs with the development of the facial skeleton. Initially, the orbital fissures are large, the orbital index (orbital height/orbital breadth × 100) is high and the volume is great so that little change occurs in overall size after 7 years of age. The orbital fissures are relatively larger, and while an infraorbital foramen is usually present at birth, the canal may not be fully formed, remaining dehiscent for some years. Resorption occurs with advancing age, leading to dehiscences and widening of the fissures. The female orbit is in general more elongated and relatively larger than that of the male.

Periorbita

The importance of the orbital periosteum lies in its ability to protect the orbital contents and resist the spread of infection and malignancy. It is adherent to the orbital margins, sutures, foramina, fissures and lacrimal fossa and is continuous with dura through the superior orbital fissure, optic canal and ethmoidal canals. It encloses the lacrimal fossa and surrounds the duct as far as the inferior meatus. It must, therefore, be dissected from its attachments with care, at the least to avoid troublesome prolapse of fat into the operative field.

The extremities of the tarsal plates in the lids are attached to the orbital margin by strong fibrous structures – the palpebral (canthal) ligaments. The medial canthal ligament is made up of the preseptal and pretarsal heads of the orbicularis oculi muscle. Each of these has a superficial and deep component. The superficial heads fuse medially to form that part of the medial canthal ligament that attaches to the anterior lacrimal crest and the deep heads attach to the posterior lacrimal crest. This invests the lacrimal sac with a muscular covering, which compresses the sac on blinking. The superficial heads may be detached without serious consequence during surgery, but complete detachment, particularly during fractures when part of the lacrimal bone is also avulsed, leads to unopposed action of the orbicularis muscle. The resulting deformity is a rounding of the medial canthus, disappearance of the caruncle and increased intercanthal distance.

The fascia bulbi (Tenon's capsule) is a thin membrane surrounding the globe from cornea to optic nerve. Inferiorly it is thickened to form the suspensory ligament of Lockwood, the importance of which becomes evident after radical maxillectomy (Manson *et al.*, 1985).

Radiological evaluation of the orbit

(Lloyd, 1975; Bilaniuk and Zimmerman, 1980; Dutton, 1984)

In addition to clinical evaluation, important information is provided by radiological assessment of this area. Techniques available include:

- Plain X-ray
- Hypocycloidal tomography
- Computerized tomography (CT)
- Magnetic resonance imaging (MRI)
- Orbital venography
- Carotid angiography
- Ultrasound.

Of these techniques, CT and to a lesser extent MRI are the most useful. Plain X-rays may show adjacent sinus pathology such as a frontoethmoidal mucocoele but are frequently associated with false negatives in respect to both the sinus and orbit (Moseley, 1991). Hypocycloidal tomography has been superseded by CT, which allows evaluation of both soft tissue and bone detail, depending upon the window widths. Direct coronal and axial sections should always be performed. Excellent detail of orbital structures is provided by this technique combined with a highly accurate assessment of paranasal sinus pathology (Lund, Howard and Lloyd, 1983). More recently, MRI has been evaluated in this area and is now an important investigative technique (Lloyd *et al.*, 1987) but requires special sequences to suppress the high fat signal which may obscure pathological change.

Sinonasal pathology and the orbit
Infection and inflammation

A variety of inflammatory and infective sinonasal conditions may impinge on the orbit, the commonest of which are the orbital complications of acute bacterial sinusitis. Gross polyposis, particularly when it begins at an early age, can produce significant hyperteliorism with widening of the intercanthal distance (Figures 24.3 and 24.4) (Lund and Lloyd, 1983). Fungal infections may also cause widening of the ethmoid complex when allergic polypoid change is provoked and in its more aggressive forms, may directly invade the orbit and gain access to the cavernous sinus and middle cranial fossa via the orbital apex (Figure 24.5).

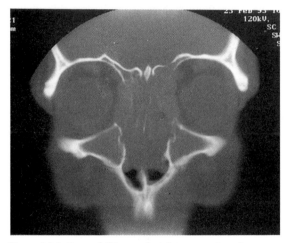

Figure 24.3 Coronal CT scan showing expansion of ethmoids with erosion of the lamina papyracea and total opacification of sinuses associated with gross polyposis.

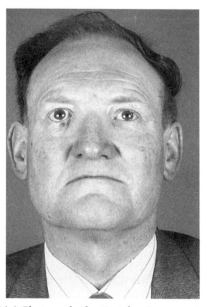

Figure 24.4 Photograph of patient showing expansion of medial canthal region and hyperteliorism associated with gross polyposis

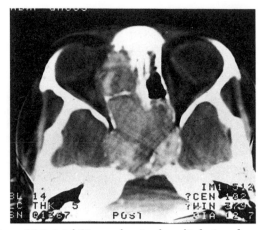

Figure 24.5 Axial CT scan showing fungal infection of sinuses invading middle cranial fossa via the cavernous sinus with typical heterogeneous signal

Orbital complications of sinusitis

The availability of antibiotics has considerably altered the frequency with which orbital complications result from sinusitis, but if they occur, the consequences are potentially disastrous. In 1969, Jarrett and Gutman reported the figures of the pre-antibiotic era in which 20% of patients with orbital infection completely lost vision, 20% died and 10% had permanent visual damage. Embryological considerations determine that sinusitis in children under 5 years is confined to the maxillary and the ethmoid sinuses, while the frontal sinus is the commonest source of orbital cellulitis in adults. Acute sphenoiditis may also result in significant orbital complications by a direct effect on the optic nerve and cavernous sinus in individuals with a dehiscent intervening lateral sphenoidal wall. In children and adolescents relatively minor upper respiratory tract infections can suddenly result in orbital complications whereas in adults the situation may become more chronic or contribute to the development of a mucocoele.

Congenital dehiscences or open suture lines in children facilitate spread through the medial, superior or inferior orbital walls. The lamina papyracea is so thin that a degree of orbital oedema can result from even early stages of sinusitis. The orbital periosteum can be readily stripped facilitating the formation of an intraorbital but extraperiosteal abscess. Complex venous drainage and the absence of valves in ophthalmic veins allows direct communication between the cavernous sinus, orbit and pterygoid plexus. Consequently, spread of infection along suture lines can result, by direct invasion through bone or retrograde thrombophlebitis leading to 159 children developing orbital infection out of 6770 with sinusitis (Fearon, Edwards and Bird, 1979).

In 1937, Hubert classified orbital complications of sinusitis into five groups:

1 Inflammatory oedema of the eyelids with or without oedema of orbital contents
2 Subperiosteal abscesses with
  a oedema of the lids or
  b spread of pus to the lids
3 Abscess of orbital tissues
4 Mild and severe orbital cellulitis with phlebitis of ophthalmic veins
5 Cavernous sinus thrombosis.

Spread into the superior orbital fissure can result in ophthalmoplegia, anaesthesia of the ophthalmic division of the trigeminal nerve and, in combination with optic nerve damage, an 'orbital apex syndrome' results.

With the formation of a *subperiosteal or extraperiosteal abscess* in the medial orbit, the globe is pushed forwards and laterally (Figure 24.6). The displacement and pain are accompanied by diplopia and chemosis of the unprotected cornea and ultimately results in visual loss due primarily to compression of the central retinal artery. Rapid administration of high-dose broad-spectrum intravenous antibiotics in combination with intranasal decongestants must be instituted. Constant careful monitoring of visual acuity is imperative (in particular of colour vision which is the first modality to be affected) and ocular mobility will indicate when surgical intervention is appropriate. Visual acuity may be difficult to assess due to swelling of the lid. Combined ophthalmic and otolaryngological assessment is thus always desirable and while CT scanning is of obvious value in determining localized collections of infection (Schramm, Myers and Kennerdell, 1978), it should not delay surgical intervention in the presence of deteriorating vision. Spontaneous discharge may occur through the upper lid from the frontal sinus or near the medial canthus from the ethmoid.

Failure to improve or any clinical deterioration requires drainage, which is most reliably accomplished by an external approach, usually combined with maxillary sinus drainage. Trephination of the frontal sinus alone with insertion of an external drain through which irrigation may be performed has been used in the past but external frontoethmoidectomy provides a more definitive procedure. Endoscopic drainage and decompression are also successful alternatives but should only be employed by those surgeons with an extensive experience in the technique. Orbital complications from sinusitis still constitute some of the surgical emergencies facing the otorhinolaryngologist and complete visual loss is almost always permanent. Young children can develop orbital complications with alarming rapidity, but have often had little effective antibiotic treatment. Consequently many improve once this is commenced parenterally, but as visual status is difficult, if not impossible, to assess, early surgical drainage is preferable to risking blindness.

Orbital cellulitis represents a potentially more serious complication with oedema of the retrobulbar orbital structures enclosed by the periorbita, leading to restriction of eye movements, chemosis with varying degrees of axial proptosis, ophthalmoplegia and rapid visual deterioration. There may be papilloedema of the optic disc and the patient is at risk of *cavernous sinus thrombosis*. There may be an associated subperiosteal abscess and/or a localized *intraperiosteal abscess* can form. Management depends upon aggressive antibiotic therapy and surgical orbital decompression.

A less common complication is that of periorbital cellulitis or *preseptal abscess* formation in the upper eyelid, anterior to the orbital septum, the fibrous layer running from the orbital margin of the tarsal plates. When the lids are opened, the eye is found to be normal, undisplaced with normal movements and vision. Treatment is again antibiotics and surgical drainage.

Frontoethmoidal mucocoeles (Table 24.1)

A mucocoele is an epithelial-lined, mucus-containing sac completely filling the sinus and capable of expansion (Natvig and Larsen, 1978). All paranasal sinuses can develop a mucocoele, with the frontal and ethmoidal sinuses most commonly affected (Rubin, Lund and Salmon, 1986; Lloyd, 1988) followed by the sphenoid and the maxillary sinus. Expansion may take place over many years or occur rapidly when secondary infection produces a pyocoele. Mucocoeles encroach on the orbit from all sinus sites. They are relatively uncommon and rarely bilateral. Only five cases out of the author's series of 135 frontoethmoidal mucocoeles have been bilateral (4%). The true incidence is difficult to determine due to patterns of referral, reporting and even ethnic variation. Sphenoidal mucocoeles may be referred to neurosurgeons and appear in the re-

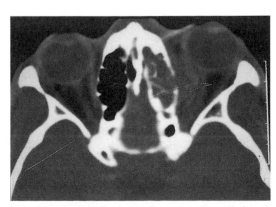

Figure 24.6 Axial CT scan showing extraperiosteal abscess associated with acute ethmoiditis

Table 24.1 Mucocoeles: review of major series

Author	No.	Male	Female	Age range	Site (%) Fronto-ethmoid	Ethmoid	Maxilla	Sphenoid	Treatment (no.)	Follow up	Recurrence (%)
Zizmour and Noyek (1968)	100	—	—	—	64	30	5	1	—	—	—
Bordley and Bosley (1973)	56	32	24	14–68	100	—	—	—	Drainage (1) Lynch-Howarth (6) Osteoplastic flap (28) Radical sinusectomy (21)	—	30: Lynch-Howarth 21: Osteoplastic flap
Canalis, Zajchuk and Jenkins (1978)	20	11	9	9–74	—	100	—	—	Lynch-Howarth (20)	2–7 years (mean 3.3 years)	20
Natvig and Larsen (1978)	112	55	57	10–70	91	6	3	—	Lynch-Howarth (60)	3–29 years (mean 11 years)	18
Hu and Lin (1982)	77	41	36	9–72	100	—	—	—	Lynch-Howarth Endonasal	—	—
Kennedy et al. (1989)	18	10	8	10–76	61	28		11	Endoscopic marsupialization	2–42 months (mean 18 months)	0
Harrison and Lund (1993)	118	74	44	10–87	92	6	1	1	Lynch-Howarth (118)	Mean 3.3 years	7

spective literature (Nugent, Sprinkle and Bloor, 1970; Diaz *et al.*, 1978; Close and O'Connor, 1983; Davis, Small and Lund, 1992). It has been suggested that the Japanese have a higher incidence of maxillary mucocoeles but it is possible that these are retention cysts rather than true mucocoeles (Hasegawa *et al.*, 1979). The majority of mucocoeles occur in patients aged between 40 and 70 years but they have been reported from 23 months (Timon and O'Dwyer, 1989) to 87 years (Harrison and Lund, 1993). There is a slight male preponderance overall but right and left sides are equally affected.

Aetiology

The formation of a mucocoele has traditionally been attributed to a combination of obstruction of the affected sinus and inflammation. The fact that the frontoethmoidal region is most commonly affected would partially support this contention but the condition is rare and generally unilateral, in contrast to the frequency with which obstruction and inflammation are encountered in this region. It is probable that many patients develop a mucus-filled sinus due to obstruction of its drainage but only a small number

progress to mucocoele formation and while factors in their clinical history may contribute to the obstruction, such as previous surgery or trauma (Lund, 1987), a significant proportion (36%) have no such factor. Development of the mucocoele would appear to depend upon the degree and duration of obstruction, the absence of alternative drainage routes and a process of bone resorption and expansion possibly initiated by infection. Histological studies confirm the presence of bone remodelling at the interface between mucocoele and sinus wall (Lund and Milroy, 1991) and recent studies on bone-resorbing factors confirm the presence of PGE_2, collagenase, and cytokines such as interleukin 1 (IL_1) and tumour necrosis factor (TNF) compared with normal controls and chronically inflamed mucosa (Lund *et al.*, 1988; Lund, Henderson and Song, 1993).

Clinical features

Expansion of the mucocoele generally follows the route of least resistance, into the orbit. The majority of patients are thus initially referred to ophthalmic surgeons because of displacement of the globe. With a frontoethmoidal mucocoele, the majority of patients (91%) exhibit some degree of proptosis (1–17 mm),

55% lateral displacement (2–13 mm), and 59% inferior displacement (1–10 mm) (Figure 24.7a). Ninety-five per cent experience diplopia but this may be minimal if the condition has developed over many years. Ocular mobility in upward gaze is limited in 55% by the mass which can often be felt in the upper medial quadrant of the orbit, sometimes with a characteristic 'egg-shell' crackling sensation due to the thinned overlying bone. Anterior ethmoidal muco coeles which can occur in quite young children may compress the nasolacrimal region, producing epiphora. Conversion to a pyocoele, with additional infection will cause rapid expansion, compromising

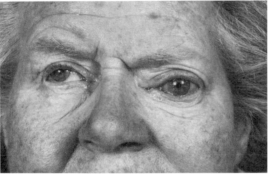

(a)

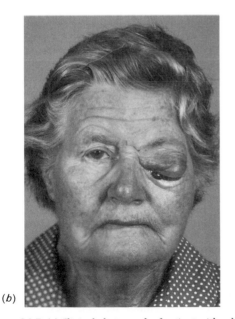

(b)

Figure 24.7 (a) Clinical photograph of patient with orbital displacement due to frontoethmoidal mucocoele. (b) Same patient with acute infection of mucocoele

vision and occasionally discharging through the upper lid (4%) (Figure 24.7b).

Mucocoeles (and pyocoeles) of the posterior ethmoid and sphenoid sinuses cause retro-orbital headaches, facial pain and orbital symptoms such as diplopia, proptosis, ophthalmoplegia and visual loss. In severe cases, intracranial extension may produce meningitis and raised intracranial pressure (Nugent, Sprinkle and Bloor, 1970; Sellars and De Villiers, 1981; Wurster, Levine and Sisson, 1986).

Radiology

Plain sinus X-rays will show the classical features of a frontethmoidal mucocoele in the majority of cases (Lloyd, 1988). These are an expanded frontal sinus, with loss of the scalloped margin and translucence, and depression or erosion of the supraorbital ridge. The loss of the scalloped margin will only be seen when the vertical portion of the frontal sinus is affected. CT scanning is now employed (direct coronal and axial sections), confirming the above features and demonstrating an homogeneous smooth-walled mass, expanding the sinus, with thinning or loss of bone (Figure 24.8). There may also be evidence of new bone formation or sclerosis. CT with intravenous contrast characteristically shows ring enhancement in the presence of a pyocoele.

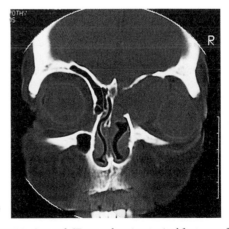

Figure 24.8 Coronal CT scan showing typical features of a frontoethmoidal mucocoele, with expansion of the frontal sinus, erosion of bone and displacement of the globe

Magnetic resonance demonstrates a high signal on T2-weighted spin echo sequences and a low signal on inversion recovery due to a long T1 relaxation time (Figure 24.9). However, if there has been any haemorrhage, either spontaneous or associated with attempts at drainage, a signal of mixed intensity is produced with some loculi of high intensity on inversion recovery, T1- and T2-weighted spin echo sequences (Gomori *et al.*, 1985).

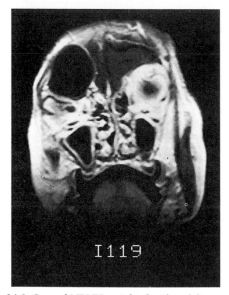

Figure 24.9 Coronal MRI T1-weighted with gadolinium DTPA showing low signal area of frontal mucocoele

Ethmoidal mucocoeles are easily missed on plain sinus X-rays (Lloyd, Bartram and Stanley, 1974) and although a lateral X-ray may show expansion of the sphenoid, with elevation or erosion of the floor of the pituitary fossa, both these and maxillary sinus mucocoeles are best seen on CT and distinguished from other pathology. This includes acute and chronic sinusitis, polyps, retention cysts, dermoids and cholesterol granuloma and the range of benign and malignant neoplasms which can affect this area.

Treatment

Until recently the majority of patients with frontoethmoidal mucocoeles were treated via an external modified Lynch-Howarth approach and radical frontoethmoidectomy. All the lining mucosa was stripped except where erosion of bone had exposed dura and the majority (92%) had a large fenestrated (1 cm diameter) silastic tube inserted from the frontal sinus to the nasal cavity. This was left in place for an average of 5 months. However, a proportion of mucocoeles can be approached endoscopically, which avoids an external incision and associated morbidity. The displacement of the globe may take several

months to resolve completely while bone remodelling occurs, though this may have the advantage of diminishing the postoperative exacerbation of diplopia often experienced by patients with rapid decompression of the orbit. This approach is particularly suitable for ethmoidal, maxillary and sphenoidal mucocoeles and in the young, but not all frontoethmoidal mucocoeles are accessible endoscopically (Kennedy *et al.*, 1989; Stammberger, 1991). Under these circumstances external and endoscopic approaches may be combined to preserve the frontonasal recess and avoid stenting which is an unphysiological solution, likely to result in circumferential stenosis. Notwithstanding this, the recurrence rate in 100 cases of frontoethmoidal mucocoeles treated by external frontoethmoidectomy was 4% with 3–27 year follow up. It is not yet possible to determine the long-term success using an endoscopic approach as insufficient numbers and follow up are available. However, in 22 cases treated endoscopically during the last 5 years, there has been no recurrence and the patency of the frontonasal recess can be regularly confirmed endoscopically.

The osteoplastic flap has also been advocated, particularly in the USA, but has few if any advantages over the external or endoscopic frontoethmoidectomy.

Orbital decompression

The otorhinolaryngologist may be required to perform orbital decompression. This may relate to the orbital contents, for which the commonest indication is thyroid eye disease, though pseudotumour, orbital infiltration in Wegener's granulomatosis and the palliation of metastatic deposits have also been reported (Thawley, 1979; Calcaterra and Thompson, 1980; Harrison, 1980; Sobol, Druck and Wolf, 1980). More recently decompression of the optic nerve has been approached endoscopically in cases of traumatic compression by fractures of the canal or a foreign body (Kennedy *et al.*, 1990; Stammberger, 1991).

Thyroid eye disease is characterized by significant global displacement, the nature of which is dependent upon the pattern of muscle and fat hypertrophy (Figure 24.10). CT will demonstrate this well, with the classical 'Coca-Cola bottle' sign apparent on the axial view. The thyroid metabolism must be stabilized and most patients have already received oral steroids and/or radiotherapy. Surgical decompression is primarily undertaken for optic neuropathy or when there is severe exposure keratopathy, rather than for cosmetic indications alone. The decompression must be seen as the first stage of surgical management, which will usually include surgery on the extraocular muscles, lid surgery and blepharoplasty at a later time. A variety of approaches has been described (Figure 24.11). In 1911, Dollinger first described decompression by removal of the lateral wall of the orbit, which allows the orbital contents to herniate

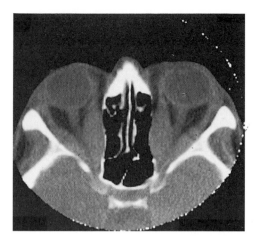

Figure 24.10 Axial CT scan showing classical extraocular muscle hypertrophy of thyroid eye disease producing 'Coca-Cola bottle' compression of lamina papyracea

orbital wall, while Hirsch (1950) later reported inferior decompression into the maxillary antrum. Ogura subsequently (1978) combined these two methods via a transantral approach. Harrison (1981) championed the Patterson's external ethmoidectomy which allows greater access and removal of the entire medial wall from the level of the ethmoidal vessels inferiorly and across the floor as far as the infraorbital nerve, and lateral to this if necessary. Between 4 and 7 mm of decompression can readily be achieved by this approach. It may also be combined with a lateral orbitotomy. A similar degree of decompression can be achieved endoscopically, though a large middle meatal antrostomy is required to reach sufficiently far laterally across the floor. The decompression can be continued most successfully as far posteriorly as the sphenoid which is of benefit in cases of significant orbital apex compression. The endoscope may also be combined with an external approach (Figure 24.12).

Where the optic canal has been traumatized by a fracture or a foreign body it may be possible to remove displaced fragments or a foreign body, and decompress the nerve. Special instrumentation including ensheathed drills are recommended though it is uncertain whether incising the optic nerve sheath is advisable.

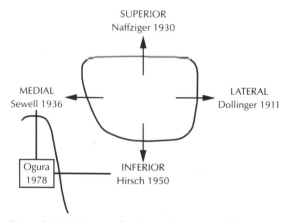

Figure 24.11 Diagram showing various approaches described for orbital decompression

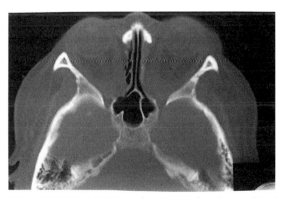

Figure 24.12 Axial CT scan showing results after combined external and endoscopic orbital decompression

into the temporal fossa. This produces only a few millimetres of improvement, so in 1931 Naffziger described decompression into the anterior cranial fossa via a transcranial route. This approach was not without morbidity and is now reserved for the most extreme cases with visual compromise unresponsive to other approaches.

Decompression via the paranasal sinuses was first described by Sewall in 1936 by removal of the medial

Dacryocystorhinostomy

Obstruction of the nasolacrimal duct has traditionally been the preserve of the ophthalmic surgeon but an endonasal approach using the microscope for magnification and illumination has been used in a number of centres for some years (El-Khoury and Rouvier, 1992). More recently the advent of endoscopic sinus surgery has widened otolaryngological interest in nasolacrimal surgery and may be undertaken with relative ease (McDonogh and Meiring, 1989). In primary cases the hard maxillary bone overlying the sac and canal must be removed by drill, curette or laser, which is not necessary in revision procedures (Figure 24.13).

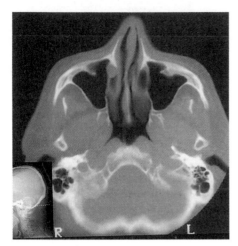

Figure 24.13 Axial CT showing expanded right nasolacrimal duct

Trauma

A sense organ enclosed within an incomplete bony box is inevitably vulnerable to trauma. Accidental trauma can occur in association with facial injury or as a complication of sinus surgery.

Facial trauma involving the orbit

The orbital margin provides a protective boundary for the globe as it is stronger than the orbital walls. If the orbit is struck with a round object, the orbital rim will withstand considerable force. However, compression of the orbital contents will produce a 'blow-out' fracture of the inferior and/or medial walls (Smith and Regan, 1957; Dodick *et al.*, 1971; Rumelt and Ernest, 1972; Mirsky and Saunders, 1979).

The zygoma itself frequently withstands direct blows, but fractures at sites of potential weakness, namely at the zygomaticofrontal and zygomaticomaxillary sutures. Clinically this fracture is evident by depression or flattening of the orbital rim, inferior deviation of the lateral canthus, localized step deformity of the inferior rim at the zygomaticomaxillary suture, tenderness over the zygomatic arch, pain with mastication and ecchymosis of the buccal mucosa. Varying degrees of floor fracture and displacement may be associated with tripod fractures and

because of the significant functional and cosmetic deformity which can result, it is important to diagnose and repair them early.

Clinical features

Early signs and symptoms of a 'blow-out' of the orbital floor are restriction of extraocular mobility (particularly in upward gaze), infraorbital anaesthesia (including the canine teeth), orbital swelling and ecchymosis. The patient with a nasoethmoid complex fracture will also present with periorbital ecchymoses, probably secondary to ethmoidal artery damage, flattening of the nasal root and widening of the intercanthal distance. Traumatic telecanthus does not always occur but should be excluded and may be difficult to establish when oedema obscures the medial palpebral angle. An alternative is to measure the interpupillary width which is normally twice the intercanthal distance. The medial canthal ligament can be further tested by traction on the lashes which should make the lid margin taut. If this does not occur, disruption of the medial ligament has probably occurred.

It is obviously important carefully to assess visual acuity, the pupils, lid and ocular movements. Surgical emphysema may be palpable and globe displacement indicates retrobulbar haemorrhage if exophthalmos is present, or orbital floor displacement if enophthalmos is found. Epiphora is not a reliable sign of nasolacrimal damage which may need separate assessment once the initial oedema has settled (Holt and Holt, 1985). Facial fractures may also be associated with cerebrospinal leaks.

Fractures of the lamina papyracea can occur alone, or with fractures of the floor (Figure 24.14), but are more often seen in association with complex midfacial

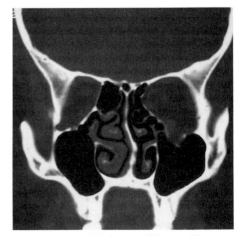

Figure 24.14 Coronal CT showing 'blow-out' fractures of medial and inferior orbital walls

fractures. They may thus be accompanied by cerebrospinal fluid leakage, lacrimal damage, visual loss and severe epistaxis from the anterior ethmoidal artery. In addition, there may be downward displacement of the medial canthus, subcutaneous or subconjunctival emphysema and limitation of lateral movement.

Radiology

Radiological examination is important in determining the site and extent of bony trauma. Waters' occipitomental and Caldwell occipitofrontal views will demonstrate orbital fractures in 70% of cases, but false positives are common and CT is recommended if a 'blow-out' fracture is suspected. This will show the classical 'tear-drop' sign in the antrum roof (Figure 24.14), though it is usually due to entrapment of fat rather than the actual inferior rectus muscle.

Treatment

Therapeutic success must be judged in terms of preservation of binocular vision, the prevention of resolution of enophthalmos and the restoration of ocular mobility. Sacks and Friedland (1979) found the commonest presenting signs or symptoms in 100 patients with orbital floor fracture to be hyperaesthesia, irregularity of the infraorbital rim, periorbital swelling and diplopia. Some symptoms such as oedema and hyperaesthesia will often resolve spontaneously, but considerable controversy surrounds the indications and timing of orbital floor exploration.

If there is no evidence of extraocular muscle restriction and no diplopia, despite a fracture on radiography, exploration is not mandatory (Putterman, Stevens and Urist, 1974). However, combinations of diplopia and enophthalmos usually require immediate exploration once other causes of diplopia such as haematoma of the inferior rectus muscle have been eliminated by a forced duction test. Enophthalmos alone only causes diplopia in extremes of gaze but is unacceptable cosmetically. It may be initially masked by oedema or haematoma so unless accompanied by changes in visual acuity, it is advisable to wait 7–10 days before deciding to operate. This is particularly pertinent as exploration in the acute situation is associated with a risk of visual loss. It is possible for late enophthalmos to develop due to secondary atrophy of orbital fat and fibrosis.

Surgical management depends on the extent of injury. Collapse of the anterior wall of the maxilla or orbital floor requires intra-antral manipulation. A variety of commercial stents and balloons is now available for this purpose which conform to the contours of the antral cavity (Figure 24.15). Alternatively Whitehead's varnish on ribbon gauze may be successfully inserted via a Caldwell-Luc approach and removed 2–3 weeks later via the sublabial incision or an intranasal antrostomy (middle or inferior). More

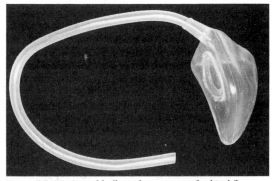

Figure 24.15 Antral balloon for support of orbital floor following reduction of fracture

formal reconstruction of the orbital floor may be indicated with significant enophthalmos, prolapse of fat or with comminuted, hinged or inferiorly displaced bone. A Patterson's approach to the inferior orbital rim will allow careful dissection of orbital periosteum and insertion of supporting material though this can be the site of infection or be absorbed/extruded. Bone, cartilage, fascia lata, tantalum, Teflon and silicone have all been used, but of the artificial materials, silastic sheeting and hydroxyapatite seem to be the best tolerated and most successful in the long term.

In fractures of the medial wall, if there is evidence of posterolateral displacement of the lacrimal bone and its attached medial canthal ligament, an open repair is indicated to reattach the bone with wires. Bilateral traumatic telecanthus requires bilateral exploration and wiring of the fractured bone. Damage to the nasolacrimal apparatus can be dealt with by insertion of silastic tubes. In these circumstances early exploration produces the best results as late reconstruction can be difficult. Late complications associated with these injuries include one eye being lower, diplopia, enophthalmos, dacrocystitis and epiphora (Reynolds, 1978). In selected cases it may be possible to apply an endoscopic endonasal approach in experienced hands (Yamaguchi *et al.*, 1991).

Iatrogenic orbital trauma

Orbital damage due to endoscopic sinus procedures is a source of much concern, however, all sinus procedures can be and have been associated with orbital damage. Maniglia (1989) reported on 18 major orbital complications secondary to a range of sinonasal operations, including polypectomy, conventional ethmoidectomy and Caldwell-Luc. During conventional *antral lavage*, particularly under general anaesthesia, incorrect angle of entry can lead to penetration of the orbital floor or, in the presence of a dehiscent infraorbital canal, excessive pressure on lavage may affect the orbital contents. For this reason the eyes should always be uncovered during the procedure and observed closely so that the operation can be abandoned at the first sign of proptosis.

In 1979 Freedman and Kern reported a 2.8% complication rate in 1000 cases undergoing *intranasal ethmoidectomy* of which less than 1% were orbital, while Eichel (1979) accepted a 25% rate of orbital ecchymosis in his series. Intranasal ethmoidectomy without present methods of illumination and visualization was a difficult operation to perform well and to teach. Our attention has been refocused by the increasing popularity of *endoscopic sinus surgery* and a number of orbital complications have received considerable publicity. However, it is clear that the endoscope makes surgery in this area neither safer nor more dangerous and it is the anatomical and pathological knowledge of the surgeon, combined with their surgical experience which will dictate the relative risk of such surgery. The anatomy may have been significantly distorted by the disease itself or previous surgery in addition to the many anatomical variants possible in this area. Thus CT scanning is mandatory preoperatively, both direct coronal and, if surgery in the posterior ethmoids or sphenoid is anticipated, axial sections. Some surgeons have advocated using local rather than general anaesthesia to increase safety, for pain may indicate penetration of the orbit, though this cannot be relied upon. The patient should, however, be questioned preoperatively with regard to visual acuity, the presence of epiphora and previous strabismus which may be temporarily exacerbated by the muscle relaxation of anaesthesia.

During the procedure, the eyes should always be *uncovered* and under direct observation when close to the orbit. The presence or absence of the lamina papyracea can be directly determined and, if orbital periosteum is uncovered, gentle pressure on the globe may reveal areas of bony dehiscence. Exposure of the periosteum is of no consequence so long as it is recognized and not penetrated. When performing the infundibulotomy, the sickle knife should be angled away from the orbit, which is often closely juxtaposed to the uncinate process anteriorly. If prolapse of fat does occur, it should be repositioned with some gelatin sponge, the patient placed on antibiotics and told not to blow the nose for 10–14 days to avoid surgical emphysema. It has been recommended that all tissue removed during surgery should be placed in normal saline or Ringer's solution to see if it floats, i.e. is fat (or brain!). This may be of value when operating in patients with extensive polyps. Any significant penetration of the orbit endangers the medial rectus muscle.

Similarly when enlarging the middle meatal antrostomy anteriorly, the nasolacrimal duct may be damaged. The bone surrounding the duct is considerably thicker than that of the uncinate process and will prove difficult to remove with the back-biting Ostrum-type forceps. This resistance should alert the operator to the potential hazard. If the duct is crushed or even transected, it is probably sufficient in most cases to adopt a conservative approach as the majority will have no long-term sequelae, though it may be worth removing the overlying fragments of bone.

Another orbital complication is haemorrhage into the orbit due to damage to the anterior ethmoidal artery. Retraction of the vessel may be associated with a rapidly developing orbital haematoma which may require immediate decompression. Although lateral canthotomy has been recommended, the otolaryngological surgeon is more familiar with an external frontoethmoidectomy decompression which may be readily accomplished (under general anaesthesia) and should be performed without delay.

A more serious complication relates to damage to the orbital apex and optic nerve in the posterior ethmoidal cells (particularly the Onodi cells running lateral to the sphenoid) and within the sphenoid itself. The bone overlying the nerve may be clinically dehiscent in 6% of the normal population and ethnic variation may place other individuals at risk. If diminished visual acuity is apparent in the immediate postoperative period which is not due to an obvious haematoma, alert ophthalmic colleagues, immediately remove any nasal packing, raise the patient's head and commence an infusion of mannitol, acetazolamide and commence parenteral dexamethasone. If after an hour there is no improvement, re-explore the surgical cavity and perform an external decompression to ensure no posterior haematoma is present.

In *Caldwell-Luc* approaches, the infraorbital nerve may be damaged and if transantral ethmoidectomy is attempted by this route, penetration of the orbit is a possible consequence. The *Lynch-Howarth* and *Patterson external frontoethmoidectomy approaches* can be associated with a number of minor orbital complications. Of greatest significance is superior oblique underaction following a Lynch-Howarth approach due to disturbance of the trochlea. This may occur in up to 30% of patients if the periosteum is not specifically reattached in this area (Lund and Rolfe, 1989). The nasolacrimal duct may be damaged in the Patterson's inferior approach and this combined with temporary oedema of orbicularis oculi renders epiphora a relatively common, though fortunately short-lived postoperative symptom. Detachment of the inferior oblique and both anterior and posterior components of the medial canthal ligament may also have an effect on ocular movements though this is often obscured by the effects of decompressing the orbital pathology.

The nasolacrimal duct is frequently transected during *lateral rhinotomy* and *craniofacial resection*. So long as this is performed obliquely, patients rarely experience problems in the long term. Only seven patients out of over 200 undergoing craniofacial resection have required a formal dacryocystorhinostomy. Similarly resection of significant amounts of orbital periosteum appear to have little deleterious effect upon orbital function. However, *midfacial degloving* may produce temporary epiphora postoperatively where the ducts are preserved but stretched during the procedure (Howard and Lund, 1992).

In *radical maxillectomy*, the bony inferior support of the orbit is removed but the fascial sling (suspensory ligament of Lockwood) is sufficient to maintain the eye in position long term and this is facilitated by the immediate insertion of a Whitehead's varnish pack and temporary prosthesis during the healing process.

Neoplasia

A wide variety of benign and malignant conditions arising in adjacent structures such as the skin, sinuses, and skull base may spread to the orbit and vice versa (Table 24.2). The involvement of the eye and the necessity to remove it raises significant psychological issues, equivalent to amputation of a limb. However, preservation of the eye must be based on an unemotional decision that it will not jeopardize prognosis and that the eye will have functional capabilities if preserved. This situation may be complicated by combined radiotherapy which may result in cataract formation, glaucoma, and occasionally retinal atrophy.

Table 24.2 Primary orbital tumours

Vascular
   capillary haemangioma
   cavernous haemangioma
   lymphangioma
Lacrimal gland
   pleomorphic adenoma
   malignant, e.g. adenoid cystic
Lymphoproliferative
   pseudotumour
   lymphoma
Rhabdomyosarcoma
Histiocytic
   Letterer-Siwe
   Hand-Schüller-Christian
   eosinophilic granuloma
Neural
   optic nerve glioma
   optic nerve meningioma
   neurofibroma
Metastases
   Children, e.g. neuroblastoma, Ewing's sarcoma,
   leukaemia
   Adults, e.g. bronchus, breast, prostate, kidney, gut

The distinction between benign and malignant disease may also be academic when benign tumours of the skull base such as meningioma, specifically associated with hyperostosis, are capable of affecting both optic canals, rendering the patient blind in both eyes.

Benign

Benign tumours of the nose and sinuses may affect the orbit. The angiofibroma, a lesion almost exclusively associated with young males, arises from the region of the sphenopalatine foramen and presents in the nasal cavity and nasopharynx as a vascular mass. However, as it enlarges, it expands the pterygopalatine fossa and dumb-bells into the infratemporal region whence it can compromise important structures in the orbital apex and impinge on the inferior orbital fissure (Figure 24.16). Consequently, occasionally patients may present with visual loss (Harrison, 1987).

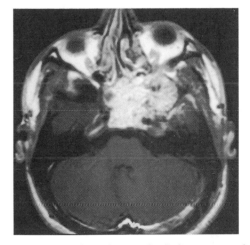

Figure 24.16 Axial MRI (T1-weighted) showing typical 'salt and pepper' appearance of angiofibroma extending into infratemporal fossa

The inverted papilloma is one of the commonest benign sinonasal tumours which characteristically arises in the middle meatus and invades the maxillary sinus. It is frequently intimately related to the nasolacrimal duct and may spread extraperiosteally into the orbit. Rarely it may be both intraorbital and intraperiosteal, which poses a difficult management problem (Figure 24.17).

Osteomas arising in the frontoethmoidal region may encroach on the orbit (Figure 24.18). These benign bony lesions can achieve large proportions, making their point of origin difficult to determine but it is said that they arise at junctional points between membranous and cartilaginous bone and are usually composed of a cancellous core with varying amounts of dense compact bone peripherally. In a series of 23 patients (Atallah and Jay, 1981) 10 presented with

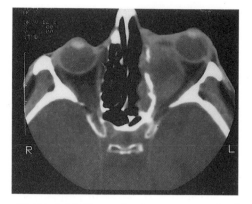

Figure 24.17 Axial CT scan showing a rare example of intraperiosteal inverted papilloma

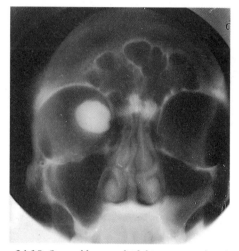

Figure 24.18 Coronal hypocycloidal tomogram showing osteoma impinging on orbit

ocular symptoms of whom six had proptosis. Osteomas are readily visualized on plain sinus X-rays and are not infrequently seen incidentally when, if small and asymptomatic, require no treatment. However, in the presence of symptoms and when associated with mucocoele formation (4%: Lund, 1987) an external frontoethmoidectomy approach is generally indicated. If greater access is required, then a lateral rhinotomy or even craniofacial approach have been utilized (Cousins, Lund and Cheesman, 1987).

Malignant

Invasion of the orbit from the anterior ethmoidal complex occurs early and in a number of ways. Visual symptoms of unilateral epiphora, proptosis and diplopia were commonly reported in a series of

patients with malignant tumours of the sinonasal region (Lund, 1983) and were present in 50% of 116 patients undergoing craniofacial surgery for malignant disease. Invasion occurs through the thin or dehiscent bone of the lamina papyracea or through the region of the infraorbital canal. Fortunately, the orbital periosteum is resistant to tumour spread but once disease has breached it, the orbital contents cannot be salvaged. In Harrison's series (1978) at least 50% of patients required orbital clearance. This is in contradistinction to orbital exenteration where the lids are also removed leaving a bony socket. This is rarely necessary with sinonasal malignancy as this does not, with a few exceptions, locally invade the superficial tissues of the lids nor drain by this route lymphatically. When orbital clearance is performed, the lids (minus tarsal plates and lash margin) are preserved, forming a skin-lined socket for a future prosthesis, a situation which is only compromised by perioperative radiotherapy (Figures 24.19 and 24.20).

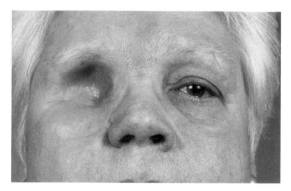

Figure 24.19 Skin-lined following orbital clearance

The craniofacial approach has allowed satisfactory assessment of the medial orbital wall as far as the apex (Cheesman, Lund and Howard, 1986). If tumour is found adjacent to the periosteum, provided frozen section control is available, this may be resected and skin grafted with little functional disability. In those cases where the tumour is found to be adherent to the periosteum, the periosteum is opened well away from the tumour margin. Obvious involvement of the inner periosteal surface makes orbital clearance mandatory. In the absence of macroscopic intraperiosteal disease, the periosteum is widely excised with a small amount of adjacent orbital fat and submitted to frozen section. Clearance of orbital contents must be performed if there is any evidence of tumour penetration. In its absence, adequate periosteal excision can be undertaken. This can include almost the entire medial aspect, from the ethmoidal vessels superiorly to the attachment of the inferior oblique muscle inferiorly without major compromise

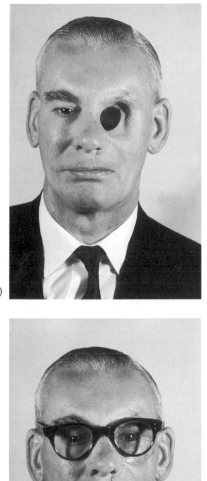

(a)

(b)

Figure 24.20 (*a*) Patient after orbital clearance and radiotherapy with breakdown of eye-lids. (*b*) Same patient with orbital prosthesis in place

of orbital function and the exposed fat is covered by a split skin graft.

As a consequence, it has been possible to preserve a number of eyes which would have been hitherto sacrificed. Between 1970 and 1980, 47% of cases of sinonasal malignancy underwent total maxillectomy with or without orbital clearance, between 1981 and 1991 this had fallen to 26% (Howard and Lund,

1993). In a series of 140 cases of malignant sinonasal disease undergoing craniofacial resection, 23% underwent primary orbital clearance. Sixteen patients had periosteal resection, three of whom underwent secondary clearance which did not appear adversely to affect prognosis. However, two patients developed massive recurrence involving the preserved eye from which they subsequently succumbed. This technique should only be employed in patients who can be followed up closely.

Once tumour has traversed the lamina, it may spread intraorbitally but extraperiosteally to the orbital apex and thence escape into the middle cranial fossa. Modern imaging techniques have enabled us to detect this with a high degree of accuracy preoperatively (Lund, Howard and Lloyd, 1983; Lund *et al.*, 1989) (Figures 24.21 and 24.22). An understanding of the natural history of the disease is also important in the management of the patient. In a similar way to meningioma (Figure 24.23), chondrosarcoma in-

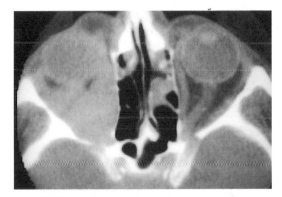

Figure 24.21 Axial CT showing malignant tumour (metastatic adenocarcinoma of breast) in orbital apex

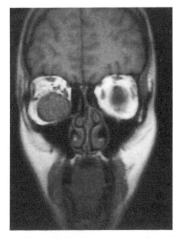

Figure 24.22 Coronal MRI showing alveolar soft part sarcoma occupying inferior left orbit

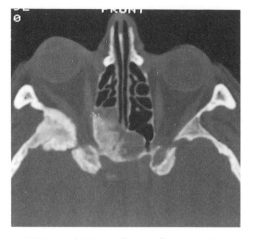

Figure 24.23 Axial CT scan showing hyperostosis associated with sphenoidal meningioma

volves the sphenoid leading to bilateral optic canal compression. Adenoid cystic carcinoma is capable of perineural lymphatic spread, both directly and by embolization (Howard and Lund, 1985) which may compromise the optic nerve (Figure 24.24).

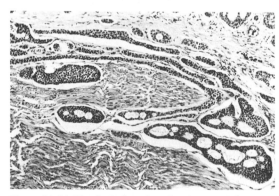

Figure 24.24 Histological section of optic nerve taken some distance from adenoid cystic carcinoma of ethmoid showing embolic deposits of tumour (haematoxylin and eosin)

Tumours arising in the skin of the medial canthus may, however, be referred for orbital exenteration, particularly when the ethmoids and cribriform plate are involved. A variety of methods of repair is available though, as many of these lesions occur in the elderly, it is one of the few circumstances where a forehead flap is still of use, being rapid, reliable and receptive to a subsequent prosthesis.

The palliative role of orbital clearance should also be considered. Painful proptosis in a blind eye can be the source of considerable misery and it may be worth removing the eye under these circumstances. Occasionally patients with significant fibrotic infiltration of the orbit in Wegener's granulomatosis may similarly benefit.

Lateral orbitotomy and craniotomy

For extensive lesions occupying the lateral portion of the orbit and/or extending superiorly into the anterior cranial fossa it may be necessary to approach the orbit from the lateral side. The lateral orbitotomy is achieved by removal of the lateral orbital rim with cuts through the frontal bone, supraorbital margin and zygoma level with the orbital floor. This bone is rewired in position at the end of the procedure. In the lateral craniotomy, a curved coronal incision is made within the hair, from hairline anteriorly to the root of the helix taking care not to damage the superficial temporal artery. The craniotomy is made in the frontal bone with a fissure burr, the size of which is dictated by the disease and the bone pedicled inferiorly on the intact periosteum and temporalis muscle (Figures 24.25 and 24.26). This approach can be used for benign cysts and tumours.

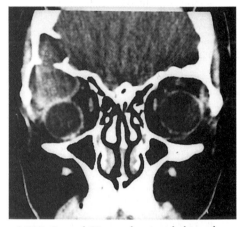

Figure 24.25 Coronal CT scan showing cholesterol granuloma affecting superolateral quadrant of orbit

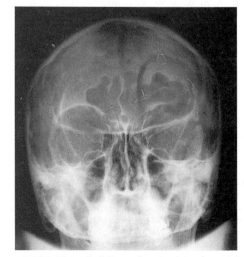

Figure 24.26 Plain skull X-ray showing lateral craniotomy osteotomy

Rehabilitation following orbital clearance and exenteration

Irrespective of whether the patient is left with a skin-lined socket or not, an orbital prosthesis is required in most cases. In the past these were attached to a pair of spectacles or were retained in the socket with tissue adhesive (Conley and Baker, 1979). More recently the advent of osseo-integrated techniques has greatly improved the retention of the prostheses. The Branemark system utilizes titanium screws which become an integral part of the skeleton and to which the prosthesis can be firmly attached. These can be implanted at the time of the resection or preferably as a secondary procedure. There must be at least 3–4 mm depth of bone and radiotherapy will interfere with integration. In the orbit it is advisable to wait at least 6 months or longer if radiotherapy has been given before exposing the fitments so it is appropriate to offer a temporary prosthesis in the interim period.

References

ATALLAH, N. and JAY, M. M. (1981) Osteomas of the paranasal sinuses. *Journal of Laryngology and Otology*, **95**, 291–304

BILANIUK, L. T. and ZIMMERMAN, R. A. (1980) Computer-assisted tomography: sinus lesions with orbital involvement. *Head and Neck Surgery*, **2**, 293–301

BORDLEY, J. E. and BOSLEY, W. R. (1973) Mucoceles of the frontal sinus: causes and treatment. *Annals of Otology, Rhinology and Laryngology*, **82**, 696–702

CALCATERRA, T. C. and THOMPSON, J. W. (1980) Antral-ethmoidal decompression of the orbit in Graves' disease: ten year experience. *Laryngoscope*, **90**, 1941–1949

CANALIS, R. F., ZAJCHUK, J. T. and JENKINS, H. A. (1978) Ethmoidal mucocoeles. *Archives of Otolaryngology*, **104**, 286–291

CHEESMAN, A. D., LUND, V. J. and HOWARD, D. J. (1986) Craniofacial resection for tumours of the nasal cavity and paranasal sinuses. *Head and Neck Surgery*, **8**, 429–435

CLOSE, L. G. and O'CONNOR, W. E. (1983) Sphenoethmoidal mucocoeles with intracranial extension. *Otolaryngology, Head and Neck Surgery*, **91**, 350–357

CONLEY, J. and BAKER, D. C. (1979) Management of the eye socket in cancer of the paranasal sinuses. *Archives of Otolaryngology*, **105**, 702–705

COUSINS, V., LUND, V. J. and CHEESMAN, A. D. (1987) Craniofacial resection for extensive lesions of the anterior skull base. *Australian and New Zealand Journal of Surgery*, **57**, 515–520

DAVIS, C. H. G., SMALL, M. and LUND, V. J. (1992) An 'empty' sphenoid mucocoele. *British Journal of Neurosurgery*, **6**, 381–384

DIAZ, F., FATCHOW, R., DUVALL, A. J., QUICK, C. A. and ERICKSON, D. L. (1978) Mucocoeles with intracranial and extracranial extensions. *Journal of Neurosurgery*, **48**, 284–288

DODICK, J. M., GALIN, M. A., LITTLETON, J. T. and SOD, L. M. (1971) Concomitant medial wall fracture and blowout fracture of the orbit. *Archives of Ophthalmology*, **85**, 273–281

DOLLINGER, J. (1911) Die Drickentlastund der Augenhokle dursh Entfernung der ausseren Orbitalwand bei Hochgradigen Exophthalmos und Koneskutwer Hornhauterkroning. *Deutsche Medizinische Wochenschrift*, **37**, 1885–1890

DOXANAS, M. T. and ANDERSON, R. L. (1984) (eds) *Clinical Orbital Anatomy*. Baltimore: Williams & Wilkins

DUTTON, J. J. (1984) Radiographic evaluation of the orbit. In: *Clinical Orbital Anatomy*, edited by M. T. Doxanas and R. L. Anderson. Baltimore: Williams & Wilkins. Ch. 3, pp. 35–56

EICHEL, B. S. (1979) The intranasal ethmoidectomy procedure: historical, technical and clinical considerations. *Laryngoscope*, **82**, 1806–1821

EL-KHOURY, J. and ROUVIER, P. (1992) Dacryocystorhinostomie endonasale. *Acta ORL Belgica*, **46**, 401–404

FEARON, B., EDWARDS, B. and BIRD, R. (1979) Orbital-facial complications of sinusitis in children. *Laryngoscope*, **89**, 947–953

FREEDMAN, H. M. and KERN, E. B. (1979) Complications of intranasal ethmoidectomy: a review of 1000 consecutive operations. *Laryngoscope*, **89**, 421–432

GORMAN, C. A. (1978) The presentation and management of endocrine ophthalmology. *Clinics in Endocrinology and Metabolism*, **7**, 67–96

GOMORI, J. M., GROSSMAN, R. I., GOLDBERG, H. I., ZIMMERMAN, R. A. and BILANIUK, L. T. (1985) Intracranial hematomas: imaging by high-field MR. *Radiology*, **157**, 87–93

HARRISON, D. F. N. (1971) Surgical anatomy of the maxillary and ethmoidal sinuses – a reappraisal. *Laryngoscope*, **81**, 1658–1664

HARRISON, D. F. N. (1978) Critical look at the classification of maxillary sinus carcinomata. *Annals of Otology, Rhinology and Laryngology*, **87**, 1–7

HARRISON, D. F. N. (1980) The ENT surgeon looks at the orbit. *Journal of Laryngology and Otology*, Suppl. 2, 1–43

HARRISON, D. F. N. (1981) Surgical approach to the medial orbital wall. *Annals of Otology, Rhinology and Laryngology*, **90**, 415–419

HARRISON, D. F. N. (1987) The natural history, pathogenesis and treatment of juvenile angiofibroma. *Archives of Otolaryngology – Head and Neck Surgery*, **113**, 936–942

HARRISON, D. F. N. and LUND, V. J. (1993) *Tumours of the Upper Jaw*. London: Churchill Livingstone

HASEGAWA, M., SAITO, Y., WATNABE, I. and EUGENE, B. (1979) Post-operative mucocoeles in the maxillary sinus. *Rhinology*, **17**, 253–256

HIRSCH, O. (1950) Surgical decompression for malignant exophthalmos. *Archives of Otolaryngology*, **51**, 325–331

HOLT, G. R. and HOLT, J. E. (1985) Nasoethmoid complex injuries. *Otolaryngologic Clinics of North America*, **18**, 87–98

HOWARD, D. J. and LUND, V. J. (1985) Reflections on the management of adenoid cystic carcinoma of the nasal cavity and paranasal sinuses. *Otolaryngology – Head and Neck Surgery*, **93**, 338–340

HOWARD, D. J. and LUND, V. J. (1992) The midfacial degloving approach to sinonasal disease. *Journal of Laryngology and Otology*, **106**, 1059–1062

HOWARD, D. J. and LUND, V. J. (1993) Surgical options in the management of nose and sinus neoplasia. In: *Tumours of the Upper Jaw*, edited by D. F. N. Harrison, and V. J. Lund. London: Churchill Livingstone. pp. 329–336

HU, X. H. and LIN, D. Z. (1982) Mucocele des sinus. *Revue de Laryngologie, Otologie et Rhinologie*, **103**, 199–201

HUBERT, L. (1937) Orbital infections due to nasal sinusitis. *New York Journal of Medicine*, **37**, 1559–1564

JARRETT, W. and GUTMAN, F. (1969) Ocular complications of infection in the paranasal sinuses. *Archives of Ophthalmology*, **81**, 683–688

KANSKI, J. J. (1989) *Clinical Ophthalmology*, 2nd edn. Oxford: Butterworth-Heinemann

KENNEDY, D. W., JOSEPHSON, J. S., ZINREICH, S. J., MATTOX, D. E. and GOLDSMITH, M. M. (1989) Endoscopic sinus surgery for mucoceles: a viable alternative. *Laryngoscope*, **99**, 885–889

KENNEDY, D. W., GOODSTEIN, M. L., MILLER, N. R. and ZINREICH, S. J. (1990) Endoscopic transnasal orbital decompression. *Archives of Otolaryngology – Head and Neck Surgery*, **116**, 275–282

LLOYD, G. A. S. (1975) *Radiology of the Orbit*. Philadelphia: W. B. Saunders

LLOYD, G. A. S. (1988) *Diagnostic Imaging of the Nose and Paranasal Sinuses*. London: Springer-Verlag

LLOYD, G. A. S., BARTRAM, C. I. and STANLEY, P. (1974) Ethmoid mucocoeles. *British Journal of Radiology*, **47**, 646–651

LLOYD, G. A. S., LUND, V. J., PHELPS, P. D. and HOWARD, D. J. (1987) Magnetic resonance imaging in the evaluation of nose and paranasal sinus disease. *British Journal of Radiology*, **60**, 957–968

LUND, V. J. (1983) Malignant tumours of the nasal cavity and paranasal sinuses. *Oto-Rhino-Laryngology*, **45**, 1–12

LUND, V. J. (1987) Anatomical considerations in the aetiology of fronto-ethmoidal mucocoeles. *Rhinology*, **25**, 83–88

LUND, V. J. and LLOYD, G. A. S. (1983) Radiological changes associated with benign nasal polyps. *Journal of Laryngology and Otology*, **97**, 503–510

LUND, V. J. and MILROY, C. M. (1991) Fronto-ethmoidal mucocoeles: a histopathological analysis. *Journal of Laryngology and Otology*, **105**, 921–923

LUND, V. J. and ROLFE, M. (1989) Ophthalmic considerations in fronto-ethmoidal mucocoeles. *Journal of Laryngology and Otology*, **103**, 667–669

LUND, V. J., HENDERSON, B. and SONG, Y. (1993) Involvement of cytokines and vascular adhesion receptors in the pathology of fronto-ethmoidal mucocoeles. *Acta Otolaryngologica*, **113**, 540–546

LUND, V. J., HOWARD, D. J. and LLOYD, G. A. S. (1983) CT evaluation of paranasal sinus tumours for craniofacial resection. *British Journal of Radiology*, **56**, 439–446

LUND, V. J., HARVEY, W., MEGHJI, S. and HARRIS, M. (1988) Prostaglandin synthesis in the pathogenesis of fronto-ethmoidal mucocoeles. *Acta Otolaryngologica*, **106**, 145–151

LUND, V. J., HOWARD, D. J., LLOYD, G. A. S. and CHEESMAN, A. D. (1989) Magnetic resonance imaging of paranasal sinus tumours for craniofacial resection. *Head and Neck Surgery*, **11**, 279–283

MCDONOGH, M. and MEIRING, J. H. (1989) Endoscopic transnasal dacrocystorhinostomy. *Journal of Laryngology and Otology*, **103**, 585–587

MANIGLIA, A. J. (1989) Fatal and major complications secondary to nasal and sinus surgery. *Laryngoscope*, **99**, 276–283

MANSON, P. W., CARMELLA, M., CLIFFORD, M. A., ILIFF, N. T. and MORGAN, R. (1985) Mechanisms of global support and post traumatic enophthalmos: I, The anatomy of the ligament sling and its relation to intramuscular cone orbital fat. *Plastic and Reconstructive Surgery*, **77**, 193–202

MIRSKY, R. G. and SAUNDERS, R. A. (1979) A case of isolated medial wall fracture with medial rectus entrapment following seemingly trivial trauma. *Journal of Pediatric Ophthalmology and Strabismus*, **16**, 287–293

MOSELEY, I. (1991) The plain radiograph in ophthalmology: a wasteful and potentially dangerous anachronism. *Journal of The Royal Society of Medicine*, **84**, 76–80

NAFFZIGER, H. (1931) Progressive exophthalmos following thyroidectomy. *Annals of Surgery*, **94**, 582–586

NATVIG, K. and LARSEN, T. E. (1978) Mucocele of the paranasal sinuses. *Journal of Laryngology and Otology*, **92**, 1075–1082

NUGENT, G. R., SPRINKLE, P. and BLOOR, B. M. (1970) Sphenoid sinus mucoceles. *Journal of Neurosurgery*, **32**, 443–451

OGURA, J. H. (1978) Surgical results of orbital decompression for malignant exophthalmos. *Journal of Laryngology and Otology*, **92**, 181–196

PUTTERMAN, A. M., STEVENS, T. and URIST, M. J. (1974) Non-surgical management of blow-out fractures of the orbital floor. *American Journal of Ophthalmology*, **77**, 232–240

REYNOLDS, J. R. (1978) Late complications versus method of treatment in a large series of mid-facial fractures. *Plastic and Reconstructive Surgery*, **61**, 871–875

RONTAL, E., RONTAL, M. and GUILDFORD, F. T. (1979) Surgical anatomy of the orbit. *Annals of Otology, Rhinology and Laryngology*, **88**, 382–386

ROPER-HALL, M. J. (1989) *Stallard's Eye Surgery*, 7th edn. London: Wright

RUBIN, J. S., LUND, V. J. and SALMON, B. (1986) Fronto-ethmoidectomy in the treatment of mucocoeles: a neglected operation. *Archives of Otolaryngology – Head and Neck Surgery*, **112**, 434–436

RUMELT, M. B. and ERNEST, J. T. (1972) Isolated blow-out fractures of the medial orbital wall with medial rectus entrapment. *American Journal of Ophthalmology*, **73**, 451–453

SACKS, A. C. and FRIEDLAND, J. A. (1979) Orbital floor fractures: should they be explored early. *Plastic and Reconstructive Surgery*. **64**, 190–193

SCHRAMM, V. L., MYERS, E. N. and KENNERDELL, J. S. (1978) Orbital complications of acute sinusitis. Evaluation, management and outcome. *Otolaryngology*, **86**, 221–230

SELLARS, S. L. and DE VILLIERS, J. C. (1981) The sphenoid sinus mucocoele. *Journal of Laryngology and Otology*, **95**, 493–502

SEWALL, E. C. (1936) Operative control of progressive exophthalmos. *Archives of Otolaryngology*, **24**, 621–624

SHAHEEN, O. H. (1967) Epistaxis in the middle-aged and elderly. *MS Thesis*, University of London

SMITH, E. C. and REGAN, W. F. (1957) Blow-out fracture of the orbit: mechanism and correction of inferior orbital fracture. *American Journal of Ophthalmology*, **44**, 733–736

SOBOL, S., DRUCK, N. S. and WOLF, M. (1980) Palliative orbital decompression for metastatic melanoma to the orbit. *Laryngoscope*, **90**, 329–333

STAMMBERGER, H. (1991) *Functional Endoscopic Sinus Surgery*. Philadelphia: BC Decker

THAWLEY, S. E. (1979) Wegeners granulomatosis: unusual indication for orbital decompression. *Laryngoscope*, **89**, 145–154

TIMON, C. I. and O'DWYER, T. P. (1989) Ethmoidal mucocoeles in children. *Journal of Laryngology and Otology*, **103**, 284–286

WOLFF, E. (1976) *Anatomy of the Eye and Orbit*, 7th edn, revised by R. Warwick. London: H. K. Lewis

WOOD JONES, F. (1939) The anterior superior alveolar nerve and vessels. *Journal of Anatomy*, **73**, 583–591

WURSTER, C., LEVINE, T. and SISSON, G. (1986) Mucocele of the sphenoid sinus causing sudden onset of blindness. *Otolaryngology – Head and Neck Surgery*, **94**, 257–259

YAMAGUCHI, N., ARAI, S., MITANI, H. and UCHIDA, Y. (1991) Endoscopic endonasal technique of the blowout fracture of the medial orbital wall. *Operative Techniques in Otolaryngology – Head and Neck Surgery*, **2**, 269–274

ZIZMOUR, J. and NOYEK, A. M. (1968) Cysts and benign tumours of the paranasal sinuses. *Seminars in Roentgenology*, **3**, 172–185

Volume index